# Critical and Intensive Care: A Survival Guide

# Critical and Intensive Care: A Survival Guide

Edited by Paul Curtis

hayle
medical

New York

Hayle Medical,
750 Third Avenue, 9th Floor,
New York, NY 10017, USA

Visit us on the World Wide Web at:
www.haylemedical.com

ISBN: 978-1-63241-595-0

**Cataloging-in-Publication Data**

Critical and intensive care : a survival guide / edited by Paul Curtis.
    p. cm.
Includes bibliographical references and index.
ISBN 978-1-63241-595-0
1. Critical care medicine. 2. Emergency medicine. 3. Intensive care units.
I. Curtis, Paul.
RC86.7 .C75 2019
616.025--dc23

# Table of Contents

# Preface

Critical and intensive care is concerned with the life support and monitoring provided to individuals with life-threatening conditions. Such care is particularly significant in patients with airway or respiratory compromise, instability, acute renal failure, multiple organ failure or potentially lethal cardiac arrhythmias. An important criterion for the facilitation of intensive care to patients is that the condition is potentially reversible and that the patient can survive. Critical care adopts a system-by-system approach to medicine with emphasis on the central nervous system, cardiovascular system, hematology, respiratory system, endocrine system, gastro-intestinal tract, renal system, etc. This book is compiled in such a manner, that it will provide in-depth knowledge about the practice of critical and intensive care. Different approaches, evaluations, methodologies and advanced studies on critical care medicine have been included in this book. For all those who are interested in critical and intensive care medicine and nursing, this book can prove to be an essential guide.

Significant researches are present in this book. Intensive efforts have been employed by authors to make this book an outstanding discourse. This book contains the enlightening chapters which have been written on the basis of significant researches done by the experts.

Finally, I would also like to thank all the members involved in this book for being a team and meeting all the deadlines for the submission of their respective works. I would also like to thank my friends and family for being supportive in my efforts.

**Editor**

# Prognostic implications of blood lactate concentrations after cardiac arrest: a retrospective study

Antonio Maria Dell'Anna[1,2], Claudio Sandroni[2], Irene Lamanna[1], Ilaria Belloni[1], Katia Donadello[1,3], Jacques Creteur[1], Jean-Louis Vincent[1*] and Fabio Silvio Taccone[1]

## Abstract

**Background:** Elevated lactate concentration has been associated with increased mortality after out-of-hospital cardiac arrest (CA). We investigated the variables associated with high blood lactate concentrations and explored the relationship between blood lactate and neurological outcome in this setting.

**Methods:** This was a retrospective analysis of an institutional database that included all adult (> 18 years) patients admitted to a multidisciplinary Department of Intensive Care between January 2009 and January 2013 after resuscitation from CA. Blood lactate concentrations were collected at hospital admission and 6, 12, 24 and 48 h thereafter. Neurological outcome was evaluated 3 months post-CA using the Cerebral Performance Category (CPC) score: a CPC of 3–5 was used to define a poor outcome.

**Results:** Of the 236 patients included, 162 (69%) had a poor outcome. On admission, median lactate concentrations (5.3[2.9–9.0] vs. 2.5[1.5–5.5], $p < 0.001$) and cardiovascular sequential organ failure assessment (cSOFA) score (3[0–4] vs. 0[0–3], $p = 0.003$) were higher in patients with poor than in those with favourable outcomes. Lactate concentrations were higher in patients with poor outcomes at all time points. Lactate concentrations were similar in patients with out-of-hospital and in-hospital CA at all time points. After adjustment, high admission lactate was independently associated with a poor neurological outcome (OR 1.18, 95% CI 1.08–1.30; $p < 0.001$). In multivariable analysis, use of vasopressors and high $PaO_2$ on admission, longer time to return of spontaneous circulation and altered renal function were associated with high admission lactate concentrations.

**Conclusions:** High lactate concentrations on admission were an independent predictor of poor neurological recovery post-CA, but the time course was not related to outcome. Prolonged resuscitation, use of vasopressors, high $PaO_2$ and altered renal function were predictors of high lactate concentrations.

**Keywords:** Neurological outcome, Cardiopulmonary resuscitation, In-hospital cardiac arrest, Hyperlactataemia

## Background

Every year, between 37 and 100 per 100,000 inhabitants have an out-of-hospital cardiac arrest (OHCA) in Western countries, with approximately 10% surviving to hospital discharge [1, 2]. Despite the more immediate availability of advanced life support, survival to hospital discharge after in-hospital CA (IHCA) does not exceed 15–20% [3, 4]. High-quality cardiopulmonary resuscitation (CPR) and early defibrillation, when indicated, are essential to achieve a good outcome [5]. However, when return of spontaneous circulation (ROSC) is achieved, there is still uncertainty about which therapeutic interventions most effectively improve the survival and neurological recovery of these patients.

Blood lactate concentrations may represent a marker of cellular hypoxia after CA. Patients with high blood lactate concentrations on admission after CA are more

*Correspondence: jlvincent@intensive.org
[1] Department of Intensive Care, Erasme Hospital, Université Libre de Bruxelles, Route de Lennik 808, 1070 Brussels, Belgium
Full list of author information is available at the end of the article

likely to die than those with lower concentrations [6, 7]. In this setting, blood lactate concentrations may be considered as a marker of prolonged hypoperfusion or poor resuscitation. Other studies have also suggested that a faster decrease in lactate concentrations during the early hours after resuscitation may be correlated with better survival [8–10]. This decrease may reflect more rapid haemodynamic stabilization with therapy. Nevertheless, these studies included only patients with OHCA and the importance of lactate concentrations in IHCA survivors remains uncertain. As the underlying causes and management of OHCA and IHCA are different (e.g. cardiac vs. non-cardiac causes, different delays for interventions, different types of initial rhythm, presence of pre-existing medical conditions), the absolute initial lactate concentrations, as well as changes in lactate concentrations over time, may vary accordingly and potentially have different prognostic value. Few data are available on the impact of lactate concentrations and their evolution on neurological recovery, and the variables associated with high blood lactate after CA have not been well studied [7].

The aims of this study were, therefore, to: (a) evaluate whether any lactate-related variable (i.e. admission value, peak lactate, decreased concentration over time, area under the curve of concentrations over 48 h) was associated with neurological outcome; (b) identify the variables associated with high lactate concentrations after CA; and (c) explore the differences in lactate concentrations between IHCA and OHCA.

## Methods

### Study population
We retrospectively reviewed prospectively collected data from all adult (> 18 years of age) patients who were admitted to the 35-bed medical/surgical Department of Intensive Care of Erasme Hospital after OHCA or IHCA (excluding patients with CA occurring in the ICU) between January 2009 and January 2013. The local Institutional Review Board approved the study and waived the need for informed consent.

### Routine post-resuscitation care
A standardized institutional protocol is used in all post-cardiac arrest patients (1). All comatose patients, irrespective of CA location and initial rhythm, are treated with targeted temperature management (TTM) for 24 h, with a target temperature of 32–34 °C. Cooling is started immediately after ICU admission with a combination of cold fluid bolus (20–30 ml/kg of a crystalloid solution in 30 min) and a circulating water blanket device (Medi-Therm II, Gaymar, USA). Body temperature is measured using invasive haemodynamic monitoring (PiCCO, Pulsion, Munich, Germany) when in place (need determined

by attending physician depending on patient condition) or a rectal temperature probe. Analgo-sedation is provided using midazolam (0.03–0.1 mg/kg/h) and morphine (0.1–0.3 mg/kg/h) infusions. Cisatracurium is administered to control shivering in the induction phase (as a bolus of 0.15 mg/kg) and, if needed, as a continuous infusion thereafter (1–3 mcg/kg/min). After 24 h of cooling, rewarming (0.3–0.5 °C/h) is performed passively and sedation discontinued when body temperature reaches 37 °C.

Patients are kept in a 30° semi-recumbent position; ventilation is set to keep $PaCO_2$ between 35 and 45 mmHg and $SpO_2$ > 94%. Transesophageal echocardiography is routinely performed within the first 6–18 h after ICU admission. Blood glucose is kept between 110 and 150 mg/dL and mean arterial pressure maintained > 65–70 mm Hg using fluids, dobutamine and/or noradrenaline. Intra-aortic balloon counterpulsation (IABP) or extracorporeal membrane oxygenation (ECMO) is used in cases of severe cardiogenic shock.

### Neurological assessment and withdrawal of life support
After rewarming and discontinuation of sedation, repeated neurological examination and standard or continuous electroencephalography (EEG) together with somatosensory evoked potentials (SSEPs) at day 3 are performed ("multimodal" approach). After the first 72 h, a decision to withdraw life support may be taken in comatose patients based on: (a) bilateral absence of the N20 wave of SSEPs; (b) presence of status myoclonus (defined as continuous and generalized myoclonus persisting for ≥ 30 min [11]) in combination with EEG abnormalities (generalized discharges or burst suppression); (c) refractory (i.e. resistant to two antiepileptic drugs and continuous intravenous sedative administration) status epilepticus occurring from a flat or burst suppression background. The medical charts of patients were reviewed to classify deaths as "non-neurological" (i.e. persistent shock or multiple organ failure in the absence of neurological injury or before neurological prognostication could be assessed) or as neurological (i.e. severe anoxic brain injury) [12].

### Data collection
We collected patient demographics, comorbidities and Utstein variables, including CA location, initial rhythm, bystander CPR and time to ROSC. After hospital admission, blood lactate concentrations are routinely measured with arterial blood gases, glucose and electrolytes every 3–4 h by point-of-care analysers (GEM Premier 4000; Instrumentation Laboratory, Bedford, MA, USA). We recorded the initial lactate concentration, measured within 1 h after hospital admission, and values measured

Prognostic implications of blood lactate concentrations after cardiac arrest: a retrospective...

3

at 6, 12, 24 and 48 h after admission, with a margin of $\pm 1$ h. At the same time points, we also recorded blood gases, heart rate (HR) and MAP and calculated a sequential organ failure assessment (SOFA) score [13] from the ICU patient data monitoring system (Picis Critical Care Manager, Picis Inc., Wakefield, USA). The SOFA score was calculated excluding the neurological component because of the confounding effect of sedation. Shock was defined as a cardiovascular SOFA (cSOFA) of 3 or 4.

All available lactate measurements during the first 48 h or until death (if the patient died within 48 h) were plotted to calculate the area under the curve ($AUC_{0-48}$). We report the highest value recorded during the first 48 h as the "peak lactate". The absolute decrease in lactate concentrations from admission was calculated at 6, 12 and 24 h, using the following formulas: [(lactate at 6 h—lactate on admission)/6] mEql/L, [(lactate at 12 h—lactate on admission)/12] mEq/L and [(lactate at 24 h—lactate on admission)/24] mEq/L. Similarly, the "relative" decrease in lactate concentrations was calculated as follows: [(lactate at 6 h—lactate on admission)/ lactate on admission $\times$ 100]%, [(lactate at 12 h—lactate on admission)/lactate on admission $\times$ 100]% and [(lactate at 24 h—lactate on admission)/lactate on admission $\times$ 100]% [8, 14].

## Outcome assessment

Outcome was assessed by the neurological outcome at 3 months, determined using the Cerebral Performance Category score (CPC; 1 = no neurological disability, 2 = mild neurological disability, 3 = severe neurological impairment, 4 = vegetative state, 5 = death) [15]. The CPC was prospectively evaluated during follow-up visits or by telephone interview with the general practitioner. A favourable outcome was defined as a CPC 1 or 2 and poor outcome as CPC 3–5.

## Statistical analysis

Statistical analyses were performed using IBM SPSS Statistics 21 for Macintosh. Descriptive statistics were computed for all study variables. A Kolmogorov–Smirnov test was used, and histograms and normal quantile plots were examined to verify the normality of distribution of continuous variables. Data are presented as count (percentage), mean ($\pm$ standard deviation) or median [25th–75th percentiles], as appropriate. Differences between groups were assessed using a Chi-square or Fisher's exact test for categorical variables, as appropriate, and a $T$ test or a Wilcoxon rank test for continuous variables. Data from repeated measures (lactate, HR, MAP, cSOFA on admission and at 6, 12, 24 and 48 h, thereafter) were analysed using a two-way ANOVA, or the Friedman ANOVA for data that were not normally distributed. Differences

between groups for each time point were explored using a Mann–Whitney $U$ test for nonparametric data. Association between continuous variables was evaluated using linear regression. Multivariable logistic regression was performed to identify factors independently associated with high blood lactate concentrations on admission. Multivariate binomial backward logistic regression was used to assess whether blood lactate on admission or decrease in lactate concentrations was independently correlated with favourable outcome. The discriminative ability of variables identified to predict neurological outcome by multivariate analysis was evaluated using receiver operating characteristic (ROC) curves with the corresponding AUC. Subgroup analyses included comparisons between IHCA and OHCA, patients with shockable and non-shockable rhythm and patients with shock (defined as cSOFA $\geq 3$) and without shock on admission. A $p < 0.05$ was considered as statistically significant.

## Results

### General characteristics of the study cohort

Among 244 consecutive patients admitted to our ICU after CA, 236 were included in the study (Additional file 1: Figure S1). The mean age of our cohort was 63 years; 155 (66%) patients were male and 137 (58%) had an OHCA; 162 (69%) patients had a poor neurological outcome at 3 months (Table 1).

### Blood lactate concentrations and outcome

The median blood lactate concentration on admission was 4.3[2.0–8.5] mEq/L. Lactate concentrations were higher on admission (5.3[2.9–9.0] vs. 2.5[1.5–5.5], $p < 0.001$) and at each time point thereafter in patients with poor than in those with favourable neurological outcome (Table 1 and Additional file 1: Figure S2). Peak lactate concentration (6.7[3.8–10.2] vs. 3.6[2.2–6.3], $p < 0.001$) and lactate $AUC_{0-48}$ (3.9[2.4–6] vs. 3.2[2.4–4.5] mEq/L*h, $p = 0.027$) were also higher in patients with poor than in those with favourable neurological outcome. There were no differences in the relative changes in blood lactate concentrations at any time point between patients with poor and those with favourable neurological outcomes (Table 1).

Blood lactate levels on admission were somewhat higher in patients who died from a non-neurological cause ($n = 72$) than in those who died of neurological causes ($n = 87$), but the differences did not reach statistical significance (6.5 [3.2–9.1] vs. 4.8 [2.4–9.4] mEq/L; $p = 0.16$). Changes in blood lactate concentrations from admission to 12 h were similar in these two groups (data not shown).

In multivariable analysis, high admission blood lactate concentration was associated with significantly higher

**Table 1  Characteristics of study population according to neurological outcome at 3 months**

| Parameter | All patients (236) | CPC 1–2 (74) | CPC 3–5 (162) | p value |
|---|---|---|---|---|
| *General* | | | | |
| Age (years) | 63 ± 15 | 59 ± 14 | 64 ± 16 | 0.03 |
| Male, n (%) | 155 (60%) | 57 (77%) | 98 (61%) | 0.02 |
| *Comorbidities* | | | | |
| COPD/asthma, n (%) | 43 (18%) | 15 (20%) | 28 (17%) | 0.59 |
| Heart disease, n (%) | 107 (46%) | 40 (54%) | 67 (42%) | 0.09 |
| Diabetes, n (%) | 50 (21%) | 21 (28%) | 29 (18%) | 0.08 |
| Chronic renal failure, n (%) | 38 (16%) | 12 (16%) | 26 (16%) | 1 |
| Liver cirrhosis, n (%) | 14 (6%) | 6 (8%) | 8 (65%) | 0.38 |
| Immunosuppression, n (%) | 28 (12%) | 5 (7%) | 23 (14%) | 0.13 |
| *Cardiac arrest* | | | | |
| OHCA, n (%) | 137 (58%) | 43 (58%) | 94 (58%) | 1 |
| VF/VT, n (%) | 100 (42%) | 57 (77%) | 43 (27%) | <0.001 |
| Bystander CPR, n (%) | 136 (58%) | 54 (73%) | 82 (52%) | 0.03 |
| Time to ROSC (min) | 19 ± 14 | 17 ± 13 | 20 ± 14 | 0.10 |
| *ABG* | | | | |
| Lactate admission (mEq/L) | 4.3 [2–8.5] | 2.5 [1.5–5.5] | 5.3 [2.9–9.0] | <0.001 |
| Lactate 6 h (mEq/L) | 2.7 [1.6–5] | 2.0 [1.3–2.9] | 3.3 [1.8–5.9] | <0.001 |
| Lactate 12 h (mEq/L) | 2.2 [1.4–4.2] | 1.6 [1.2–2.3] | 2.8 [1.6–5.3] | <0.001 |
| Lactate 24 h (mEq/L) | 1.5 [1.1–2.8] | 1.3 [1.0–1.7] | 1.8 [1.3–3.2] | <0.001 |
| Lactate 48 h (mEq/L) | 1.4 [1.0–2.0] | 1.1 [0.8–1.7] | 1.6 [1.1–2.5] | 0.001 |
| $aDLC_{0-6}$ (mEq/L*h) | 0.2 [0–0.6] | 0.1 [0–0.5] | 0.2 [0–0.6] | 0.16 |
| $aDLC_{0-12}$ (mEq/L*h) | 0.1 [0–0.3] | 0.1 [0–0.2] | 0.2 [0–0.4] | 0.006 |
| $aDLC_{0-24}$ (mEq/L*h) | 0.1 [0–0.3] | 0.1 [0–0.1] | 0.1 [0–0.3] | 0.008 |
| $rDLC_{0-6}$ (%) | 25 [−5 to 54] | 24 [−8 to 56] | 24 [−5 to 53] | 0.98 |
| $rDLC_{0-12}$ (%) | 37 [2–62] | 28 [−7 to 59] | 40 [33–47] | 0.08 |
| $rDLC_{0-24}$ (%) | 53 [18–71] | 48 [25–68] | 55 [17–77] | 0.64 |
| $AUC_{0-48}$, mEq/L*h | 4.7 ± 4.2 | 3.74 ± 2.53 | 5.17 ± 4.72 | 0.016 |
| Peak lactate, mEq/L | 5 [3–9] | 3.6 [2.2–6.3] | 6.7 [3.8–10.2] | <0.001 |
| pH on admission | 7.25 [7.16–7.36] | 7.27 [7.18–7.37] | 7.25 [7.15–7.34] | 0.09 |
| $PaO_2$ on admission (mmHg) | 121 [77–228] | 143 [84–220] | 118 [77–232] | 0.54 |
| $PaCO_2$ on admission (mmHg) | 42 ± 14 | 43 ± 12 | 42 ± 15 | 0.41 |
| *Haemodynamics* | | | | |
| HR on admission (bpm) | 89 ± 21 | 89 ± 19 | 88 ± 22 | 0.75 |
| MAP on admission (mmHg) | 90 ± 24 | 98 ± 23 | 88 ± 24 | 0.004 |
| Vasopressors/inotropes on admission | 130 (55%) | 30 (40%) | 100 (62%) | 0.003 |
| Vasopressors/inotropes at 6 h | 139 (59%) | 32 (43%) | 107 (66%) | 0.01 |
| Vasopressors/inotropes at 12 h | 150 (64%) | 37 (50%) | 113 (70%) | 0.003 |
| Vasopressors/inotropes at 24 h | 129 (60%) | 37 (50%) | 92 (66%) | 0.03 |
| Vasopressors/inotropes at 48 h | 131 (61%) | 32 (43%) | 99 (71%) | <0.001 |
| *SOFA scores* | | | | |
| SOFA score on admission | 4 [2–7] | 4 [2–5] | 4 [2–8] | 0.08 |
| cSOFA admission | 2 [0–4] | 0 [0–3] | 3 [0–4] | 0.003 |
| hSOFA admission | 0 [0–0] | 0 [0–0] | 0 [0–1] | 0.001 |
| hSOFA maximum | 0 [0–0] | 0 [0–0] | 0 [0–1] | 0.001 |
| *Interventions* | | | | |
| IABP, n (%) | 18 (8%) | 9 (12%) | 9 (5.6%) | 0.19 |
| ECMO, n (%) | 15 (6%) | 2 (3%) | 13 (8%) | 0.15 |
| CRRT, n (%) | 32 (14%) | 3 (4%) | 29 (18%) | 0.004 |

Prognostic implications of blood lactate concentrations after cardiac arrest: a retrospective...

5

**Table 1 continued**

| Parameter | All patients (236) | CPC 1–2 (74) | CPC 3–5 (162) | p value |
|---|---|---|---|---|
| *Outcomes* | | | | |
| ICU LOS (days) | 3 [1–6] | 5 [3–11] | 2 [1–4] | <0.001 |
| Neurological cause of death | 87 (36%) | – | 87 (54%) | <0.001 |

CPC Cerebral Performance Category, CPC 1–2 favourable outcome, CPC 3–5 poor outcome, MAP mean arterial pressure, SOFA sequential organ failure assessment (without the neurological subscore), cSOFA cardiovascular SOFA score, ICU intensive care unit, LOS length of stay, HR heart rate, ABG arterial blood gas analysis, aDLC absolute decrease in lactate concentration over time expressed as mEq/L*h, rDLC relative decrease in lactate concentration over time expressed as %, $AUC_{0-48}$ area under the curve of lactate concentrations for the first 48 h after admission, COPD chronic obstructive pulmonary disease, IABP intra-aortic balloon counterpulsation, ECMO extracorporeal membrane oxygenation, CRRT continuous renal replacement therapy, hSOFA hepatic SOFA subscore, VF/VT ventricular fibrillation/ventricular tachycardia, OHCA out-of-hospital cardiac arrest, CPR cardiopulmonary resuscitation, ROSC return of spontaneous circulation

**Table 2 Logistic regression analysis to identify predictors of poor neurological outcome (CPC 3–5) at 3 months**

| Parameter | OR | 95% CI | p value |
|---|---|---|---|
| Bystander CPR | 0.30 | 0.14–0.64 | 0.002 |
| Shockable rhythm | 0.11 | 0.05–0.23 | <0.001 |
| Lactate on admission, mEq/L | 1.18 | 1.08–1.30 | <0.001 |

OR odds ratio, CI confidence interval, CPR cardiopulmonary resuscitation

odds of poor neurological outcome (OR 1.18[1.08–1.30], $p < 0.001$) (Table 2). Using an ROC curve, blood lactate on admission had a predictive accuracy of 0.69 (95% CI 0.62–0.75) for poor neurological outcome (Additional file 1: Figure S3).

### Subgroup analyses

Lactate concentrations were similar in IHCA and OHCA patients on admission and at subsequent time points (Table 3). In patients with IHCA, but not in those with OHCA, blood lactate concentrations were higher in patients with a poor neurological outcome than in those with a favourable outcome at all time points (Additional file 1: Table S1). Lactate concentrations on admission and at subsequent time points were similar in patients with shockable than those with non-shockable rhythms (Additional file 1: Table S2). Blood lactate concentrations were higher on admission and throughout the study period in patients with shock on admission than in those without (Additional file 1: Table S3).

### Predictors of lactate concentrations and correlation with other haemodynamic variables

There was a weak correlation between blood lactate concentrations on admission and time to ROSC ($r = 0.29$, $p < 0.001$) and MAP on admission ($r = -0.39$, $p < 0.001$, Fig. 1). There was also a significant correlation between initial blood lactate concentration and absolute decrease in lactate concentrations at 6 and 24 h (Additional file 1: Figure S4). In a linear regression model, the use of vasopressors on admission, time to ROSC, initial $PaO_2$ and renal SOFA on admission were independently associated

with high admission lactate levels (Table 4); however, the model explained only 32% of the variance.

### Discussion

Patients with a poor neurological outcome after CA had higher lactate values on admission and over the first 2 days than patients with a favourable outcome. Blood lactate concentration on admission remained a significant predictor of poor outcome even after adjustment for major confounders. Nonetheless, the relative decrease in lactate at 6, 12 and 24 h was not related to neurological outcome. In a linear regression model, use of vasopressors, $PaO_2$, time to ROSC and renal SOFA were independently associated with high admission blood lactate concentration.

The pathophysiology of hyperlactataemia is complex and can involve tissue hypoperfusion, adrenergic hyperstimulation [16] and altered lactate clearance by the liver [17]. Interestingly, high lactate concentrations in our study were associated with renal dysfunction, which was probably a marker of organ failure [18] more than the kidney's inability to clear lactate [16]. There was no association between lactate levels and the intensity of therapy (i.e. ECMO or IABP), although the number of treated patients was relatively limited. There was also no association of lactate on admission and hepatic dysfunction as assessed by the hepatic SOFA subscore. Moreover, increased $PaO_2$ values were predictive of high lactate concentration on admission. Recent studies have suggested that very high $PaO_2$ values (> 300 mmHg) may aggravate post-anoxic brain injury [19]. However, a specific threshold for oxygen toxicity has not yet been identified in clinical practice and the mechanisms relating oxygen toxicity to lactate production need to be further evaluated in this setting.

A high blood lactate concentration on admission was significantly correlated with poor neurological outcome. Similarly, in a large cohort of 443 patients, Lee et al. reported that a high blood lactate measured within 1 h of ROSC was correlated with CPC 3–5 at hospital discharge [7]. In 394 CA survivors enrolled over a 10-year period,

**Table 3 Characteristics of patients according to arrest location (out of hospital [OHCA] vs. in hospital [IHCA])**

| Parameter | OHCA (137) | IHCA (99) | P value |
|---|---|---|---|
| *General* | | | |
| Age | 61 ± 15 | 63 ± 15 | 040 |
| Male | 92 (67%) | 64 (64%) | 0.78 |
| *Comorbidities* | | | |
| COPD/asthma, n (%) | 24 (17%) | 19 (19%) | 0.74 |
| Heart disease, n (%) | 62 (45%) | 45 (45%) | 1.00 |
| Diabetes, n (%) | 31 (23%) | 19 (19%) | 0.63 |
| Chronic renal failure, n (%) | 21 (15%) | 17 (17%) | 0.51 |
| Liver cirrhosis, n (%) | 6 (4%) | 8 (8%) | 0.27 |
| Immunosuppression, n (%) | 17 (12%) | 11 (11%) | 0.84 |
| *Cardiac arrest* | | | |
| VF/VT | 65 (47%) | 35 (35%) | 0.086 |
| Bystander CPR | 57 (42%) | 79 (80%) | <0.001 |
| Time to ROSC (min) | 21.4 ± 12.8 | 16.7 ± 14.3 | 0.011 |
| *ABG* | | | |
| Lactate admission (mEq/L) | 4.3 [2.2–7.9] | 4.8 [1.9–8.6] | 0.81 |
| Lactate 6 h (mEq/L) | 2.7 [1.7–4.7] | 2.7 [1.6–5.5] | 0.51 |
| Lactate 12 h (mEq/L) | 2.2 [1.5–4.2] | 2.3 [1.4–4.1] | 0.78 |
| Lactate 24 h (mEq/L) | 1.5 [1.1–3.0] | 1.4 [1.0–2.5] | 0.605 |
| Lactate 48 h (mEq/L) | 1.4 [1.0–2.0] | 1.4 [1.0–2.3] | 0.415 |
| $aDLC_{0-6}$ (mEq/L*h) | .150 [−.03 to .583] | .167 [0–.517] | 0.88 |
| $aDLC_{0-12}$ (mEq/L*h) | 0.14 [0–0.3] | 0.12 [0–0.3] | 0.55 |
| $aDLC_{0-24}$ (mEq/L*h) | .075 [.004–.192] | .073 [.018–.228] | 0.469 |
| $rDLC_{0-6}$ (%) | 28 [−9 to 55] | 22 [0–50] | 0.75 |
| $rDLC_{0-12}$ (%) | 38 [0–64] | 33 [7–61] | 0.65 |
| $rDLC_{0-24}$ (%) | 51.6 [10.5–75.3] | 56 [25.5–70.5] | 0.558 |
| $AUC_{0-48}$, mEq/L*h | 4.6 ± 4 | 4.7 ± 4.4 | 0.901 |
| Peak lactate, mEq/L | 6.4 ± 3.8 | 6.9 ± 5.2 | 0.001 |
| pH admission | 7.25 [7.16–7.34] | 7.27 [7.19–7.40] | 0.038 |
| $PaO_2$ admission (mmHg) | 124 [82–228] | 116 [70–234] | 0.289 |
| $PaCO_2$ admission (mmHg) | 43.5 ± 14.8 | 40.4 ± 12.7 | 0.101 |
| *Haemodynamics* | | | |
| HR admission | 87 ± 22 | 91 ± 19 | 0.120 |
| MAP admission (mmHg) | 96 ± 25 | 84 ± 20 | <0.001 |
| Vasopressors/inotropes admission | 60 (44%) | 70 (71%) | <0.001 |
| Vasopressors/inotropes 6 h | 67 (49%) | 72 (73%) | <0.001 |
| Vasopressors/inotropes 12 h | 75 (55%) | 75 (75%) | 0.001 |
| Vasopressors/inotropes 24 h | 66 (52%) | 63 (73%) | 0.002 |
| Vasopressors/inotropes 48 h | 68 (53%) | 63 (73%) | 0.004 |
| *SOFA score* | | | |
| SOFA admission | 3.5 [2–5] | 5 [3–8] | <0.001 |
| cSOFA admission | 0 [0–4] | 3 [0–4] | <0.001 |

**Table 3 continued**

| Parameter | OHCA (137) | IHCA (99) | P value |
|---|---|---|---|
| hSOFA baseline | 0 [0–0] | 0 [0–1] | <0.001 |
| hSOFA maximum | 0 [0–0] | 0 [0–1] | 0.002 |
| *Interventions* | | | |
| IABP, n (%) | 9 (7%) | 9 (9%) | 0.47 |
| ECMO, n (%) | 7 (5%) | 8 (8%) | 0.42 |
| CRRT, n (%) | 19 (14%) | 13 (13%) | 1 |
| *Outcomes* | | | |
| ICU LOS (days) | 2 [1–6] | 4 [1–7] | 0.23 |
| Neurological cause of death, n (%) | 61 (44%) | 26 (26%) | 0.008 |
| Poor outcome at 3 months | 94 (69%) | 68 (69%) | 0.711 |

*MAP* mean arterial pressure, *SOFA* sequential organ failure assessment (without the neurological subscore), *cSOFA* cardiovascular SOFA score, *ICU* intensive care unit, *LOS* length of stay, *HR* heart rate, *aDLC* absolute decrease in lactate concentration over time expressed as mEq/L*h, *rDLC* relative decrease in lactate concentration over time expressed as %; $AUC_{0-48}$ area under the curve of lactate concentrations for the first 48 h since admission, *COPD* chronic obstructive pulmonary disease, *IABP* intra-aortic balloon counterpulsation, *ECMO* extracorporeal membrane oxygenation, *CRRT* continuous renal replacement therapy, *hSOFA* hepatic SOFA subscore, *VF/VT* ventricular fibrillation/ventricular tachycardia, *OHCA* out-of-hospital cardiac arrest, *CPR* cardiopulmonary resuscitation, *ROSC* return of spontaneous circulation

Kliegel et al. [20] found a significant correlation between lactate at baseline, 24 and 48 h and neurological outcome. Moreover, blood lactate concentrations have been included, along with initial rhythm, estimated no-flow and low-flow intervals and creatinine levels, in a hospital admission predictive score for good neurological recovery after successful resuscitation from OHCA [21].

A decrease in lactate concentrations over time is a reliable marker of effective treatment in critically ill patients with shock [22–25]. As expected, we found that the higher the lactate on admission, the greater the decrease over time [26]. However, there was no relationship between lactate decrease and neurological outcome. Our findings contrast with those of Donnino et al. [14] who reported that lactate decrease at 6 and 12 h was more pronounced in survivors than in non-survivors, but no data on neurological recovery were available. Two studies have reported that the decrease in lactate at 12 h was an independent marker of good neurological outcome [8, 9]. The differences between these studies and our results may be explained by a lower median lactate on admission in our study (4.3 mEq/L in our study vs. 6 to 15 mEq/L in [8, 9, 14]), which is probably explained by a shorter duration of CA in our cohort of patients.

Of note, we also reported data in patients with IHCA, whereas most previous studies included only OHCA patients. Only Karagiannis et al. [27], in a small group of 28 patients after IHCA, described higher lactate concentrations at 6, 18 and 24 h after ROSC in non-survivors

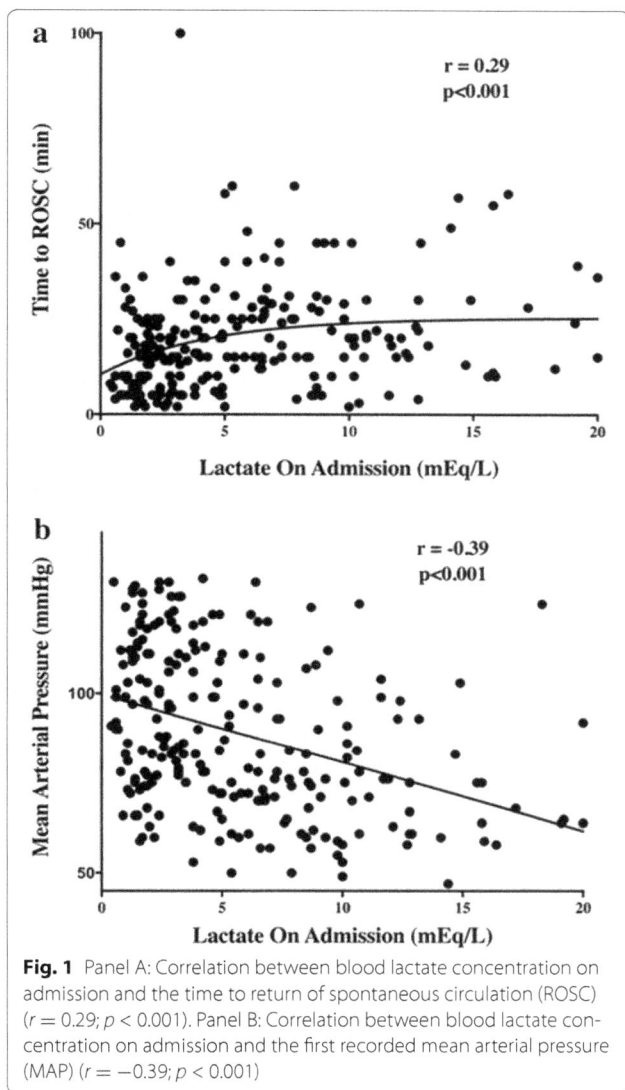

**Fig. 1** Panel A: Correlation between blood lactate concentration on admission and the time to return of spontaneous circulation (ROSC) ($r = 0.29$; $p < 0.001$). Panel B: Correlation between blood lactate concentration on admission and the first recorded mean arterial pressure (MAP) ($r = -0.39$; $p < 0.001$)

**Table 4 Linear regression analysis for admission blood lactate**

| Parameter | Coefficient | p value |
|---|---|---|
| Renal SOFA | $0.94 \pm 0.23$ | <0.001 |
| PaO$_2$ on admission | $0.006 \pm 0.002$ | 0.001 |
| Time to ROSC (min) | $0.067 \pm 0.021$ | 0.001 |
| Vasopressors on admission | $1.78 \pm 0.62$ | 0.004 |

*SOFA* sequential organ failure assessment, *ROSC* return of spontaneous circulation

than in survivors, and a significantly lower percentage decrease in lactate at 6 and 12 h in non-survivors. In our cohort, lactate levels were similar in IHCA and OHCA patients at all time points. This is of interest because IHCA is usually secondary to different aetiologies than

OHCA and associated with severe pre-existing comorbidities, which may alter the generalizability of outcome predictors for OHCA to the IHCA setting. Blood lactate values were also similar regardless of the initial rhythm, despite the fact that patients with non-shockable rhythms are more likely to have prior hypoxia or hypotension and, in general, a longer time from arrest to CPR [28, 29]. This suggests that the prognostic value of lactate levels on admission is independent of these CA characteristics and applicable to a wide CA population.

Our study has some limitations. First, given the retrospective design, we could not reliably account for some variables that may have influenced lactate concentrations, especially on admission, particularly CPR quality, total doses of adrenaline during CPR and fluid administration or fluid balance. However, consistent management in a single centre can reasonably exclude important differences in treatment strategies among patients. Moreover, we provided time to ROSC, but could not differentiate between "no-flow" and "low-flow" times, which could further influence the initial lactate levels (e.g. prolonged "no-flow" times should be associated with higher lactate values). Second, we evaluated a limited cohort of patients, including a heterogeneous population of patients with IHCA and OHCA, which may limit the generalizability of our findings. Third, our model could account for only one-third of the variability in lactate concentrations on admission, indicating that other factors that we did not account for—e.g. no-flow period, total dose of adrenaline given during CPR, vasopressors given during the ICU stay—may be involved in the pathophysiology of high lactate concentrations in this setting. Fourth, baseline lactate concentration may be related to the quality of resuscitation during CA, whereas lactate concentration at 12 or 24 h may be related more to the quality of critical care provided. Although this statement sounds logical, we have almost no data in the literature to confirm this hypothesis and the retrospective nature of our study precludes any additional analysis. Furthermore, the interpretation of baseline lactate could also be confounded by underlying conditions (e.g. sepsis) and/or aetiology of arrest (e.g. prolonged hypoxaemia before arrest). Fifth, lactate concentrations were available to the treating clinicians; although lactate concentrations are not used as a marker of poor prognosis in this setting, we cannot exclude that persistently high lactate concentrations may have encouraged limitation of invasive therapies in some of these patients, thus raising the risk of "self-fulfilling prophecy". Finally, we evaluated liver function using the hepatic SOFA subscore, which is based on total bilirubin levels. Hypoxic hepatitis, as observed after CA, is, however, defined as an elevation of aminotransferases; nevertheless, the occurrence of hypoxic hepatitis is rare [30] and generally occurs 1–2 days after CA, which would be of limited interest for interpretation of admission lactate levels.

## Conclusions

Blood lactate concentrations in patients after CA were significantly higher in those with worse short- and long-term outcomes. However, decrease in lactate over time was not correlated with outcome. Interpretation of high lactate concentrations in CA survivors is complex and multifactorial.

### Abbreviations

CA: cardiac arrest; CPR: cardiopulmonary resuscitation; EEG: electroencephalogram; HR: heart rate; IHCA: in-hospital cardiac arrest; MAP: mean arterial pressure; OHCA: out-of-hospital cardiac arrest; ROSC: return of spontaneous circulation; SOFA: sequential organ failure assessment; SSEP: somatosensory evoked potential; TTM: therapeutic temperature management; VF/VT: ventricular fibrillation/ventricular tachycardia.

### Author details

[1] Department of Intensive Care, Erasme Hospital, Université Libre de Bruxelles, Route de Lennik 808, 1070 Brussels, Belgium. [2] Department of Anesthesiology and Intensive Care, Catholic University School of Medicine, Largo Agostino Gemelli 8, 00168 Rome, Italy. [3] Anaesthesia and Intensive Care B, Department of Surgery, Dentistry, Paediatrics and Gynaecology, University of Verona, AOUI-University Hospital Integrated Trust of Verona, P.le L.A. Scuro 10, 37134 Verona, Italy.

### Authors' contributions

FST, KD and AMD conceived the study protocol; AMD, IB, IL, KD and FST participated in the design and coordination of the study; AMD, IB, IL and FST and MH were responsible for data collection; JC and JLV supervised data collection; AMD, IB, IL, CS, JC and JLV participated in data interpretation; AMD, IL, CS and FST carried out the literature search; AMD, KD, IB, IL and FST drafted the present manuscript; CS, JC and JLV critically revised the manuscript. All authors read and approved the final manuscript.

### Competing interests

The authors declare that they have no competing interests.

### References

1. Mozaffarian D, Benjamin EJ, Go AS, Arnett DK, Blaha MJ, Cushman M, et al. Heart disease and stroke statistics-2016 update: a report from the American Heart Association. Circulation. 2016;133:e38–360.
2. Atwood C, Eisenberg MS, Herlitz J, Rea TD. Incidence of EMS-treated out-of-hospital cardiac arrest in Europe. Resuscitation. 2005;67:75–80.
3. Sandroni C, Nolan J, Cavallaro F, Antonelli M. In-hospital cardiac arrest: incidence, prognosis and possible measures to improve survival. Intensive Care Med. 2007;33:237–45.
4. Nolan JP, Soar J, Smith GB, Gwinnutt C, Parrott F, Power S, et al. Incidence and outcome of in-hospital cardiac arrest in the United Kingdom National Cardiac Arrest Audit. Resuscitation. 2014;85:987–92.
5. Deakin CD, Nolan JP, Soar J, Sunde K, Koster RW, Smith GB, et al. European resuscitation council guidelines for resuscitation 2010 section 4. Adult advanced life support. Resuscitation. 2010;81:1305–52.
6. Mullner M, Sterz F, Domanovits H, Behringer W, Binder M, Laggner AN. The association between blood lactate concentration on admission,

7. Lee DH, Cho IS, Lee SH, Min YI, Min JH, Kim SH, et al. Correlation between initial serum levels of lactate after return of spontaneous circulation and survival and neurological outcomes in patients who undergo therapeutic hypothermia after cardiac arrest. Resuscitation. 2015;88:143–9.
8. Donnino MW, Andersen LW, Giberson T, Gaieski DF, Abella BS, Peberdy MA, et al. Initial lactate and lactate change in post-cardiac arrest: a multi-center validation study. Crit Care Med. 2014;42:1804–11.
9. Lee TR, Kang MJ, Cha WC, Shin TG, Sim MS, Jo IJ, et al. Better lactate clearance associated with good neurologic outcome in survivors who treated with therapeutic hypothermia after out-of-hospital cardiac arrest. Crit Care. 2013;17:R260.
10. Hayashida K, Suzuki M, Yonemoto N, Hori S, Tamura T, Sakurai A, et al. Early lactate clearance is associated with improved outcomes in patients with postcardiac arrest syndrome: a prospective, multicenter observational study (SOS-KANTO 2012 Study). Crit Care Med. 2017;45:e559–66.
11. Sandroni C, Cariou A, Cavallaro F, Cronberg T, Friberg H, Hoedemaekers C, et al. Prognostication in comatose survivors of cardiac arrest: an advisory statement from the European Resuscitation Council and the European Society of Intensive Care Medicine. Intensive Care Med. 2014;40:1816–31.
12. Lemiale V, Dumas F, Mongardon N, Giovanetti O, Charpentier J, Chiche JD, et al. Intensive care unit mortality after cardiac arrest: the relative contribution of shock and brain injury in a large cohort. Intensive Care Med. 2013;39:1972–80.
13. Vincent JL, Moreno R, Takala J, Willatts S, De MA, Bruining H, et al. The SOFA (Sepsis-related Organ Failure Assessment) score to describe organ dysfunction/failure. On behalf of the Working Group on Sepsis-Related Problems of the European Society of Intensive Care Medicine. Intensive Care Med. 1996;22:707–10.
14. Donnino MW, Miller J, Goyal N, Loomba M, Sankey SS, Dolcourt B, et al. Effective lactate clearance is associated with improved outcome in post-cardiac arrest patients. Resuscitation. 2007;75:229–34.
15. Jennett B, Bond M. Assessment of outcome after severe brain damage. Lancet. 1975;1:480–4.
16. Adeva-Andany M, Lopez-Ojen M, Funcasta-Calderon R, Ameneiros-Rodriguez E, Donapetry-Garcia C, Vila-Altesor M, et al. Comprehensive review on lactate metabolism in human health. Mitochondrion. 2014;17:76–100.
17. Tapia P, Soto D, Bruhn A, Alegria L, Jarufe N, Luengo C, et al. Impairment of exogenous lactate clearance in experimental hyperdynamic septic shock is not related to total liver hypoperfusion. Crit Care. 2015;19:188.
18. Sandroni C, Dell'Anna AM, Tujjar O, Geri G, Cariou A, Taccone FS. Acute Kidney Injury (AKI) after cardiac arrest: a systematic review and meta-analysis of clinical studies. Minerva Anestesiol. 2016;82:989–99.
19. Dell'anna AM, Lamanna I, Vincent JL, Taccone FS. How much oxygen in adult cardiac arrest? Crit Care. 2014;18:555.
20. Kliegel A, Losert H, Sterz F, Holzer M, Zeiner A, Havel C, et al. Serial lactate determinations for prediction of outcome after cardiac arrest. Medicine (Baltimore). 2004;83:274–9.
21. Adrie C, Cariou A, Mourvillier B, Laurent I, Dabbane H, Hantala F, et al. Predicting survival with good neurological recovery at hospital admission after successful resuscitation of out-of-hospital cardiac arrest: the OHCA score. Eur Heart J. 2006;27:2840–5.
22. Jansen TC, van Bommel J, Schoonderbeek FJ, Sleeswijk Visser SJ, van der Klooster JM, Lima AP, et al. Early lactate-guided therapy in intensive care unit patients: a multicenter, open-label, randomized controlled trial. Am J Respir Crit Care Med. 2010;182:752–61.
23. Jones AE, Shapiro NI, Trzeciak S, Arnold RC, Claremont HA, Kline JA. Lactate clearance vs central venous oxygen saturation as goals of early sepsis therapy: a randomized clinical trial. JAMA. 2010;303:739–46.
24. Gu WJ, Zhang Z, Bakker J. Early lactate clearance-guided therapy in patients with sepsis: a meta-analysis with trial sequential analysis of randomized controlled trials. Intensive Care Med. 2015;41:1862–3.
25. Vincent JL, Quintairos e Silva AQ, Couto L Jr, Taccone FS. The value of blood lactate kinetics in critically ill patients: a systematic review. Crit Care. 2016;20:257.

26. De Backer DP, Donadello K. Lactate change after cardiopulmonary resuscitation: everything is in the baseline value! Crit Care Med. 2014;42:e805–6.

27. Karagiannis C, Georgiou M, Kouskouni E, Iacovidou N, Xanthos T. Association of lactate levels with outcome after in-hospital cardiac arrest. Resuscitation. 2012;83:e175–6.

28. Roberts-Thomson KC, Lau DH, Sanders P. The diagnosis and management of ventricular arrhythmias. Nat Rev Cardiol. 2011;8:311–21.

29. Murakoshi N, Aonuma K. Epidemiology of arrhythmias and sudden cardiac death in Asia. Circ J. 2013;77:2419–31.

30. Champigneulle B, Geri G, Bougouin W, Dumas F, Arnaout M, Zafrani L, et al. Hypoxic hepatitis after out-of-hospital cardiac arrest: Incidence, determinants and prognosis. Resuscitation. 2016;103:60–5.

# 2

# Plasma microRNAs levels are different between pulmonary and extrapulmonary ARDS patients: a clinical observational study

Yi Zheng[1,2], Song-qiao Liu[1], Qin Sun[1], Jian-feng Xie[1], Jing-yuan Xu[1], Qing Li[1], Chun Pan[1], Ling Liu[1] and Ying-zi Huang[1*]

## Abstract

**Background:** Mesenchymal stem cells (MSC) obviously alleviate the damage of the structure and function of pulmonary vascular endothelial cells (VEC). The therapeutic effects of MSC are significantly different between pulmonary ARDS (ARDSp) and extrapulmonary ARDS (ARDSexp). MicroRNAs (miRNAs), as important media of MSC regulating VEC, are not studied between ARDSp and ARDSexp. We aimed to explore the plasma levels difference of miRNAs that regulate VEC function and are associated with MSC (*MSC-VEC*-miRNAs) between ARDSp and ARDSexp patients.

**Methods:** *MSC-VEC*-miRNAs were obtained through reviewing relevant literatures screened in PubMed database. We enrolled 57 ARDS patients within 24 h of admission to the ICU and then collected blood samples, extracted plasma supernatant. Patients' clinical data were collected. Then, plasma expression of *MSC-VEC*-miRNAs was measured by real-time fluorescence quantitative PCR. Simultaneously, plasma endothelial injury markers VCAM-1, vWF and inflammatory factors TNF-α, IL-10 were detected by ELISA method.

**Results:** Fourteen miRNAs were picked out after screening. A total of 57 ARDS patients were included in this study, among which 43 cases pertained to ARDSp group and 14 cases pertained to ARDSexp group. Plasma miR-221 and miR-27b levels in ARDSexp group exhibited significantly lower than that in ARDSp group (miR-221, 0.22 [0.12–0.49] vs. 0.57 [0.22–1.57], $P = 0.008$, miR-27b, 0.34 [0.10–0.46] vs. 0.60 [0.20–1.46], $P = 0.025$). Plasma vWF concentration in ARDSexp group exhibited significantly lower than that in ARDSp group (0.77 [0.29–1.54] vs. 1.80 [0.95–3.51], $P = 0.048$). Significant positive correlation was found between miR-221 and vWF in plasma levels ($r = 0.688$, $P = 0.022$). Plasma miR-26a and miR-27a levels in non-survival group exhibited significantly lower than that in survival group (miR-26a, 0.17 [0.08–0.20] vs. 0.69 [0.24–2.33] $P = 0.018$, miR-27a, 0.23 [0.16–0.58] vs. 1.45 [0.38–3.63], $P = 0.021$) in ARDSp patients.

**Conclusion:** Plasma miR-221, miR-27b and vWF levels in ARDSexp group are significantly lower than that in ARDSp group. Plasma miR-26a and miR-27a levels in non-survival group are significantly lower than that in survival group in ARDSp patients.

**Keywords:** Pulmonary ARDS, Extrapulmonary ARDS, MicroRNA, Vascular endothelial cell

## Background

Acute respiratory distress syndrome (ARDS) is a common critical disease in intensive care unit (ICU). In recent years, although mechanical ventilation, liquid management, extracorporeal membrane oxygenation and other therapeutic technologies have improved significantly, ARDS is associated with high morbidity and mortality in critically ill patients [1]. Endothelial dysfunction is a key characteristic of ARDS, giving rise to increasing vascular permeability and then pulmonary edema and respiratory failure [2, 3]. The biological underpinnings

*Correspondence: yz_huang@126.com
[1] Department of Critical Care Medicine, Zhongda Hospital, School of Medicine, Southeast University, No. 87, Dingjiaqiao Road, Gulou District, Nanjing 210009, China
Full list of author information is available at the end of the article

manipulating the development of endothelial dysfunction in ARDS are incompletely cognized and represent the inevitable course to precision diagnosis and treatment.

Patients with ARDS which is a heterogeneous syndrome have variant etiologies and pathologies and respond differently to therapeutic interventions [4]. One approach to reducing ARDS heterogeneity is to subclassify patients as ARDSp (originating from pulmonary disease) or ARDSexp (originating from extrapulmonary disease) [5]. In the early stages of ARDS, there were significant differences in damage degree of endothelial cells between ARDSp and ARDSexp [6, 7]. When lung morphology was analyzed by computed tomography (CT), ARDSp was characterized by prominent consolidation, while ARDSexp was characterized by prominent ground-glass opacification [8]. The two subtypes of ARDS respond differently to therapeutic interventions such as alterations in positive end-expiratory pressure, prone ventilation, and recruitment maneuvers [9–13]. Nevertheless, the underlying mechanism governing this difference needs further research.

Mesenchymal stem cells (MSC), protecting adherens junction (VE-cadherin and β-catenin), reducing the lung endothelial cell apoptosis, improve pulmonary vascular endothelial cells (VEC) permeability of ARDS [14–18]. However, the therapeutic effects of MSC are significantly different between ARDSp and ARDSexp [19]. This is similar to bone marrow-derived mononuclear cell more effectively improving survival, lung mechanics and histology in ARDSexp than these in ARDSp [20]. The mechanism of difference is not entirely clear.

MicroRNAs (miRNAs), a group of small (19–25 nucleotides) non-coding segments of RNA, regulate gene expression by binding to target mRNA to inhibit their translation. MiRNAs also play an important role in the regulation of gene expression in the pathogenesis of ARDS. Previous studies [21, 22] showed that MSC control activity of pulmonary VEC through regulating microRNAs (miRNAs) levels. Herein, we tentatively defined *MSC-VEC*-miRNAs as a group of miRNAs which are associated with MSC, have regulatory effects on VEC and have previously been studied in ARDS. Then, levels of *MSC-VEC*-miRNAs can be different in patients with ARDSp and ARDSexp.

Yet, so far, no study has tested whether *MSC-VEC*-miRNAs may serve as biomarkers distinguish between ARDSp and ARDSexp. In this study, 14 *MSC-VEC*-miRNAs were filtrated through relevant literatures. Further, we have examined the expression levels of these *MSC-VEC*-miRNAs in plasma collected from patients diagnosed as ARDSp and ARDSexp. Our purpose is to explore the plasma levels difference of *MSC-VEC*-miRNAs between ARDSp and ARDSexp which is probably

helpful for the study in pathogenesis and clinical diagnosis of ARDSp and ARDSexp.

## Methods
### Screening of *MSC-VEC*-miRNA
Using the combination of keywords and MeSH terms for "endothelial cell" and "microRNA", we searched PubMed for articles that describe associations between the miRNAs and endothelial cell. Each article was reviewed and associated miRNAs ("miRNAs cluster 1") were recorded. Then, we searched each miRNA in "miRNAs cluster 1" individually in conjunction with mesenchymal stromal cell (e.g., "miR-21" and "mesenchymal stromal cell") and reviewed each article to get miRNAs ("miRNAs cluster 2") associated with mesenchymal stromal cell from "miRNAs cluster 1". Using the same method, we obtained *MSC-VEC*-miRNAs, eligible microRNAs that were associated with MSC, has regulatory effects on VEC and has previously been studied in ARDS (Additional file 1: Table S1).

### Subject recruitment and sample acquisition
All new ICU admissions at Zhongda Hospital Affiliated to Southeast University from January 2016 to September 2016 were screened for the presence of ARDS based on acute respiratory distress syndrome: the Berlin Definition [23]. Additional inclusion criteria included 18 years $\leq$ age $\leq$ 89 years and admission into the ICU within the previous 24 h. We excluded immunocompromised patients including history of stem cell transplant, immunosuppressive medication using and excluded patients with malignant tumor and pregnant women.

After signing informed consent, subjects had blood drawn via venipuncture or from pre-existing intravascular catheters. Blood samples from enrolled patients were obtained within 24 h of admission to the ICU. Samples were centrifuged at 1900$g$ for 10 min, and the plasma supernatant was extracted and stored in refrigeratory at − 80 degrees Celsius.

### Patients data collection
Demographic and clinical data from eligible patients was abstracted from the electronic medical record. Demographic data: gender, age, actual height, actual weight, etc. Patient's condition: main diagnosis, acute physiology and chronic health evaluation (APACHE) II scores, sequential organ failure assessment (SOFA) scores, ARDS etiology. ARDS severity: arterial blood $PO_2/FiO_2$ ratio, Murray lung injury score. The style of oxygen therapy and parameters: noninvasive ventilation, invasive ventilation and ventilator parameters. Clinical outcomes: ICU and hospital length of stay, 28-day mortality, occurrence of shock (defined by clinician), occurrence of acute

kidney injury [KDIGO Clinical Practice Guideline for Acute Kidney Injury].

### RNA isolation

The frozen plasma was taken out from refrigeratory and incubated at 37 °C in a water bath until samples are completely thawed. Prolonged incubation should be avoided, which may compromise RNA integrity. RNAs were isolated from plasma samples using miRNeasy serum/plasma kits (Qiagen). The miRNeasy Serum/Plasma Spike-In Control, a *Caenorhabditis elegans* miR-39 miRNA mimic, was chosen as the normalized internal control. 3.5 µl miRNeasy Serum/Plasma Spike-In Control ($1.6 \times 10^8$ copies/µl working solution) was added to the tube containing the lysate before adding chloroform in the RNA extraction process.

### Real-time PCR

After total RNA isolation, quantitative real-time PCR (qRT-PCR) was performed with a miScript System (Qiagen, USA). All procedures were performed according to the instructions provided by the manufacturer. Reverse transcription (RT) was done in a reaction component of 20 µl, which contained 2 µl miScript Reverse Transcriptase Mix, 2 µl miScript Nucleics Mix, 4 µl miScript HiSpec Buffer, a certain volume of template RNA containing 100 ng total RNA and a little RNase-free water increasing reaction volume to 20 µl. The mixture was incubated 37 °C for 60 min and 95 °C for 5 min. The 20 µl RT product was diluted into 100 µl. Reaction system of quantitative real-time PCR contained 10 µl SYBR Green PCR Master Mix, 2 µl miScript specific primer, 2 µl miScript universal primer, 2 µl cDNA and 4 µl RNase-free water. qRT-PCR used an Applied Biosystems StepOne detection system at 95 °C for 15 min, followed by 40 cycles of 95 °C for 15 s, 55 °C for 30 s, 70 °C for 30 s. All qRT-PCRs were performed in triplicate, and the raw Ct (threshold cycle) of each sample was the mean value of three Ct values. The data were analyzed by the $2^{-\Delta\Delta CT}$ method.

### Statistical analysis

Baseline characteristics and clinical condition indicator of human subjects were compared between ARDSp and ARDSexp. Expression levels of selected miRNAs detected by qRT-PCR were normalized to miR-39 and analyzed using the $2^{-\Delta\Delta CT}$ method. Results for normally distributed continuous variables are presented as mean ± SD and compared between groups by Student's *t* tests. Results for non-normally distributed continuous variables are summarized as medians [interquartile ranges] and were compared by Mann–Whitney *U* tests. Results for categorical variables are presented as sample

rate (constituent ratio) and were compared Chi-squared test or Fisher exact test. Logistic regression analysis was carried out to determine the variables that were associated independently with the death of ARDSp patients. We examined whether miR-26a and miR-27a were independent risk factors for the death after adjustment for age and APACHE II score. All tests were two-sided, and *P* values < 0.05 were considered statistically significant.

## Results

### Screening result of *MSC-VEC*-miRNA

Fourteen miRNAs were picked out which include miR-15a, miR-16, miR-21, miR-24, miR-26a, miR-27a, miR-27b, miR-126, miR-146a, miR-150, miR-155, miR-221, miR-223, miR-320. Relevant references were presented with PubMed Unique Identifier in Additional file 2: Table S2. The detail information of these miRNAs is shown in Table 1.

### General characteristics of the patients with ARDS

A total of 101 patients admitted to the ICU of Zhongda Hospital Affiliated to Southeast University from January 2016 to September 2016; diagnosed ARDS were inspected. Ultimately, 44 patients were excluded (30 malignant tumor patients, six patients administered glucocorticoid in the past 6 months, five patients older than 90 years old and three pregnant women). Fifty-seven were included in the study: 43 cases in ARDSp group and 14 cases in ARDSexp group. Age, BMI, APACHE II score, SOFA score, lactic acid, 28-day mortality rate had no statistical difference (*P* > 0.05) between ARDSp and ARDSexp. General data of the 57 ARDS are listed in Table 2.

### Comparison of patient's clinical condition indexes between ARDSp and ARDSexp

Indicators from clinical monitoring and laboratory detection were compared between ARDSp and ARDSexp. Oxygenation index ($PO_2/FiO_2$) in ARDSp was lower than that in ARDSexp (145 [119–203] vs. 206 [184–253], *P* = 0.012). Murray lung injury score in ARDSp was significantly higher than ARDSexp (2.7 [2–3.3] vs. 1.8 [1.3–2.4], *P* = 0.008). $FiO_2$ and PEEP had no statistical difference between ARDSp and ARDSexp (*P* > 0.05). The proportion of ECMO, CRRT and invasive mechanical ventilation treatment had no statistical difference between ARDSp and ARDSexp (*P* > 0.05). Indexes related to infection and shock had no statistical difference between two groups (*P* > 0.05) (Table 3).

### Comparison of plasma *MSC-VEC*-miRNAs levels between ARDSp and ARDSexp

Plasma miR-221 and miR-27b levels in ARDSexp group exhibited significantly lower than that in ARDSp group

**Table 1　Summary of candidate *MSC-VEC*-miRNAs Regulation in vascular endothelial cells**

| MiRNAs | Function on angiogenic process | Gene targets | Adjusting direction |
|---|---|---|---|
| miR-15a | Inhibits angiogenesis through direct targeting of VEGF and FGF | FGF2, FGFR1, VEGF, VEGFR2 | − |
| miR-16 | Inhibits tumor angiogenesis and EC-mediated angiogenesis in vitro and in vivo | FGF2, FGFR1, VEGF, VEGFR2 | − |
| miR-21 | Induces tumor angiogenesis in vitro | PTEN | + |
| miR-24 | Decreases endothelial cell proliferation | Sp1 | − |
| miR-26a | Prevents endothelial cell apoptosis | TRPC6 | + |
| miR-27a | Promotes EC angiogenesis in vitro | SEMA6A, Spry2, Dll4 | + |
| miR-27b | Promotes EC angiogenesis in vitro | SEMA6A, Spry2, Dll4 | + |
| miR-126 | Promotes EC angiogenesis in vitro and in vivo | Spred-1, PIK3R2, VCAM-1 | + |
| miR-150 | Restores vascular barrier function | Ang2 | + |
| miR-146a | Promotes senescence of endothelial cells | NOX4 | − |
| miR-155 | Promotes tumor angiogenesis | VHL | + |
| miR-221 | Inhibits EC-mediated angiogenesis in vitro | c-kit, eNOS | − |
| miR-223 | Prevents endothelial cell proliferation | β1 integrin, IGF-1R | − |
| miR-320 | Inhibits diabetic angiogenesis in vitro | IGF-1 | − |

miR: microRNA, −: Negative regulation, +: Positive adjustment

**Table 2　General data comparison between ARDSp and ARDSexp**

| Variable | Total ($n = 57$) | $ARDS_p$(1) ($n = 43$) | $ARDS_{exp}$(2) ($n = 14$) | P value (1) versus (2) |
|---|---|---|---|---|
| *General condition* | | | | |
| Age (years) | 59.0 ± 17.5 | 56.6 ± 20.4 | 63.7 ± 12.6 | 0.13 |
| Male n (%) | 41 (71.9%) | 30 (69.8%) | 11 (78.6%) | 0.52 |
| BMI | 23.9 ± 3.6 | 24.0 ± 3.8 | 23.6 ± 3.0 | 0.70 |
| APACHE II score | 21.3 ± 8.4 | 21.8 ± 8.5 | 20.0 ± 8.4 | 0.50 |
| SOFA score | 10.4 ± 4.9 | 10.4 ± 4.6 | 10.3 ± 5.7 | 0.93 |
| 28-day mortality | 18 (31.6%) | 14 (32.6%) | 4 (22.2%) | 1.00 |
| *Basic diseases* | | | | |
| COPD n (%) | 1 (1.8%) | 0 (0%) | 1 (7.1%) | 0.25 |
| Hypertension n (%) | 16 (28.1%) | 13 (30.2%) | 3 (21.4%) | 0.77 |
| CHD n (%) | 8 (14.0%) | 7 (16.3%) | 1 (7.1%) | 0.68 |
| CVD n (%) | 8 (14.0%) | 8 (18.6%) | 0 (0%) | 0.19 |
| DM n (%) | 12 (21.1%) | 10 (23.3%) | 2 (14.3%) | 0.74 |
| HBD n (%) | 7 (12.3%) | 1 (2.3%) | 6 (42.9%) | 0.001 |
| ISD n (%) | 0 (%) | 0 (%) | 0 (%) | 1.00 |
| *ARDS etiology* | | | | |
| PI n (%) | 36 (63.2%) | 36 (83.7%) | 0 (0%) | < 0.001 |
| Inhalation n (%) | 3 (5.3%) | 3 (7.0%) | 0 (0%) | 0.57 |
| PC n (%) | 4 (7.0%) | 4 (9.5%) | 0 (0%) | 0.515 |
| Sepsis n (%) | 3 (5.3%) | 0 (0%) | 3 (20%) | 0.016 |
| Pancreatitis n (%) | 4 (7.0%) | 0 (0%) | 4 (26.7%) | 0.004 |
| EPT n (%) | 5 (8.8%) | 0 (0%) | 5 (33.3%) | 0.001 |
| Others n (%) | 2 (3.5%) | 0 (0%) | 2 (14.3%) | 0.057 |
| *Organ dysfunction* | | | | |
| Septic shock n (%) | 22 (38.6%) | 17 (39.5%) | 5 (35.7%) | 0.23 |
| AKI n (%) | 14 (24.6%) | 10 (23.3%) | 4 (28.6%) | 0.97 |

*BMI* body mass index, *COPD* chronic obstructive pulmonary disease, *ARDS* acute respiratory distress syndrome, *AKI* acute kidney injury, *APACHE* acute physiology and chronic health evaluation, *SOFA* sequential organ failure assessment, *CHD* coronary heart disease, *CVD* cerebrovascular disease, *DM* diabetes mellitus, *HBD* hepatobiliary diseases, *ISD* immune system disease, *PI* pulmonary infection, *PC* pulmonary contusion, *EPT* extrapulmonary trauma

**Table 3  Comparison of patient's clinical condition indexes between ARDSp and ARDSexp**

| Variable | Total (n = 57) | ARDS$_p$(1) (n = 43) | ARDS$_{exp}$(2) (n = 14) | P value (1) versus (2) |
|---|---|---|---|---|
| *Lung injury severity* | | | | |
| PH | 7.4 [7.35–7.45] | 7.41 [7.36–7.46] | 7.37 [7.32–7.43] | 0.26 |
| FiO$_2$ | 0.5 [0.4–0.6] | 0.5 [0.4–0.6] | 0.4 [0.4–0.5] | 0.06 |
| PEEP(cmH2O) | 8 [5–12] | 8 [5–12] | 5 [5–12] | 0.54 |
| PO$_2$/FiO$_2$(mmHg) | 165 [112–211] | 145 [110–203] | 206 [184–253] | 0.012 |
| Murray score | 2.3 [1.7–3.1] | 2.7 [2–3.3] | 1.8 [1.3–2.4] | 0.008 |
| *Infection index* | | | | |
| Leukocyte count | 10.4 [6–16.7] | 10.4 [6.4–14.5] | 11.8 [5.5–18.3] | 0.81 |
| Platelet count | 134 [90–188] | 134 [107–195] | 128 [49–184] | 0.38 |
| CRP | 74 [25–128] | 74 [31–121] | 75 [15–141] | 0.87 |
| PCT | 1.3 [0.2–12.9] | 1. 0 [0.2–13.1] | 1.86 [0.7–10.4] | 0.60 |
| *Shock index* | | | | |
| HR | 73 [63–121] | 72 [63–120] | 76 [63–125] | 0.66 |
| NE | 5 [0–27.5] | 4 [0–20] | 5 [0–85] | 0.21 |
| Lactic acid | 2.1 [1–3.1] | 2.0 [0.9–2.9] | 2.2[1.2–5.4] | 0.11 |
| *Organ supporting* | | | | |
| IMV n (%) | 40 (70.2%) | 32 (74.4%) | 8 (57.1%) | 0.37 |
| ECMO n (%) | 12 (21.1%) | 12 (27.9%) | 0 (0%) | 0.065 |
| CRRT n (%) | 10 (17.5%) | 7 (16.3%) | 3 (21.4%) | 0.97 |

*PH* arterial blood pH value, *PO$_2$* arterial partial pressure of oxygen, *FiO$_2$* oxygen concentration, *PEEP* positive end expiratory pressure, *Murray score* lung injury score used for ARDS patients, *CRP* C reactive protein, *PCT* procalcitonin, *IMV* invasive mechanical ventilation, *ECMO* extracorporeal membrane oxygenation, *CRRT* continuous renal replacement therapy, *HR* heart rate, *NE* norepinephrine. P < 0.05 suggests statistical difference

(0.22 [0.12–0.49] vs. 0.57 [0.22–1.57], $P = 0.008$), (0.34 [0.10–0.46] vs. 0.60 [0.20–1.46], $P = 0.025$). Other 12 kinds of plasma miRNAs levels between two groups showed no statistical difference. Plasma levels of *MSC-VEC*-miRNAs between ARDSp and ARDSexp are shown in Fig. 1.

### Comparison of plasma vWF, VCAM-1, IL10, TNFα concentration between ARDSp and ARDSexp

Plasma vWF concentration in ARDSexp group exhibited significantly lower than that in ARDSp group (0.77 [0.29–1.54] vs. 1.80 [0.95–3.51], $P = 0.048$). However, VCAM-1, IL10, TNFα concentration between two groups showed no statistical difference. Plasma concentration of VCAM-1, IL10, TNFα between ARDSp and ARDSexp is shown in Fig. 2.

### The correlation of plasma levels between miR-27b/miR-221 and vWF

As plasma miR-27b/miR-221 and vWF levels were significant different between ARDSp and ARDSexp groups, we analyzed the correlation of plasma levels between miR-27b/miR-221 and vWF. We found significant positive correlation between miR-221 and vWF in plasma levels ($r = 0.688$, $P = 0.022$). However, there was no significant correlation between miR-27b and vWF in plasma levels (Fig. 3).

### Comparison of plasma patient's clinical illness condition data between survival and non-survival group in ARDSp patients

APACHE II score, SOFA score, P/F, Murray score, CRP, Lactic acid were used as common indicators to evaluate ARDS patients' clinical illness condition. This study showed that APACHE II score, SOFA score and lactic acid in survival group were significantly lower than that in non-survival group (APACHE II score: $18.7 \pm 7.6$ vs. $28.1 \pm 7.6$, $P<0.001$; SOFA score: $8.8 \pm 4.1$ vs. $14.0 \pm 3.8$, $P<0.001$; lactic acid: 1.7 [0.9–2.2] vs. 2.9 [1.2–3.3], $P = 0.015$) in ARDSp patients. P/F, Murray score and CRP between two groups showed no statistical difference (Table 4).

### Comparison of plasma *MSC-VEC*-miRNAs levels between survival and non-survival group in ARDSp patients

In our research, extrapulmonary ARDS was caused by sepsis, pancreatitis, extrapulmonary trauma etc. We just analyzed plasma *MSC-VEC*-miRNAs and vWF, VCAM-1, IL10, TNFα levels between 28 days survival and 28 days non-survival group in ARDSp patients in order to reduce the heterogeneity between patients. Plasma miR-26a and miR-27a levels in non-survival group exhibited significantly lower than that in survival group (miR-26a: 0.17 [0.08–0.20] vs. 0.69 [0.24–2.33] $P = 0.018$; miR-27a: 0.23

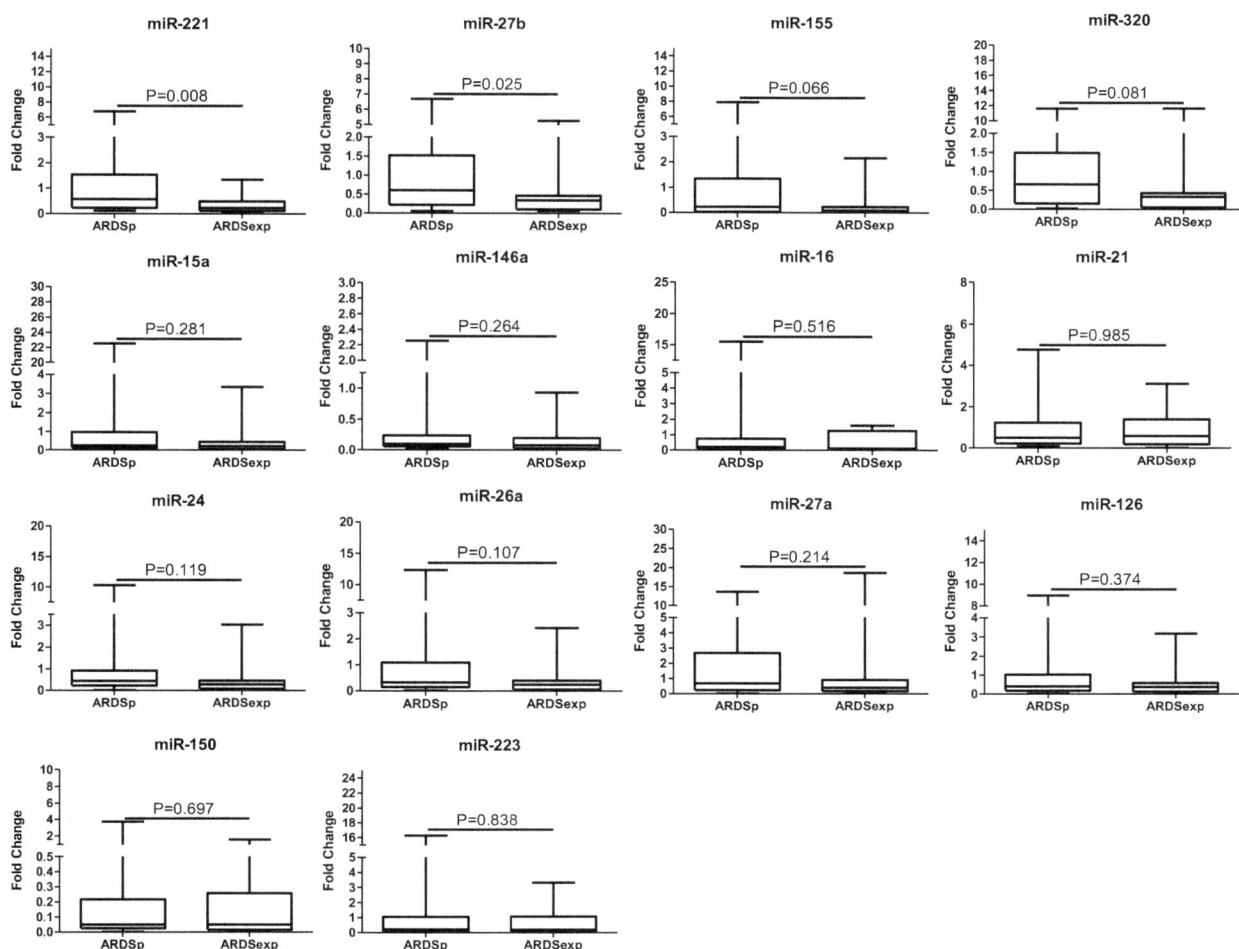

**Fig. 1** Comparison of *MSC-VEC*-miRNAs between ARDSp and ARDSexp. Data presented as a relative fold change between ARDSp and ARDSexp for each miRNA. Box plots are displayed where the horizontal bar represents the median, the box represents the IQR, and the whiskers represent the maximum and minimum values. Comparisons made by Mann–Whitney *U* test. *miRNA* microRNA, *IQR* interquartile range

[0.16–0.58] vs. 1.45 [0.38–3.63], $P = 0.021$) in ARDSp patients. Other 12 kinds of miRNAs and vWF, VCAM-1, IL10, TNFα levels in plasma between two groups showed no statistical difference (Figs. 4, 5).

**The predictive value of miR-26a and miR-27a for prognosis of ARDSp patients**

As APACHE II score, SOFA score, lactic acid, miR-26a and miR-27a were significantly different between non-survival and survival groups in ARDSp patients, ROC curves were drawn and the area under the curve (AUC) values for APACHE II score, SOFA score, lactic acid, miR-26a and miR-27a were, respectively, 0.808 (95%CI: 0.673–0.943), 0.828 (95%CI: 0.693–0.962), 0.782 (95%CI: 0.564–0.897), 0.787 (95%CI: 0.650–0.925), 0.782 (95%CI: 0.650–0.918) (Fig. 6). We also divided the patients into two groups according to median miR-26a

or miR-27a value. Survival curve analysis showed that ARDSp patients with lower concentration of miR-26a/miR-27a had higher mortality (Fig. 7). Tables 5 and 6 show the results of the multivariate logistic regression analysis for the death of ARDSp patients. MiR-26a (OR: 1.483, 95% CI: 0.999–2.200, $P = 0.050$), miR-27a (OR: 1.425, 95% CI: 1.008–2.015, $P = 0.045$) were may independently associated with the death of ARDSp patients.

**Discussion**

The results of this study demonstrate that the expression of plasma miR-221, miR-27b and endothelial markers vWF is significantly different between ARDSp and ARDSexp patients. Plasma miR-26a and miR-27a levels showed significantly different between non-survival group and survival group in ARDSp patients.

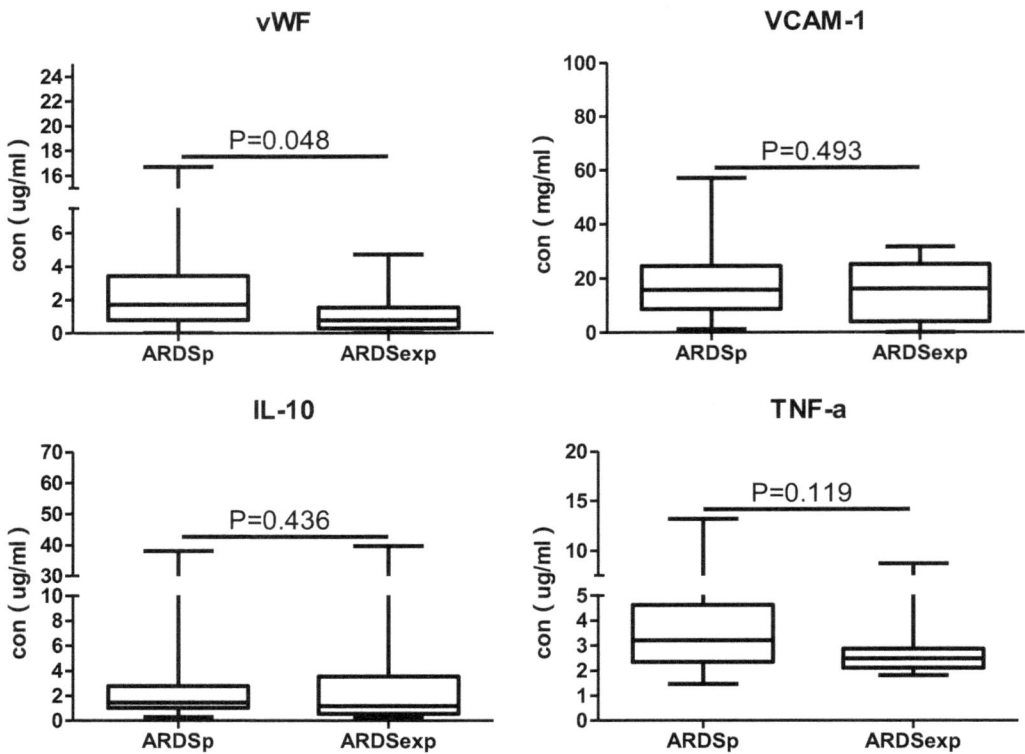

**Fig. 2** Comparison of plasma vWF, VCAM-1, IL10, TNFα concentration between ARDSp and ARDSexp. The concentration unit of vWF, IL10, TNFα is ug/ml. The concentration unit of VCAM-1 is mg/ml. Box plots are displayed where the horizontal bar represents the median, the box represents the IQR and the whiskers represent the maximum and minimum values. Comparisons made by Mann–Whitney $U$ test

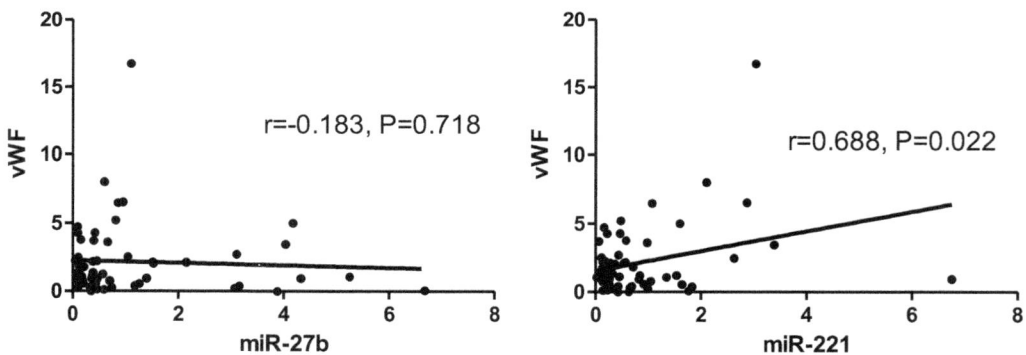

**Fig. 3** Correlation between vWF and miR-27b/miR-221

The characteristics of the enrolled patients in this study may impact research results. The ARDSp patients are more serious than the ARDSexp patients in the local lung injury and lung function lesion. The ARDSp patients owned higher Murray lung injury score and lower $PO_2/FiO_2$ than the ARDSexp patients and included all 12 patients received ECMO treatment. But indicators

related to the overall illness condition, such as APACHE II scores, SOFA scores, blood lactate levels, doses of norepinephrine and the proportion of complicating sepsis, septic shock, AKI showed no statistical difference between ARDSp and ARDSexp patients. There was no difference in the 28-day mortality between the two groups, probably because the overall illness condition

## Table 4 Comparison of patient's clinical illness condition data in ARDSp patients

| Variable | Survival (n = 29) | Non-survival (n = 14) | P value |
|---|---|---|---|
| APACHE II score | 18.7 ± 7.6 | 28.1 ± 7.6 | < 0.001 |
| SOFA score | 8.8 ± 4.1 | 14.0 ± 3.8 | < 0.001 |
| P/F(mmHg) | 150 [113–203] | 130 [100–195] | 0.39 |
| Murray score | 2.6 [2.0–3.0] | 3.0 [2.3–3.7] | 0.09 |
| CRP | 73.7 [31.0–111] | 91.3 [33.3–121] | 0.76 |
| Lactic acid | 1.7 [0.9–2.2] | 2.9 [1.2–3.3] | 0.015 |

had no difference between the two groups. Therefore, the survival rate depends on overall illness severity or, say, the systematic condition of the whole organ rather than single organ lesions. We should pay attention to primary disease treatment and, meanwhile, systematic organ maintenance to prevent multiple organ dysfunction on critically ill patients.

In our study, pulmonary vascular endothelium lesion in ARDSp patients may be more serious than that in ARDSexp patients which embody in Murray lung injury score and $PO_2/FiO_2$. The result is in agreement with the previous research [24–26]. Previous studies show that miR-27b promotes vascular endothelial cell angiogenesis, yet miR-221 inhibits vascular endothelial cell-mediated angiogenesis. So, we deem ARDSp patients will express higher levels of miR-221 and, conversely, express reduced levels of miR-27b than ARDSexp patients. However, our research shows that plasma miR-221 and miR-27b levels

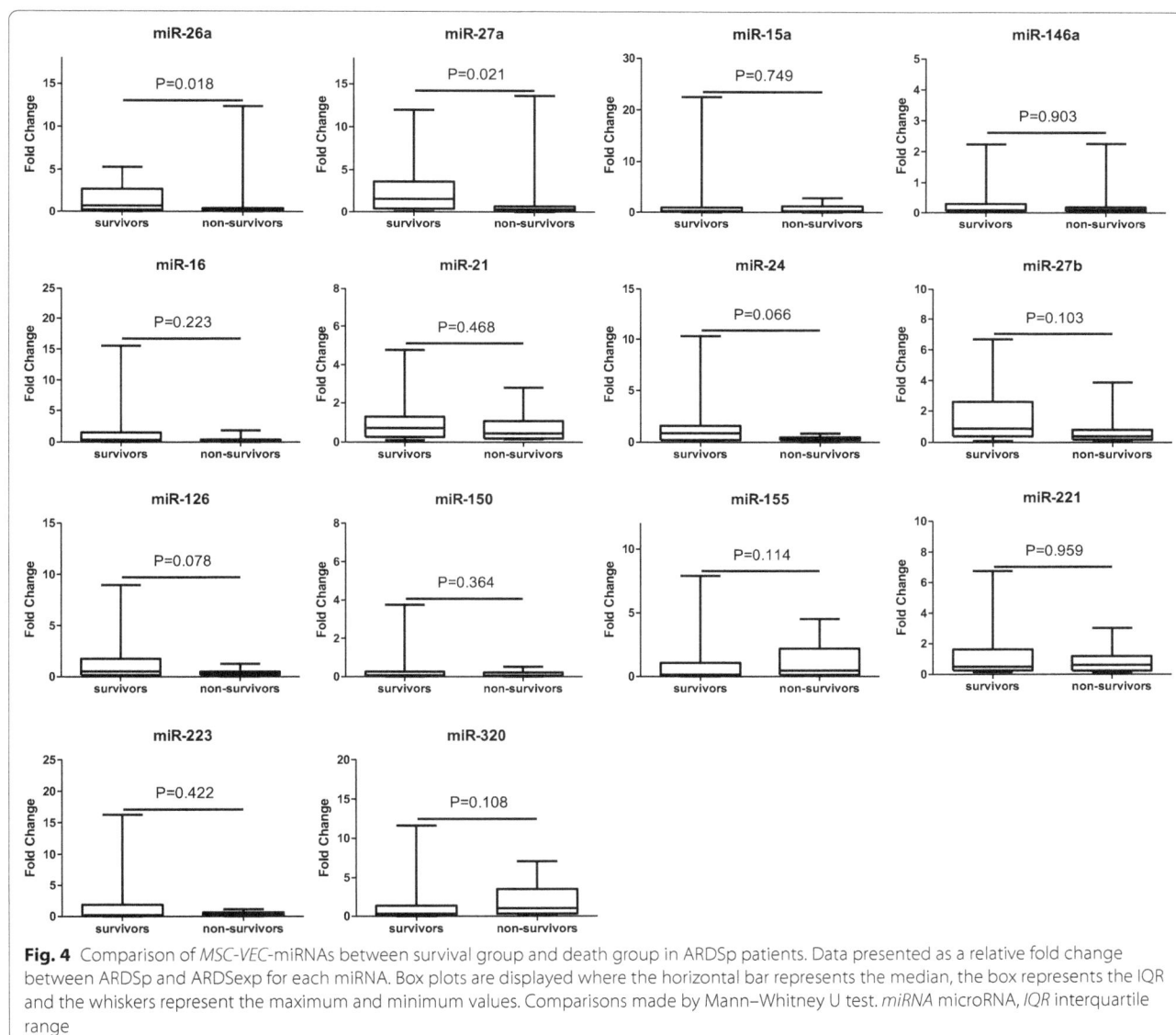

**Fig. 4** Comparison of *MSC-VEC*-miRNAs between survival group and death group in ARDSp patients. Data presented as a relative fold change between ARDSp and ARDSexp for each miRNA. Box plots are displayed where the horizontal bar represents the median, the box represents the IQR and the whiskers represent the maximum and minimum values. Comparisons made by Mann–Whitney U test. *miRNA* microRNA, *IQR* interquartile range

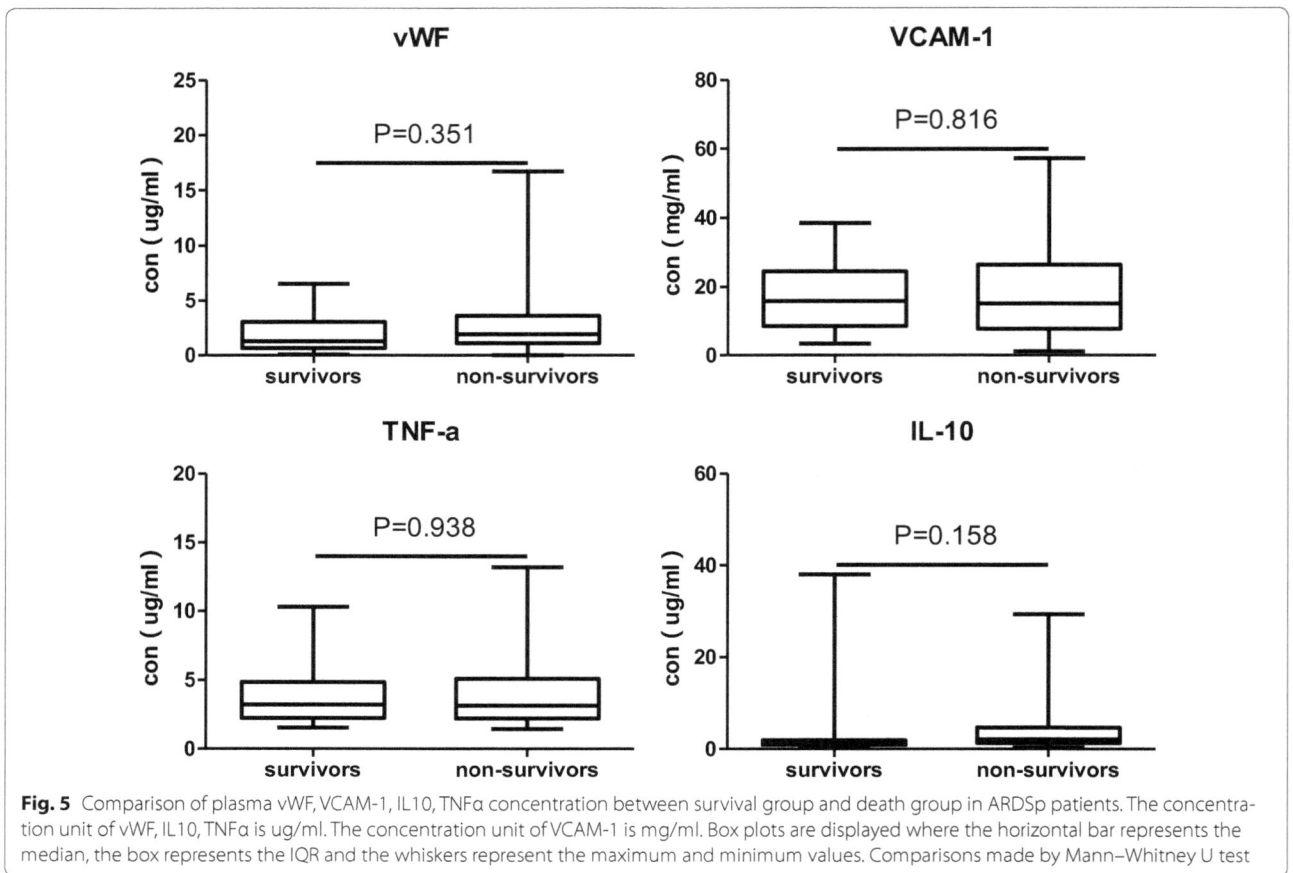

**Fig. 5** Comparison of plasma vWF, VCAM-1, IL10, TNFα concentration between survival group and death group in ARDSp patients. The concentration unit of vWF, IL10, TNFα is ug/ml. The concentration unit of VCAM-1 is mg/ml. Box plots are displayed where the horizontal bar represents the median, the box represents the IQR and the whiskers represent the maximum and minimum values. Comparisons made by Mann–Whitney U test

in ARDSexp group exhibited significantly lower than that in ARDSp group which is inconsistent with expected results. We reviewed forepassed clinical researches and acquired contradictory results with each other. Significant increase in miR-27b expression was observed in the serum samples of patients with peripheral artery disease and arteriosclerosis obliterans when compared to the controls [27, 28]. Coskunpinar et al. [29] reported an increased plasma expression level of miR-221 in acute myocardial infarction compared with healthy controls. However, Tsai et al. presented that stroke patients and atherosclerosis subjects had significantly lower miR-221 serum levels than healthy controls [30]. These conclusions give us a hint that the expression of miRNAs is complex in different diseases originating from the similar pathological change.

Meanwhile, this research explored endothelial markers vWF, VCAM-1 and inflammatory cytokines IL10, TNFα. Plasma vWF concentration in ARDSexp group exhibited significantly lower than that in ARDSp group; however, plasma VCAM-1, IL10, TNFα concentration showed no statistical difference between two groups. As far as we know, endothelium can release vWF which

forms additional links between the platelets' glycoprotein and the collagen fibrils. To a certain extent, elevated vWF concentration reflected vascular endothelium lesion. But there was much controversy as to whether vWF could serve as a biomarker for ARDS. VWF is considered as in vivo and in vitro marker of endothelial injury in patients with ARDS [31]. It has previously been reported that high plasma level of vWF was associated with a greater risk of developing ARDS in sepsis patients and was associated with higher mortality in patients with established ARDS [31–34]. It also was reported that plasma levels of vWF did not appear to serve as useful markers for predicting ARDS in patients at risk and mortality in ARDS patients [35–37]. The vWF studies in ARDSp and ARDSexp are rare. Calfee et al. [38] reported that plasma vWF levels were significantly lower in ARDSp than that in ARDSexp which was not consistent with our result. It may be because patients in ARDSexp group were severer with higher APACHE III score and mortality in this study which was not consistent with our research, too. Upregulation of VCAM-1 in endothelial cells by cytokines partly occurs as a result of increased gene TNFα transcription. So, in our results,

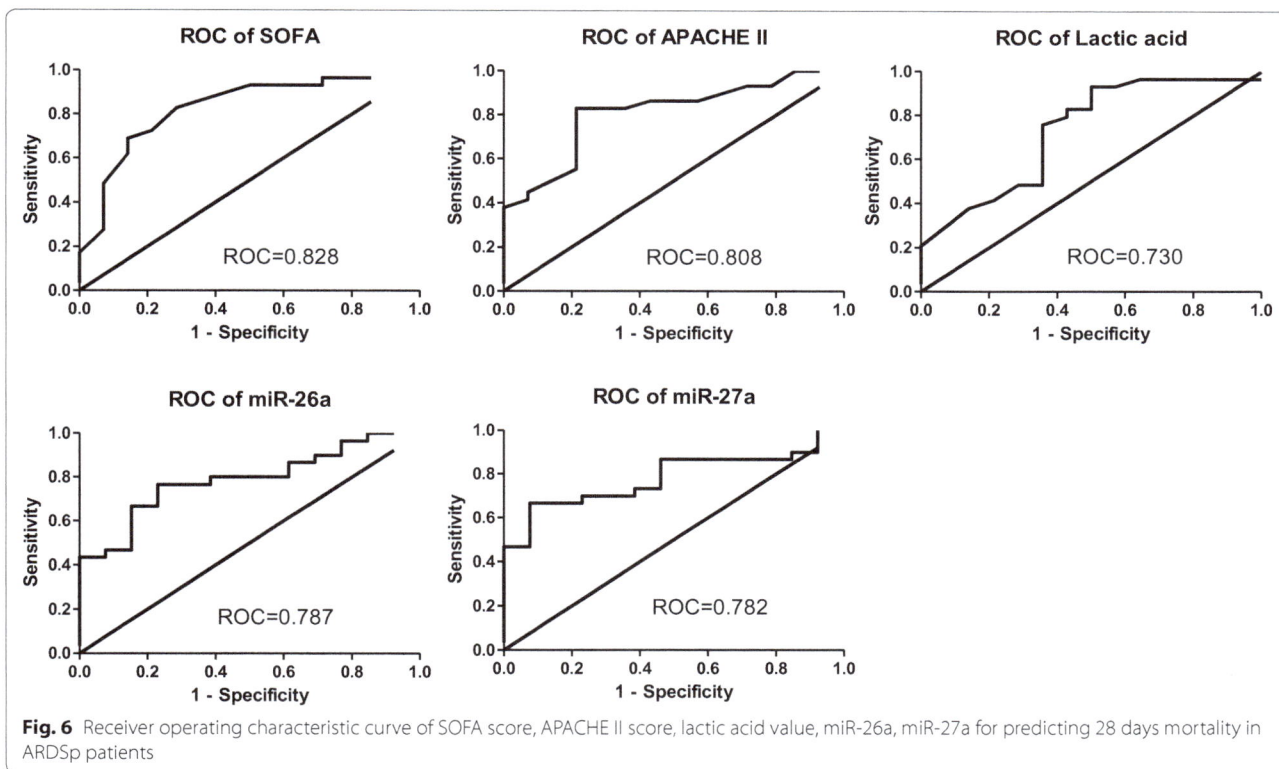

**Fig. 6** Receiver operating characteristic curve of SOFA score, APACHE II score, lactic acid value, miR-26a, miR-27a for predicting 28 days mortality in ARDSp patients

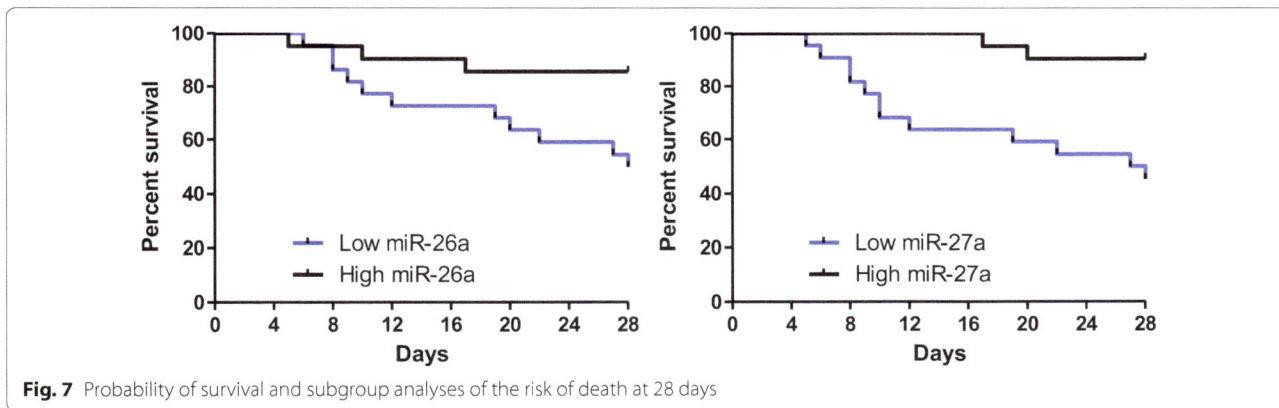

**Fig. 7** Probability of survival and subgroup analyses of the risk of death at 28 days

**Table 5 Multivariable analysis (miR-26a included) of the death of ARDSp patients**

|  | Odds ratio | 95% CI | P value |
|---|---|---|---|
| (Intercept) | 3931.707 | – | 0.004 |
| Age | 0.959 | 0.908–1.013 | 0.133 |
| APACHE II score | 0.791 | 0.679–0.921 | 0.003 |
| miR-26a | 1.483 | 0.999–2.200 | 0.050 |

VCAM-1 and TNFα change in the same direction. In our study, leukocyte count, PCT, CRP showed no statistical difference between two groups, which is consistent with the change direction of IL10, TNFα.

Significant positive correlation between miR-221 and vWF in plasma levels was found in our study. Circulating is mostly released constitutively from endothelial storage organelles, Weibel–Palade bodies (WPBs) [39, 40]. WPBs are released from endothelial cells in response to a large

**Table 6 Multivariable analysis (miR-27a included) of the death of ARDSp patients**

|  | Odds ratio | 95% CI | P value |
|---|---|---|---|
| (Intercept) | 1673.348 | – | 0.007 |
| Age | 0.964 | 0.914–1.017 | 0.185 |
| APACHE II score | 0.803 | 0.679–0.926 | 0.002 |
| miR-27a | 1.425 | 1.008–2.015 | 0.045 |

number of agonists which include two distinct groups: those that act by elevating intracellular calcium ion ($Ca^{2+}$) levels and those that act by raising cAMP levels in the cell [41–44]. Xiang et al. [45] identified that miR-24 and miR-335 targeted human vWF 3'UTR. Previous studies with regard to miR-221 regulating vWF production are absent. However, miR-221 increases free $Ca^{2+}$ level of mast cells by PI3 K/Akt/PLCγ/$Ca^{2+}$ signaling pathway [46]. MiR-221 may have the same regulatory role in vascular endothelial cells. The reasons of the positive correlation between miR-221 and vWF in plasma levels need to be studied further.

Because the etiology of extrapulmonary ARDS is diverse, we just analyzed plasma *MSC-VEC*-miRNAs and vWF, VCAM-1, IL10, TNFα levels between 28 days survival and 28 days non-survival group in ARDSp patients in order to reduce the heterogeneity between patients. In ARDSp patients, plasma miR-26a and miR-27a levels in non-survival group exhibited significant statistical differences. Plasma levels of miR-26a and miR-27a were lower in non-survival group, which might be because the two miRNAs were protective factors of vascular endothelial cell. APACHE II score, SOFA score, and lactic acid value showed significant statistical differences between two groups. Receiver operating characteristic curve (ROC curve) showed that SOFA score, APACHE II score, lactic acid value, miR-26a, miR-27a roughly equally predict the prognosis of ARDSp patients. Survival curve intuitively points out that plasma miR-26a and miR-27a levels were associated with mortality in ARDSp patients. So, miR-26a and miR-27a may be potential biomarkers for predicting the prognosis of ARDSp patients, the molecular mechanisms behind this which need to be further studied.

There are limitations in this study. Firstly, as stated above, our candidate miRNAs limited to the *MSC-VEC*-miRNAs, which is associated with MSC, has regulatory effects on VEC and has previously been studied in ARDS. The broader miRNA spectrum needs to be involved in future research. Secondly, this study is a clinical observational study, but not involved the molecular mechanism of miRNA regulation in cell. So, we cannot determine where the differential expression of plasma miR-221 and miR-27b come from and which results the difference contributes to. Thirdly, the sample size is relatively small

which may have limited the power of statistical difference in this study.

In conclusion, ARDSp patients have higher Murray lung injury score and worse oxygenation index than ARDSexp patients in our study. Plasma miR-221, miR-27b and vWF levels in ARDSexp patients exhibited significantly lower than that in ARDSp patients. Significant positive correlation was found between miR-221 and vWF in plasma levels. In addition, we found plasma miR-26a and miR-27a levels in non-survival group exhibited significantly lower than that in survival group in ARDSp patients.

**Abbreviations**
ARDS: acute respiratory distress syndrome; MSC: mesenchymal stem cells; VEC: vascular endothelial cells; ARDSp: pulmonary ARDS; ARDSexp: extrapulmonary ARDS; miRNAs: microRNAs, miR microRNA; ICU: intensive care unit; vWF: von Willebrand factor; APACHE: acute physiology and chronic health evaluation; SOFA: sequential organ failure assessment; KDIGO: kidney disease improving global outcomes; ECMO: extracorporeal membrane oxygenation; CRRT: continuous renal replacement therapy; VCAM-1: vascular cell adhesion molecule 1; IL: interleukin; TNFα: tumor necrosis factor α; CRP: c-Reactive protein; PCT: procalcitonin; ROC: receiver operating characteristic; AUC: area under the curve; AKI: acute kidney injury; IQR: interquartile range.

**Authors' contributions**
YZH and YZ designed the study. YZ, QS, QL, JFX, and CP conducted experimental operation, performed statistical analyses and interpretation of the data. YZ, SQL collect clinical data and wrote the manuscript. LL, YZH commented on the manuscript. All authors read and approved the final manuscript.

**Author details**
[1] Department of Critical Care Medicine, Zhongda Hospital, School of Medicine, Southeast University, No. 87, Dingjiaqiao Road, Gulou District, Nanjing 210009, China. [2] Department of Critical Care Medicine, The First Affiliated Hospital of Medical School of Zhejiang University, 79 Qingchun Road, Shangcheng District, Hangzhou 310003, China.

**Acknowledgements**
The authors thank Hai-bo Qiu, Yi Yang, Ming Xue, Sen Lu, and Rong-rong Huang for their support in the realization of this study.

**Competing interests**
The authors declare that they have no competing interests

**Funding**
The study was sponsored by Natural Science Foundation of Jiangsu Province (CN) (BK20141344).

# References

1. Bellani G, Laffey JG, Pham T, Fan E, Brochard L, Esteban A, Gattinoni L, van Haren F, Larsson A, McAuley DF, et al. Epidemiology, patterns of care, and mortality for patients with acute respiratory distress syndrome in intensive care units in 50 countries. JAMA. 2016;315(8):788–800.
2. Orfanos SE, Mavrommati I, Korovesi I, Roussos C. Pulmonary endothelium in acute lung injury: from basic science to the critically ill. Intensive Care Med. 2004;30(9):1702–14.
3. Gill SE, Rohan M, Mehta S. Role of pulmonary microvascular endothelial cell apoptosis in murine sepsis-induced lung injury in vivo. Respir Res. 2015;16:109.
4. Gattinoni L, Pelosi P, Suter PM, Pedoto A, Vercesi P, Lissoni A. Acute respiratory distress syndrome caused by pulmonary and extrapulmonary disease. Different syndromes? Am J Respir Crit Care Med. 1998;158(1):3–11.
5. Bernard GR, Artigas A, Brigham KL, Carlet J, Falke K, Hudson L, Lamy M, Legall JR, Morris A, Spragg R. The American–European consensus conference on ARDS. Definitions, mechanisms, relevant outcomes, and clinical trial coordination. Am J Respir Crit Care Med. 1994;149(3 Pt 1):818–24.
6. Rocco PR, Pelosi P. Pulmonary and extrapulmonary acute respiratory distress syndrome: myth or reality? Curr Opin Crit Care. 2008;14(1):50–5.
7. Hoeper MM, Spiekerkoetter E, Westerkamp V, Gatzke R, Fabel H. Intravenous iloprost for treatment failure of aerosolised iloprost in pulmonary arterial hypertension. Eur Respir J. 2002;20(2):339–43.
8. Goodman LR, Fumagalli R, Tagliabue P, Tagliabue M, Ferrario M, Gattinoni L, Pesenti A. Adult respiratory distress syndrome due to pulmonary and extrapulmonary causes: CT, clinical, and functional correlations. Radiology. 1999;213(2):545–52.
9. Rialp G, Betbese AJ, Perez-Marquez M, Mancebo J. Short-term effects of inhaled nitric oxide and prone position in pulmonary and extrapulmonary acute respiratory distress syndrome. Am J Respir Crit Care Med. 2001;164(2):243–9.
10. Lim CM, Kim EK, Lee JS, Shim TS, Lee SD, Koh Y, Kim WS, Kim DS, Kim WD. Comparison of the response to the prone position between pulmonary and extrapulmonary acute respiratory distress syndrome. Intensive Care Med. 2001;27(3):477–85.
11. Riva DR, Oliveira MB, Rzezinski AF, Rangel G, Capelozzi VL, Zin WA, Morales MM, Pelosi P, Rocco PR. Recruitment maneuver in pulmonary and extrapulmonary experimental acute lung injury. Crit Care Med. 2008;36(6):1900–8.
12. Kloot TE, Blanch L, Melynne Youngblood A, Weinert C, Adams AB, Marini JJ, Shapiro RS, Nahum A. Recruitment maneuvers in three experimental models of acute lung injury. Effect on lung volume and gas exchange. Am J Respir Crit Care Med. 2000;161(5):1485–94.
13. Tugrul S, Akinci O, Ozcan PE, Ince S, Esen F, Telci L, Akpir K, Cakar N. Effects of sustained inflation and postinflation positive end-expiratory pressure in acute respiratory distress syndrome: focusing on pulmonary and extrapulmonary forms. Crit Care Med. 2003;31(3):738–44.
14. Pati S, Gerber MH, Menge TD, Wataha KA, Zhao Y, Baumgartner JA, Zhao J, Letourneau PA, Huby MP, Baer LA, et al. Bone marrow derived mesenchymal stem cells inhibit inflammation and preserve vascular endothelial integrity in the lungs after hemorrhagic shock. PLoS ONE. 2011;6(9):e25171.
15. Yang Y, Chen QH, Liu AR, Xu XP, Han JB, Qiu HB. Synergism of MSC-secreted HGF and VEGF in stabilising endothelial barrier function upon lipopolysaccharide stimulation via the Rac1 pathway. Stem Cell Res Ther. 2015;6:250.
16. Hu S, Li J, Xu X, Liu A, He H, Xu J, Chen Q, Liu S, Liu L, Qiu H, et al. The hepatocyte growth factor-expressing character is required for mesenchymal stem cells to protect the lung injured by lipopolysaccharide in vivo. Stem Cell Res Ther. 2016;7(1):66.
17. Wang H, Zheng R, Chen Q, Shao J, Yu J, Hu S. Mesenchymal stem cells microvesicles stabilize endothelial barrier function partly mediated by hepatocyte growth factor (HGF). Stem Cell Res Ther. 2017;8(1):211.
18. Potter DR, Miyazawa BY, Gibb SL, Deng X, Togaratti PP, Croze RH, Srivastava AK, Trivedi A, Matthay M, Holcomb JB, et al. Mesenchymal stem cell derived extracellular vesicles attenuate pulmonary vascular permeability and lung injury induced by hemorrhagic shock and trauma. J Trauma Acute Care Surg. 2017;84(2):245–56.
19. Liu L, He H, Liu A, Xu J, Han J, Chen Q, Hu S, Xu X, Huang Y, Guo F, et al. Therapeutic effects of bone marrow-derived mesenchymal stem cells in models of pulmonary and extrapulmonary acute lung injury. Cell Transplant. 2015;24(12):2629–42.
20. Araujo IM, Abreu SC, Maron-Gutierrez T, Cruz F, Fujisaki L, Carreira H Jr,

Ornellas F, Ornellas D, Vieira-de-Abreu A, Castro-Faria-Neto HC, et al. Bone marrow-derived mononuclear cell therapy in experimental pulmonary and extrapulmonary acute lung injury. Crit Care Med. 2010;38(8):1733–41.
21. Zhou Z, You Z. Mesenchymal stem cells alleviate LPS-induced acute lung injury in mice by MiR-142a-5p-controlled pulmonary endothelial cell autophagy. Cell Physiol Biochem. 2016;38(1):258–66.
22. Bao H, Gao F, Xie G, Liu Z. Angiotensin-converting enzyme 2 inhibits apoptosis of pulmonary endothelial cells during acute lung injury through suppressing MiR-4262. Cell Physiol Biochem. 2015;37(2):759–67.
23. Force ADT, Ranieri VM, Rubenfeld GD, Thompson BT, Ferguson ND, Caldwell E, Fan E, Camporota L, Slutsky AS. Acute respiratory distress syndrome: the Berlin definition. JAMA. 2012;307(23):2526–33.
24. Kim SJ, Oh BJ, Lee JS, Lim CM, Shim TS, Lee SD, Kim WS, Kim DS, Kim WD, Koh Y. Recovery from lung injury in survivors of acute respiratory distress syndrome: difference between pulmonary and extrapulmonary subtypes. Intensive Care Med. 2004;30(10):1960–3.
25. Morisawa K, Fujitani S, Taira Y, Kushimoto S, Kitazawa Y, Okuchi K, Ishikura H, Sakamoto T, Tagami T, Yamaguchi J, et al. Difference in pulmonary permeability between indirect and direct acute respiratory distress syndrome assessed by the transpulmonary thermodilution technique: a prospective, observational, multi-institutional study. J Intensive Care. 2014;2(1):24.
26. Luo L, Shaver CM, Zhao Z, Koyama T, Calfee CS, Bastarache JA, Ware LB. Clinical predictors of hospital mortality differ between direct and indirect ARDS. Chest. 2017;151(4):755–63.
27. Signorelli SS, Volsi GL, Pitruzzella A, Fiore V, Mangiafico M, Vanella L, Parenti R, Rizzo M, Volti GL. Circulating miR-130a, miR-27b, and miR-210 in patients with peripheral artery disease and their potential relationship with oxidative stress. Angiology. 2016;67(10):945–50.
28. Li T, Cao H, Zhuang J, Wan J, Guan M, Yu B, Li X, Zhang W. Identification of miR-130a, miR-27b and miR-210 as serum biomarkers for atherosclerosis obliterans. Clin Chim Acta. 2011;412(1–2):66–70.
29. Coskunpinar E, Cakmak HA, Kalkan AK, Tiryakioglu NO, Erturk M, Ongen Z. Circulating miR-221-3p as a novel marker for early prediction of acute myocardial infarction. Gene. 2016;591(1):90–6.
30. Tsai PC, Liao YC, Wang YS, Lin HF, Lin RT, Juo SH. Serum microRNA-21 and microRNA-221 as potential biomarkers for cerebrovascular disease. J Vasc Res. 2013;50(4):346–54.
31. Ware LB, Eisner MD, Thompson BT, Parsons PE, Matthay MA. Significance of von Willebrand factor in septic and nonseptic patients with acute lung injury. Am J Respir Crit Care Med. 2004;170(7):766–72.
32. Rubin DB, Wiener-Kronish JP, Murray JF, Green DR, Turner J, Luce JM, Montgomery AB, Marks JD, Matthay MA. Elevated von Willebrand factor antigen is an early plasma predictor of acute lung injury in nonpulmonary sepsis syndrome. J Clin Invest. 1990;86(2):474–80.
33. Ware LB, Conner ER, Matthay MA. von Willebrand factor antigen is an independent marker of poor outcome in patients with early acute lung injury. Crit Care Med. 2001;29(12):2325–31.
34. Siemiatkowski A, Kloczko J, Galar M, Czaban S. von Willebrand factor antigen as a prognostic marker in posttraumatic acute lung injury. Haemostasis. 2000;30(4):189–95.
35. Bajaj MS, Tricomi SM. Plasma levels of the three endothelial-specific proteins von Willebrand factor, tissue factor pathway inhibitor, and thrombomodulin do not predict the development of acute respiratory distress syndrome. Intensive Care Med. 1999;25(11):1259–66.
36. Moss M, Ackerson L, Gillespie MK, Moore FA, Moore EE, Parsons PE. von Willebrand factor antigen levels are not predictive for the adult respiratory distress syndrome. Am J Respir Crit Care Med. 1995;151(1):15–20.
37. Cartin-Ceba R, Hubmayr RD, Qin R, Peters S, Determann RM, Schultz MJ, Gajic O. Predictive value of plasma biomarkers for mortality and organ failure development in patients with acute respiratory distress syndrome. J Crit Care. 2015;30(1):219.e1–7.
38. Calfee CS, Janz DR, Bernard GR, May AK, Kangelaris KN, Matthay MA, Ware LB. Distinct molecular phenotypes of direct vs indirect ARDS in single-center and multicenter studies. Chest. 2015;147(6):1539–48.
39. Valentijn KM, Eikenboom J. Weibel–Palade bodies: a window to von Willebrand disease. J Thromb Haemost. 2013;11(4):581–92.
40. van den Biggelaar M, Hernandez-Fernaud JR, van den Eshof BL, Neilson LJ, Meijer AB, Mertens K, Zanivan S. Quantitative phosphoproteomics unveils temporal dynamics of thrombin signaling in human endothelial cells. Blood. 2014;123(12):e22–36.
41. Vischer UM, Barth H, Wollheim CB. Regulated von Willebrand factor

secretion is associated with agonist-specific patterns of cytoskeletal remodeling in cultured endothelial cells. Arterioscler Thromb Vasc Biol. 2000;20(3):883–91.

42. van den Eijnden-Schrauwen Y, Atsma DE, Lupu F, de Vries RE, Kooistra T, Emeis JJ. Involvement of calcium and G proteins in the acute release of tissue-type plasminogen activator and von Willebrand factor from cultured human endothelial cells. Arterioscler Thromb Vasc Biol. 1997;17(10):2177–87.

43. Vischer UM, Wollheim CB. Epinephrine induces von Willebrand factor release from cultured endothelial cells: involvement of cyclic AMP-dependent signalling in exocytosis. Thromb Haemost. 1997;77(6):1182–8.

44. Kaufmann JE, Oksche A, Wollheim CB, Gunther G, Rosenthal W, Vischer UM. Vasopressin-induced von Willebrand factor secretion from endothelial cells involves V2 receptors and cAMP. J Clin Invest. 2000;106(1):107–16.

45. Xiang Y, Cheng J, Wang D, Hu X, Xie Y, Stitham J, Atteya G, Du J, Tang WH, Lee SH, et al. Hyperglycemia repression of miR-24 coordinately upregulates endothelial cell expression and secretion of von Willebrand factor. Blood. 2015;125(22):3377–87.

46. Xu H, Gu LN, Yang QY, Zhao DY, Liu F. MiR-221 promotes IgE-mediated activation of mast cells degranulation by PI3 K/Akt/PLCgamma/Ca(2+) pathway. J Bioenerg Biomembr. 2016;48(3):293–9.

# 3

# Frequency and prognostic impact of basic critical care echocardiography abnormalities in patients with acute respiratory distress syndrome

Kay Choong See[1,2]*, Jeffrey Ng[1,2], Wen Ting Siow[1,2], Venetia Ong[1,2] and Jason Phua[1,2]

## Abstract

**Background:** Among intensive care unit (ICU) patients with acute respiratory distress syndrome (ARDS), apart from acute cor pulmonale (ACP), the frequency and prognostic impact of basic critical care echocardiography (BCCE) abnormalities are not well defined.

**Methods:** Observational study of patients with ARDS, admitted from September 2012 to May 2014, who underwent BCCE within 48 h of admission to a 20-bed medical ICU. We examined the association of two major BCCE-detected abnormalities (left ventricular ejection fraction < 40% and severe ACP) with ICU/hospital mortality and ICU/hospital length of stay. Multivariable models adjusted for age and illness severity.

**Results:** Of 234 patients with ARDS (age 62.3 ± 14.3 years; 88/37.6% female; APACHE II 26.8 ± 8.3; 26.5% ICU mortality; 32.1% hospital mortality), 94 (40.2%) had at least one major BCCE-detected abnormality. The more common major BCCE abnormality found was severe ACP (28.2%), followed by left ventricular ejection fraction < 40% (16.2%). On multivariate analysis, only severe ACP remained significantly associated with ICU/hospital mortality. Hospital mortality for mild, moderate and severe ARDS was 17.0, 27.9 and 50.0%, respectively (without severe ACP), and was 29.2, 48.3 and 53.8%, respectively (with severe ACP).

**Conclusions:** BCCE abnormalities were common, but only severe ACP had prognostic significance in ARDS, identifying patients who are at increased risk of ICU and hospital mortality. The presence of severe ACP appears to upstage ARDS severity by one level.

**Keywords:** Echocardiography, Intensive care units, Respiratory distress syndrome, adult, Cor pulmonale, Ventricular dysfunction, left

## Background

Acute respiratory distress syndrome (ARDS) is a common critical illness with high mortality [1]. Patients may develop cardiac complications as the result of severe illness or as a side effect of treatment. In particular, patients with ARDS may develop right ventricular overload and acute cor pulmonale (ACP) [2–4]. The pathophysiology of ACP is complex and is related to pulmonary vasoconstriction, permissive hypercapnia, intrapulmonary microthrombi and positive pressure mechanical ventilation [4–6].

The spread of basic critical care echocardiography (BCCE) technology and expertise will allow intensive care unit (ICU) physicians to incorporate BCCE into routine clinical practice. For instance, BCCE has been recognized as a useful tool for hemodynamic optimization of patients known to have shock [7, 8]. BCCE can also be used to detect two major echocardiographic abnormalities: left ventricular ejection fraction and severe ACP [9].

*Correspondence: kay_choong_see@nuhs.edu.sg
[1] Division of Respiratory and Critical Care Medicine, University Medicine Cluster, National University Health System, 1E Kent Ridge Road, NUHS Tower Block Level 10, Singapore 119228, Singapore
Full list of author information is available at the end of the article

Apart from ACP, there is uncertainty over the frequency and prognostic significance of the above-mentioned two major BCCE abnormalities in newly admitted ICU patients with ARDS. Knowing this information would be useful for delineating the potential role of BCCE screening for such critically ill patients, which is currently unclear [10]. We therefore aimed to investigate the frequency of BCCE-detected abnormalities in patients with ARDS and to elucidate any associations with ICU and hospital mortality, or with increased ICU or hospital length of stay.

## Methods
### Participants and setting

We conducted a prospective observational study of patients with ARDS admitted to our 20-bed medical ICU from September 2012 to May 2014, who underwent BCCE within 48 h of admission. Due to manpower constraints, BCCE was routinely scheduled on three weekdays (Monday, Wednesday and Friday) and was done on an ad hoc basis over weekends and public holidays for newly admitted patients. BCCE was not done if patients discharged or died before it could be done. Three patients, who had surgical dressings over the chest/abdomen precluding satisfactory transthoracic echocardiographic windows, were excluded. No other exclusion criteria were used. Only the first ICU admission for each patient was analysed. The presence and severity of ARDS were determined on the day of BCCE.

Our Ethics Review Board (National Healthcare Group Domain-Specific Review Board) permitted waiver of informed consent (DSRB B/2013/00132). Although we reported some of our data in a prior study on BCCE training [9], our current study has different aims, the number of ARDS patients has been doubled and we have collected new information pertaining to ARDS.

### Scanning procedure and clinical care

BCCE was only performed by competent attending physicians or fellows, or by fellows under supervision, using the Sparq Ultrasound System (Philips Healthcare, Andover, MA) equipped with a 2–4 MHz broadband sector, phased array transducer. Physicians were deemed to be competent if they had at least 1 year of daily experience with BCCE performance and interpretation. At least seven standard views (acoustic windows) were obtained and recorded for each BCCE scan: parasternal long axis, parasternal short axis, apical four-chamber (three views), subcostal and inferior vena cava (IVC) [9]. For this study, we considered two major abnormalities because these are reliably detected by bedside echocardiography: visually estimated left ventricular ejection fraction < 40% and severe ACP (right ventricular dilatation with the

right-to-left ventricular size (area) ratio $\geq$ 1 in end diastole at the papillary muscle level and interventricular septal straightening/paradoxical motion using the parasternal short axis view) [9, 11, 12]. The presence of ACP was determined by visually examining the relative sizes of the right and left ventricles in both the parasternal short axis views and the apical four-chamber views. We chose the parasternal short axis view as the main view to assess the relative sizes of the right and left ventricles and to assess for septal straightening/paradoxical motion (see Fig. 1 for an example), as this view had a fixed landmark (papillary muscles) and was not prone to foreshortening or rotational error. Since we relied on a ratio of 1 between the right and left ventricle sizes, we also found that visual comparison was rapid and accurate without routine manual tracing of the endocardial borders. We used the apical four-chamber as a secondary safeguard against false ACP determination, which in our experience did not occur. Conversely, if we had used the apical four-chamber view as the main view, potential foreshortening or rotational error would lead to under-recognition of RV dilatation and ACP. We determined that the cor pulmonale was acute, rather than chronic, if there was no significant right ventricular dysfunction noted previously, either clinically or from prior echocardiography.

Usage of BCCE findings and clinical care were left to the discretion of the attending physicians. During the time period of the study, we did not enforce any protocol with regard to specific BCCE abnormalities or mandate repeat scanning. For hemodynamic management, our ICU relied on arterial line blood pressure [13], with the option of FloTrac/Vigileo (Edwards Lifesciences, Irvine, CA) continuous arterial pressure waveform-based

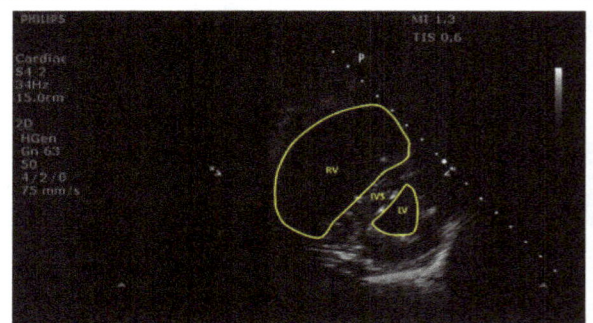

**Fig. 1** An example of acute cor pulmonale. 82-year-old woman with myelodysplastic syndrome was intubated for severe community-acquired pneumonia. She had no known cardiac problems or chronic lung disease. On admission to the intensive care unit, basic echocardiography was done. The parasternal short axis view showed a dilated right ventricle (RV) in end diastole at the papillary muscle level and interventricular septum (IVS) straightening, indicating acute cor pulmonale. The RV and left ventricle (LV) areas may be determined via endocardial tracing as shown, though in many cases, an RV/LV ratio of $\geq$ 1 can be determined visually without routine manual tracing

cardiac output measurements and echocardiography. Noradrenaline was the preferred vasopressor, particularly for septic shock [14]. For ventilator management, patients received low tidal volume ventilation with minimal analgesia and sedation, but not high-frequency oscillatory ventilation [15] or nitric oxide [16]. None of the patients received prone positioning as this was not usual practice for our ICU during the study period. Sepsis was treated with early, broad-spectrum antibiotics and source control.

## Data collection

Clinical data were extracted from the ICU computerized database and medical records. The latest arterial blood gas measurement, which was taken on the day of the BCCE scan, was used to compute the arterial oxygen partial pressure (in mmHg) to inspired oxygen fraction (PF ratio). Respiratory parameters extracted from the database included tidal volume, respiratory rate and positive end-expiratory pressure at the time of BCCE. We did not routinely perform inspiratory pause manoeuvres at the time of BCCE. These manoeuvres were nonetheless done routinely for mechanically ventilated patients every morning by our respiratory therapists, and we recorded plateau pressures and respiratory compliance readings taken on the morning of the BCCE scan.

ARDS was defined using the Berlin Definition [17]. To diagnose ARDS, patients needed a PF ratio < 300 mmHg, a positive end-expiratory pressure $\geq$ 5 cm $H_2O$ (may be non-invasively delivered for mild ARDS), no predominant cardiac failure or fluid overload and bilateral infiltrates on chest radiography. These features must also develop within 1 week of a known clinical insult or new or worsening respiratory symptoms. The severity of ARDS was classified as mild (PF ratio 201–300 mmHg), moderate (PF ratio 101–200 mmHg) and severe (PF ratio 100 mmHg or less).

## Statistical analysis

Univariate comparisons of proportions, means and medians were, respectively, done using Fisher exact, Student t and Wilcoxon rank-sum tests. Confidence intervals of binomial probability distributions were computed using the Clopper–Pearson (exact) method. We examined the association of major BCCE-detected abnormalities with ICU/hospital mortality and ICU/hospital length of stay. Logistic regression was used to analyse mortality as an outcome. Linear regression was used to analyse length of stay (log-transformed to achieve normality) as an outcome. Both the logistic regression and linear regression models corrected for age, and Acute Physiology and Chronic Health Evaluation (APACHE) II score. Statistical significance was taken as $P < 0.05$.

## Results

During the study period, 1218 patients (1371 admissions; age 61.8 ± 16.5 years; 492/40.4% female; APACHE II 22.7 ± 9.0) were treated in our ICU. We performed BCCE for 651 patients (709 admissions; age 61.0 ± 16.6 years; 251/38.6% female; APACHE II 24.0 ± 8.2). Although we did not collect information on the presence or absence of ARDS for patients who did not receive BCCE, these patients did not differ from the whole ICU population in terms of age ($P = 0.973$), gender ($P = 0.448$) and APACHE II score ($P = 0.915$).

Among patients who received BCCE, 234 patients fulfilled the Berlin Definition of ARDS (age 62.3 ± 14.3 years; 88/37.6% female; APACHE II 26.8 ± 8.3) (Table 1). Ninety-four patients (40.2%) had at least one major BCCE-detected abnormality. The more common major BCCE abnormality found was severe ACP (28.2%), followed by left ventricular ejection fraction < 40% (16.2%). Among our 66 patients with ACP, no patient had any clinical cor pulmonale at baseline. Additionally, of 42 (63.6% of 66) patients who had prior transthoracic echocardiography, no patient had moderate or severe right ventricular dysfunction noted, and only 3 (4.6% of 66) patients had mild right ventricular dysfunction noted. Hospital mortality was 20.5% (83 patients, 95% CI 12.4–30.8) for mild ARDS, 33.3% (108 patients, 95% CI 24.6–43.1) for moderate ARDS and 51.2% (43 patients, 95% CI 35.5–66.7%) for severe ARDS (Table 2).

On multivariate analysis, among the major BCCE abnormalities, only severe ACP was associated with ICU and hospital mortality (Table 3). No associations between major BCCE abnormalities and ICU/hospital length of stay existed (Table 4). Hospital mortality for mild, moderate and severe ARDS was 17.0, 27.9 and 50.0%, respectively (without severe ACP), and was 29.2, 48.3 and 53.8%, respectively (with severe ACP) (Table 2).

## Discussion

The main findings of our study are as follows: firstly, BCCE abnormalities in ARDS patients were common, affecting 40% of the patients. Secondly, the presence of severe ACP—but not moderate/severe left ventricular dysfunction—within 48 h of ICU admission identified patients who were at increased risk of ICU and hospital mortality. Thirdly, both the BCCE-detected major abnormalities were not associated with ICU or hospital length of stay. Finally, the presence of severe ACP appears to upstage ARDS severity by one level.

Our study provided new information on the relative frequency of two major BCCE abnormalities in ARDS patients. We found that the more common abnormality was severe ACP, at 28.2%, which was around the same frequency demonstrated in another smaller study [18]

**Table 1 Patient characteristics and outcomes**

| Patient characteristic or outcome | All patients with ARDS (N = 234) | Patients with ARDS, without severe ACP (N = 168) | Patients with ARDS, with severe ACP (N = 66) | P value |
|---|---|---|---|---|
| Age (years) (mean ± SD) | 62.3 ± 14.3 | 62.0 ± 14.7 | 64.8 ± 12.9 | 0.180 |
| Female sex (%) | 88 (37.6) | 65 (38.7) | 23 (34.9) | 0.654 |
| APACHE II score (mean ± SD) | 26.8 ± 8.3 | 26.7 ± 8.1 | 27.3 ± 8.7 | 0.615 |
| Arterial blood gas measurement | | | | |
| PF ratio (mmHg) (mean ± SD) | 171 ± 67 | 172 ± 69 | 169 ± 63 | 0.801 |
| pH (mean ± SD) | 7.33 ± 0.12 | 7.34 ± 0.11 | 7.31 ± 0.13 | 0.065 |
| $PaCO_2$ (mmHg) (mean ± SD) | 43 ± 14 | 42 ± 13 | 47 ± 16 | 0.001 |
| ARDS[a] (%) | | | | |
| Mild | 83 (35.5) | 59 (35.1) | 24 (36.4) | 0.892 |
| Moderate | 108 (46.2) | 79 (47.0) | 29 (43.9) | |
| Severe | 43 (18.4) | 30 (17.9) | 13 (19.7) | |
| Primary diagnosis (%) | | | | |
| Pneumonia | 208 (88.9) | 151 (89.9) | 57 (86.4) | 0.489 |
| Non-pneumonia sepsis | 26 (11.1) | 17 (10.1) | 9 (13.6) | |
| Comorbidities (%) | | | | |
| Diabetes mellitus | 81 (34.6) | 61 (36.3) | 20 (30.3) | 0.446 |
| Hypertension | 115 (49.2) | 86 (51.2) | 29 (43.9) | 0.384 |
| Ischaemic heart disease | 55 (23.5) | 43 (25.6) | 12 (18.2) | 0.304 |
| Chronic heart failure | 9 (3.9) | 7 (4.2) | 2 (3.0) | 1.000 |
| Asthma | 14 (6.0) | 10 (6.0) | 4 (6.1) | 1.000 |
| COPD | 17 (7.3) | 13 (7.7) | 4 (6.1) | 0.785 |
| Bronchiectasis | 10 (4.3) | 7 (4.2) | 3 (4.6) | 1.000 |
| Chronic renal failure | 38 (16.2) | 27 (16.1) | 11 (16.7) | 1.000 |
| Chronic liver disease | 10 (4.3) | 8 (4.8) | 2 (3.0) | 0.729 |
| Stroke | 16 (6.8) | 13 (7.7) | 3 (4.6) | 0.566 |
| Cancer | 39 (16.7) | 31 (18.5) | 8 (12.1) | 0.330 |
| Actual body weight (kg) (mean ± SD) | 63.3 ± 17.2 | 63.4 ± 16.6 | 62.9 ± 18.6 | 0.840 |
| Ventilation modes (%) | | | | |
| Nil ventilation | 0 (0.0) | 0 (0.0) | 0 (0.0) | 0.942 |
| CPAP | 17 (7.3) | 13 (7.7) | 4 (6.1) | |
| NIV | 10 (4.3) | 7 (4.2) | 3 (4.6) | |
| Invasive | 207 (88.5) | 148 (88.1) | 59 (89.4) | |
| Respiratory parameters at time of BCCE | | | | |
| Respiratory rate (breaths/min) (mean ± SD) | 24 ± 3 | 24 ± 4 | 24 ± 2 | 0.274 |
| Tidal volume (ml) (mean ± SD) | 408 ± 113 | 409 ± 113 | 407 ± 112 | 0.931 |
| Tidal volume (ml/kg IBW) (mean ± SD) | 7 ± 2 | 7 ± 2 | 7 ± 3 | 0.276 |
| PEEP (cm H2O) (mean ± SD) | 7 ± 3 | 6 ± 3 | 7 ± 3 | 0.089 |
| Plateau pressure[b] (cm $H_2O$) (mean ± SD) | 21 ± 3 | 21 ± 2 | 21 ± 5 | 0.507 |
| Compliance[b] (ml/cm $H_2O$) (mean ± SD) | 31 ± 14 | 29 ± 12 | 34 ± 18 | 0.047 |
| On vasoactive agents (%) | | | | |
| Any agent[c] | 77 (32.9) | 55 (32.7) | 22 (33.3) | 1.000 |
| Dopamine | 4 (1.7) | 2 (1.2) | 2 (3.0) | 0.316 |
| Noradrenaline | 73 (31.2) | 52 (31.0) | 21 (31.8) | 1.000 |
| Dobutamine | 2 (0.9) | 2 (1.2) | 0 (0.0) | 1.000 |
| Vasopressin | 1 (0.4) | 1 (0.6) | 0 (0.0) | 1.000 |

**Table 1 continued**

| Patient characteristic or outcome | All patients with ARDS (N = 234) | Patients with ARDS, without severe ACP (N = 168) | Patients with ARDS, with severe ACP (N = 66) | P value |
|---|---|---|---|---|
| BCCE-detected major abnormalities (%) | | | | |
| Left ventricular ejection fraction < 40% | 38 (16.2) | 28 (16.7) | 10 (15.2) | 0.846 |
| Severe acute cor pulmonale | 66 (28.2) | 0 (0.0) | 66 (100.0) | < 0.001 |
| Any major abnormalities | 94 (40.2) | 28 (16.7) | 66 (100.0) | < 0.001 |
| LOS, ICU (days), median (IQR) | 7 (4–12) | 7 (4–12) | 7 (3–13) | 0.931 |
| LOS, hospital (days), median (IQR) | 17.5 (9–28) | 18 (9–26) | 17 (8–31) | 0.837 |
| Mortality, ICU (%) | 62 (26.5) | 37 (22.0) | 25 (37.9) | 0.021 |
| Mortality, hospital (%) | 75 (32.1) | 47 (28.0) | 28 (42.4) | 0.043 |

ACP Acute cor pulmonale (severe ACP is defined as right ventricular dilatation with the right-to-left ventricular size ratio ≥ 1 in end diastole at the papillary muscle level and interventricular septal straightening/paradoxical motion), APACHE II Acute Physiology and Chronic Health Evaluation II, ARDS acute respiratory distress syndrome, BCCE basic critical care echocardiography, COPD chronic obstructive pulmonary disease, CPAP continuous positive airway pressure, IBW ideal body weight. For males, IBW = 50 + 2.3 kg for each increment of 2.54 cm (1 inch) in length over 152.4 cm (5 feet). For females, IBW = 45.5 + 2.3 kg for each increment of 2.54 cm (1 inch) in length over 152.4 cm (5 feet), ICU intensive care unit, IQR interquartile range, LOS length of stay, PEEP positive end-expiratory pressure, SD standard deviation, NIV non-invasive ventilation

[a] ARDS severity according to the Berlin Definition: mild (PF ratio 201–300 mmHg), moderate (PF ratio 101–200 mmHg) and severe (PF ratio 100 mmHg or less), where PF ratio is the ratio of arterial oxygen partial pressure (mmHg) to inspired oxygen fraction

[b] Data only for the intubated patients (N = 207)

[c] Patients could be on more than one vasoactive agent

**Table 2 Hospital mortality of patients with acute respiratory distress syndrome, with or without severe acute cor pulmonale**

| Hospital mortality | All ARDS patients (N = 234) | ARDS patients without severe ACP (N = 168) | ARDS patients with severe ACP (N = 66) | P value[b] |
|---|---|---|---|---|
| Severity of ARDS[a] (%, CI) | | | | |
| Mild | 17/83 (20.5, 12.4–30.8) | 10/59 (17.0, 8.4–29.0) | 7/24 (29.2, 12.6–51.1) | 0.239 |
| Moderate | 36/108 (33.3, 24.6–43.1) | 22/79 (27.9, 18.3–39.1) | 14/29 (48.3, 29.4–67.5) | 0.065 |
| Severe | 22/43 (51.2, 35.5–66.7) | 15/30 (50.0, 31.3–68.7) | 7/13 (53.8, 25.1–80.8) | 1.000 |
| Overall cohort (%, CI) | 75/234 (32.1, 26.1–38.4) | 47/168 (28.0, 21.3–35.4) | 28/66 (42.4, 30.3–55.2) | 0.043* |

ACP Acute cor pulmonale (severe ACP is defined as right ventricular dilatation with the right-to-left ventricular size ratio ≥ 1 in end diastole at the papillary muscle level and interventricular septal straightening/paradoxical motion), ARDS acute respiratory distress syndrome, CI 95% confidence interval

*P < 0.05

[a] ARDS severity according to the Berlin Definition: mild (PF ratio 201–300 mmHg), moderate (PF ratio 101–200 mmHg) and severe (PF ratio 100 mmHg or less), where PF ratio is the ratio of arterial oxygen partial pressure (mmHg) to inspired oxygen fraction

[b] Computed for the mortality difference between patients with and without severe acute cor pulmonale, using the Fisher exact test

**Table 3 Association of basic critical care echocardiography screening-derived abnormalities with mortality in patients with acute respiratory distress syndrome**

| Major BCCE-detected abnormalities | ICU mortality | | Hospital mortality | |
|---|---|---|---|---|
| | Univariate OR (95% CI)[a] | Multivariate OR (95% CI)[b] | Univariate OR (95% CI)[a] | Multivariate OR (95% CI)[b] |
| Screened patients with acute respiratory distress syndrome (Berlin Definition) | | | | |
| Left ventricular ejection fraction < 40% | 2.37 (1.15–4.89)* | 2.10 (0.99–4.43) | 2.19 (1.08–4.45)* | 2.00 (0.95–4.18) |
| Severe acute cor pulmonale | 2.16 (1.17–4.00)* | 2.14 (1.13–4.04)* | 1.90 (1.05–3.43)* | 1.89 (1.02–3.50)* |

BCCE Basic critical care echocardiography, CI confidence interval, ICU intensive care unit, OR odds ratio

*P < 0.05

[a] Odds ratio (with 95% confidence interval) derived using logistic regression on mortality, unadjusted

[b] Odds ratio (with 95% confidence interval) derived using multiple logistic regression on mortality, adjusted for age and Acute Physiology and Chronic Health Evaluation II score

**Table 4** **Association of basic critical care echocardiography screening-derived abnormalities with log(length of stay) in patients with acute respiratory distress syndrome**

| Major BCCE-detected abnormalities | Log (length of stay, ICU) | | Log (length of stay, hospital) | |
|---|---|---|---|---|
| | Univariate ratio (95% CI)[a] | Multivariate ratio (95% CI)[b] | Univariate ratio (95% CI)[a] | Multivariate ratio (95% CI)[b] |
| Screened patients with acute respiratory distress syndrome (Berlin Definition) | | | | |
| Left ventricular ejection fraction < 40% | 1.00 (0.75–1.33) | 1.00 (0.74–1.34) | 0.84 (0.62–1.15) | 0.86 (0.63–1.17) |
| Severe acute cor pulmonale | 1.07 (0.84–1.36) | 1.10 (0.87–1.39) | 1.04 (0.81–1.34) | 1.06 (0.82–1.37) |

*BCCE* Basic critical care echocardiography, *CI* Confidence interval, *ICU* Intensive care unit

[a] Exponentiated coefficient (with 95% confidence interval) derived using linear regression on the log-transformed LOS, unadjusted

[b] Exponentiated coefficient (with 95% confidence interval) derived using multiple linear regression on the log-transformed LOS, adjusted for age and Acute Physiology and Chronic Health Evaluation II score

and in a separate study focusing on severe H1N1 infection [19]. Nonetheless, this frequency was higher than the prevalence of severe ACP of 7% found in a prior multicentre study by Mekontso-Dessap and colleagues [3], which could be due to our non-adoption of strategies such as prone positioning to off-load the right ventricle and a higher proportion (89 vs. 40%) of pneumonia (pneumonia being a risk factor for ACP) in our cohort [5]. Across the ARDS severity gradient, ACP was fairly consistently found in 28.9, 26.9 and 30.2% of mild, moderate and severe ARDS cases. This would imply that, in our setting of high pneumonia prevalence, there was little interaction between ACP and ARDS severity. It is possible that ACP may be more a consequence of treatment strategies than disease manifestation, which would then make ACP potentially modifiable. Interestingly, among patients with ARDS, patients with ACP had slightly better respiratory system compliance compared to patients without ACP. This could reflect the lung recruitment effect of slightly higher positive end-expiratory pressure applied in cases of ACP.

Moderate/severe left ventricular dysfunction was less common in our study population, occurring in 16.2% of patients. Although previously published ARDS-specific data are not available, the frequency of left ventricular dysfunction in our cohort is consistent with prior data derived from patients with septic shock [20]. Similarly, our finding that left ventricular dysfunction had no association with mortality is also consistent with the lack of association in septic patients [21–23]. Given that we saw no increased mortality even though we only used inotropic medications very sparingly, our findings do not support the need to treat isolated left ventricular dysfunction in ARDS.

In contrast to left ventricular dysfunction, we found the presence of severe ACP to be particularly important for predicting mortality [3, 4, 11, 12]. Our definition of severe ACP involved a right-to-left ventricular size ratio

$\geq 1$ on transthoracic echocardiography, which corresponds to the definition of severe ACP on trans*esophageal* echocardiography in a recent study [3]. The latter study also found that less severe ACP (i.e. right-to-left ventricular size ratio > 0.6 and < 1) was conversely *not* associated with mortality. The increased mortality engendered by severe ACP may be due to an increased incidence of circulatory failure in ARDS patients [4]. In our experience, such patients are harmed by fluid administration and often require moderate-to-high doses of noradrenaline support [5]. Separately, the absence of any relationship between BCCE findings and ICU/hospital length of stay is in line with prior data for ACP [4] and with our earlier study [9], which implies that length of stay may be more influenced by non-cardiac factors. Moreover, although ACP could be contributed by volume overload, we feel that this would be partially mitigated by our ICU's fluid management protocol, which we had established since 2011 [13]. Also, although we cannot completely exclude a cardiac contribution to ACP, the overlap between left ventricular ejection fraction < 40% and ACP was only 10 patients, which was 15.2% of the 66 patients with ACP. We also did a sensitivity analysis for the presence or absence of left ventricular ejection fraction < 40%, using logistic regression with respect to ICU and hospital mortality, adjusted for age and APACHE II score. Including patients with left ventricular ejection fraction < 40%, ACP was associated with ICU and hospital mortality with an adjusted odds ratio of 2.14 (95% CI 1.13–4.04) and 1.89 (1.02–3.50), respectively. Excluding patients with left ventricular ejection fraction < 40%, ACP was associated with ICU and hospital mortality with an adjusted odds ratio of 2.38 (95% CI 1.17–4.84) and 1.88 (0.95–3.71), respectively. Therefore, the presence of left ventricular ejection fraction < 40% did not substantially alter the conclusions of our study.

Knowledge of the presence of ACP may be key to improving the survival of ARDS patients [5, 24]. To this

Frequency and prognostic impact of basic critical care echocardiography abnormalities...

29

end, Mekontso-Dessap and colleagues found that four variables could be used to risk-stratify ARDS patients for the presence of ACP (as determined by transesophageal echocardiography within three days of ARDS diagnosis): pneumonia as a cause of ARDS, driving pressure $\geq 18$ cm H2O, PF ratio $< 150$ mmHg and arterial carbon dioxide partial pressure $\geq 48$ mmHg [3]. Among our patients (Table 1), arterial carbon dioxide partial pressure was indeed significantly higher in patients with severe ACP, though we did not detect significant differences in PF ratio, pneumonia diagnosis or driving pressure. Nonetheless, to use this four-variable risk stratification method, arterial blood gases must be drawn and that patients had to be well sedated or even paralyzed for accurate measurement of driving pressure. Furthermore, after risk stratification, confirmation by echocardiography would still be required. Based on our study, we suggest an alternative approach of directly screening *all* ARDS patients with BCCE, which we believe can be done quickly at the bedside.

In addition, we found that the presence of severe ACP can significantly add to the Berlin Definition for ARDS, and should not be taken as a mere marker of ARDS severity. Previously, the ARDS Definition Task Force reported that using the Berlin Definition, mild, moderate and severe ARDS were associated with hospital or 90-day mortality of 27% (95% CI 24–30%), 32% (95% CI 29–34%) and 45% (95% CI 42–48%), respectively [17]. In our cohort of patients with ARDS, the presence of severe ACP appears to upstage ARDS severity by one level— this may have implications on treatment thresholds and patient recruitment for future studies.

Our results suggest that screening of patients on admission, rather than waiting for clinical deterioration, would be preferable for early identification and treatment of abnormalities. For instance, the detection of severe ACP in ARDS patients should prompt strategies to protect the right ventricle. Such strategies include targeting plateau pressures below 27 cm $H_2O$, maintaining adequate oxygenation and avoiding hypercarbia beyond 60 mmHg [2, 5]. Prone positioning to off-load the right ventricle and extracorporeal carbon dioxide removal to allow tidal volume (and hence plateau pressure) reduction could also be considered [5, 6]. However, while we encourage BCCE, it should only be done if frontline physicians are competent in its use and interpretation [25]. Moreover, it is a complementary modality and does not replace good clinical acumen and practice.

We acknowledge limitations for our study. Firstly, we performed a single-centre observational study, and our results require external validation. Secondly, due to resource limitations, we only managed to screen patients once within 48 h of admission and do not know whether a narrower screening interval (e.g. within 24 h of admission) or repeated screening after that would yield further information. Thirdly, we did not utilize transesophageal echocardiography as our ICU physicians have not acquired this level of expertise, and transesophageal echocardiography may improve the detection of severe ACP compared to using transthoracic echocardiography. Fourthly, although we checked that no patient had any pre-existing cor pulmonale clinically or on prior echocardiography (which was available for 63.6% of ACP cases), some patients might have developed subclinical cor pulmonale after their last echocardiography. Fifthly, we concede that determination of both LVEF and ACP may be imperfect. Nonetheless, in our experience, accuracy of visual LVEF grading and visual estimation of RV/LV size ratio were fairly good, even for trainees when compared with an experienced supervisor (correct grading achieved in 85% of cases for visual LVEF and in 92.5% of cases for visual estimation of RV/LV size ratio, after performing 30 echo examinations) [9]. Finally, we did not mask BCCE findings from clinicians, which meant that BCCE could have changed management. We did not study specific treatments administered, but should they improve survival, the association of BCCE-detected abnormalities with mortality would then be biased towards the null.

In conclusion, severe ACP—but not left ventricular dysfunction—may help identify ARDS patients at elevated risk of ICU and hospital mortality. BCCE, when used as a screening tool, can then alert the treating physician to the presence of ACP, allowing prompt institution of measures that may alter ARDS outcomes. While further validation is required, we believe that our study should encourage ICU physicians to incorporate BCCE into routine screening of ARDS patients admitted to ICU.

**Abbreviations**
ACP: acute cor pulmonale; APACHE: acute physiology and chronic health evaluation; BCCE: basic critical care echocardiography; ICU: intensive care unit; PF ratio: ratio of arterial oxygen partial pressure to inspired oxygen fraction.

**Authors' contributions**
KCS, JN, WTS, VO and JP jointly conceived the study and prepared the manuscript; KCS, JN, WTS and VO performed the data extraction; KCS performed the data analysis; JP supervised the analysis and edited the manuscript. All authors read and approved the final manuscript.

**Author details**
[1] Division of Respiratory and Critical Care Medicine, University Medicine Cluster, National University Health System, 1E Kent Ridge Road, NUHS Tower Block Level 10, Singapore 119228, Singapore. [2] Department of Medicine, Yong Loo Lin School of Medicine, National University of Singapore, Singapore, Singapore.

**Acknowledgements**
The authors thank Dr. Chan Yiong Huak, Yong Loo Lin School of Medicine, National University of Singapore, for providing independent statistical review of this manuscript.

**Competing interests**
The authors declare that they have no competing interests.


**Funding**
No funding was required for this study.


**References**
1. Bellani G, Laffey JG, Pham T, Fan E, Brochard L, Esteban A, Gattinoni L, van Haren F, Larsson A, McAuley DF, et al. Epidemiology, patterns of care, and mortality for patients with acute respiratory distress syndrome in intensive care units in 50 Countries. JAMA. 2016;315(8):788–800.
2. Vieillard-Baron A, Price LC, Matthay MA. Acute cor pulmonale in ARDS. Intensive Care Med. 2013;39(10):1836–8.
3. Mekontso Dessap A, Boissier F, Charron C, Begot E, Repesse X, Legras A, Brun-Buisson C, Vignon P, Vieillard-Baron A. Acute cor pulmonale during protective ventilation for acute respiratory distress syndrome: prevalence, predictors, and clinical impact. Intensive Care Med. 2016;42(5):862–70.
4. Boissier F, Katsahian S, Razazi K, Thille AW, Roche-Campo F, Leon R, Vivier E, Brochard L, Vieillard-Baron A, Brun-Buisson C, et al. Prevalence and prognosis of cor pulmonale during protective ventilation for acute respiratory distress syndrome. Intensive Care Med. 2013;39(10):1725–33.
5. Repesse X, Charron C, Vieillard-Baron A. Acute cor pulmonale in ARDS: rationale for protecting the right ventricle. Chest. 2015;147(1):259–65.
6. Guerin C, Matthay MA. Acute cor pulmonale and the acute respiratory distress syndrome. Intensive Care Med. 2016:42(5):934–6.
7. Kanji HD, McCallum J, Sirounis D, MacRedmond R, Moss R, Boyd JH. Limited echocardiography-guided therapy in subacute shock is associated with change in management and improved outcomes. J Crit Care. 2014;29(5):700–5.
8. Jones AE, Tayal VS, Sullivan DM, Kline JA. Randomized, controlled trial of immediate versus delayed goal-directed ultrasound to identify the cause of nontraumatic hypotension in emergency department patients. Crit Care Med. 2004;32(8):1703–8.
9. See KC, Ong V, Ng J, Tan RA, Phua J. Basic critical care echocardiography by pulmonary fellows: learning trajectory and prognostic impact using a minimally resourced training model. Crit Care Med. 2014;42(10):2169–77.
10. Via G, Hussain A, Wells M, Reardon R, ElBarbary M, Noble VE, Tsung JW, Neskovic AN, Price S, Oren-Grinberg A, et al. International evidence-based recommendations for focused cardiac ultrasound. J Am Soc Echocardiogr. 2014;27(7):683.e1–683.e33.
11. Vieillard-Baron A. Assessment of right ventricular function. Curr Opin Crit Care. 2009;15(3):254–60.
12. Vieillard-Baron A, Prin S, Chergui K, Dubourg O, Jardin F. Echo–Doppler demonstration of acute cor pulmonale at the bedside in the medical intensive care unit. Am J Respir Crit Care Med. 2002;166(10):1310–9.
13. See KC, Mukhopadhyay A, Lau SC, Tan SM, Lim TK, Phua J. Shock in the first 24 h of intensive care unit stay: observational study of protocol-based fluid management. Shock. 2015;43(5):456–62.
14. De Backer D, Aldecoa C, Njimi H, Vincent JL. Dopamine versus norepinephrine in the treatment of septic shock: a meta-analysis. Crit Care Med. 2012;40(3):725–30.
15. Ferguson ND, Cook DJ, Guyatt GH, Mehta S, Hand L, Austin P, Zhou Q, Matte A, Walter SD, Lamontagne F, et al. High-frequency oscillation in early acute respiratory distress syndrome. N Engl J Med. 2013;368(9):795–805.
16. Afshari A, Brok J, Moller AM, Wetterslev J. Inhaled nitric oxide for acute respiratory distress syndrome (ARDS) and acute lung injury in children and adults. Cochrane Database Syst Rev. 2010;(7):CD002787.
17. ARDS Definition Task Force, Ranieri VM, Rubenfeld GD, Thompson BT, Ferguson ND, Caldwell E, Fan E, Camporota L, Slutsky AS. Acute respiratory distress syndrome: the Berlin Definition. JAMA. 2012;307(23):2526–33.
18. Guervilly C, Forel JM, Hraiech S, Demory D, Allardet-Servent J, Adda M, Barreau-Baumstark K, Castanier M, Papazian L, Roch A. Right ventricular function during high-frequency oscillatory ventilation in adults with acute respiratory distress syndrome. Crit Care Med. 2012;40(5):1539–45.
19. Brown SM, Pittman J, Miller Iii RR, Horton KD, Markewitz B, Hirshberg E, Jones J, Grissom CK. Right and left heart failure in severe H1N1 influenza A infection. Eur Respir J. 2011;37(1):112–8.
20. Boissier F, Razazi K, Seemann A, Bedet A, Thille AW, de Prost N, Lim P, Brun-Buisson C, Mekontso Dessap A. Left ventricular systolic dysfunction during septic shock: the role of loading conditions. Intensive Care Med. 2017;43(5):633–42.
21. Sevilla Berrios RA, O'Horo JC, Velagapudi V, Pulido JN. Correlation of left ventricular systolic dysfunction determined by low ejection fraction and 30-day mortality in patients with severe sepsis and septic shock: a systematic review and meta-analysis. J Crit Care. 2014;29(4):495–9.
22. Huang SJ, Nalos M, McLean AS. Is early ventricular dysfunction or dilatation associated with lower mortality rate in adult severe sepsis and septic shock? A meta-analysis. Crit Care. 2013;17(3):R96.
23. Vieillard-Baron A, Caille V, Charron C, Belliard G, Page B, Jardin F. Actual incidence of global left ventricular hypokinesia in adult septic shock. Crit Care Med. 2008;36(6):1701–6.
24. Biswas A. Right heart failure in acute respiratory distress syndrome: an unappreciated albeit a potential target for intervention in the management of the disease. Indian J Crit Care Med. 2015;19(10):606–9.
25. Mayo PH, Maury E. Echography is mandatory for the initial management of critically ill patients: we are not sure. Intensive Care Med. 2014;40(11):1760–2.

# 4

# Epidemiology, causes, evolution and outcome in a single-center cohort of 1116 critically ill patients with hypoxic hepatitis

Astrid Van den broecke[1,3*†] ⓘ, Laura Van Coile[1†], Alexander Decruyenaere[1,2], Kirsten Colpaert[1,3], Dominique Benoit[1,3], Hans Van Vlierberghe[1,4] and Johan Decruyenaere[1,3]

## Abstract

**Background:** Hypoxic hepatitis (HH) is a type of acute hepatic injury that is histologically characterized by centrilobular liver cell necrosis and that is caused by insufficient oxygen delivery to the hepatocytes. Typical for HH is the sudden and significant increase of aspartate aminotransferase (AST) in response to cardiac, circulatory or respiratory failure. The aim of this study is to investigate its epidemiology, causes, evolution and outcome.

**Methods:** The screened population consisted of all adults admitted to the intensive care unit (ICU) at the Ghent University Hospital between January 1, 2007 and September 21, 2015. HH was defined as peak AST > 5 times the upper limit of normal (ULN) after exclusion of other causes of liver injury. Thirty-five variables were retrospectively collected and used in descriptive analysis, time series plots and Kaplan–Meier survival curves with multi-group log-rank tests.

**Results:** HH was observed in 4.0% of the ICU admissions at our center. The study cohort comprised 1116 patients. Causes of HH were cardiac failure (49.1%), septic shock (29.8%), hypovolemic shock (9.4%), acute respiratory failure (6.4%), acute on chronic respiratory failure (3.3%), pulmonary embolism (1.4%) and hyperthermia (0.5%). The 28-day mortality associated with HH was 45.0%. Mortality rates differed significantly ($P = 0.007$) among the causes, ranging from 33.3% in the hyperthermia subgroup to 52.9 and 56.2% in the septic shock and pulmonary embolism subgroups, respectively. The magnitude of AST increase was also significantly correlated ($P < 0.001$) with mortality: 33.2, 44.4 and 55.4% for peak AST 5–10× ULN, 10–20× ULN and > 20× ULN, respectively.

**Conclusion:** This study surpasses by far the largest cohort of critically ill patients with HH. HH is more common than previously thought with an ICU incidence of 4.0%, and it is associated with a high all-cause mortality of 45.0% at 28 days. The main causes of HH are cardiac failure and septic shock, which include more than 3/4 of all episodes. Clinicians should search actively for any underlying hemodynamic or respiratory instability even in patients with moderately increased AST levels.

**Keywords:** Critical care medicine, Critically ill, Epidemiology, Hypoxic hepatitis, Intensive care medicine, Ischemic hepatitis, Liver failure, Mortality, Outcome, Shock liver

## Background

Hypoxic hepatitis (HH), also referred to as "ischemic hepatitis" or "shock liver," is a type of acute hepatic injury that is histologically characterized by centrilobular liver cell necrosis and that is caused by insufficient oxygen delivery to the hepatocytes [1]. Typical for this form of liver cell necrosis is the sudden and significant increase of aspartate aminotransferase (AST) in response to cardiac, circulatory or respiratory failure [1]. Although often missed, HH is a fairly common cause of hepatic dysfunction in an intensive care unit (ICU) with a pooled incidence of 2.5% from a recent meta-analysis of 1782

*Correspondence: Astrid.Vandenbroecke@UGent.be
†Astrid Van den broecke and Laura Van Coile have contributed equally to this study and are the joint first authors
3 Department of Intensive Care Medicine, Ghent University Hospital, De Pintelaan 185, 9000 Ghent, Belgium
Full list of author information is available at the end of the article

patients [2]. Its incidence varies widely among published studies, ranging from 0.16 to 12%, depending upon institution, population studied and definition used [1–8]. However, a high associated mortality of approximately 50% has been consistently observed in all studies [2–6, 8].

The major causes of HH are septic shock, respiratory failure and cardiogenic shock [1, 2]. Possible pathophysiological mechanisms include (1) ischemia due to reduced blood supply (forward failure) or due to right heart failure (backward failure) with venous congestion, (2) hypoxemia due to reduced blood oxygenation and (3) increased oxygen consumption due to elevated metabolic demand (e.g., in severe hyperthermia or septic shock) [1, 9]. Patients with comorbidities are more likely to develop HH, as they have an increased vulnerability even to minor hemodynamic or respiratory insults, such as short periods of hypotension or hypoxemia. These comorbidities contribute substantially to the high mortality associated with HH [4, 7, 8].

HH is reflected by a typical pattern of liver enzyme alterations. It presents with a sudden and significant increase of AST, alanine aminotransferase (ALT) and lactate dehydrogenase (LDH), reaching their peak levels around 24 h after ICU admission [4] and declining steadily to baseline within 10–15 days [1]. Initially, AST exceeds ALT, but as ALT declines more slowly, a reversal of the AST/ALT ratio is observed within 3 days after the peak [5, 6, 8, 10]. Although this biochemical pattern is highly suggestive of HH, it is not pathognomonic and warrants further evaluation [1]. Other common causes of significant increases in aminotransferase levels are drug-induced liver injury (e.g., acetaminophen toxicity) and acute viral hepatitis. However, studies have shown that a sudden and significant increase of AST is caused by HH in more than 50% of the cases [11, 12]. Furthermore, HH is frequently associated with a prolonged prothrombin time and accompanied by additional evidence of end-organ hypoperfusion, such as impaired renal function and increased lactate level [3–6]. A rapid rise and subsequent fall in aminotransferase levels with reversal of the initial AST/ALT ratio, a prolongation of prothrombin time and an increase in serum creatinine level comprise a triad of biochemical abnormalities that can suggest the diagnosis of HH, as proposed by Raurich et al. [6].

Currently, only limited data from small retrospective studies are available, making HH an understudied disease. The largest cohort described to date was recently published and included 565 patients [8]. The aim of this study is to investigate in detail the epidemiology, causes, evolution and outcome of HH in a large single-center cohort. More insight in HH may improve awareness and facilitate earlier diagnosis.

## Methods
### Study cohort and data collection
The screened population consisted of all consecutive adults ($\geq$ 18 years, $n = 29,874$) who were admitted to the surgical, cardiac or medical ICU at the Ghent University Hospital between January 1, 2007 and September 21, 2015. HH was defined as a significant but transient increase in AST level above 5 times the upper limit of normal (ULN) after exclusion of other potential causes of liver injury. Different AST cutoff values for defining HH are used in the literature [2]. As HH has been histologically proven to occur even in patients with moderately elevated AST levels (at AST levels of 252 and 300 IU/L in the cohort of Cohen et al. [13] and Bynum et al. [14], respectively), a cutoff of at least 5 times the ULN was used in this study, i.e., 155 and 185 U/L for females and males, respectively. The 4012 identified patients whose AST level exceeded our cutoff value were evaluated for the presence of HH by three independent experts based on the pattern of liver enzyme alterations, the daily clinical notes and the discharge summaries. The sine qua non was the exposure to a hemodynamic or respiratory insult preceding the AST increase and the exclusion of other potential causes of liver injury. A flow diagram of the exclusion criteria is shown in Fig. 1. Reasons for exclusion were (1) acute liver failure, (2) chronic liver failure, (3) other conditions associated with abnormal liver tests such as cholangitis and pancreatitis, (4) liver surgery, (5) surgery near the liver, (6) hepatic vessel injury or thrombosis, (7) rhabdomyolysis, (8) an unclear increase of creatine kinase (CK), (9) post-anesthesia without overt evidence of an acute cardiac or respiratory event perioperatively, (10) missing data and (11) duplicate patients. (In patients having developed multiple episodes of HH during the study period, only the first episode is eligible for analysis.) Rhabdomyolysis was defined as serum CK exceeding 5 times the ULN (i.e., 850 and 974 U/L for females and males, respectively) with a CK-MB/CK ratio below 6% [6]. Patients with elevated CK levels but with unknown CK-MB value were excluded due to the uncertain CK increase. This study was approved by the Ethics Committee of the Ghent University Hospital (project numbers 2015/0796-0797). Due to the retrospective nature of this study, the need for informed consent was waived.

Routinely available biochemical parameters were recorded, including AST (U/L), ALT (U/L), LDH (U/L), bilirubin (mg/dL), alkaline phosphatase (AP) (U/L), gamma-glutamyl transpeptidase (U/L), lipase (U/L), international normalized ratio (INR), platelet count ($10^3$/µL), white blood cell count ($10^3$/µL), hemoglobin (g/dL), CK (U/L), creatinine (mg/dL), urea (mg/dL) and lactate (mg/dL). Values at specific time points were estimated

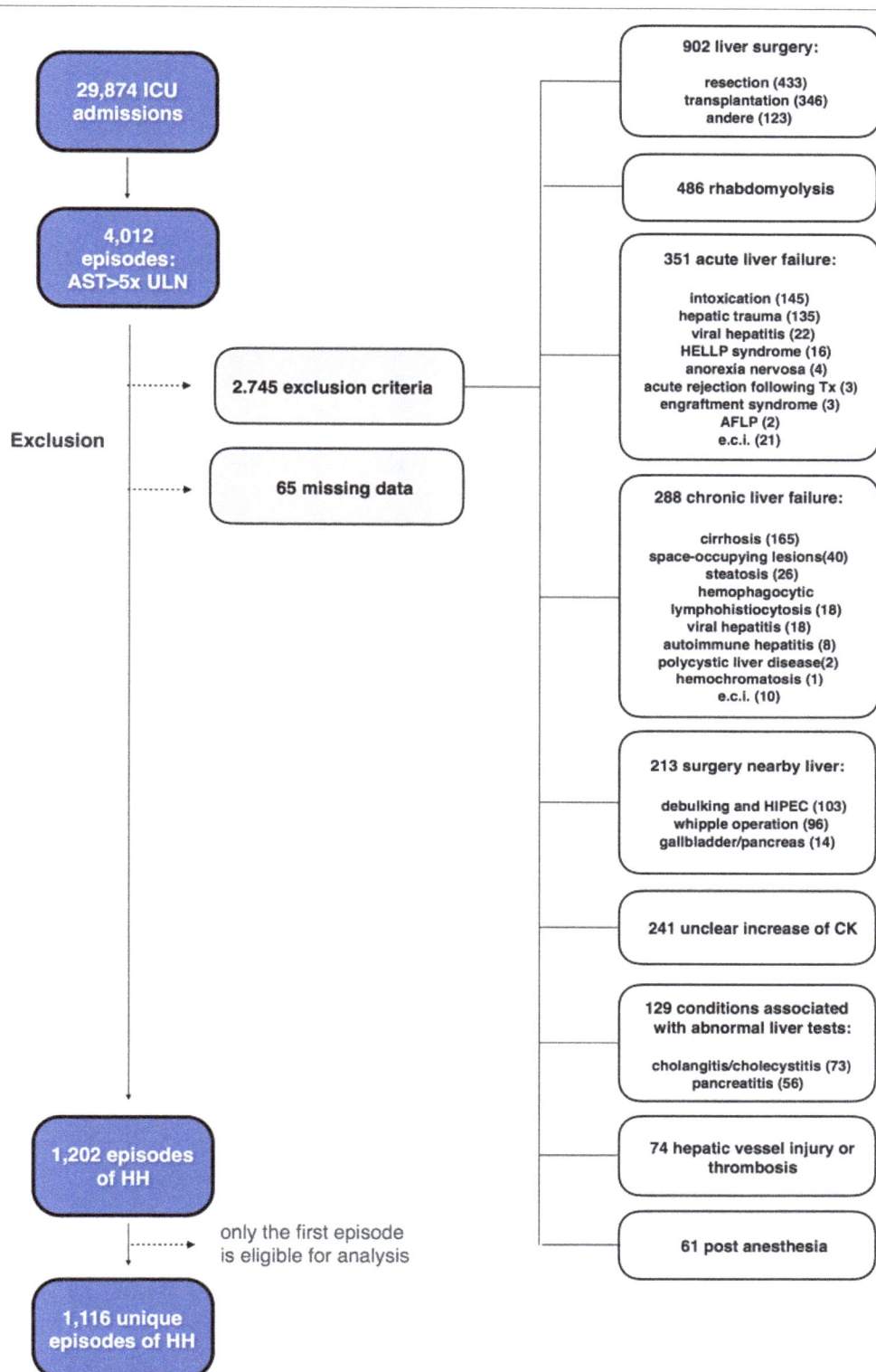

**Fig. 1** Flow diagram of the exclusion criteria. *AFLP* acute fatty liver of pregnancy, *AST* aspartate aminotransferase, *CK* creatine kinase, *e.c.i* e causa ignota, *HELLP* hemolysis, elevated liver enzymes and low platelet count, *HH* hypoxic hepatitis, *HIPEC* hyperthermic intraperitioneal chemotherapy, *ICU* intensive care unit

using linear interpolation between consecutive recorded values. Parameters related to patient characteristics included sex, age, body mass index (BMI) and comorbidities (diabetes mellitus, cardiac function and chronic respiratory disease). Parameters related to the episode of HH included cause, severity of illness scores [acute physiology II score (APS-II) and the simplified acute physiology II score (SAPS-II)], supportive therapy (inotropic agents, vasopressor agents, mechanical ventilation, intra-aortic balloon pump (IABP) and need for dialysis), ICU and hospital length of stay, duration of the HH episode, and ICU and in-hospital mortality at 28 days. The peak of HH was defined as the point in time (T-ASTmax) when AST reached its peak value (ASTmax). In this study, the time origin was set to T-ASTmax (designated as time 0) and all recorded values are expressed in time relative to T-ASTmax for optimal comparison. Severity of illness scores were recorded over a time span of 24 h around T-ASTmax. Three categories for severity of HH were used: "5–10× ULN", "10–20× ULN" and "> 20× ULN". Seven underlying causes of HH were defined: cardiac failure, septic shock, hypovolemic shock, pulmonary embolism, acute respiratory failure, acute on chronic respiratory failure and hyperthermia.

### Statistical analysis

Categorical data are reported as counts and percentages. Continuous data are reported as the median with the first (Q1) and third (Q3) quartiles. For categorical variables, comparisons between groups are performed using the Pearson's Chi square test for contingency. For continuous variables, a permutation test based on difference in medians between groups is used. A Tukey-like approach with permutation resampling is applied to adjust $P$ values for multiple pairwise comparisons. All statistical tests are performed as two-sided tests at a significance level of 0.05. The time trend of laboratory variables is graphically assessed using time series plots and stacked bar charts. Kaplan–Meier survival curves until 28 days after T-ASTmax and multi-group log-rank tests are used to compare the all-cause mortality between groups. Statistical analysis is performed using R version 3.3.2 [15].

## Results
### Patient and episode characteristics

During the study period, 29,874 adult patients with a male-to-female ratio of approximately 3:2 were admitted to the ICU at our center, of whom 4012 patients had peak AST levels exceeding 5 times the ULN. In 30.0% (1202/4012) of the cases, the elevation of AST was caused by HH, resulting in an overall ICU incidence of 4.0% (1202/29,874). As only the first episode was eligible for analysis in patients with multiple episodes of HH during the study period, the final study cohort comprised 1116 patients.

The all-cause mortality of patients admitted to the ICU at our center during the study period was 7.7% (2302/29,874). Among these non-survivors, 19.8% (455/2302) had developed HH during their ICU stay. The all-cause mortality associated with HH was 45.0% (502/1116) at 28 days, of which 90.6% occurred during ICU stay. The survival curves by cause of HH are presented in Fig. 2.

In our study cohort, the median age was 66.0 (Q1–Q3 55.0–74.0) years with a male-to-female ratio of 3:2. The median SAPS-II score at T-ASTmax was 66.0 (Q1–Q3

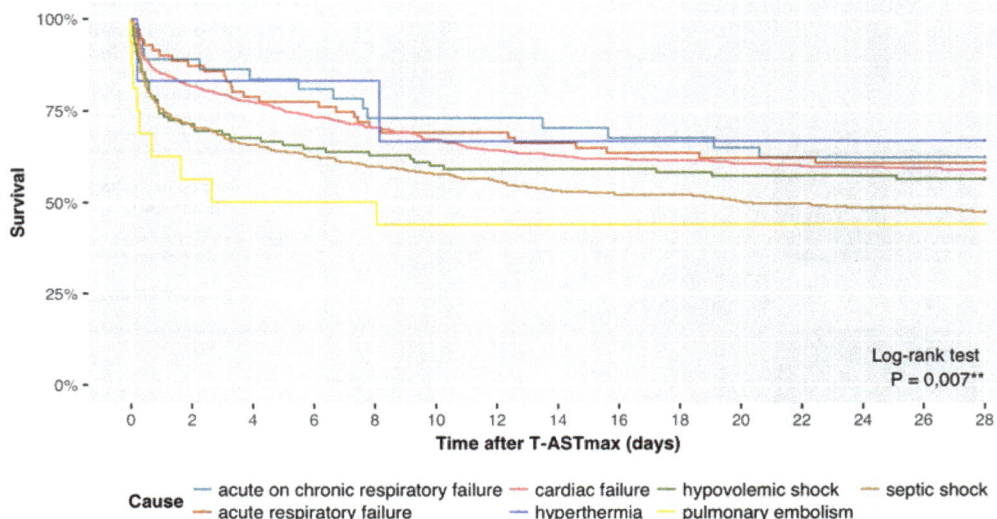

**Fig. 2** Survival curves by cause of hypoxic hepatitis. T-ASTmax is designated as the time 0. *T-ASTmax* time point of maximum AST value

43.0–81.0). 74.9% of patients required mechanical ventilation. Vasopressor and inotropic agents were used in 60.8 and 43.2%, respectively, and 9.5% were on dialysis at T-ASTmax. The causes of HH, in decreasing order of frequency, were cardiac failure (49.1%), septic shock (29.8%), hypovolemic shock (9.4%), acute respiratory failure (6.4%), acute on chronic respiratory failure (3.3%), pulmonary embolism (1.4%) and hyperthermia (0.5%). An episode of HH (length of time that AST levels are exceeding 5 times the ULN) had a median duration of 54.3 (Q1–Q3 26.4–94.2) h, during which the median recovery time (duration from peak AST to levels below 5 times the ULN) was 34.7 (Q1–Q3 14.6–67.2) h.

Survivors had significantly lower severity of illness scores (median SAPS-II score of 54.0 vs. 76.0, $P < 0.001$ and median APS-II score 25.0 vs. 30.0, $P = 0.005$) as compared to non-survivors. They were less likely to have septic shock (25.6 vs. 35.1%, $P = 0.003$). Peak AST levels above 20 times ULN were less commonly seen in survivors (33.4 vs. 50.8%, $P < 0.001$). More characteristics, classified according to survival status, are presented in Table 1.

The three ASTmax subgroups ("5–10× ULN" vs. "10–20× ULN" vs. "> 20× ULN") were also compared with each other. The causes of HH were equally represented within each subgroup. Patients with higher peak AST levels had higher severity of illness scores (median SAPS-II score of 57.0 vs. 60.0 vs. 73.0, $P < 0.001$; median APS-II score of 24.0 vs. 26.5 vs. 32.0, $P < 0.001$) and a higher need for supportive therapy, such as inotropic agents (38.5 vs. 37.9 vs. 50.2%, $P < 0.001$), vasopressor agents (50.9 vs. 59.4 vs. 70.0%, $P < 0.001$), dialysis (4.8 vs. 8.4 vs. 14.1%, $P < 0.001$) and IABP (13.7 vs. 20.7% vs. 18.9%, $P = 0.041$). In addition, higher peak AST levels were associated with higher 28-day mortality rates (33.2 vs. 44.4 vs. 55.4%, $P < 0.001$). More characteristics, classified according to severity of HH and to cause of HH, are presented in Tables 2 and 3, respectively.

**Trend of liver tests**

The time trend of the liver tests is illustrated in Fig. 3. Once the AST level exceeded 5 times the ULN (designated as start of HH), it reached a median peak level of 521.2 (Q1–Q3 269.1–1581.6) U/L within a median of 16.3 (Q1–Q3 7.9–26.8) h. Subsequently, AST started to decline, dropping below 5 times the ULN after a median time of 34.7 (Q1–Q3 14.6–67.2) h and normalizing after a median time of 6.4 (Q1–Q3 3.9–10.9) days in survivors. ALT and LDH peaked at median values of 332.0 (Q1–Q3 149.4–953.6) U/L and 1180.6 (Q1–Q3 684.1–2770.8) U/L within a median time of 22.0 (Q1–Q3 9.7–43.0) and 21.4 (Q1–Q3 10.0–43.6) h after start of HH, respectively. In survivors, LDH returned to baseline

(< 233 U/L) within a median of 5.1 (Q1–Q3 1.3–15.9) days after its peak. ALT declined more slowly, returning to baseline (< 31 and < 40 U/L for females and males, respectively) within 8.6 (Q1–Q3 3.9–16.5) days after its peak. When considering all patients, including those with AST already exceeding 5 times the ULN at ICU admission, ALT and LDH peaked at T-ASTmax in the majority of patients (65.5 and 53.1%, respectively) and to a lesser extent after T-ASTmax (26.2 and 29.8%, respectively).

The median relative increase of AST, ALT and LDH at T-ASTmax was 15.0, 8.7 and 4.7 times their ULN, respectively. LDH exceeded both AST and ALT at all time points in more than 80% of patients. The median AST/ALT ratio was 1.6 at the start of HH, increased to 1.8 at T-ASTmax and subsequently declined, reversing within a median of 32.5 h after T-ASTmax.

In addition, Fig. 3 illustrates that the median INR, creatinine and bilirubin levels also peaked at T-ASTmax, albeit to a much less extent, with median bilirubin level never exceeding the ULN. This is also illustrated in Fig. 4. Both in survivors and non-survivors, the proportion of patients with bilirubin level above the ULN increased mildly at T-ASTmax and then gradually decreased again. The proportion of survivors with bilirubin above 3 times the ULN was limited and increased slightly later during ICU stay. Likewise, AP remained stable during HH, except for a mild increase later during ICU stay, as illustrated in Figs. 3 and 4.

The pattern of liver enzyme alterations described above was found in all ASTmax subgroups (see Appendix Figs. 5, 6, 7). Median values of other laboratory tests at start of HH and at T-ASTmax are presented in Table 4.

**28-day mortality**

HH was associated with high mortality rates, especially early in its course. 18.5% died within 24 h after T-ASTmax. After this first day, the hazard declined dramatically, but remained quite high, resulting in 40.2 and 45.0% all-cause mortality at 14 and 28 days, respectively. 90.6% of deaths occurred during ICU stay.

Twenty-eight-day mortality rates differed significantly among the causes of HH ($P = 0.007$). The high number of early deaths in the pulmonary embolism, septic shock and hypovolemic shock subgroups mainly accounted for the early mortality associated with HH. 37.5, 24.3, 25.7% of these patients died within 24 h after T-ASTmax. The mortality rate in the pulmonary embolism subgroup exceeded at all times those of other subgroups and ultimately resulted in 56.2% mortality at 28 days. The septic shock and hypovolemic shock subgroups had a 28-day mortality of 52.9 and 43.8%, respectively. While the early mortality in the cardiac failure subgroup was less pronounced, yet still considerable as 14.8% of these patients

**Table 1 Characteristics of patients with HH classified by in-hospital 28-day mortality**

| Variable | Patients Total (n = 1116) | In-hospital 28-day mortality No (n = 614) | Yes (n = 502) | P |
|---|---|---|---|---|
| Sex[a] | | | | |
| Male | 61.3% (684) | 62.2% (382) | 60.2% (302) | 0.483 |
| Age[b] (year) | 66.0 (55.0–74.0) | 63.0 (53.0–73.0) | 68.0 (58.0–76.8) | <0.001 |
| BMI[b] (kg/m²) | 25.4 (22.9–28.9) | 25.4 (23.0–28.5) | 25.4 (22.9–29.4) | 0.774 |
| Cause[a] | | | | |
| Cardiac failure | 49.1% (548) | 52.3% (321) | 45.2% (227) | 0.103 |
| Septic shock | 29.8% (333) | 25.6% (157) | 35.1% (176) | 0.003 |
| Hypovolemic shock | 9.4% (105) | 9.6% (59) | 9.2% (46) | 0.999 |
| Acute respiratory failure | 6.4% (71) | 7.0% (43) | 5.6% (28) | 0.927 |
| Acute on chronic respiratory failure | 3.3% (37) | 3.7% (23) | 2.8% (14) | 0.956 |
| Pulmonary embolism | 1.4% (16) | 1.1% (7) | 1.8% (9) | 0.945 |
| Hyperthermia | 0.5% (6) | 0.7% (4) | 0.4% (2) | 0.995 |
| Comorbidities | | | | |
| Echocardio[a] | | | | |
| Overall | | | | 0.406 |
| Normal | 40.0% (446) | 42.0% (258) | 37.5% (188) | — |
| LV dysfunction | 25.1% (280) | 23.5% (144) | 27.1% (136) | — |
| Missing | 22.2% (248) | 22.5% (151) | 23.3% (117) | — |
| LV and RV dysfunction | 8.0% (89) | 8.0% (49) | 8.0% (40) | — |
| RV dysfunction | 4.7% (53) | 5.2% (32) | 4.2% (21) | — |
| DM[a] | 18.7% (209) | 17.4% (107) | 20.3% (102) | 0.218 |
| Chronic respiratory failure[a] | 11.4% (127) | 10.7% (66) | 12.2% (61) | 0.287 |
| SOI scores[c] | | | | |
| APS-II[b] | 28.0 (21.0–34.0) | 25.0 (18.0–32.0) | 30.0 (24.0–35.2) | 0.005 |
| SAPS-II[b] | 66.0 (46.0–81.0) | 54.0 (36.0–71.0) | 76.0 (58.0–89.0) | <0.001 |

| Variable | Patients Total (n = 1116) | In-hospital 28-day mortality No (n = 614) | Yes (n = 502) | P |
|---|---|---|---|---|
| ASTmax[a] | | | | |
| 5–10× ULN | 35.4% (395) | 43.0% (264) | 26.1% (131) | <0.001 |
| 10–20× ULN | 23.4% (261) | 23.6% (145) | 23.1% (116) | 0.985 |
| >20× ULN | 41.2% (460) | 33.4% (205) | 50.8% (255) | <0.001 |
| Supportive therapy[c] | | | | |
| Ventilation[a] | 74.9% (836) | 66.4% (408) | 85.3% (428) | <0.001 |
| Medication | | | | |
| Inotropic agents[a] | 43.2% (482) | 39.3% (241) | 48.0% (241) | 0.003 |
| Vasopressor agents[a] | 60.8% (678) | 51.1% (314) | 72.5% (364) | <0.001 |
| Dialysis[a] | 9.5% (106) | 6.8% (42) | 12.7% (64) | <0.001 |
| IABP[a] | 17.5% (195) | 19.5% (120) | 14.9% (75) | 0.044 |
| LOS | | | | |
| ICU[b] (day) | 4.4 (1.2–11.7) | 6.4 (2.7–17.7) | 1.8 (0.4–7.1) | <0.001 |
| Hospital[b] (day) | 12.1 (3.0–28.9) | 25.7 (13.9–48.1) | 2.1 (0.4–8.1) | <0.001 |
| Duration | | | | |
| Episode of HH[b] (h) | 54.3 (26.4–94.2) | 53.4 (23.9–94.2) | 56.7 (30.7–94.1) | 0.527 |
| Recovery of HH[b] (h) | 34.7 (14.6–67.2) | 35.5 (14.1–68.0) | 32.6 (16.2–61.4) | 0.393 |
| 28-day mortality | | | | |
| ICU[a] | 40.8% (455) | 0.0% (0) | 90.6% (455) | <0.001 |
| In-hospital[a] | 45.0% (502) | 0.0% (0) | 100.0% (502) | <0.001 |

*APS-II* acute physiology II, *AST* aspartate aminotransferase, *ASTmax* maximum AST value, *BMI* body mass index, *HH* hypoxic hepatitis, *IABP* intra-aortic balloon pump, *ICU* intensive care unit, *LOS* length of stay, *LV* left ventricle, *P P* value, *Q1* first quartile, *Q3* third quartile, *RV* right ventricle, *SAPS-II* simplified acute physiology II, *SOI* severity of illness, *T-ASTmax* time point of maximum AST value, *ULN* upper limit of normal

Italics indicate the significant P values

[a] % (n)

[b] Median (Q1–Q3)

[c] At T-ASTmax ± 12 h

**Table 2 Characteristics of patients with HH classified by ASTmax subgroup**

| Variable | Patients | | | P |
|---|---|---|---|---|
| | ASTmax subgroup | | | |
| | 5× ULN–10× ULN (n = 395) | 10× ULN–20× ULN (n = 261) | >20× ULN (n = 460) | |
| Sex[a] | | | | |
| Male | 60.5% (239) | 62.5% (163) | 61.3% (282) | 0.882 |
| Age[b] (year) | 63.0 (45.0–73.5) | 66.0 (56.0–75.0) | 67.0 (55.8–75.0) | 0.014 |
| BMI[b] (kg/m²) | 25.5 (23.1–28.7) | 25.5 (22.9–29.2) | 25.1 (22.9–28.9) | 0.647 |
| Cause[a] | | | | |
| Overall | | | | 0.135 |
| Cardiac failure | 50.6% (200) | 49.8% (130) | 47.4% (218) | – |
| Septic shock | 29.4% (116) | 26.1% (68) | 32.4% (149) | – |
| Hypovolemic shock | 7.6% (30) | 10.3% (27) | 10.4% (48) | – |
| Acute respiratory failure | 7.1% (28) | 9.2% (24) | 4.1% (19) | – |
| Acute on chronic respiratory failure | 3.3% (13) | 1.9% (5) | 4.1% (19) | – |
| Pulmonary embolism | 1.5% (6) | 1.5% (4) | 1.3% (6) | – |
| Hyperthermia | 0.5% (2) | 1.1% (3) | 0.2% (1) | – |
| Comorbidities | | | | |
| Echocardio[a] | | | | |
| Normal | 43.8% (173) | 34.5% (90) | 39.8% (183) | 0.234 |
| LV dysfunction | 20.5% (81) | 27.6% (72) | 27.1% (136) | 0.136 |
| Missing | 25.3% (100) | 26.8% (70) | 17.0% (78) | 0.008 |
| LV and RV dysfunction | 5.8% (23) | 8.4% (22) | 9.6% (44) | 0.452 |
| RV dysfunction | 4.6% (18) | 2.7% (7) | 6.1% (28) | 0.422 |
| DM[a] | 14.9% (59) | 21.1% (55) | 20.7% (95) | 0.055 |
| Chronic respiratory failure[a] | 12.2% (48) | 10.7% (28) | 11.1% (51) | 0.826 |

| Variable | Patients | | | P |
|---|---|---|---|---|
| | ASTmax subgroup | | | |
| | 5× ULN–10× ULN (n = 395) | 10× ULN–20× ULN (n = 261) | >20× ULN (n = 460) | |
| SOI scores[c] | | | | |
| APS-II[b] | 24.0 (18.0–31.0) | 26.5 (20.0–32.2) | 32.0 (24.0–37.9) | <0.001 |
| SAPS-II[b] | 57.0 (36.2–74.0) | 60.0 (41.0–78.2) | 73.0 (56.0–86.5) | <0.001 |
| Supportive therapy[c] | | | | |
| Ventilation[a] | 71.9% (284) | 72.4% (189) | 78.9% (363) | 0.035 |
| Medication | | | | |
| Inotropic agents[a] | 38.5% (152) | 37.9% (99) | 50.2% (231) | <0.001 |
| Vasopressor agents[a] | 50.9% (201) | 59.4% (155) | 70.0% (322) | <0.001 |
| Dialysis[a] | 4.8% (19) | 8.4% (22) | 14.1% (65) | <0.001 |
| IABP[a] | 13.7% (54) | 20.7% (54) | 18.9% (87) | 0.041 |
| LOS | | | | |
| ICU[b] (day) | 4.6 (1.6–11.2) | 4.8 (1.4–11.2) | 4.0 (0.7–12.4) | 0.325 |
| Hospital[b] (day) | 12.5 (6.5–29.5) | 13.1 (4.1–27.6) | 10.2 (0.9–29.8) | 0.250 |
| Duration | | | | |
| Episode of HH[b] (h) | 23.6 (11.4–37.2) | 56.8 (40.5–79.6) | 104.7 (78.1–132.0) | <0.001 |
| Recovery of HH[b] (h) | 12.6 (6.1–22.2) | 36.2 (22.7–52.0) | 77.7 (56.6–102.4) | <0.001 |
| 28-day mortality | | | | |
| ICU[a] | 29.4% (116) | 38.3% (100) | 52.0% (239) | <0.001 |
| In-hospital[a] | 33.2% (131) | 44.4% (116) | 55.4% (255) | <0.001 |

APS-II acute physiology II, AST aspartate aminotransferase, ASTmax maximum AST value, BMI body mass index, HH hypoxic hepatitis, IABP intra-aortic balloon pump, ICU intensive care unit, LOS length of stay, LV left ventricle, P P value, Q1 first quartile, Q3 third quartile, RV right ventricle, SAPS-II simplified acute physiology II, SOI severity of illness, T-ASTmax time point of maximum AST value, ULN upper limit of normal

Italics indicate the significant P values

[a] % (n)

[b] Median (Q1–Q3)

[c] At T-ASTmax ± 12 h

**Table 3  Characteristics of patients with HH classified by clinical cause**

| Variable | Cause | | | | | | | |
|---|---|---|---|---|---|---|---|---|
| | Cardiac failure (n = 548) | Septic shock (n = 333) | Hypov-olemic shock (n = 105) | Acute res-piratory failure (n = 71) | Acute on chronic res-piratory failure (n = 37) | Pulmonary embolism (n = 16) | Hyperthermia (n = 6) | P |
| Sex[a] | | | | | | | | |
| Male | 63.1% (346) | 61.6 (205) | 57.1% (60) | 54.9% (39) | 54.1% (20) | 62.5 (10) | 66.7% (4) | 0.721 |
| Age[b] (year) | 68.0 (58.0–76.0) | 64.0 (52.0–74.0) | 64.0 (56.0–73.0) | 59.0 (48.5–71.5) | 65.0 (61.0–72.0) | 57.5 (47.5–61.5) | 54.5 (35.8–64.2) | 0.003 |
| BMI[b] (kg/m²) | 25.5 (23.3–28.7) | 25.0 (22.1–29.3) | 26.2 (23.4–28.9) | 24.2 (22.0–27.8) | 24.6 (22.1–27.3) | 27.8 (25.1–31.0) | 27.6 (23.7–29.3) | 0.202 |
| Comorbidities | | | | | | | | |
| Echocardio[a] | | | | | | | | |
| Normal | 32.7% (179) | 51.1% (170) | 43.8% (46) | 36.6% (26) | 48.6% (18) | 18.8% (3) | 66.7% (4) | < 0.001 |
| LV dysf. | 36.5% (200) | 15.9% (53) | 5.7% (6) | 21.1% (15) | 10.8% (4) | 6.2% (1) | 16.7% (1) | < 0.001 |
| Missing | 13.3% (73) | 26.1% (87) | 46.7% (49) | 35.2% (25) | 24.3% (9) | 25.0% (4) | 16.7% (1) | < 0.001 |
| LV and RV dysf. | 13.0% (71) | 3.3% (11) | 1.0% (1) | 4.2% (3) | 2.7% (1) | 12.5% (2) | 0.0% (0) | < 0.001 |
| RV dysf. | 4.6% (25) | 3.6% (12) | 2.9% (3) | 2.8% (2) | 13.5% (5) | 37.5% (6) | 0.0% (0 | < 0.001 |
| DM[a] | 20.8% (114) | 19.2% (64) | 10.5% (11) | 12.7% (9) | 24.3% (9) | 12.5% (2) | 0.0% (0) | 0.103 |
| Chronic respiratory failure[a] | 8.4% (46) | 9.6% (32) | 9.5% (10) | 0.0% (%) | 100.0% (37) | 12.5% (2) | 0.0% (0) | < 0.001 |
| SOI scores[c] | | | | | | | | |
| APS-II[b] | 28.0 (23.0–35.0) | 26.0 (21.0–35.0) | 26.0 (18.5–32.5) | 30.0 (28.0–34.0) | 26.5 (24.2–30.8) | 36.5 (36.2–36.8) | 21.5 (19.2–25.0) | 0.590 |
| SAPS-II[b] | 66.0 (44.0–79.0) | 67.0 (49.0–84.0) | 65.0 (48.0–82.0) | 63.0 (31.0–79.0) | 67.5 (55.0–73.5) | 83.0 (69.2–99.2) | 41.5 (34.0–48.2) | 0.171 |
| ASTmax[a] | | | | | | | | |
| Overall | | | | | | | | 0.135 |
| 5–10× ULN | 36.5% (200) | 34.8% (116) | 28.6% (30) | 39.4% (28) | 35.1% (13) | 37.5% (6) | 33.3% (2) | – |
| 10–20× ULN | 23.7% (130) | 20.4% (68) | 25.7% (27) | 33.8% (24) | 13.5% (5) | 25.0% (4) | 50.0% (3) | – |
| > 20× ULN | 39.8% (218) | 44.7% (149) | 45.7% (48) | 26.8% (19) | 51.4% (19) | 37.5% (6) | 16.7% (1) | – |
| Supportive therapy[c] | | | | | | | | |
| Ventilation[a] | 79.2% (434) | 73.0% (243) | 70.5% (74) | 60.6% (43) | 64.9 (24) | 75.0% (12) | 100.0% (6) | 0.004 |
| Medication | | | | | | | | |
| Inotropic agents[a] | 63.1% (346) | 26.4% (88) | 21.0% (22) | 12.7% (9) | 21.6% (8) | 43.8% (7) | 33.3% (2) | < 0.001 |
| Vasopressor agents[a] | 58.6% (321) | 69.1% (230)[d] | 61.9% (65) | 46.5% (33) | 43.2% (16) | 75.0% (12) | 16.7% (1) | < 0.001 |
| Dialysis[a] | 10.4% (57) | 11.1% (37) | 2.9% (3) | 9.9% (7) | 2.7% (1) | 0.0% (0) | 16.7% (1) | 0.090 |
| IABP[a] | 32.8% (180) | 4.2% (14) | 0.0% (0) | 1.4% (1) | 0.0% (0) | 0.0% (0) | 0.0% (0) | < 0.001 |
| LOS | | | | | | | | |
| ICU[b] (day) | 4.6 (1.4–10.5) | 4.7 (0.9–15.8) | 2.6 (0.7–7.8) | 6.3 (2.3–15.0) | 3.2 (1.4–7.8) | 2.2 (0.3–4.1) | 7.7 (6.6–14.2) | 0.135 |
| Hospital[b] (day) | 11.1 (4.6–25.7) | 12.3 (1.1–37.9) | 11.2 (0.9–28.8) | 14.3 (5.2–30.2) | 20.6 (7.6–27.7) | 5.4 (0.3–19.4) | 43.4 (10.2–97.4) | 0.037 |
| Duration | | | | | | | | |
| Episode of HH[b] (h) | 50.6 (24.9–99.3) | 54.5 (25.1–87.2) | 69.4 (36.8–89.5) | 71.3 (39.0–90.0) | 28.4 (15.1–77.2) | 69.5 (28.0–139.0) | 54.6 (35.4–74.0) | 0.137 |

died within 24 h, its 28-day mortality of 41.4% ranked fourth among all subgroups. The acute respiratory failure and acute on chronic respiratory failure subgroups had similar survival curves and outcome, with 39.4 and 37.8% mortality at 28 days. The lowest mortality rate of 33.3% at 28 days was observed in the hyperthermia subgroup. The survival curves by cause of HH are presented in Fig. 2.

The 28-day mortality also increased significantly (P < 0.001) with severity of HH, ranging from 33.2% in the "5–10× ULN" subgroup to 55.4% in the "> 20× ULN"

**Table 3 continued**

| Variable | Cause | | | | | | | |
| --- | --- | --- | --- | --- | --- | --- | --- | --- |
| | Cardiac failure (*n* = 548) | Septic shock (*n* = 333) | Hypov-olemic shock (*n* = 105) | Acute res-piratory failure (*n* = 71) | Acute on chronic res-piratory failure (*n* = 37) | Pulmonary embolism (*n* = 16) | Hyperthermia (*n* = 6) | *P* |
| Recovery of HH<sup>b</sup> (h) | 33.8 (3.4–67.5) | 34.3 (14.3–60.9) | 41.7 (21.1–65.1) | 31.0 (16.2–62.1) | 39.9 (11.6–89.3) | 35.3 (10.5–65.4) | 29.6 (21.7–43.3) | 0.810 |
| 28-day mortality | | | | | | | | |
| ICU<sup>a</sup> | 37.8% (207) | 48.3% (161) | 40.0% (42) | 33.8% (24) | 27.0% (10) | 56.2% (9) | 33.3% (2) | *0.012* |
| In-hospital<sup>a</sup> | 41.4% (227) | 52.9% (176) | 43.8% (46) | 39.4% (28) | 37.8% (14) | 56.2% (9) | 33.3% (2) | *0.029* |

*APS-II* acute physiology II, *AST* aspartate aminotransferase, *ASTmax* maximum AST value, *BMI* body mass index, *HH* hypoxic hepatitis, *IABP* intra-aortic balloon pump, *ICU* intensive care unit, *LOS* length of stay, *LV* left ventricle, *P* P value, *Q1* first quartile, *Q3* third quartile, *RV* right ventricle, *SAPS-II* simplified acute physiology II, *SOI* severity of illness, *T-ASTmax* time point of maximum AST value, *ULN* upper limit of normal

<sup>a</sup> % (*n*)

<sup>b</sup> Median (Q1–Q3)

<sup>c</sup> At T-ASTmax ± 12 h

<sup>d</sup> A condition for septic shock was the need of vasopressor agents. In this table, the proportion of patients receiving vasopressor agents only at T-ASTmax is given

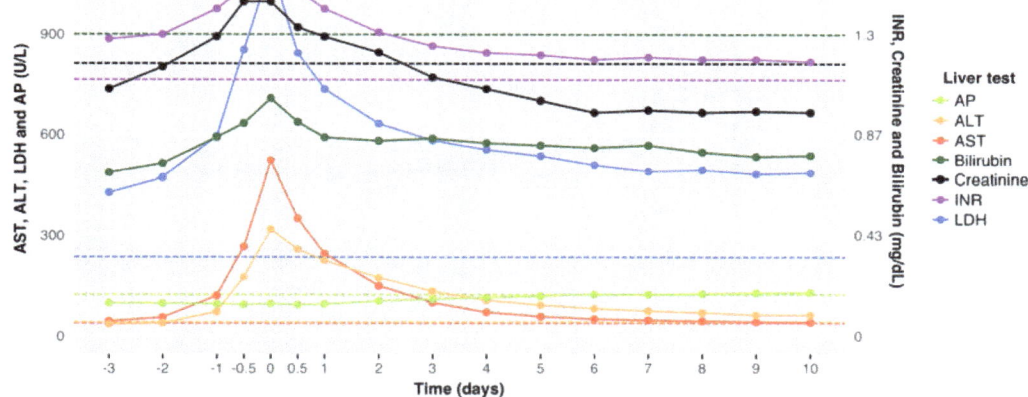

**Fig. 3** Time trend of liver tests in hypoxic hepatitis. Time trend of the median AP, ALT, AST, bilirubin, creatinine, INR and LDH levels in hypoxic hepatitis. T-ASTmax is designated as time 0. AST, ALT, LDH and AP levels are measured in U/L and are plotted using the left y-axis. Bilirubin and creatinine levels are measured in mg/dL and plotted using the right y-axis. INR has no unit, but is also plotted using the right y-axis. *AP* alkaline phosphatase, *ALT* alanine aminotransferase, *AST* aspartate aminotransferase, *INR* international normalized ratio, *LDH* lactate dehydrogenase

subgroup. There was no significant difference (*P* = 0.363) in 28-day mortality between men (39.8%) and women (42.4%).

## Discussion

Hypoxic hepatitis is a type of acute hepatic injury in critically ill patients caused by cardiac, circulatory or respiratory failure. While commonly known and referred to as "shock liver" in daily clinical practice, little research has been done. However, early recognition of HH and

management of its underlying cause and complications may improve ultimate outcome. For a long time, only studies with a relatively small number of patients have been conducted. In 2015, a meta-analysis of 24 studies that included 1782 patients summarized the available evidence, but still lacked detailed information on important patient characteristics, biochemical findings and clinical course [2]. To overcome these shortcomings, Aboelsoud et al. recently performed an extensive analysis of the Medical Information Mart for Intensive Care III

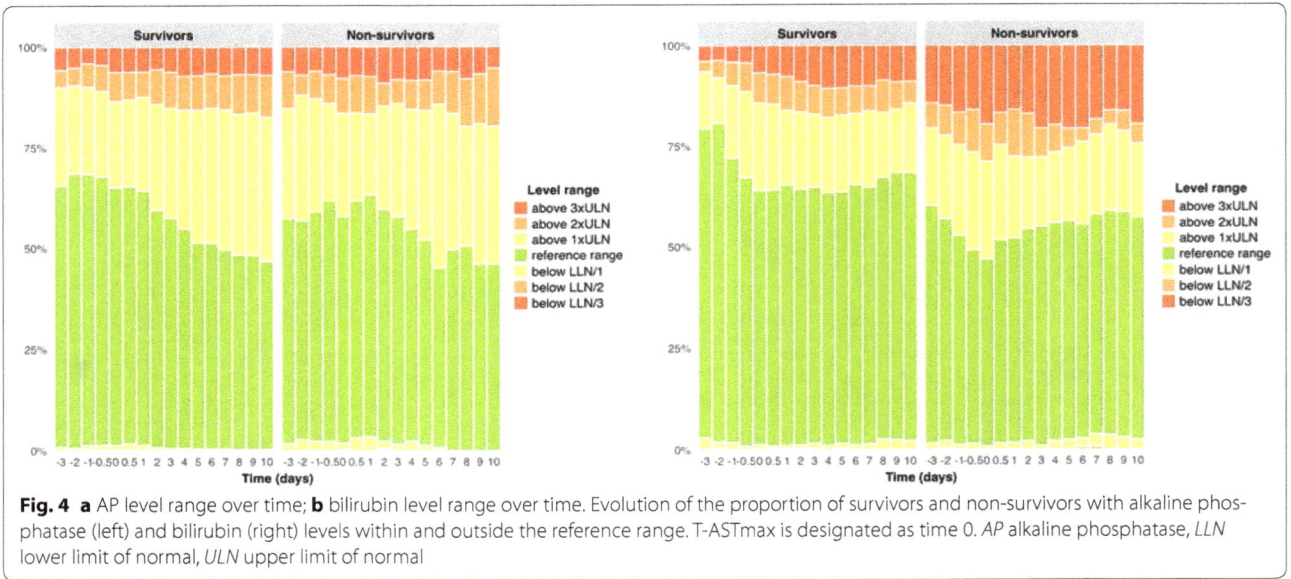

**Fig. 4  a** AP level range over time; **b** bilirubin level range over time. Evolution of the proportion of survivors and non-survivors with alkaline phosphatase (left) and bilirubin (right) levels within and outside the reference range. T-ASTmax is designated as time 0. *AP* alkaline phosphatase, *LLN* lower limit of normal, *ULN* upper limit of normal

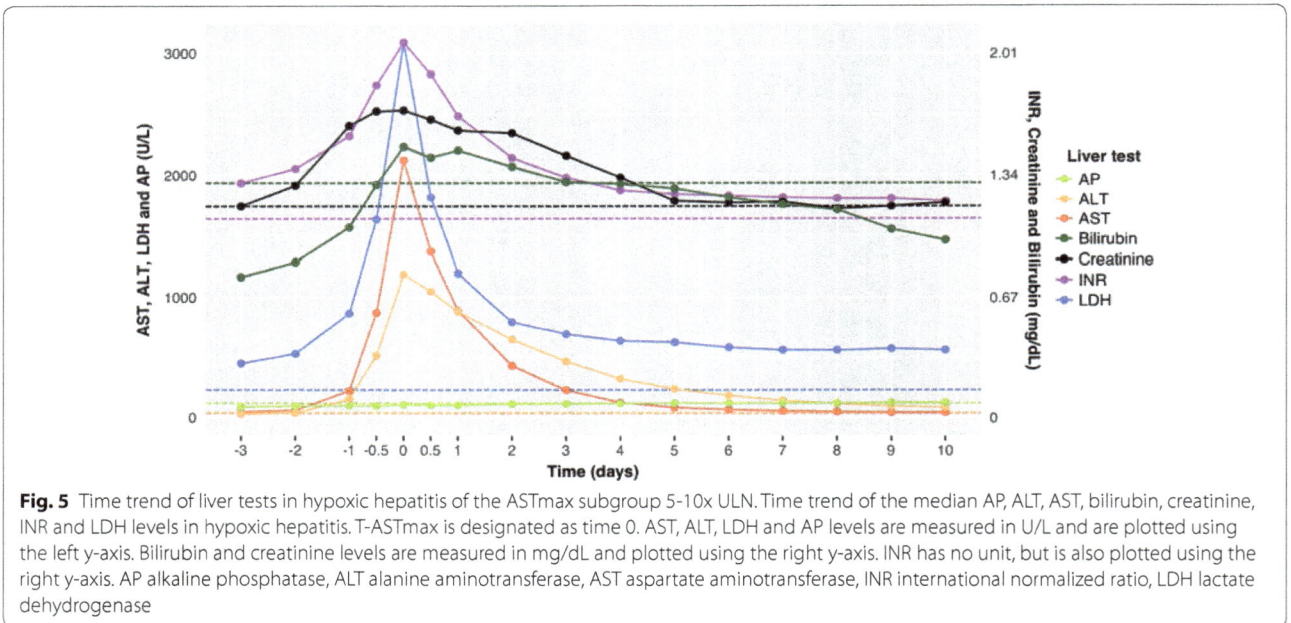

**Fig. 5**  Time trend of liver tests in hypoxic hepatitis of the ASTmax subgroup 5-10x ULN. Time trend of the median AP, ALT, AST, bilirubin, creatinine, INR and LDH levels in hypoxic hepatitis. T-ASTmax is designated as time 0. AST, ALT, LDH and AP levels are measured in U/L and are plotted using the left y-axis. Bilirubin and creatinine levels are measured in mg/dL and plotted using the right y-axis. INR has no unit, but is also plotted using the right y-axis. AP alkaline phosphatase, ALT alanine aminotransferase, AST aspartate aminotransferase, INR international normalized ratio, LDH lactate dehydrogenase

(MIMIC-III) research database. Their study comprised 565 patients with HH and was the largest cohort study published to date [8].

In our study of 1116 critically ill patients with HH, we investigated in detail its incidence, causes, evolution and outcome. We used an AST cutoff of at least 5 times the ULN (i.e., 155 and 185 U/L for females and males, respectively) to define HH, while other studies have used higher cutoff values ranging from 400 to 3000 U/L [2]. HH has been histologically proven to occur even in patients with

moderately elevated AST levels (at AST levels of 252 and 300 IU/L in the cohort of Cohen et al. [13] and Bynum et al. [14], respectively). Additionally, by using a lower cutoff, the sensitivity to identify patients with HH could be increased. However, this approach could also result in a lower specificity, leading to an increased number of patients that are falsely diagnosed as having HH. In order to maintain a high specificity, we have thoroughly reviewed the clinical notes, the time trend of liver tests and the discharge summaries of the 4012 identified

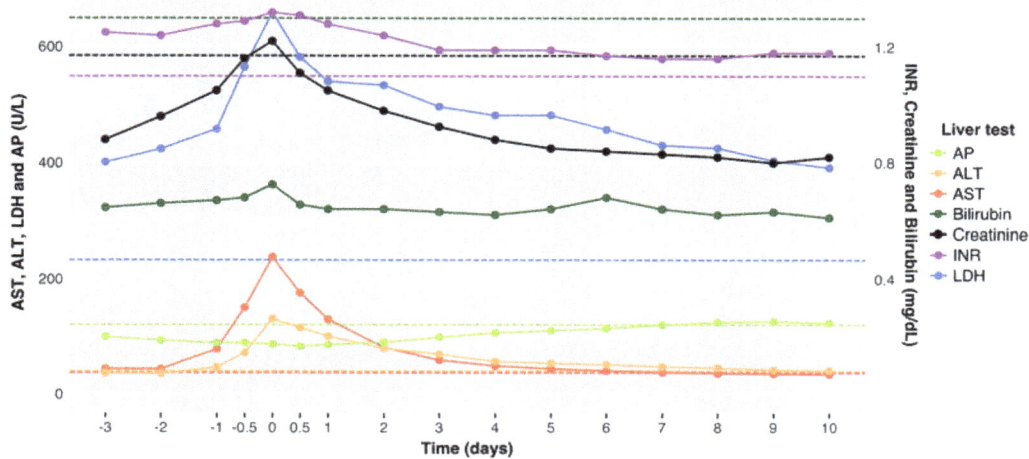

**Fig. 6** Time trend of liver tests in hypoxic hepatitis of the ASTmax subgroup 10-20x ULN. Time trend of the median AP, ALT, AST, bilirubin, creatinine, INR and LDH levels in hypoxic hepatitis. T-ASTmax is designated as time 0. AST, ALT, LDH and AP levels are measured in U/L and are plotted using the left y-axis. Bilirubin and creatinine levels are measured in mg/dL and plotted using the right y-axis. INR has no unit, but is also plotted using the right y-axis. AP alkaline phosphatase, ALT alanine aminotransferase, AST aspartate aminotransferase, INR international normalized ratio, LDH lactate dehydrogenase

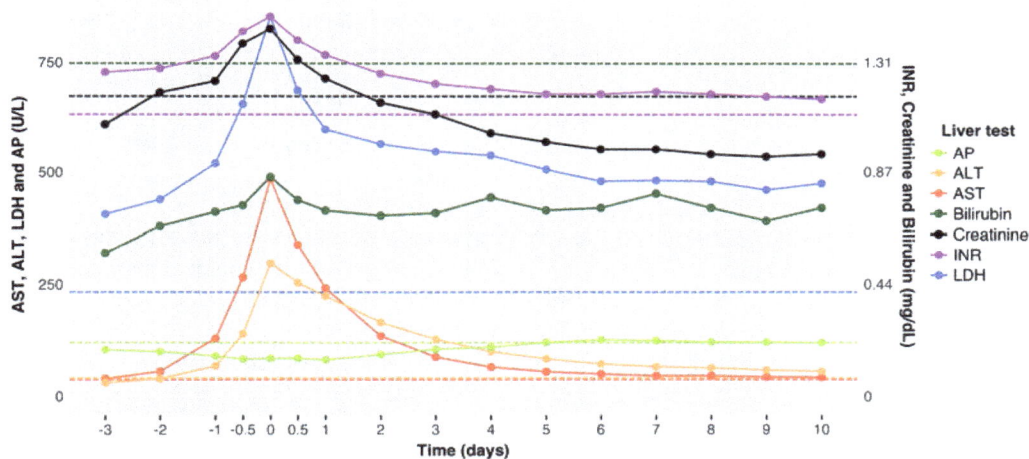

**Fig. 7** Time trend of liver tests in hypoxic hepatitis of the ASTmax subgroup >20x ULN. Time trend of the median AP, ALT, AST, bilirubin, creatinine, INR and LDH levels in hypoxic hepatitis. T-ASTmax is designated as time 0. AST, ALT, LDH and AP levels are measured in U/L and are plotted using the left y-axis. Bilirubin and creatinine levels are measured in mg/dL and plotted using the right y-axis. INR has no unit, but is also plotted using the right y-axis. AP alkaline phosphatase, ALT alanine aminotransferase, AST aspartate aminotransferase, INR international normalized ratio, LDH lactate dehydrogenase

patients whose AST level exceeded our cutoff value. Our high number of excluded patients (70.0%) after applying extensive exclusion criteria may reflect a high specificity. In contrast, Aboelsoud et al. [8] used a cutoff of 800 U/L for both AST and ALT to include patients, but only excluded 24.3% of these patients based on evidence of acetaminophen poisoning, acute viral hepatitis or liver surgery.

Our study uncovered interesting results. Firstly, it indicated that HH may be more common than previously thought. In our study, an incidence of 4.0% was observed, which is higher than the pooled incidence of 2.5% from a meta-analysis of 1782 patients [2] and the incidence of 1.5% in the MIMIC-III cohort [8]. Moreover, approximately one in five critically ill patients that have died during their ICU stay had developed HH. This

**Table 4 Median laboratory values (Q1–Q3) at different time stages**

| Variable | At start of HH | At T-ASTmax |
|---|---|---|
| AST (U/L) | 185.0 (155.0–185.0) | 521.2 (269.1–1581.6) |
| ALT (U/L) | 120.8 (70.1–193.5) | 317.0 (143.5–924.5) |
| LDH (U/L) | 691.8 (465.8–1025.7) | 1106.4 (624.8–2602.8) |
| Bilirubin (mg/dL) | 0.8 (0.5–1.6) | 1.0 (0.6–2.0) |
| GGT (U/L) | 73.1 (36.2–160.4) | 82.5 (41.7–167.0) |
| AP (U/L) | 88.2 (61.8–150.9) | 94.0 (62.9–167.0) |
| Lipase (U/L) | 32.4 (18.9–58.9) | 33.5 (18.5–66.4) |
| INR | 1.4 (1.2–1.8) | 1.6 (1.3–2.2) |
| PC ($10^3$/μL) | 165.7 (103.6–241.0) | 146.0 (79.5–218.0) |
| WBC ($10^3$/μL) | 12.5 (8.8–17.6) | 13.2 (9.0–18.5) |
| Hb (g/dL) | 10.1 (8.8–12.0) | 9.8 (8.6–11.5) |
| CK (U/L) | 214.0 (77.2–747.2) | 322.2 (105.1–1102.9) |
| Creatinine (mg/dL) | 1.4 (0.9–2.1) | 1.4 (0.9–2.2) |
| Urea (mg/dL) | 57.1 (38.9–91.3) | 61.6 (40.6–96.4) |
| Lactate (mg/dL) | 31.3 (16.2–62.2) | 27.4 (14.7–56.2) |

*AP* alkaline phosphatase, *ALT* alanine aminotransferase, *AST* aspartate aminotransferase, *CK* creatine kinase, *GGT* gamma-glutamyl transpeptidase, *Hb* hemoglobin, *INR* international normalized ratio, *LDH* lactate dehydrogenase, *PC* platelet count, *WBC* white blood cell count

higher incidence observed in our study is of course a direct consequence of the lower AST cutoff used. However, it should be noted that the underlying conditions, the typical liver test pattern and the considerable mortality of 33.2% at 28 days in patients with a less pronounced rise of AST (peak AST level between 5 and 10 times the ULN) are just as much compatible with the diagnosis of HH as in patients with higher peak AST level. Any sudden increase in aminotransferases above 5 times the ULN should therefore prompt the clinician to actively search for any changes in physiological parameters and maintain strict hemodynamic and respiratory control.

Secondly, the typical liver test pattern that suggests diagnosis of HH was observed in all subgroups of our study cohort. HH was characterized by (1) a sudden and significant increase of aminotransferases with an AST/ALT ratio greater than 1, (2) a similar rise in LDH mostly exceeding both AST and ALT and (3) a steady decline of aminotransferases with reversal of the AST/ALT ratio approximately 1.5 days after T-ASTmax. In survivors, LDH normalized first, followed by AST and finally ALT (median of 5.1, 6.4 and 8.6 days after T-ASTmax, respectively). Bilirubin followed a similar pattern as the aminotransferases, but the magnitude of its increase was much less pronounced, with median levels never exceeding the ULN. The associated prolongation of INR and impairment of renal function as described by Raurich et al. [6] were also confirmed in this study.

Finally, we observed a 28-day mortality of 45.0%, which is in line with the reported mortality of 49% from

a meta-analysis of 1782 patients [2] and the mortality of 44.1% in the MIMIC-III cohort [8]. HH was especially associated with high mortality rates early in its course, with roughly 40% of deaths occurring within 24 h after T-ASTmax. This was mainly driven by the severity of the underlying causes [2], although the ultimate cause of death was not inferred in this study. The magnitude of AST increase also appeared to be correlated with mortality on univariate analysis.

Our study has a number of strengths. To our knowledge, it is by far the largest cohort study of patients with HH ($n = 1116$). It comprises twice as many patients as the second largest cohort study, which was recently published and included 565 patients [8]. Additionally, by using a low AST cutoff of 5 times the ULN while simultaneously excluding many conditions that could mimic HH, we are confident that we could identify nearly all patients with HH at our center with a low risk of misdiagnosis. Our study may have some limitations inherent in its retrospective design. However, we believe that the retrospective design had little to no impact on our results given the entirely computerized monitoring and management at our ICU, the detailed review of patient records and the high number of patients included. Nevertheless, we should be careful to generalize these results to a broader patient population since only critically ill patients older than 18 years and only from a single university hospital ICU were included.

## Conclusions

This study surpasses by far the largest cohort of critically ill patients with hypoxic hepatitis. HH is more common than previously thought with an ICU incidence of 4.0%, and it is associated with a high all-cause mortality of 45.0% at 28 days. The main causes of HH are cardiac failure and septic shock, which include more than 3/4 of all episodes. Clinicians should search actively for any underlying hemodynamic or respiratory instability even in patients with moderately increased AST levels.

**Abbreviations**
HH: hypoxic hepatitis; AST: aspartate aminotransferase; ICU: intensive care unit; ALT: alanine aminotransferase; LDH: lactate dehydrogenase; ULN: upper limit of normal; CK: creatine kinase; AP: alkaline phosphatase; INR: international normalized ratio; BMI: body mass index; APS-II: acute physiology II; SAPS-II: simplified acute physiology II; T-ASTmax: time point of maximum AST value; ASTmax: maximum AST value; Q1: first quartile; Q3: third quartile; MIMIC-III: Medical Information Mart for Intensive Care III.

**Authors' contributions**
AV and LV designed the study, collected data, performed and interpreted statistical analysis, and drafted the manuscript. Both authors contributed equally to this study and are the joint first authors. AD performed and interpreted statistical analysis, and drafted the manuscript. KC, HV and DB designed the study and revised the manuscript. JD designed the study, interpreted

statistical analysis and revised the manuscript. All authors read and approved the final manuscript.

**Author details**
[1] Faculty of Medicine and Health Sciences, Ghent University, Ghent, Belgium.
[2] Department of Internal Medicine, Ghent University Hospital, Ghent, Belgium.
[3] Department of Intensive Care Medicine, Ghent University Hospital, De Pintelaan 185, 9000 Ghent, Belgium. [4] Department of Hepatology and Gastro-Enterology, Ghent University Hospital, Ghent, Belgium.

**Acknowledgements**
Not applicable.

**Competing interests**
The authors declare that they have no competing interests.

**Funding**
None.

**References**
1. Henrion J. Hypoxic hepatitis. Liver Int. 2012;32(7):1039–52.
2. Tapper EB, Sengupta N, Bonder A. The incidence and outcomes of ischemic hepatitis: a systematic review with meta-analysis. Am J Med. 2015;128(12):1314–21.
3. Henrion J, Schapira M, Luwaert R, Colin L, Delannoy A, Heller FR. Hypoxic hepatitis: clinical and hemodynamic study in 142 consecutive cases. Medicine (Baltimore). 2003;82(6):392–406.
4. Birrer R, Takuda Y, Takara T. Hypoxic hepatopathy: pathophysiology and prognosis. Intern Med. 2007;46(14):1063–70.
5. Fuhrmann V, Kneidinger N, Herkner H, Heinz G, Nikfardjam M, Bojic A, et al. Hypoxic hepatitis: underlying conditions and risk factors for mortality in critically ill patients. Intensive Care Med. 2009;35(8):1397–405.
6. Raurich JM, Llompart-Pou JA, Ferreruela M, Colomar A, Molina M, Royo C, et al. Hypoxic hepatitis in critically ill patients: incidence, etiology and risk factors for mortality. J Anesth. 2011;25(1):50–6.
7. Fuchs S, Bogomolski-Yahalom V, Paltiel O, Ackerman Z. Ischemic hepatitis: clinical and laboratory observations of 34 patients. J Clin Gastroenterol. 1998;26(3):183–6.
8. Aboelsoud MM, Javaid AI, Al-Qadi MO, Lewis JH. Hypoxic hepatitis—its biochemical profile, causes and risk factors of mortality in critically-ill patients: a cohort study of 565 patients. J Crit Care. 2017;41:9–15.
9. Dunn GD, Hayes P, Breen KJ, Schenker S. The liver in congestive heart failure: a review. Am J Med Sci. 1973;265(3):174–89.
10. Ebert EC. Hypoxic liver injury. Mayo Clin Proc. 2006;81(9):1232–6.
11. Whitehead MW, Hawkes ND, Hainsworth I, Kingham JG. A prospective study of the causes of notably raised aspartate aminotransferase of liver origin. Gut. 1999;45(1):129–33.
12. Johnson RD, O'Connor ML, Kerr RM. Extreme serum elevations of aspartate aminotransferase. Am J Gastroenterol. 1995;90(8):1244–5.
13. Bynum TE, Boitnott JK, Maddrey WC. Ischemic hepatitis. Dig Dis Sci. 1979;24(2):129–35.
14. Cohen JA, Kaplan MM. Left-sided heart failure presenting as hepatitis. Gastroenterology. 1978;74(3):583–7.
15. Core Team R. R: a language and environment for statistical computing. Vienna: R Foundation for Statistical Computing; 2016.

# 5

# Physiological predictors of respiratory and cough assistance needs after extubation

Nicolas Terzi[1,2,3*], Frédéric Lofaso[4,5,6], Romain Masson[3], Pascal Beuret[7], Hervé Normand[8,9,10], Edith Dumanowski[10], Line Falaize[11,12], Bertrand Sauneuf[3,13], Cédric Daubin[3], Jennifer Brunet[3], Djillali Annane[14], Jean-Jacques Parienti[15] and David Orlikowski[4,5,16,17]

## Abstract

**Background:** Identifying patients at high risk of post-extubation acute respiratory failure requiring respiratory or mechanical cough assistance remains challenging. Here, our primary aim was to evaluate the accuracy of easily collected parameters obtained before or just after extubation in predicting the risk of post-extubation acute respiratory failure requiring, at best, noninvasive mechanical ventilation (NIV) and/or mechanical cough assistance and, at worst, reintubation after extubation.

**Methods:** We conducted a multicenter prospective, open-label, observational study from April 2012 through April 2015. Patients who passed a weaning test after at least 72 h of endotracheal mechanical ventilation (MV) were included. Just before extubation, spirometry and maximal pressures were measured by a technician. The results were not disclosed to the bedside physicians. Patients were followed until discharge or death.

**Results:** Among 3458 patients admitted to the ICU, 730 received endotracheal MV for longer than 72 h and were then extubated; among these, 130 were included. At inclusion, the 130 patients had mean ICU stay and endotracheal MV durations both equal to 11 ± 4.2 days. After extubation, 36 patients required curative NIV, 7 both curative NIV and mechanical cough assistance, and 8 only mechanical cough assistance; 6 patients, all of whom first received NIV, required reintubation within 48 h. The group that required NIV after extubation had a significantly higher proportion of patients with chronic respiratory disease ($P = 0.015$), longer endotracheal MV duration at inclusion, and lower Medical Research Council (MRC) score ($P = 0.02$, $P = 0.01$, and $P = 0.004$, respectively). By multivariate analysis, forced vital capacity (FVC) and peak cough expiratory flow (PCEF) were independently associated with (NIV) and/or mechanical cough assistance and/or reintubation after extubation. Areas under the ROC curves for pre-extubation PCEF and FVC were 0.71 and 0.76, respectively.

**Conclusion:** In conclusion, FVC measured before extubation correlates closely with FVC after extubation and may serve as an objective predictor of post-extubation respiratory failure requiring NIV and/or mechanical cough assistance and/or reintubation in heterogeneous populations of medical ICU patients.

ClinicalTrials.gov as #NCT01564745

## Background

Weaning patients off endotracheal positive-pressure ventilation involves two steps: separation of the patient from the ventilator and extubation. The day of extubation is a critical time during an intensive care unit (ICU) stay, as extubation failure occurs in 10–20% of patients and is associated with up to 50% hospital mortality [1–6]. There is some evidence that extubation failure can directly worsen patient outcomes independently of underlying illness severity [5]. Several factors may contribute to extubation failure, including cough impairment and presence of thick and/or excessive mucus, in addition to hypoventilation [4]. Cough assistance and noninvasive

*Correspondence: nterzi@chu-grenoble.fr
[3] Service de réanimation médicale, Centre Hospitalier Universitaire Grenoble - Alpes, CS10217, Grenoble Cedex 09, France
Full list of author information is available at the end of the article

mechanical ventilation (NIV) can help to prevent post-extubation respiratory failure. However, as these techniques are time-consuming, criteria for selecting those patients most likely to benefit would be useful. Ideally, these criteria would be objective, easily measured parameters obtained immediately before and/or after extubation. Adequate respiratory muscle strength is essential to generate the pressures and flows needed to clear airway secretions during coughing. Accordingly, peak cough expiratory flow (PCEF) was found in many studies to predict successful decannulation and extubation [7–12]. However, the tracheal tube can alter PCEF values via two mechanisms: it elevates airway resistance [13]; and it eliminates the role of the glottis in coughing [14].

Here, our objective was to evaluate the accuracy of parameters easily collected before versus after extubation in predicting the risk of post-extubation respiratory failure requiring, at best, NIV and/or mechanical cough assistance and, at worst, reintubation. We assessed cough performance and other easily collected respiratory parameters obtained before and after extubation, with the goal of determining which parameters and measurement conditions best identified patients who would require NIV and/or mechanical cough assistance after extubation.

## Methods

### Study population

We conducted a multicenter, prospective, observational study in two university-affiliated hospitals (Caen and Garches) and one general hospital (Roanne) in France from April 2012 through April 2015. The appropriate ethics committee (CPP Nord-Ouest III) approved the study (#2011-A00849-32), which was registered on ClinicalTrials.gov (#NCT01564745). All patients provided written informed consent.

Patients 18 years of age or older and sufficiently cooperative without sedation were eligible if they were admitted to the ICU and received invasive mechanical ventilation (MV) for at least 72 h then passed a weaning test performed according to recommendations [4, 15, 16]. Exclusion criteria were previous long-term NIV at home and unavailability of an lung function test (LFT) technician.

### Study procedures

Weaning from the ventilator was performed following a standardized protocol. Patients were screened daily for predefined weaning-readiness criteria, i.e., improvement in clinical signs, peripheral capillary oxygen saturation ($SpO_2$) > 92% with fraction of inspired oxygen < 50% and positive end-expiratory pressure < 5 cm $H_2O$, no infusion of vasopressor agents or sedatives, and adequate responses to simple commands. When these criteria were

met, a spontaneous breathing test (SBT) was performed, by having the patient either breathe spontaneously from the ventilator on a T piece or receive pressure-support ventilation with an inspiratory pressure of 7 $cmH_2O$ and zero end-expiratory pressure. The test was interrupted if any of the following signs of poor tolerance was observed: respiratory rate > 35/min, $SpO_2$ < 90%, heart rate > 140/min, and arterial systolic blood pressure > 180 mmHg or < 90 mmHg. Patients who successfully completed the test were considered for a trial of extubation. Decisions to perform a cuff-leak test and/or give corticosteroid therapy were based on standard practice at each study center.

Patients who passed an SBT and were considered for extubation underwent lung function testing (LFT) (see Additional file 1). After extubation, the patients breathed spontaneously with an oxygen flow titrated to maintain $SpO_2$ > 90%.

Physicians were blinded to LFT results. Patients were followed until ICU discharge or death.

### Lung function testing (LFT)

LFT was repeated after extubation provided and there was no laryngeal edema (see Additional file 1).

### Clinical data

At ICU admission, we recorded the following: comorbidities, MV duration at inclusion, number of tracheal aspirates within 24 h before extubation, Glasgow Coma Scale score, Medical Research Council (MRC) scale combined score for muscle strength [17], and Borg Scale [18] score for subjective dyspnea.

### Extubation care and definitions

According to guidelines, patients were extubated by the physician if they passed an SBT [4, 15, 16]. We evaluated the accuracy of easily collected parameters obtained before or just after extubation in predicting weaning failure defined as a need for NIV and/or mechanical cough assistance and/or reintubation within 48 h after extubation.

Patients received NIV if they met at least one of the following predefined criteria: respiratory rate > 30 breaths/min; $SpO_2$ < 90%; ≥ 20% variation in heart rate or blood pressure; clinical signs of respiratory distress (i.e., cyanosis, sweating, involvement of accessory respiratory muscles, paradoxical abdominal motion, consciousness impairment); $PaO_2$ < 60 mm Hg with ≥ 6 L/min $O_2$; and hypercapnia with respiratory acidosis (i.e., $PaCO_2$ > 45 mm Hg and pH < 7.35). All patients received chest physiotherapy twice daily to promote secretion clearance, with deep inspiration and manual cough assistance. Mechanical cough assistance was used, alone or with NIV, when conventional chest physiotherapy failed to prevent secretion accumulation with severe hypoxemia defined as $SaO_2 < 90\%$ with $\geq 6$ L/min $O_2$ or $FiO_2 > 50\%$. Reintubation was considered when there was no improvement within 2 h and was performed according to guidelines [15, 16].

## Statistical analysis
Quantitative variables were described as mean $\pm$ SD and qualitative variables as number (%). To compare demographics, clinical data, and LFT results between groups with and without weaning failure as defined above (NIV and/or mechanical cough assistance and/or reintubation, within 48 h after extubation), we used the Chi-square test for categorical variables and the Wilcoxon $t$ test for quantitative co-variables. Multivariate logistic regression was performed to identify pre-extubation measurements independently associated with weaning failure. The close correlations among respiratory parameters precluded the use of a single multivariate model. Therefore, we built a separate multivariate logistic regression model to assess the ability of each LFT variable to predict weaning failure. All models were adjusted for MV duration (< 7 vs. $\geq 7$ days), MRC scale score (< 48 vs. $\geq 48$), and previous chronic respiratory failure. Model discrimination was assessed by the concordance index (c-index) and plotted on a receiver operating characteristic (ROC) curve. For each LFT variable, we identified the cutoff that maximized the Youden index, and we computed the sensitivity and specificity of this cutoff for predicting weaning failure. In addition, correlations between each LFT parameter before and after extubation were assessed by Pearson's correlation coefficient.

All $P$ values were two-tailed with no adjustment for multiple comparisons. $P$ values < 0.05 were considered significant. The statistical analyses were performed using SAS statistical software, version 9.4 (SAS Institute Inc., Cary, NC, USA).

## Results
### Study population
Among 3458 patients admitted to the study ICUs, 730 received MV for more than 72 h and were then extubated; among these, 130 were included in the study (Fig. 1). Table 1 reports their main characteristics at ICU admission. At study inclusion, mean values for ICU stay and MV duration were both $11.0 \pm 4.2$ days. Five patients were excluded from the analysis because they required immediate reintubation due to either laryngeal edema ($n = 3$) or acute coma ($n = 2$) and consequently could not undergo post-extubation testing.

After extubation, 36 patients required curative NIV, including 7 who also needed mechanical cough assistance, and 8 required only mechanical cough assistance.

Reintubation was performed within 2 days after extubation in 6 patients and on day 6 in 1 patient. All reintubated patients received NIV within 2 days following extubation, and none died in the ICU. Patients who were reintubated were significantly younger and had a lower BMI than those who received only NIV and/or mechanical cough assistance.

## Comparison of lung function parameters before and after extubation
Vital capacity (VC), forced vital capacity (FVC), peak expiratory flow (PEF), and PCEF were significantly higher after than before extubation. Maximal inspiratory pressure (MIP) and maximal expiratory pressure (MEP) were significantly higher before than after extubation (all $P$ values < 0.001). As shown in Table 2, the pre-extubation and post-extubation values correlated with each other for all variables (all $P$ values < 0.0001); the correlation was strongest for FVC ($R = 0.89$).

## Comparison of patients who did ($n = 44$) and did not (81) require NIV or mechanical cough assistance after extubation
As shown in Table 3, the group that required post-extubation NIV or mechanical cough assistance had a significantly higher proportion of patients with chronic respiratory disease, longer ICU stay and MV durations at study inclusion, and lower MRC scores compared to the other group.

By univariate analysis, pre-extubation LFT variables significantly associated with post-extubation NIV and/or mechanical cough assistance were $PaCO_2$, VC, FVC, MIP, MEP, PEF, and PCEF (Table 2). Post-extubation LFT variables significantly associated with post-extubation NIV and/or mechanical cough assistance were VC, FVC, MEP, PEF, and PCEF (Table 2).

By multivariate logistic regression adjusted for MV duration, MRC score, and the existence of chronic respiratory failure, variables independently associated with post-extubation NIV and/or mechanical cough assistance were VC, FVC, MIP, MEP, PEF, and PCEF (Table 4).

## ROC curve analysis of performance of the independent predictors
As shown in Fig. 2, the areas under the ROC curves for pre-extubation PCEF, PEF, FVC, MIP, and MEP were 0.71, 0.67, 0.76, 0.61, and 0.69, respectively. The cutoffs that performed best in predicting post-extubation NIV and/or mechanical cough assistance were 85 L/min for PCEF, 62 L/min for PEF, and 1412 mL for FVC. The PCEF cutoff had 74% sensitivity and 62% specificity, the PEF cutoff 51% sensitivity and 76% specificity, and the FVC cutoff 65% sensitivity and 81% specificity.

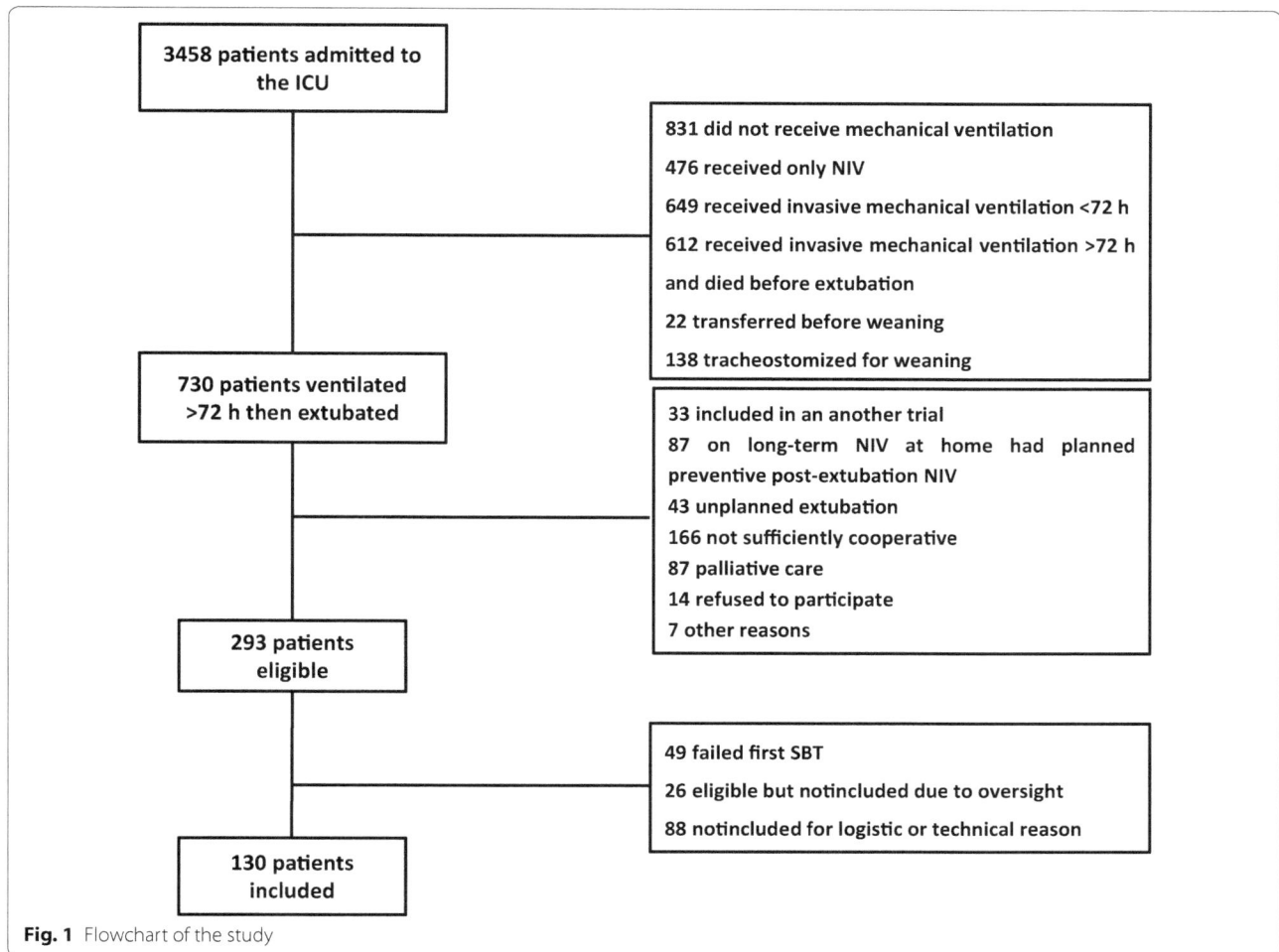

**Fig. 1** Flowchart of the study

As shown in Fig. 3, the areas under the ROC curves for post-extubation PCEF, PEF, FVC, MIP, and MEP were 0.76, 0.68, 0.80, 0.62, and 0.73, respectively. The cutoffs that performed best in predicting post-extubation NIV and/or mechanical cough assistance were 113 L/min for PCEF, 151 L/min for PEF, and 1430 mL for FVC. The PCEF cutoff had 56% sensitivity and 90% specificity, the PEF cutoff 57% sensitivity and 76% specificity, and the FVC cutoff 72% sensitivity and 85% specificity.

## Discussion

The main finding from this study is that the parameter with the closet correlation between pre- and post-extubation values was FVC. FVC may be an objective marker for identifying patients in whom NIV and/or mechanical cough assistance might prevent reintubation. Hypoventilation, cough impairment, and presence of thick and/or excessive mucus can contribute to extubation failure. Most of the previous studies evaluating cough efficiency before extubation focused on PCEF. However, the PCEF

cutoffs varied widely [9, 12], perhaps due to differences in study populations and MV durations. Moreover, the diversity of devices used to measure PCEF, presence of a cannula used to bypass the upper airway [19], and differences in the degree of patient coordination and cooperation during measurements may influence the results [12, 20, 21]. In our study, the optimal PCEF cutoff was 85 L/min before extubation and 113 L/min just after extubation. Our pre-extubation PCEF cutoff was higher than in earlier studies. However, our objective was to predict a need for post-extubation NIV and/or mechanical cough assistance, whereas previous studies [12, 20] sought to predict reintubation. Furthermore, the correlation between pre- and post-extubation PCEF values was weak. Several hypotheses can be suggested to explain this finding. The inability of intubated patients to close their glottis limits the pressure generated during coughing and therefore limits the PCEF values compared to those measured without the tube. Also, resistances are higher with than without the endotracheal tube. Finally, in a

### Table 1 Characteristics of the patients at ICU admission

| Parameters | Mean ± SD or n (%) |
|---|---|
| Total (n = 130) | |
| Age (years) | 59.4 ± 15.6 |
| Male | 71 (54.6) |
| BMI | 27.2 ± 6.7 |
| Chronic disease | |
| Chronic obstructive pulmonary disease | 16 (12.3%) |
| Chronic restrictive pulmonary disease | 11 (8.4%) |
| Chronic heart disease | 13 (10%) |
| SAPS II | 45 ± 21 |
| SOFA | 7 ± 5 |
| Main reason for ICU admission | |
| Acute respiratory failure | 91 (70) |
| Heart failure | 14 (10.8) |
| Neurologic failure | 9 (6.9) |
| Septic shock | 12 (9.2) |
| Postoperative | 1 (0.8) |
| Other | 3 (2.3) |

BMI body mass index, SAPS II Simplified Acute Physiology Score II [30], SOFA Sequential Organ Failure Assessment

recent study in tracheostomized patients with neuromuscular disease, PCEF was higher after than before decannulation [13, 22].

Interestingly, Bach and Saporito [7] were the first to use PCEF as a criterion for extubation in patients with neuromuscular disease. However, they measured PCEF immediately after extubation and enhanced performance by combining maximal insufflation with an abdominal thrust timed to glottis opening. The results showed that PCEF > 160 L/min predicted successful extubation. More recently, they challenged their previous PCEF cutoff by demonstrating that professionals who had extensive experience with the noninvasive management of respiratory failure were able to extubate continuously ventilator-dependent patients who had severe cough impairment [8]. Finally, they demonstrated that using noninvasive techniques to improve cough performance and minute ventilation could drastically modify the outcomes of extubated patients, including those dependent on a ventilator [8]. These studies and our data suggest that identifying both the optimal PCEF value and the best PCEF measurement conditions in critically ill patients remains

### Table 2 Correlations between physiological parameters before and after extubation

| | VC<br>Before extubation | FVC<br>Before extubation | MIP<br>Before extubation | MEP<br>Before extubation | PEF<br>Before extubation | PECF<br>Before extubation |
|---|---|---|---|---|---|---|
| VC<br>After extubation | | | | | | |
| R | 0.61 | | | | | |
| P value | < 0.0001 | | | | | |
| FVC<br>After extubation | | | | | | |
| R | | 0.89 | | | | |
| P value | | < 0.0001 | | | | |
| MIP<br>After extubation | | | | | | |
| R | | | 0.70 | | | |
| P value | | | < 0.0001 | | | |
| MEP<br>After extubation | | | | | | |
| R | | | | 0.66 | | |
| P value | | | | < 0.0001 | | |
| PEF<br>After extubation | | | | | | |
| R | | | | | 0.60 | |
| P value | | | | | < 0.0001 | |
| PCEF<br>After extubation | | | | | | |
| R | | | | | | 0.58 |
| P value | | | | | | < 0.0001 |

For each parameter, the table shows the correlation coefficient and P value

Italics indicate significant data

VC vital capacity, FVC forced vital capacity, MIP maximal inspiratory pressure, MEP maximal expiratory pressure, PEF peak expiratory flow, PCEF peak cough expiratory flow

**Table 3  Univariate analyses**

| Parameters | No NIV or mechanical cough assistance after extubation ($n = 81$)<br>Mean ± SD or n (%) | NIV or mechanical cough assistance after extubation | | | P value* |
|---|---|---|---|---|---|
| | | All patients ($n = 44$)<br>Mean ± SD or n (%) | Patients who required NIV ($n = 36$)<br>Mean ± SD or n (%) | Patients who required Mechanical cough assistance ($n = 8$)<br>Mean ± SD or n (%) | |
| Age, years | 58.8 ± 14.8 | 59.8 ± 16.4 | 59.6 ± 15.7 | 60.8 ± 20.3 | 0.71 |
| SOFA at admission | 7.7 ± 5 | 7.2 ± 4.2 | 7.5 ± 4.1 | 5.9 ± 4.8 | 0.59 |
| Coma Glasgow Scale score | 15 ± 0 | 15 ± 0 | 15 ± 0 | 15 ± 0 | 1.00 |
| Chronic respiratory failure | 11 (14%) | 14 (32%) | 14 (39%) | 0 | *0.015* |
| Chronic heart disease | 10 (12%) | 3 (7%) | 3 (8%) | 0 | 0.34 |
| Duration of MV, days | 12.7 ± 8.8 | 17.8 ± 15.6 | 17.4 ± 14.4 | 19.8 ± 21.2 | *0.02* |
| Diameter of the endotracheal tube, mm | 7.5 ± 0.3 | 7.4 ± 0.3 | 7.3 ± 0.3 | 7.6 ± 0.3 | 0.17 |
| MRC score | 51.1 ± 12 | 43 ± 15.5 | 43.2 ± 12.2 | 42.2 ± 12.2 | *0.004* |
| Tracheal aspiration before extubation ($n$/24 h) | 7.8 ± 3 | 7.7 ± 2.7 | 7.7 ± 2.5 | 7.6 ± 3.6 | 0.89 |
| Respiratory rate (breaths/min) | 23.2 ± 11.8 | 24.5 ± 5.6 | 24.8 ± 5.9 | 23.4 ± 4.2 | 0.50 |
| Borg Scale score (/10) | 1.9 ± 2.3 | 2.1 ± 2.2 | 2 ± 2 | 2.3 ± 3.5 | 0.60 |
| $PaCO_2$ before extubation | 5.0 ± 0.6 | 5.6 ± 1 | 5.8 ± 1 | 4.9 ± 0.7 | *0.00007* |
| VC (mL) before extubation | 1574 ± 498 | 1281 ± 536 | 1220 ± 513 | 1558 ± 586 | *0.003* |
| FVC (mL) before extubation | 1571 ± 520 | 1146 ± 457 | 1121 ± 464 | 1257 ± 439 | *0.00002* |
| MIP ($cmH_2O$) before extubation | 37 ± 15 | 31 ± 15 | 32 ± 15 | 26 ± 12 | *0.025* |
| MEP ($cmH_2O$) before extubation | 53 ± 28 | 41 ± 24 | 44 ± 25 | 30 ± 16 | *0.021* |
| PEF (L/min) before extubation | 80 ± 32 | 62 ± 30 | 60 ± 29 | 71 ± 36 | *0.004* |
| PCEF (L/min) before extubation | 97 ± 36 | 72 ± 33 | 71 ± 33 | 75 ± 36 | *0.0003* |
| VC (mL) after extubation | 1838 ± 637 | 1364 ± 499 | 1343 ± 511 | 1463 ± 464 | *0.00017* |
| FVC (mL) after extubation | 1766 ± 554 | 1284 ± 433 | 1284 ± 440 | 1282 ± 441 | *0.00003* |
| MIP ($cmH_2O$) after extubation | 28 ± 13 | 23 ± 11 | 23 ± 11 | 22 ± 10 | *0.07* |
| MEP ($cmH_2O$) after extubation | 43 ± 22 | 29 ± 17 | 31 ± 17 | 21 ± 12 | *0.002* |
| PEF (L/min) after extubation | 142 ± 77 | 107 ± 63 | 109 ± 66 | 95 ± 47 | *0.02* |
| PCEF (L/min) after extubation | 166 ± 76 | 107 ± 66 | 110 ± 72 | 94 ± 39 | *0.0001* |

Italics indicate significant data

*SOFA* Sequential Organ Failure Assessment, *MRC* Medical Research Council sum score, *PaO₂* partial pressure of $O_2$ in arterial blood, *PaCO₂* partial pressure of $CO_2$ in arterial blood, *FiO₂* fraction of inspired $O_2$, *VC* vital capacity, *FVC* forced vital capacity, *MIP* maximal inspiratory pressure, *MEP* maximal expiratory pressure, *PEF* peak expiratory flow, *PCEF* peak cough expiratory flow, *NS* nonsignificant

*P values compare patients with and without NIV and/or mechanical cough assistance

challenging because many factors, including the use of assistive devices, can influence the measurement result.

We tested the usefulness of various LFT parameters for evaluating voluntary cough at the bedside. PCEF and PEF were significantly higher in the successfully extubated group, and low PCEF and PEF values independently predicted post-extubation NIV and/or mechanical cough assistance.

As described previously [23–25], expiratory muscle strength as assessed by the MEP correlated with PCEF. MIP and MEP measurements require a static maneuver with maintenance of a maximal pressure for at least 1.5 s [26]. Nevertheless, contrary to FVC and PCEF, MIP and MEP cannot be measured easily in all mechanically ventilated patients without a specific device.

**Table 4  Multivariate analysis of extubation predictors**

| Model | Odds Ratio (IC 95%) | P value |
|---|---|---|
| Model 1 FVC | 0.998 (0.997–0.999) | 0.0005 |
| Model 2 VC | 0.999 (0.998–1.000) | 0.0078 |
| Model 2 MIP | 0.973 (0.947–1.000) | 0.05 |
| Model 3 MEP | 0.983 (0.967–0.999) | 0.043 |
| Model 4 PEF | 0.980 (0.965–0.996) | 0.012 |
| Model 5 PCEF | 0.980 (0.967–0.993) | 0.0022 |

One separate model was used for each predictor. All the models were used in multivariable analysis adjusting for the duration of mechanical ventilation (< 7-day vs. 7 days or more), chronic respiratory failure (Yes/No) and MRC (< 48 vs. 48 or more). An odds ratio (OR) > 1 signified an increased probability of necessity of mechanical ventilator assistance

Italics indicate significant data

*VC* vital capacity, *FVC* forced vital capacity, *MIP* maximal inspiratory pressure, *MEP* maximal expiratory pressure, *PEF* peak expiratory flow, *PCEF* peak cough expiratory flow

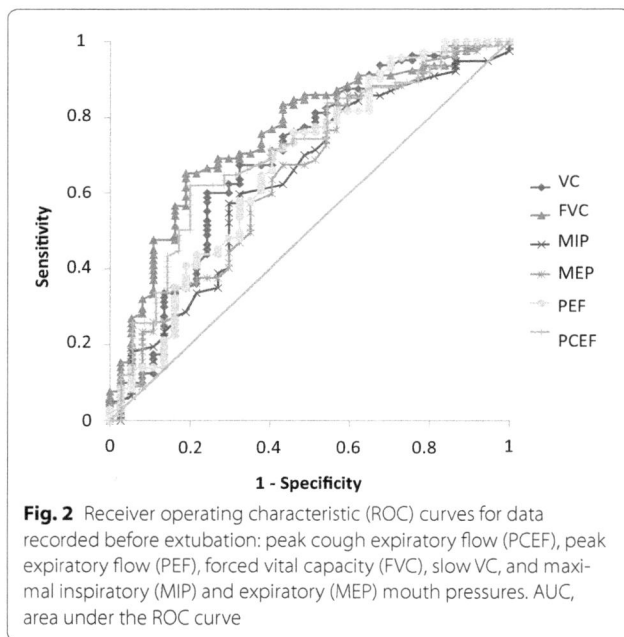

**Fig. 2**  Receiver operating characteristic (ROC) curves for data recorded before extubation: peak cough expiratory flow (PCEF), peak expiratory flow (PEF), forced vital capacity (FVC), slow VC, and maximal inspiratory (MIP) and expiratory (MEP) mouth pressures. AUC, area under the ROC curve

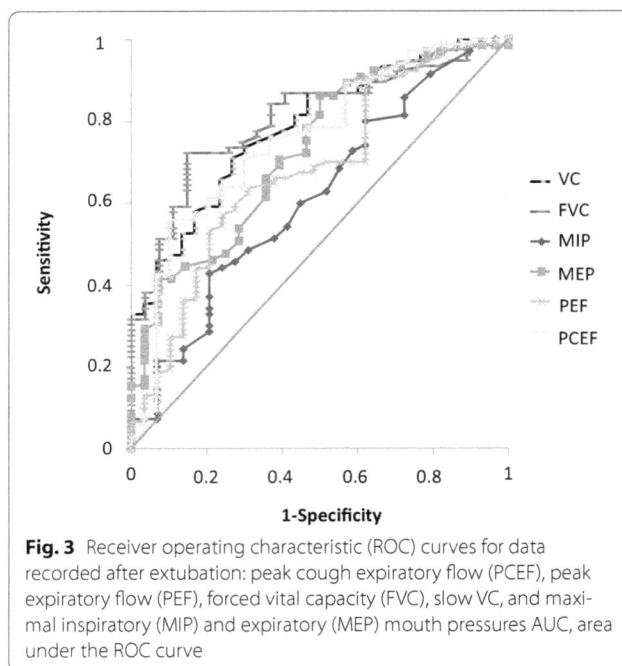

**Fig. 3**  Receiver operating characteristic (ROC) curves for data recorded after extubation: peak cough expiratory flow (PCEF), peak expiratory flow (PEF), forced vital capacity (FVC), slow VC, and maximal inspiratory (MIP) and expiratory (MEP) mouth pressures AUC, area under the ROC curve

Our study provides the first evidence that FVC correlates well with PCEF and outperforms PCEF for predicting a need for NIV and/or mechanical cough assistance after extubation. In addition, FVC was the parameter least affected by the presence of a tracheal tube, so that pre-extubation FVC < 1420 mL was 64% sensitive and 81% specific, with improvements to 72 and 85%, respectively, when FVC remained < 1420 mL after extubation.

This is not surprising given that FVC diminishes only in the event of air trapping, which is generally due to peripheral airway obstruction and not to increased central airway resistance due, for instance, to a tracheal tube.

Several limitations of our study should be addressed. First, we included only those patients who were sufficiently cooperative and were extubated at a time when the technician was available for pre-extubation LFT. This requirement decreased the number of included patients but allowed the physicians to remain blinded to LFT findings, thereby minimizing bias. Thus, of the 730 patients extubated during the study period, 130 (18%) were included. Second, we did not assess involuntary cough. However, recent work indicates that, in cooperative patients, voluntary PCEF is far more accurate than involuntary PCEF in predicting reintubation, due to underestimation of cough strength by involuntary PCEF in patients with high voluntary PCEF [21]. We deliberately confined our study to cooperative patients, since we used noninvasive but volitional measurement techniques. Third, we excluded patients with MV for less than 72 h, since extubation failure is rare in this situation. Fourth, we did not measure the rapid shallow breathing index or fluid balance, two variables significantly associated with extubation failure in a previous study [27]. However, all study patients passed an SBT. Surprisingly, maximal pressures decreased after extubation, whereas the other parameters increased. This finding may be ascribable to the difference in patient-measurement device interface between pre- and post-extubation [28, 29]. In addition, upper-airway muscle activation and coordination are usually required when using a flanged mouthpiece but are not required when a tracheal tube bypasses the upper airway, which allows the patient to concentrate the effort on the inspiratory or expiratory muscles. Finally, a tracheal tube may diminish airway compliance and, therefore, the volume change during breathing, resulting in higher pressures for the same effort. Fifth, as this study used a prospective observational design, we did not change the practices in each center regarding the use of preventive NIV. The percentage of reintubated patients was surprisingly small in our study, i.e., 3 times lower than in the study by Esteban et al. among patients receiving NIV (48 vs. 16%). This difference may be ascribable to the high prevalence in our study of patients with COPD or restrictive pulmonary disease (20.7%), who may derive particularly large benefits from NIV [30]. Although ERS/ATS guidelines do not recommend using NIV to avoid reintubation in patients with overt respiratory distress and/or respiratory failure after planned extubation, this recommendation is not considered definitive and may not apply to patients with COPD [31]. Furthermore, reported benefits of curative NIV include improved oxygenation and alveolar ventilation, better alveolar recruitment in patients with atelectasis, improved left ventricular function in patients with heart failure, and decreases in intrinsic PEEP and work of breathing [32].

A legitimate issue is whether postponing extubation might have decreased the reintubation rate in our patients, who had longer MV durations before extubation compared to those in recent studies [5, 33, 34]. This difference is due to the inclusion in our study of only those patients already on MV for 72 h. However, our patients were extubated as soon as the daily conventional SBT was successful, in keeping with recent guidelines about the optimal assessment of weaning readiness [35].

Another factor that may have contributed to the low reintubation rate in our population is the considerable experience of our staff in the noninvasive treatment of patients with chronic and complete ventilator dependency [36–38]. We share this high level of experience with teams specialized in neuromuscular diseases [39]. Moreover, the addition to NIV of mechanical insufflation-exsufflation when appropriate may have further decreased the reintubation needs, as shown in a recent randomized trial [40]. Given the persistent challenges in identifying patients at high risk of post-extubation respiratory failure requiring, at best, NIV or mechanical cough assistance and, at worst, reintubation, we chose weaning failure defined as the use of NIV, cough assistance, and/or reintubation as the study endpoint.

Finally, as demonstrated by Thille et al. [41] the ability of healthcare staff to predict extubation failure is poor. The results reported here should help to identify patients likely to benefit from preventive NIV or cough assistance, using simple physiological parameters. These results need to be confirmed in a large epidemiological study including clinical and physiological variables [33].

## Conclusion

In conclusion, our main finding is that FVC measurements before and after extubation are well correlated. FVC may serve as an objective predictor of post-extubation respiratory failure requiring NIV and/or mechanical cough assistance and/or reintubation in heterogeneous populations of medical ICU patients. FVC measurement may deserve consideration as an inexpensive tool to be used in combination with easily identified risk factors for assessing patients after a successful SBT, with the goal of identifying those likely to require prophylactic post-extubation NIV and/or mechanical cough assistance. However, further studies are necessary to confirm our results in different conditions and populations.

**Abbreviations**
FVC: Forced vital capacity; ICU: Intensive care unit; LFT: Lung function testing; MEP: Maximal expiratory pressure; MIP: Maximal inspiratory pressure; MRC sum score: Medical Research Council sum score; MV: Endotracheal mechanical ventilation; NIV: Noninvasive ventilation; PaO$_2$: Partial pressure of O$_2$ in arterial blood; PaCO$_2$: Partial pressure of CO$_2$ in arterial blood; PCEF: Peak cough expiratory flow; PEF: Peak expiratory flow; ROC curve: Receiver operating characteristic curve; SBT: Spontaneous breathing trial; SOFA: Sequential Organ Failure Assessment; VC: Vital capacity.

**Authors' contributions**
NT, FL, and DO conceived the original protocol then initiated and conducted the study. RM, ED, LF, and PB recorded the data. JJP and NT performed the statistical analysis. NT analyzed the data and drafted the manuscript. RM, PB, HN, BS, CD, JB, and DA helped to conduct the study and to draft the final manuscript. HN, NT, FL, DO, DA, and PB participated in coordinating the study. All authors read and approved the final manuscript.

**Author details**
[1] INSERM, Université Grenoble-Alpes, U1042, HP2, 38000 Grenoble, France. [2] CHU Grenoble Alpes, Service de réanimation médicale, 38000 Grenoble, France. [3] Service de réanimation médicale, Centre Hospitalier Universitaire Grenoble - Alpes, CS10217, Grenoble Cedex 09, France. [4] Université de Versailles Saint Quentin en Yvelines, INSERM U1179, Garches, France. [5] CIC 1429, INSERM, AP-HP, Hôpital Raymond Poincaré, 92380 Garches, France. [6] Service d'Explorations Fonctionnelles Respiratoires, AP-HP, Hôpital Raymond Poincaré, 92380 Garches, France. [7] Service de Réanimation, Centre Hospitalier de Roanne, 42300 Roanne, France. [8] INSERM, U1075, 14000 Caen, France. [9] Université de Caen, 14000 Caen, France. [10] CHRU Caen, Service d'Explorations Fonctionnelles Respiratoire, 14000 Caen, France. [11] INSERM U 1179, Université de Versailles-Saint Quentin en Yvelines, 104 Bd Raymond Poincaré, 92380 Garches, France. [12] CIC 1429, Inserm-APHP, Hôpital Raymond Poincaré, 104 Bd Raymond Poincaré, 92380 Garches, France. [13] Service de Réanimation Médicale Polyvalente, Centre Hospitalier Public du Cotentin, BP 208,

50102 Cherbourg-en-Cotentin, France. [14] General Intensive Care Unit, Raymond Poincaré Hospital (AP-HP), Laboratory of Inflammation and Infection, U1173, INSERM and University of Versailles SQY, 92380 Garches, France. [15] Unité de Biostatistique et de Recherche Clinique, Centre Hospitalier Universitaire de Caen, Avenue de la Côte de Nacre, 14033 Caen, France. [16] Pôle de ventilation à domicile, AP-HP, Hôpital Raymond Poincaré, 92380 Garches, France. [17] Service de Santé Publique, AP-HP, Hôpital Raymond Poincaré, 92380 Garches, France.

## Acknowledgements
The authors are indebted to all the ICU physicians who participated in the study. We thank Damien du Cheyron, Amélie Seguin, Xavier Valette for contributing to the study as well as A Wolfe, MD, for revising the manuscript.

## Competing interests
The authors declare that they have no competing interests related to this manuscript.

## Sources of support
The study was supported by the publicly funded teaching hospital *CHU de Caen*. Dr. Nicolas TERZI received a grant from the nonprofit scientific society SRLF–SPLF (*Société de Réanimation de Langue Française–Société de Pneumologie de Langue Française*).

## References
1. Epstein SK. Decision to extubate. Intensive Care Med. 2002;28(5):535–46.
2. Esteban A, Anzueto A, Frutos F, Alia I, Brochard L, Stewart TE, Benito S, Epstein SK, Apezteguia C, Nightingale P, Arroliga AC, Tobin MJ. Characteristics and outcomes in adult patients receiving mechanical ventilation: a 28-day international study. JAMA. 2002;287(3):345–55.
3. Esteban A, Frutos F, Tobin MJ, Alia I, Solsona JF, Valverdu I, Fernandez R, de la Cal MA, Benito S, Tomas R, Carriedo D, Macias S, Blanco J. A comparison of four methods of weaning patients from mechanical ventilation. Spanish Lung Failure Collaborative Group. N Engl J Med. 1995;332(6):345–50.
4. Thille AW, Cortes-Puch I, Esteban A. Weaning from the ventilator and extubation in ICU. Curr Opin Crit Care. 2013;19(1):57–64.
5. Thille AW, Harrois A, Schortgen F, Brun-Buisson C, Brochard L. Outcomes of extubation failure in medical intensive care unit patients. Crit Care Med. 2011;39(12):2612–8.
6. Vallverdu I, Calaf N, Subirana M, Net A, Benito S, Mancebo J. Clinical characteristics, respiratory functional parameters, and outcome of a two-hour T-piece trial in patients weaning from mechanical ventilation. Am J Respir Crit Care Med. 1998;158(6):1855–62.
7. Bach JR, Saporito LR. Criteria for extubation and tracheostomy tube removal for patients with ventilatory failure. A different approach to weaning. Chest. 1996;110(6):1566–71.
8. Bach JR, Goncalves MR, Hamdani I, Winck JC. Extubation of patients with neuromuscular weakness: a new management paradigm. Chest. 2010;137(5):1033–9.
9. Beuret P, Roux C, Auclair A, Nourdine K, Kaaki M, Carton MJ. Interest of an objective evaluation of cough during weaning from mechanical ventilation. Intensive Care Med. 2009;35(6):1090–3.
10. Khamiees M, Raju P, DeGirolamo A, Amoateng-Adjepong Y, Manthous CA. Predictors of extubation outcome in patients who have successfully completed a spontaneous breathing trial. Chest. 2001;120(4):1262–70.
11. Su WL, Chen YH, Chen CW, Yang SH, Su CL, Perng WC, Wu CP, Chen JH. Involuntary cough strength and extubation outcomes for patients in an ICU. Chest. 2010;137(4):777–82.
12. Smina M, Salam A, Khamiees M, Gada P, Amoateng-Adjepong Y, Manthous CA. Cough peak flows and extubation outcomes. Chest. 2003;124(1):262–8.
13. McKim DA, Hendin A, LeBlanc C, King J, Brown CR, Woolnough A. Tracheostomy decannulation and cough peak flows in patients with neuromuscular weakness. Am J Phys Med Rehabil. 2012;91(8):666–70.
14. McCool FD. Global physiology and pathophysiology of cough:
    ACCP evidence-based clinical practice guidelines. Chest. 2006;129(1 Suppl):48S–53S.
15. Perren A, Brochard L. Managing the apparent and hidden difficulties of weaning from mechanical ventilation. Intensive Care Med. 2013;39(11):1885–95.
16. Boles JM, Bion J, Connors A, Herridge M, Marsh B, Melot C, Pearl R, Silverman H, Stanchina M, Vieillard-Baron A, Welte T. Weaning from mechanical ventilation. Eur Respir J. 2007;29(5):1033–56.
17. Kress JP, Hall JB. ICU-acquired weakness and recovery from critical illness. N Engl J Med. 2014;370(17):1626–35.
18. Borg GA. Psychophysical bases of perceived exertion. Med Sci Sports Exerc. 1982;14(5):377–81.
19. Lofaso F, Louis B, Brochard L, Harf A, Isabey D. Use of the Blasius resistance formula to estimate the effective diameter of endotracheal tubes. Am Rev Respir Dis. 1992;146(4):974–9.
20. Salam A, Tilluckdharry L, Amoateng-Adjepong Y, Manthous CA. Neurologic status, cough, secretions and extubation outcomes. Intensive Care Med. 2004;30(7):1334–9.
21. Duan J, Liu J, Xiao M, Yang X, Wu J, Zhou L. Voluntary is better than involuntary cough peak flow for predicting re-intubation after scheduled extubation in cooperative subjects. Respir Care. 2014;59(11):1643–51.
22. Kang SW, Choi WA, Won YH, Lee JW, Lee HY, Kim DJ. Clinical Implications of Assisted Peak Cough Flow Measured with an External Glottic Control Device for Tracheostomy Decannulation in Patients with Neuromuscular Diseases and Cervical Spinal Cord Injuries: A Pilot Study. Arch Phys Med Rehabil. 2016;97(9):1509–14.
23. Mahajan RP, Singh P, Murty GE, Aitkenhead AR. Relationship between expired lung volume, peak flow rate and peak velocity time during a voluntary cough manoeuvre. Br J Anaesth. 1994;72(3):298–301.
24. Suleman M, Abaza KT, Gornall C, Kinnear WJ, Wills JS, Mahajan RP. The effect of a mechanical glottis on peak expiratory flow rate and time to peak flow during a peak expiratory flow manoeuvre: a study in normal subjects and patients with motor neurone disease. Anaesthesia. 2004;59(9):872–5.
25. Park JH, Kang SW, Lee SC, Choi WA, Kim DH. How respiratory muscle strength correlates with cough capacity in patients with respiratory muscle weakness. Yonsei Med J. 2010;51(3):392–7.
26. American Thoracic Society/European Respiratory Society. ATS/ERS statement on respiratory muscle testing. Am J Respir Crit Care. 2002;166:518–624.
27. Frutos-Vivar F, Ferguson ND, Esteban A, Epstein SK, Arabi Y, Apezteguia C, Gonzalez M, Hill NS, Nava S, D'Empaire G, Anzueto A. Risk factors for extubation failure in patients following a successful spontaneous breathing trial. Chest. 2006;130(6):1664–71.
28. Montemezzo D, Vieira DS, Tierra-Criollo CJ, Britto RR, Velloso M, Parreira VF. Influence of 4 interfaces in the assessment of maximal respiratory pressures. Respir Care. 2012;57(3):392–8.
29. Koulouris N, Mulvey DA, Laroche CM, Green M, Moxham J. Comparison of two different mouthpieces for the measurement of Pimax and Pemax in normal and weak subjects. Eur Respir J. 1988;1(9):863–7.
30. Peter JV, Moran JL, Phillips-Hughes J, Warn D. Noninvasive ventilation in acute respiratory failure—a meta-analysis update. Crit Care Med. 2002;30(3):555–62.
31. Rochwerg B, Brochard L, Elliott MW, Hess D, Hill NS, Nava S, Navalesi PMOTSC, Antonelli M, Brozek J, Conti G, Ferrer M, Guntupalli K, Jaber S, Keenan S, Mancebo J, Mehta S, Raoof SMOTTF. Official ERS/ATS clinical practice guidelines: noninvasive ventilation for acute respiratory failure. Eur Respir J. 2017;50(2):1602426.
32. Vitacca M, Ambrosino N, Clini E, Porta R, Rampulla C, Lanini B, Nava S. Physiological response to pressure support ventilation delivered before and after extubation in patients not capable of totally spontaneous autonomous breathing. Am J Respir Crit Care Med. 2001;164(4):638–41.
33. Thille AW, Boissier F, Ben-Ghezala H, Razazi K, Mekontso-Dessap A, Brun-Buisson C, Brochard L. Easily identified at-risk patients for extubation failure may benefit from noninvasive ventilation: a prospective before-after study. Crit Care (London, England). 2016;20:48.
34. Beduneau G, Pham T, Schortgen F, Piquilloud L, Zogheib E, Jonas M, Grelon F, Runge I, Nicolas T, Grange S, Barberet G, Guitard PG, Frat JP, Constan A, Chretien JM, Mancebo J, Mercat A, Richard JM, Brochard L, Group WS,

The RNdd. Epidemiology of weaning outcome according to a new definition. The WIND Study. Am J Respir Crit Care Med. 2017;195(6):772–83.

35. Quintard H, l'Her E, Pottecher J, Adnet F, Constantin JM, De Jong A, Diemunsch P, Fesseau R, Freynet A, Girault C, Guitton C, Hamonic Y, Maury E, Mekontso-Dessap A, Michel F, Nolent P, Perbet S, Prat G, Roquilly A, Tazarourte K, Terzi N, Thille AW, Alves M, Gayat E, Donetti L. Intubation and extubation of the ICU patient. Anaesth Crit Care Pain Med. 2017;36(5):327–41.

36. Nardi J, Leroux K, Orlikowski D, Prigent H, Lofaso F. Home monitoring of daytime mouthpiece ventilation effectiveness in patients with neuromuscular disease. Chronic Respir Dis. 2016;13(1):67–74.

37. Lacombe M, Del Amo Castrillo L, Bore A, Chapeau D, Horvat E, Vaugier I, Lejaille M, Orlikowski D, Prigent H, Lofaso F. Comparison of three cough-augmentation techniques in neuromuscular patients: mechanical insufflation combined with manually assisted cough, insufflation-exsufflation alone and insufflation-exsufflation combined with manually assisted cough. Respir Int Rev Thorac Dis. 2014;88(3):215–22.

38. Lofaso F, Prigent H, Tiffreau V, Menoury N, Toussaint M, Monnier AF, Stremler N, Devaux C, Leroux K, Orlikowski D, Mauri C, Pin I, Sacconi S, Pereira C, Pepin JL, Fauroux B, Association Francaise Contre les Myopathies research g. Long-term mechanical ventilation equipment for neuromuscular patients: meeting the expectations of patients and prescribers. Respir Care. 2014;59(1):97–106.

39. Bach JR. Noninvasive respiratory management of patients with neuromuscular disease. Ann Rehabil Med. 2017;41(4):519–38.

40. Goncalves MR, Honrado T, Winck JC, Paiva JA. Effects of mechanical insufflation-exsufflation in preventing respiratory failure after extubation: a randomized controlled trial. Crit Care (London, England). 2012;16(2):48.

41. Thille AW, Boissier F, Ben Ghezala H, Razazi K, Mekontso-Dessap A, Brun-Buisson C. Risk factors for and prediction by caregivers of extubation failure in ICU patients: a prospective study. Crit Care Med. 2015;43(3):613–20.

# 6

# Effect of inspiratory synchronization during pressure-controlled ventilation on lung distension and inspiratory effort

Nuttapol Rittayamai[1,2,3], François Beloncle[1,2,4], Ewan C. Goligher[1,5,6,7], Lu Chen[1,2], Jordi Mancebo[8,9], Jean-Christophe M. Richard[10,11] and Laurent Brochard[1,2]*

## Abstract

**Background:** In pressure-controlled (PC) ventilation, tidal volume ($V_T$) and transpulmonary pressure ($P_L$) result from the addition of ventilator pressure and the patient's inspiratory effort. PC modes can be classified into fully, partially, and non-synchronized modes, and the degree of synchronization may result in different $V_T$ and $P_L$ despite identical ventilator settings. This study assessed the effects of three PC modes on $V_T$, $P_L$, inspiratory effort (esophageal pressure–time product, $PTP_{es}$), and airway occlusion pressure, $P_{0.1}$. We also assessed whether $P_{0.1}$ can be used for evaluating patient effort.

**Methods:** Prospective, randomized, crossover physiologic study performed in 14 spontaneously breathing mechanically ventilated patients recovering from acute respiratory failure (1 subsequently withdrew). PC modes were fully (PC-CMV), partially (PC-SIMV), and non-synchronized (PC-IMV using airway pressure release ventilation) and were applied randomly; driving pressure, inspiratory time, and set respiratory rate being similar for all modes. Airway, esophageal pressure, $P_{0.1}$, airflow, gas exchange, and hemodynamics were recorded.

**Results:** $V_T$ was significantly lower during PC-IMV as compared with PC-SIMV and PC-CMV ($387 \pm 105$ vs $458 \pm 134$ vs $482 \pm 108$ mL, respectively; $p < 0.05$). Maximal $P_L$ was also significantly lower ($13.3 \pm 4.9$ vs $15.3 \pm 5.7$ vs $15.5 \pm 5.2$ cmH$_2$O, respectively; $p < 0.05$), but $PTP_{es}$ was significantly higher in PC-IMV ($215.6 \pm 154.3$ vs $150.0 \pm 102.4$ vs $130.9 \pm 101.8$ cmH$_2$O $\times$ s $\times$ min$^{-1}$, respectively; $p < 0.05$), with no differences in gas exchange and hemodynamic variables. $PTP_{es}$ increased by more than 15% in 10 patients and by more than 50% in 5 patients. An increased $P_{0.1}$ could identify high levels of $PTP_{es}$.

**Conclusions:** Non-synchronized PC mode lowers $V_T$ and $P_L$ in comparison with more synchronized modes in spontaneously breathing patients but can increase patient effort and may need specific adjustments.

**Keywords:** Airway pressure release ventilation, Lung-protective ventilation, Spontaneous ventilation, Transpulmonary pressure, Ventilator-induced lung injury

## Background

To date, volume-controlled ventilation is the most commonly employed mode during the first few days of mechanical ventilation [1]. The use of pressure-controlled (PC) modes has steadily increased, and they are now preferentially used. Under passive conditions in PC mode, the ventilator is the only respiratory pump and $V_T$ depends entirely on the set pressure, inspiratory time, and the respiratory system mechanics [2]. Inactivity of the respiratory muscles results in rapid muscle weakness [3, 4], whereas allowing spontaneous breathing improves gas exchange [5] and might prevent ventilator-induced diaphragm dysfunction (VIDD) [6, 7]. When patients

*Correspondence: BrochardL@smh.ca
[2] Keenan Research Centre and Li Ka Shing Knowledge Institute, St. Michael's Hospital, 30 Bond St, Toronto, ON M5B 1W8, Canada
Full list of author information is available at the end of the article

make spontaneous breathing efforts, however, the total driving pressure will be the sum of the pressure generated by the ventilator ($P_{aw}$) and the patient's respiratory muscles. Therefore, transpulmonary pressure ($P_L$) and $V_T$ are more difficult to control and may exceed safe limits in patients who require lung-protective ventilation, such as acute respiratory distress syndrome (ARDS).

Pressure-controlled modes can be classified according to the degree of inspiratory synchronization as fully, partially, and non-synchronized modes (Fig. 1). The nomenclature of each mode, however, varies with ventilator brand making sometimes difficult for the clinician to appreciate this distinction (Additional file 1: Table S1). In fully synchronized mode or PC continuous mandatory ventilation (PC-CMV), mechanically assisted breaths are triggered every time the patient generates spontaneous efforts. In partially synchronized mode or PC synchronized intermittent mandatory ventilation (PC-SIMV), there is a synchronization time window allowing the patient to trigger an assisted breath within the time window or to take a breath without assistance if efforts occur outside the synchronization window. Finally, in non-synchronized mode or PC intermittent mandatory

ventilation (PC-IMV), low and high pressure levels are alternately delivered for fixed intervals and patient inspiratory efforts are possible but do not trigger any additional assistance and are not intentionally synchronized. Several breath types can be observed during PC-IMV, which will result in different breathing patterns (Additional file 1: Fig. S1) [8]. A study by Richard and colleagues comparing three PC types of modes in a bench model suggested that non-synchronized modes resulted in lower $P_L$ and $V_T$ than the two other modes despite identical settings and simulated effort [9]. Though these effects are potentially attractive for offering a better lung-protective strategy, using a non-synchronized mode may also lead to unpredictable effects on patient's inspiratory effort. Because we don't know if the risk of having large $V_T$ and $P_L$ is better represented by the average values, the variability of the values needs to be also examined.

The pressure–time product (PTP) and work of breathing using Campbell's diagram are the standard methods for assessing patient inspiratory effort during mechanical ventilation [10]. However, these techniques need complex calculations based on esophageal manometry. The airway occlusion pressure at 0.1 s ($P_{0.1}$), an index of

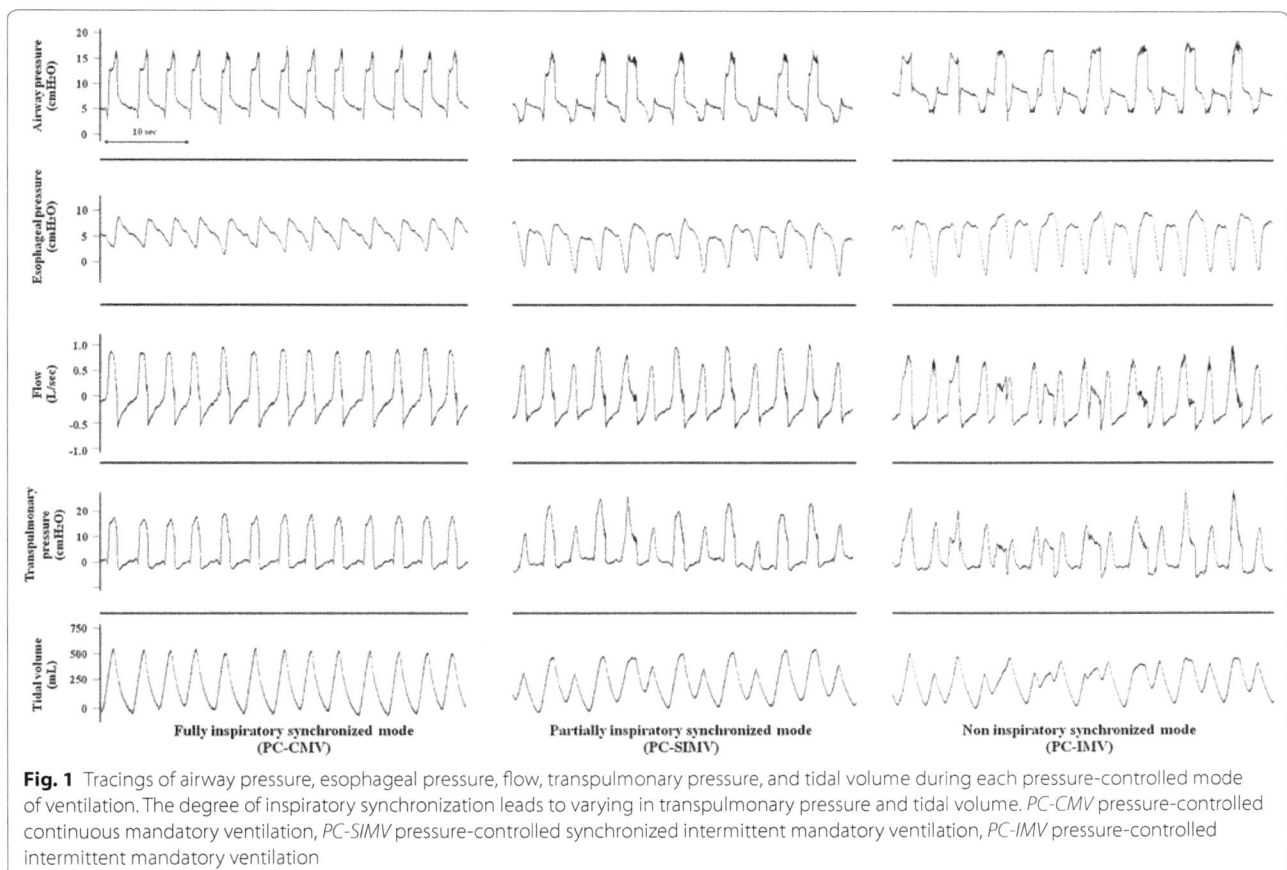

**Fig. 1** Tracings of airway pressure, esophageal pressure, flow, transpulmonary pressure, and tidal volume during each pressure-controlled mode of ventilation. The degree of inspiratory synchronization leads to varying in transpulmonary pressure and tidal volume. *PC-CMV* pressure-controlled continuous mandatory ventilation, *PC-SIMV* pressure-controlled synchronized intermittent mandatory ventilation, *PC-IMV* pressure-controlled intermittent mandatory ventilation

respiratory drive available on modern ventilators, could be an alternative method for assessing inspiratory effort.

The primary objective of this study was to assess whether non-synchronized modes of ventilation result in more protective ventilation strategy over the two other PC modes as evaluated by $V_T$ and $P_L$; secondary objectives included the effect of different degree of inspiratory synchronization on inspiratory effort determined by esophageal pressure–time product ($PTP_{es}$) and by $P_{0.1}$.

## Methods
### Study population and settings
The study was conducted in Medical–Surgical Intensive Care Units at two academic hospitals in Toronto, Canada (Clinicaltrial.gov # NCT02071277). The Research Ethics Board at St. Michael's Hospital and Mt. Sinai Hospital approved the study protocol, and informed consent was obtained from patients or their substitute decision makers prior to enrollment.

Patients were eligible for enrollment if they were spontaneously breathing under mechanical ventilation with a pressure assist-control mode or pressure support ventilation (PSV) with a ventilator driving pressure level of at least 10 cmH$_2$O (to ensure that patients were not yet on minimal support). Patients were not included if they had hemodynamic instability (> 20% variation of mean arterial pressure and/or heart rate or need doses of norepinephrine higher than 0.2 mcg/kg/min), a set positive end-expiratory pressure (PEEP) above 12 cmH$_2$O, a fractional oxygen concentration (FiO$_2$) above 0.6, a severe acid–base disturbance (arterial pH < 7.30 or > 7.55). There should be no contraindication to insert esophageal balloon catheter, chronic neuromuscular disease, intracranial hypertension, or pregnancy.

### Ventilators and equipment
A Dräger Evita-XL or a Dräger V500 ventilator (Dräger, Lubeck, Germany) which provided the three different synchronized PC modes was used. We used PCV+ assist, PCV+, and APRV modes on the Evita-XL and PC-AC, PC-SIMV+, and APRV on the V500 ventilator to represent PC-CMV, PC-SIMV, and PC-IMV, respectively. Of note, we used the mode called APRV as the only available non-synchronized mode, but the settings were similar to other classical PC-CMV modes and not to "usual" approaches using APRV with prolonged high pressure–time.

Airflow was measured with a Fleisch No. 2 pneumotachograph placed between the endotracheal tube and the Y-piece of the ventilator, connected to a differential pressure transducer (MP 150, Biopac Systems, Goleta, California, USA). Airway pressure ($P_{aw}$) was measured between the endotracheal tube and the

pneumotachograph via a pressure transducer (MP 150). Esophageal pressure ($P_{es}$) was measured using a Nutrivent catheter (Sidam, Mirandola, Italy) connected to pressure transducers (MP 150). The correct position of the esophageal balloon was assessed by an occlusion test [11, 12].

The analog signals of airflow, $P_{aw}$, and $P_{es}$ were digitized at a sampling rate of 100 Hz and stored in a laptop for subsequent calculations and analyzes using AcqKnowledge software (Biopac Systems). Volume was obtained by integration of airflow signal over time, regardless of the mode. Tidal volume variability was assessed by the coefficients of variation of tidal volume (calculated as the standard deviation divided by the mean value). $P_L$ was calculated by subtraction of $P_{aw}$ from $P_{es}$ and presented as the maximal and minimal values; mean $P_L$ was calculated as the quotient of the area under the $P_L$-time tracing divided by total cycle duration. $\Delta P_L$ was measured as the difference between maximal and minimal $P_L$ at the end of inspiration. $PTP_{es}$ was calculated as the surface enclosed within the $P_{es}$ and the relaxation line of the chest wall over inspiratory time [13, 14] and expressed in cmH$_2$O × s × min$^{-1}$ using a dedicated software (Sistema Respiratorio, Barcelona, Spain). Algorithm to calculate $PTP_{es}$ is detailed in Additional file 1: Fig. S2.

$P_{0.1}$ was measured using AcqKnowledge software from the fall in $P_{aw}$ during the first 100 ms of an occluded (zero flow) spontaneous inspiration using the end-expiratory hold function.

### Study protocol
Patients were studied in a semi-recumbent position. Three different PC modes were applied for 20 min each in random order as determined by a blind envelope pull. The ventilator settings (inspiratory pressure, PEEP, set respiratory rate, FiO$_2$, and inspiratory time) were kept unchanged and similar across all modes. These settings were as close as possible to those previously chosen by the responsible clinician, using the same driving pressure; if the patient was put on PSV mode, then the set respiratory rate during the study was set to reach the same total minute ventilation. No pressure support was added during PC-SIMV and PC-IMV. The first 15 min was devoted to ensure patient's full adaptation to the mode, and signal acquisition was done during the following 5 min. The last 2 min of the recording was analyzed offline and presented as the average values over the selected period. Sedation assessed by RASS was left to the discretion of the attended physician and not modified for the duration of the study. The occlusions to measure $P_{0.1}$ were performed and recorded every minute during 5 min of data acquisition. Arterial blood gases were collected before starting the protocol and at the end of the three studied

periods. Hemodynamic variables (mean arterial pressure and heart rate) were also recorded during the study.

### Statistical analysis

Statistical analysis was performed with Statistical Package for the Social Sciences (version 20.0, IBM SPSS, Chicago, IL, USA). Continuous variables are reported as mean ± SD, and categorical variables are reported as number and percentage. We used an analysis of variance with repeated measures followed by a post hoc pairwise test to compare the difference between the three modes.

We also performed a correlation analysis between the individual changes in $P_{0.1}$ and the individual changes in $PTP_{es}$ in order to determine whether $P_{0.1}$ could reliably indicate the direction of the changes in patients' effort. Receiver operating characteristic (ROC) curve was used to evaluate a cutoff point for $P_{0.1}$ in predicting excess patient's inspiratory effort determined as $PTP_{es} > 200$ cmH$_2$O × s × min$^{-1}$. This value was chosen as the upper value, i.e., mean value plus one standard deviation, tolerated by patients passing a successful spontaneous breathing trial [14]. A $p$ value < 0.05 was considered as statistically significant.

### Results

We enrolled 14 patients from March 2014 to July 2015. Mean age was 58 ± 12 years, and APACHE II score was 18.0 ± 5.1. Other baseline characteristics are shown in Table 1. The majority of patients (62%) had been ventilated for ARDS, and 46% were still under light levels of continuous intravenous sedation at the time of the measurements. (Average RASS score of these patients was −2 ± 1.) All but one patient tolerated the three PC modes. The latter patient was in respiratory acidosis before the study, worsened just after starting the study, and was secondarily excluded.

### Effect on breathing pattern and transpulmonary pressure

The main results are shown in Table 2 and Figs. 2 and 3. The percentage of spontaneous breathing during PC-SIMV and PC-IMV was 6.8 and 17.4% of total minute ventilation. We found that average $V_T$ and $V_T$ per predicted body weight were significantly lower during PC-IMV in comparison with the two other modes (PC-IMV vs PC-CMV, $p < 0.001$; PC-IMV vs PC-SIMV, $p = 0.049$). Tidal volume variability was significantly higher during PC-IMV as compared with the other modes (PC-IMV vs PC-CMV, p = 0.001; PC-IMV vs PC-SIMV, $p = 0.028$) (Fig. 2). Total respiratory rate also significantly increased during PC-IMV in comparison with PC-SIMV and PC-CMV (PC-IMV vs PC-CMV, $p = 0.007$; PC-IMV vs PC-SIMV, $p = 0.025$).

Average values of maximal $P_L$ and the mean $P_L$ during PC-IMV were significantly lower when compared to PC-CMV ($p = 0.006$) and PC-SIMV ($p = 0.004$), but no difference in minimum $P_L$ during each mode of ventilation was found (Fig. 3). There was a nonsignificant trend toward a decreased $\Delta P_L$ at the end of inspiration with decreasing degree of inspiratory synchronization (PC-IMV vs PC-CMV, $p = 0.144$; PC-IMV vs PC-SIMV, $p = 0.152$). No difference in minute ventilation, PaO$_2$/FiO$_2$, PaCO$_2$, and arterial pH was found between modes. In addition, no significant differences in mean arterial pressure and heart rate were found between the three PC modes (Table 2).

### Effect on patient's inspiratory effort

Patient's inspiratory effort determined by $PTP_{es}$ was higher during PC-IMV in comparison with the two other modes (PC-IMV vs PC-CMV, $p = 0.005$; PC-IMV vs PC-SIMV, $p = 0.023$), as shown in Table 3. Compared to the two other modes, $PTP_{es}$ increased by more than 15% in 10 patients and by more than 50% in 5 patients.

We found that $P_{0.1}$, measured during manual occlusions, significantly increased from 2.6 ± 1.7 cmH$_2$O during PC-CMV to 3.7 ± 2.3 cmH$_2$O during PC-IMV ($p = 0.048$) (Additional file 1: Fig. S3). We observed a strong correlation between $P_{0.1}$ and $PTP_{es}$ with a correlation coefficient of 0.754 ($p < 0.001$). In addition, the area under the ROC curve for $P_{0.1}$ to predict excess patient's inspiratory effort was 0.93 (95% confidence interval, 0.85–1.00) (Additional file 1: Fig. S4). A cutoff value for $P_{0.1}$ above 3.5 cmH$_2$O had a sensitivity of 92% and specificity of 89% in predicting $PTP_{es} > 200$ cmH$_2$O × s × min$^{-1}$.

### Discussion

We found that spontaneous efforts during different PC modes with identical ventilator settings have very different effects on $V_T$ and $P_L$. PC-IMV has no synchronization and provides less $V_T$ and $P_L$ and more $V_T$ variability than either PC-CMV or PC-SIMV, which have full or partial synchronization. No differences in terms of gas exchange and hemodynamics were found between the modes in this short-term study. The non-synchronized mode was, however, often associated with higher levels of patients' effort. Inspiratory effort was strongly correlated with $P_{0.1}$. In this context, $P_{0.1}$ might be used to detect excessive inspiratory effort.

Patients with acute respiratory failure, in particular ARDS, should be ventilated with a lung-protective strategy to reduce the risk of ventilator-induced lung injury (VILI) and to improve survival [15–17]. Using low $V_T$ and optimum PEEP to minimize $P_L$ can mitigate VILI [18]. Although neuromuscular blocking agents can be used initially, allowing spontaneous breathing can reduce

Critical and Intensive Care: A Survival Guide

**Table 1  Patient characteristics and ventilator settings**

| Patient | Gender | Age (years) | Cause of acute respiratory failure | Intubation days | APACHE II score | RASS score | Inspiratory pressure above PEEP (cmH₂O) | PEEP (cmH₂O) | Inspiratory time (s) | Set rate (breath/min) | FiO₂ | Discharge status |
|---|---|---|---|---|---|---|---|---|---|---|---|---|
| 1 | M | 62 | Sepsis, ARDS | 14 | 12 | −2 | 10 | 8 | 1 | 15 | 0.5 | Alive |
| 2* | F | 65 | COPD with exacerbation | 2 | 13 | 0 | 12 | 5 | 0.9 | 26 | 0.45 | Alive |
| 3 | M | 80 | COPD with exacerbation | 15 | 13 | 0 | 10 | 8 | 1.1 | 19 | 0.3 | Alive |
| 4 | M | 66 | Sepsis, ARDS | 3 | 16 | −2 | 16 | 8 | 1 | 20 | 0.4 | Alive |
| 5 | M | 68 | Congestive heart failure | 4 | 16 | −2 | 12 | 10 | 1 | 20 | 0.5 | Alive |
| 6 | M | 48 | Pneumonia, ARDS | 13 | 17 | −2 | 10 | 10 | 0.9 | 14 | 0.4 | Dead |
| 7 | M | 38 | Multiple trauma | 7 | 11 | −3 | 12 | 8 | 1 | 16 | 0.4 | Alive |
| 8 | F | 41 | Seizure, ARDS | 7 | 20 | −3 | 10 | 8 | 1 | 18 | 0.4 | Alive |
| 9 | M | 69 | Sepsis, ARDS | 9 | 18 | −3 | 18 | 10 | 0.8 | 25 | 0.5 | Dead |
| 10 | M | 46 | IPF exacerbation, ARDS | 10 | 19 | −3 | 20 | 8 | 0.8 | 24 | 0.5 | Alive |
| 11 | F | 67 | Cardiac arrest | 7 | 19 | −3 | 14 | 12 | 1 | 20 | 0.5 | Alive |
| 12 | M | 49 | Sepsis, ARDS | 8 | 24 | −3 | 14 | 12 | 1 | 22 | 0.4 | Alive |
| 13 | M | 63 | Pneumonia, ARDS | 2 | 25 | −1 | 16 | 10 | 0.9 | 13 | 0.4 | Dead |
| 14 | F | 51 | Pneumonia | 11 | 29 | −3 | 16 | 10 | 1.2 | 14 | 0.45 | Dead |

*ARDS* acute respiratory distress syndrome, *COPD* chronic obstructive pulmonary disease, *IPF* idiopathic pulmonary fibrosis, *PEEP* positive end-expiratory pressure, *RASS* Richmond Agitation Sedation Scale

\* Patient #2 was excluded from the data analysis due to termination of the study

**Table 2** Breathing pattern, respiratory and hemodynamic variables during three pressure-controlled modes

|  | PC-CMV | PC-SIMV | PC-IMV |
|---|---|---|---|
| Tidal volume (mL) | 482 ± 107 | 457 ± 133 | 387 ± 104*,# |
| Tidal volume per predicted body weight (mL/kg) | 7.3 ± 1.4 | 7.0 ± 2.1 | 5.9 ± 1.5*,# |
| Tidal volume variability (%) | 13.7 ± 13.7 | 21.6 ± 13.1 | 36.0 ± 18.0*,# |
| Maximal $P_L$ (cmH$_2$O) | 15.5 ± 5.2 | 15.3 ± 5.7 | 13.3 ± 4.9*,# |
| Mean $P_L$ (cmH$_2$O) | 9.8 ± 3.0 | 8.8 ± 3.3$^Y$ | 7.0 ± 3.0*,# |
| Minimum $P_L$ (cmH$_2$O) | −3.2 ± 2.8 | −3.5 ± 3.4 | −3.5 ± 3.2 |
| $\Delta P_L$ (cmH$_2$O) | 12.0 ± 6.9 | 11.9 ± 7.0 | 10.3 ± 4.6 |
| Total respiratory rate (breaths/min) | 22 ± 4 | 23 ± 6 | 27 ± 7*,# |
| Minute ventilation (L/min) | 10.2 ± 2.1 | 9.8 ± 1.9 | 9.9 ± 2.0 |
| PaO$_2$/FiO$_2$ ratio | 216 ± 60 | 223 ± 55 | 218 ± 63 |
| PaCO$_2$ (mmHg) | 48 ± 10 | 49 ± 11 | 50 ± 10 |
| Arterial pH | 7.37 ± 0.06 | 7.37 ± 0.07 | 7.36 ± 0.07 |
| Mean arterial pressure (mmHg) | 80 ± 10 | 80 ± 11 | 85 ± 14 |
| Heart rate (beats/min) | 96 ± 14 | 95 ± 13 | 96 ± 15 |

*PC-CMV* pressure-controlled continuous mandatory ventilation, *PC-SIMV* pressure-controlled synchronized intermittent mandatory ventilation, *PC-IMV* pressure-controlled intermittent mandatory ventilation

* $p < 0.05$, PC-CMV versus PC-IMV; # $p < 0.05$, PC-SIMV versus PC-IMV; $^Y$ $p < 0.05$, PC-CMV versus PC-SIMV

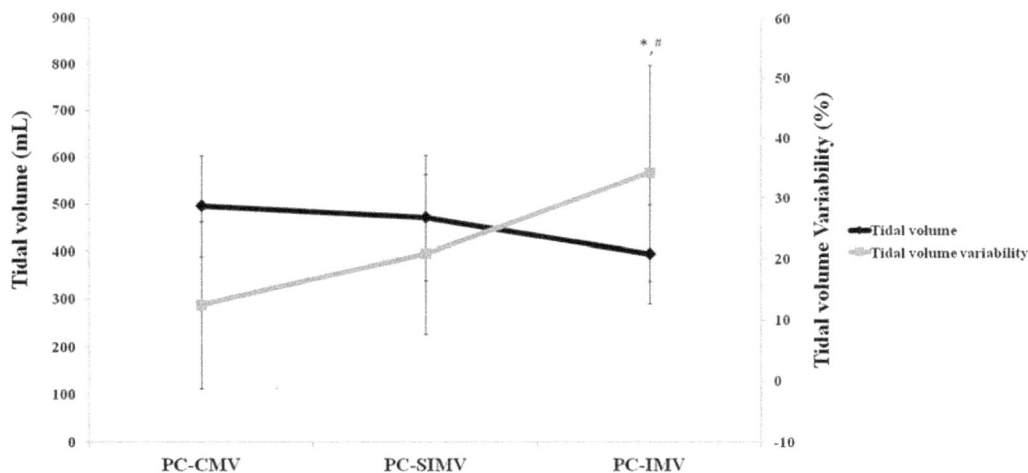

**Fig. 2** Tidal volume and tidal volume variability during fully, partially, and non inspiratory synchronized pressure-controlled modes (*$p < 0.05$; PC-IMV vs PC-CMV and #$p < 0.05$; PC-IMV vs PC-SIMV). *PC-CMV* pressure-controlled continuous mandatory ventilation, *PC-SIMV* pressure-controlled synchronized intermittent mandatory ventilation, *PC-IMV* pressure-controlled intermittent mandatory ventilation

VIDD [6, 7, 19], improves lung aeration and oxygenation [5, 20–22], and may attenuate VILI especially when the degree of lung injury is moderate [23, 24]. PC modes have been increasingly used, in particular, after 48 h of mechanical ventilation [1] because it provides a variable flow rate and may well respond to patient's demand and reduce work of breathing [2]. However, when patients breathe spontaneously during PC modes, the patient's inspiratory effort can increase $P_L$ and $V_T$ which has the potential to worsen lung injury [25, 26].

Our study shows that the level of inspiratory synchronization should be considered when using a PC mode and probably individualized. Richard et al. [9] demonstrated on a bench that $V_T$ and $P_L$ significantly increased when the degree of synchronization increased. These findings are confirmed by the present study in that non-synchronized mode lowers the average $V_T$ and $P_L$ in comparison with synchronized mode. Variation in $V_T$ and $P_L$ may occur because of different breath types during PC-IMV, and higher distending pressure may develop during some breath types such as type B breath (Additional file 1: Fig.

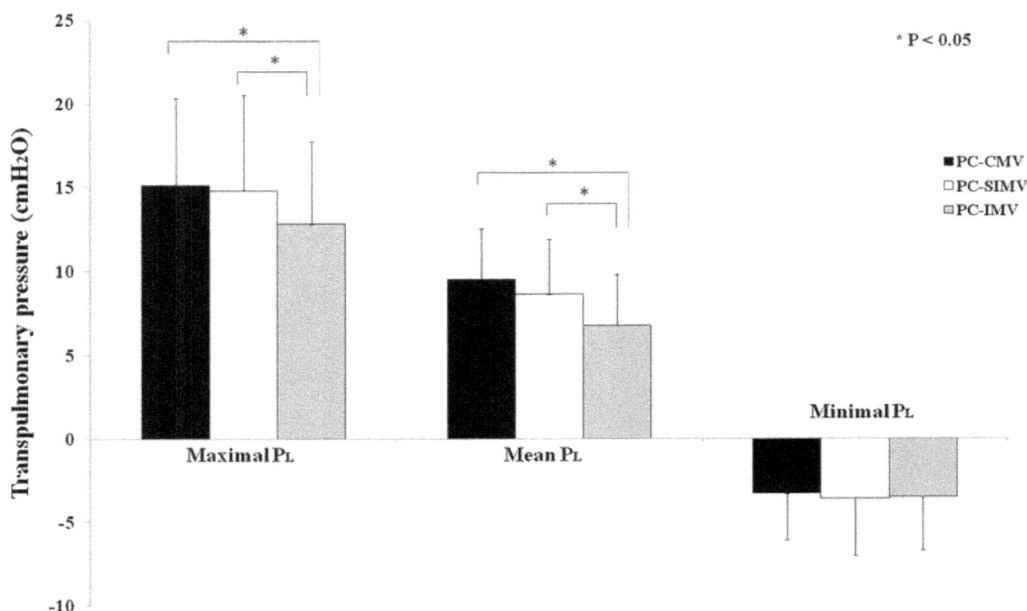

**Fig. 3** Maximal, mean, and minimum transpulmonary pressure ($P_L$) during the three pressure-controlled modes of ventilation. *PC-CMV* pressure-controlled continuous mandatory ventilation, *PC-SIMV* pressure-controlled synchronized intermittent mandatory ventilation, *PC-IMV* pressure-controlled intermittent mandatory ventilation

**Table 3 Patient inspiratory effort [esophageal pressure–time product (PTP$_{es}$)] and respiratory drive [airway occlusion pressure at 0.1 s ($P_{0.1}$)] during three pressure-controlled modes**

|  | PC-CMV | PC-SIMV | PC-IMV |
|---|---|---|---|
| PTP$_{es}$ (cmH$_2$O × s × min$^{-1}$) | 130 ± 101 | 150 ± 102 | 215 ± 154*,# |
| $P_{0.1}$ (cmH$_2$O) | 2.6 ± 1.7 | 2.9 ± 1.9 | 3.7 ± 2.3* |

*PC-CMV* pressure-controlled continuous mandatory ventilation, *PC-SIMV* pressure-controlled synchronized intermittent mandatory ventilation, *PC-IMV* pressure-controlled intermittent mandatory ventilation

* $p < 0.05$, PC-CMV versus PC-IMV; # $p < 0.05$, PC-SIMV versus PC-IMV

S1). However, the average inspiratory time in our study was around 1 s and patients had little chances to breathe at high pressure level. Furthermore, we did not add pressure support during PC-SIMV and PC-IMV limiting the chance of higher $V_T$ and $P_L$. In addition, variable $V_T$ during non-synchronized modes may mimic a more natural breathing pattern and higher variability has been associated with improved respiratory mechanics and outcomes [27–30]. Calzia et al. [31] compared PC-SIMV with PSV in 19 patients after coronary artery bypass grafting. The results showed that $V_T$ was lower during PC-SIMV (called "biphasic CPAP") than during PSV (which could be considered as fully synchronized PC mode). Gama de Abreu and colleagues [32] also compared PC-SIMV to PSV in 10 anesthetized pigs with acute lung injury. They

found that average $V_T$ was higher during PSV compared to PC-SIMV, with no differences in terms of gas exchange and hemodynamics. These findings are in line with the results of our study. In contrast, a study by Yoshida et al. [33] conducted in 18 patients with ARDS compared a non-synchronized mode with PSV set to deliver equal mean Paw. Authors showed that lung aeration and oxygenation improved during the non-synchronized mode and no differences in hemodynamics were found between modes. Our results suggest that a non-synchronized mode may be considered to be used as a transition mode between fully controlled ventilation and the resumption of spontaneous efforts in order to reduce the risk of VILI in patients with ARDS or at high risk of ARDS.

PC-IMV provided less $V_T$ and $P_L$ than the other modes, but patient inspiratory effort frequently increased either because of the lack of synchronization between the patient and the ventilator or, more likely in some patients, because insufficient setting of mechanical ventilation was provided, increasing the drive to breathe [34, 35]. Calzia et al. [31] also found that PTP$_{es}$ increased during PC-SIMV in comparison with PSV. Appropriate titration of sedative/analgesic drugs and/or adaptation of the level of ventilation (i.e. using higher respiratory rate) may alleviate the patient's high inspiratory drive. This strategy should be considered when using partially or non-synchronized modes. Other approaches for alleviating patient inspiratory effort such as using higher PEEP, extracorporeal carbon dioxide removal, or partial neuro-muscular blockade [36] may need to be explored in the future. In our study, we did not modify the backup respiratory rate, which was probably insufficient during this mode in some patients. Strong spontaneous efforts may worsen lung injury and overstretch the dependent lung zones because of a pendelluft phenomenon, especially when severe lung injury is present [25, 37]. A study by Güldner et al. [38] demonstrated that spontaneous ventilation during APRV improved oxygenation and reduced lung stress and strain regardless of the level of spontaneous effort. This latter finding may be explained by lowering $V_T$ and $P_L$ with non-synchronized mode. Spontaneous breathing during non-synchronized mode is recommended to be in the range of 10–30% of total minute ventilation to improve ventilation/perfusion matching and gas exchange and to avoid excessive work of breathing [39, 40]. In our study 16.7% of spontaneous breathing during PC-IMV is consistent with this suggestion to keep spontaneous breathing less than 30%. Thus, maintaining the advantages of non-synchronized modes while avoiding high respiratory effort merits to be attempted.

Of note, calculations of work of breathing using Campbell's diagram and $PTP_{es}$ are the gold standard for evaluating patient's inspiratory effort but these techniques are not available at the bedside. $P_{0.1}$ is a simple and noninvasive method, available on most modern ventilators, which evaluates the respiratory center drive [41]. Our study showed a good correlation between $P_{0.1}$ and $PTP_{es}$, confirming the results of previous studies conducted in different populations and with various ventilator modes [42–44]. We need to confirm that $P_{0.1}$ can be a good surrogate marker of patient's excessive inspiratory effort but it shows promising results to be used by clinicians to indicate when excessive levels of effort occur.

Our study is a short-term physiologic study and clinical outcomes were not evaluated, which limit the clinical conclusions that can be inferred from the study. The APRV mode used in this study was set to mimic the conventional ventilator setting. We did not measure respiratory mechanics to avoid sedation that may affect spontaneous breathing. We also did not measure biomarkers to assess the effect of inspiratory synchronization on lung injury. We need investigation in larger clinical studies and for longer periods of time to evaluate the impact of different types of PC mode, but we believe these data are useful to better understand how these modes can be used.

## Conclusions

Non-synchronized PC ventilation provides less $V_T$, lower $P_L$ and more breath to breath variability than partially and fully synchronized modes, despite identical ventilator settings. In this regard, this mode may help to protect the lungs and its use as a transition mode, between fully controlled ventilation and the resumption of spontaneous efforts. The risk is to increase patient's effort, and therefore, a close monitoring of respiratory drive as well as acid–base and ventilation status is needed.

### Abbreviations

ARDS: acute respiratory distress syndrome; APRV: airway pressure release ventilation; $P_{aw}$: airway pressure; PC: pressure-controlled; PC-CMV: PC continuous mandatory ventilation; PC-IMV: PC intermittent mandatory ventilation; PC-SIMV: PC synchronized intermittent mandatory ventilation; PEEP: positive end-expiratory pressure; $P_{es}$: esophageal pressure; $P_L$: transpulmonary pressure; PSV: pressure support ventilation; $PTP_{es}$: esophageal pressure–time product; $P_{0.1}$: airway occlusion pressure at 0.1 s; ROC: receiver operating characteristic; VIDD: ventilator-induced diaphragmatic dysfunction; VILI: ventilator-induced lung injury; $V_T$: tidal volume.

### Authors' contributions

NR, FB, ECG, JCMR, and LB contributed to the study conception and design. NR, FB, ECG, and LC contributed to data collection. NR, JM, and LB contributed to the data analysis and interpretation and prepared the first draft of the manuscript. All authors contributed to the critical revision and final approval of the manuscript. LB had full access to all the data in the study and takes responsibility for the content of the manuscript. All authors read and approved the final manuscript.

### Author details

Interdepartmental Division of Critical Care Medicine, University of Toronto, Toronto, ON, Canada. [2] Keenan Research Centre and Li Ka Shing Knowledge Institute, St. Michael's Hospital, 30 Bond St, Toronto, ON M5B 1W8, Canada. Division of Respiratory Diseases and Tuberculosis, Department of Medicine, Faculty of Medicine Siriraj Hospital, Bangkok, Thailand. [4] Medical Intensive Care Unit, Hospital of Angers, University of Angers, Angers, France. [5] Department of Medicine, University of Toronto, Toronto, Canada. [6] Department of Physiology, University of Toronto, Toronto, Canada. [7] Division of Respirology, Department of Medicine, University Health Network and Mount Sinai Hospital, Toronto, Canada. [8] Centre de recherche du Centre Hospitalier de l, Université de Montréal (CRCHUM), University of Montreal', Montreal, Canada. [9] Servei de Medicina Intensiva, Hospital Sant Pau, Barcelona, Spain. [10] Emergency Department, General Hospital of Annecy, Annecy, France. [11] INSERM UMR 955 eq 13, Créteil, France.

### Acknowledgements

The authors thank Dr. RabiaWaheed for considerable help with the measurements.

Funding was provided by Keenan Chair in Critical Care and Acute respiratory Failure.

This study was presented as an oral presentation at the 28th Annual Congress of the European Society of Intensive Care Medicine (October 3–7, 2015) in Berlin, Germany.

### Competing interests

NR was receiving a grant from his home institution in Thailand. FB was receiving a grant from his home institution in France. LB's laboratory has received research grants and/or equipment from the following companies: Covidien (PAV), General Electric (lung volume measurement), Fisher Paykel (Optiflow), Philips (sleep), Air Liquide (Helium, CPR). LB has received consultant fees from Covidien and Air Liquide. JM research institute has received research grants from Covidien (PAV), General Electric (lung volume measurement). JM has received speaker's honoraria from Covidien and Hamilton. JCMR has received speaker's honoraria from Covidien and Vygon. JCMR received consultant salary from Air Liquide Medical Systems. ECG and LC declare that they have no competing interests.

## References

1. Esteban A, Frutos-Vivar F, Muriel A, Ferguson ND, Peñuelas O, Abraira V, et al. Evolution of mortality over time in patients receiving mechanical ventilation. Am J Respir Crit Care Med. 2013;188(2):220–30.
2. Rittayamai N, Katsios CM, Beloncle F, Friedrich JO, Mancebo J, Brochard L. Pressure-controlled vs volume-controlled ventilation in acute respiratory failure: a physiology-based narrative and systematic review. Chest. 2015;148(2):340–55.
3. Levine S, Nguyen T, Taylor N, Friscia ME, Budak MT, Rothenberg P, et al. Rapid disuse atrophy of diaphragm fibers in mechanically ventilated humans. N Engl J Med. 2008;358(13):1327–35.
4. Jaber S, Petrof BJ, Jung B, Chanques G, Berthet J-P, Rabuel C, et al. Rapidly progressive diaphragmatic weakness and injury during mechanical ventilation in humans. Am J Respir Crit Care Med. 2011;183(3):364–71.
5. Putensen C, Mutz NJ, Putensen-Himmer G, Zinserling J. Spontaneous breathing during ventilatory support improves ventilation–perfusion distributions in patients with acute respiratory distress syndrome. Am J Respir Crit Care Med. 1999;159(4 Pt 1):1241–8.
6. Sassoon CSH, Zhu E, Caiozzo VJ. Assist-control mechanical ventilation attenuates ventilator-induced diaphragmatic dysfunction. Am J Respir Crit Care Med. 2004;170(6):626–32.
7. Futier E, Constantin J-M, Combaret L, Mosoni L, Roszyk L, Sapin V, et al. Pressure support ventilation attenuates ventilator-induced protein modifications in the diaphragm. Crit Care Lond Engl. 2008;12(5):R116.
8. Kallet RH. Patient-ventilator interaction during acute lung injury, and the role of spontaneous breathing: part 2: airway pressure release ventilation. Respir Care. 2011;56(2):190–203 **(discussion 203–206)**.
9. Richard JCM, Lyazidi A, Akoumianaki E, Mortaza S, Cordioli RL, Lefebvre JC, et al. Potentially harmful effects of inspiratory synchronization during pressure preset ventilation. Intensive Care Med. 2013;39(11):2003–10.
10. Brochard L, Martin GS, Blanch L, Pelosi P, Belda FJ, Jubran A, et al. Clinical review: respiratory monitoring in the ICU—a consensus of 16. Crit Care Lond Engl. 2012;16(2):219.
11. Baydur A, Behrakis PK, Zin WA, Jaeger M, Milic-Emili J. A simple method for assessing the validity of the esophageal balloon technique. Am Rev Respir Dis. 1982;126(5):788–91.
12. Akoumianaki E, Maggiore SM, Valenza F, Bellani G, Jubran A, Loring SH, et al. The application of esophageal pressure measurement in patients with respiratory failure. Am J Respir Crit Care Med. 2014;189(5):520–31.
13. Sassoon CS, Light RW, Lodia R, Sieck GC, Mahutte CK. Pressure–time product during continuous positive airway pressure, pressure support ventilation, and T-piece during weaning from mechanical ventilation. Am Rev Respir Dis. 1991;143(3):469–75.
14. Jubran A, Tobin MJ. Pathophysiologic basis of acute respiratory distress in patients who fail a trial of weaning from mechanical ventilation. Am J Respir Crit Care Med. 1997;155(3):906–15.
15. Acute Respiratory Distress Syndrome Network, Brower RG, Matthay MA, Morris A, Schoenfeld D, Thompson BT, et al. Ventilation with lower tidal volumes as compared with traditional tidal volumes for acute lung injury and the acute respiratory distress syndrome. N Engl J Med. 2000;342(18):1301–8.
16. Determann RM, Royakkers A, Wolthuis EK, Vlaar AP, Choi G, Paulus F, et al. Ventilation with lower tidal volumes as compared with conventional tidal volumes for patients without acute lung injury: a preventive randomized controlled trial. Crit Care Lond Engl. 2010;14(1):R1.
17. Serpa Neto A, Simonis FD, Barbas CSV, Biehl M, Determann RM, Elmer J, et al. Association between tidal volume size, duration of ventilation, and sedation needs in patients without acute respiratory distress syndrome: an individual patient data meta-analysis. Intensive Care Med. 2014;40(7):950–7.
18. Samary CS, Santos RS, Santos CL, Felix NS, Bentes M, Barboza T, et al. Biological impact of transpulmonary driving pressure in experimental acute respiratory distress syndrome. Anesthesiology. 2015;123(2):423–33.
19. Gayan-Ramirez G, Testelmans D, Maes K, Rácz GZ, Cadot P, Zádor E, et al.

20. Intermittent spontaneous breathing protects the rat diaphragm from mechanical ventilation effects. Crit Care Med. 2005;33(12):2804–9.
20. Varelmann D, Muders T, Zinserling J, Guenther U, Magnusson A, Hedenstierna G, et al. Cardiorespiratory effects of spontaneous breathing in two different models of experimental lung injury: a randomized controlled trial. Crit Care Lond Engl. 2008;12(6):R135.
21. Wrigge H, Zinserling J, Neumann P, Defosse J, Magnusson A, Putensen C, et al. Spontaneous breathing improves lung aeration in oleic acid-induced lung injury. Anesthesiology. 2003;99(2):376–84.
22. McMullen SM, Meade M, Rose L, Burns K, Mehta S, Doyle R, et al. Partial ventilatory support modalities in acute lung injury and acute respiratory distress syndrome—a systematic review. PLoS ONE. 2012;7(8):e40190.
23. Xia J, Zhang H, Sun B, Yang R, He H, Zhan Q. Spontaneous breathing with biphasic positive airway pressure attenuates lung injury in hydrochloric acid-induced acute respiratory distress syndrome. Anesthesiology. 2014;120(6):1441–9.
24. Xia J, Sun B, He H, Zhang H, Wang C, Zhan Q. Effect of spontaneous breathing on ventilator-induced lung injury in mechanically ventilated healthy rabbits: a randomized, controlled, experimental study. Crit Care Lond Engl. 2011;15(5):R244.
25. Yoshida T, Uchiyama A, Matsuura N, Mashimo T, Fujino Y. Spontaneous breathing during lung-protective ventilation in an experimental acute lung injury model: high transpulmonary pressure associated with strong spontaneous breathing effort may worsen lung injury. Crit Care Med. 2012;40(5):1578–85.
26. Yoshida T, Uchiyama A, Matsuura N, Mashimo T, Fujino Y. The comparison of spontaneous breathing and muscle paralysis in two different severities of experimental lung injury. Crit Care Med. 2013;41(2):536–45.
27. Ma B, Suki B, Bates JHT. Effects of recruitment/derecruitment dynamics on the efficacy of variable ventilation. J Appl Physiol Bethesda Md 1985. 2011;110(5):1319–26.
28. Lefevre GR, Kowalski SE, Girling LG, Thiessen DB, Mutch WA. Improved arterial oxygenation after oleic acid lung injury in the pig using a computer-controlled mechanical ventilator. Am J Respir Crit Care Med. 1996;154(5):1567–72.
29. Suki B, Alencar AM, Sujeer MK, Lutchen KR, Collins JJ, Andrade JS, et al. Life-support system benefits from noise. Nature. 1998;393(6681):127–8.
30. Kiss T, Silva PL, Huhle R, Moraes L, Santos RS, Felix NS, et al. Comparison of different degrees of variability in tidal volume to prevent deterioration of respiratory system elastance in experimental acute lung inflammation. Br J Anaesth. 2016;116(5):708–15.
31. Calzia E, Lindner KH, Witt S, Schirmer U, Lange H, Stenz R, et al. Pressure–time product and work of breathing during biphasic continuous positive airway pressure and assisted spontaneous breathing. Am J Respir Crit Care Med. 1994;150(4):904–10.
32. de Abreu MD, Cuevas M, Spieth PM, Carvalho AR, Hietschold V, Stroszczynski C, et al. Regional lung aeration and ventilation during pressure support and biphasic positive airway pressure ventilation in experimental lung injury. Crit Care Lond Engl. 2010;14(2):R34.
33. Yoshida T, Rinka H, Kaji A, Yoshimoto A, Arimoto H, Miyaichi T, et al. The impact of spontaneous ventilation on distribution of lung aeration in patients with acute respiratory distress syndrome: airway pressure release ventilation versus pressure support ventilation. Anesth Analg. 2009;109(6):1892–900.
34. Marini JJ, Smith TC, Lamb VJ. External work output and force generation during synchronized intermittent mechanical ventilation. Effect of machine assistance on breathing effort. Am Rev Respir Dis. 1988;138(5):1169–79.
35. Viale JP, Duperret S, Mahul P, Delafosse B, Delpuech C, Weismann D, et al. Time course evolution of ventilatory responses to inspiratory unloading in patients. Am J Respir Crit Care Med. 1998;157(2):428–34.
36. Doorduin J, Nollet JL, Roesthuis LH, van Hees HWH, Brochard LJ, Sinderby CA, et al. Partial neuromuscular blockade during partial ventilatory support in sedated patients with high tidal volumes. Am J Respir Crit Care Med. 2017;195(8):1033–42.
37. Yoshida T, Torsani V, Gomes S, De Santis RR, Beraldo MA, Costa ELV, et al. Spontaneous effort causes occult pendelluft during mechanical ventilation. Am J Respir Crit Care Med. 2013;188(12):1420–7.
38. Güldner A, Braune A, Carvalho N, Beda A, Zeidler S, Wiedemann B, et al. Higher levels of spontaneous breathing induce lung recruitment and

Effect of inspiratory synchronization during pressure-controlled ventilation on lung...

63

reduce global stress/strain in experimental lung injury. Anesthesiology. 2014;120(3):673–82.

39. Carvalho NC, Güldner A, Beda A, Rentzsch I, Uhlig C, Dittrich S, et al. Higher levels of spontaneous breathing reduce lung injury in experimental moderate acute respiratory distress syndrome. Crit Care Med. 2014;42(11):e702–15.

40. Putensen C, Zech S, Wrigge H, Zinserling J, Stüber F, Von Spiegel T, et al. Long-term effects of spontaneous breathing during ventilatory support in patients with acute lung injury. Am J Respir Crit Care Med. 2001;164(1):43–9.

41. Conti G, Antonelli M, Arzano S, Gasparetto A. Measurement of occlusion pressures in critically ill patients. Crit Care Lond Engl. 1997;1(3):89–93.

42. Mancebo J, Albaladejo P, Touchard D, Bak E, Subirana M, Lemaire F, et al. Airway occlusion pressure to titrate positive end-expiratory pressure in patients with dynamic hyperinflation. Anesthesiology. 2000;93(1):81–90.

43. Alberti A, Gallo F, Fongaro A, Valenti S, Rossi A. P0.1 is a useful parameter in setting the level of pressure support ventilation. Intensive Care Med. 1995;21(7):547–53.

44. Berger KI, Sorkin IB, Norman RG, Rapoport DM, Goldring RM. Mechanism of relief of tachypnea during pressure support ventilation. Chest. 1996;109(5):1320–7.

# 7

# Lung volumes and lung volume recruitment in ARDS: a comparison between supine and prone position

Hernan Aguirre-Bermeo, Marta Turella, Maddalena Bitondo, Juan Grandjean, Stefano Italiano, Olimpia Festa, Indalecio Morán and Jordi Mancebo[*]

## Abstract

**Background:** The use of positive end-expiratory pressure (PEEP) and prone position (PP) is common in the management of severe acute respiratory distress syndrome patients (ARDS). We conducted this study to analyze the variation in lung volumes and PEEP-induced lung volume recruitment with the change from supine position (SP) to PP in ARDS patients.

**Methods:** The investigation was conducted in a multidisciplinary intensive care unit. Patients who met the clinical criteria of the Berlin definition for ARDS were included. The responsible physician set basal PEEP. To avoid hypoxemia, $FiO_2$ was increased to 0.8 1 h before starting the protocol. End-expiratory lung volume (EELV) and functional residual capacity (FRC) were measured using the nitrogen washout/washin technique. After the procedures in SP, the patients were turned to PP and 1 h later the same procedures were made in PP.

**Results:** Twenty-three patients were included in the study, and twenty were analyzed. The change from SP to PP significantly increased FRC (from $965 \pm 397$ to $1140 \pm 490$ ml, $p = 0.008$) and EELV (from $1566 \pm 476$ to $1832 \pm 719$ ml, $p = 0.008$), but PEEP-induced lung volume recruitment did not significantly change ($269 \pm 186$ ml in SP to $324 \pm 188$ ml in PP, $p = 0.263$). Dynamic strain at PEEP decreased with the change from SP to PP ($0.38 \pm 0.14$ to $0.33 \pm 0.13$, $p = 0.040$).

**Conclusions:** As compared to supine, prone position increases resting lung volumes and decreases dynamic lung strain.

**Keywords:** ARDS, Lung volumes, Lung strain, Prone, PEEP recruitment, Mechanical ventilation

## Background

Acute respiratory distress syndrome (ARDS) is a permeability pulmonary edema, characterized by hypoxemia and a decrease in lung volumes and respiratory system compliance [1, 2]. In patients with ARDS, prone position (PP) produces a more homogeneous distribution of the inspired gas [3] and a better matching between ventilation and perfusion, thereby improving arterial oxygenation [3–5]. Positive end-expiratory pressure (PEEP)

and PP have also shown to decrease the percentage of non-aerated and poorly aerated lung tissue and attenuate the regional recruitment–derecruitment phenomena [5–7]. In selected ARDS patients, PP has been proposed to further improve the outcomes [8]. The benefit on survival of PP is not related only to the improvement in gas exchange [9, 10], and the protective effect on ventilator-induced lung injury [3, 9, 11, 12] could also play a role. As compared to supine position (SP), the PP reduces the steep transpulmonary pressure gradient across the vertical axis of the lung, leading to a more homogeneous distribution of pulmonary stress and strain [2, 3, 13].

However, data analyzing the variation in lung volumes with the change from SP to PP in ARDS patients

*Correspondence: jmancebo@santpau.cat
Servei de Medicina Intensiva, Hospital de la Santa Creu i Sant Pau, Universitat Autònoma de Barcelona (UAB), Sant Quintí, 89, 08041 Barcelona, Spain

are scarce and conflicting [4, 14–17]. We hypothesized that in ARDS patients, PP increases lung volumes (i.e., functional residual capacity and end-expiratory lung volume) and might decrease lung strain [16, 18]. Because the measurement of functional residual capacity (FRC) requires to be made at zero end-expiratory pressure (ZEEP), our study included a lung derecruitment maneuver from baseline PEEP to zero PEEP [19–21] subsequently followed by the reinstitution of the basal PEEP level. These allowed to analyze the variation in lung volumes and to estimate lung volume recruitment and lung strain in both supine and prone positions in patients with ARDS.

## Methods

The study was performed in the Intensive Care Department at Hospital de la Santa Creu i Sant Pau, Barcelona (Spain). This study was conducted in accordance with the amended Declaration of Helsinki.

### Patients

Patients were considered eligible for the study if they met the Berlin definition criteria for ARDS [22] and had an indication for PP in accordance with our department's protocol ($PaO_2/FiO_2$ ratio of < 150 mm Hg and $FiO_2$ of ≥ 0.6 with PEEP of at least 5 cm $H_2O$). We recommend to use protective ventilation with individualized low tidal volume (Vt) and moderate PEEP levels. Essentially, PEEP is titrated according to the gas exchange (Sat $O_2$, measured by pulse oxymeter, around 95%) with end-inspiratory plateau airway pressure (Pplat) not higher than 28 cm $H_2O$ and without hemodynamic instability (mean arterial pressure above 65 mm Hg and no need for fluid replacement). Our detailed ventilatory strategy is included in Additional file 1. Hence, all our patients had been turned in PP before inclusion in the study. To be included, patients had to present an improvement in gas exchange ($FiO_2$ ≤ 0.6 and PEEP ≤ 12 cm $H_2O$) in SP in order to avoid severe hypoxemia because of the derecruitment (induced by PEEP withdrawal and ventilation at ZEEP) during the measurement of FRC. Exclusion criteria were: age < 18 years, tracheostomy, pregnancy, major trauma, barotrauma (presence of extra-alveolar air during mechanical ventilation as assessed by daily chest X ray) and hemodynamic instability (systolic blood pressure < 80 or > 160 mm Hg, heart rate < 50 bpm or > 130 bpm or changes in ± 20% from baseline).

All patients were under continuous sedation and analgesia with intravenous perfusion of midazolam and/or propofol and opioids. During the study period, all patients received neuromuscular blocking agents.

### Protocol

The following data were collected: age, height, simplified acute physiology score III at admission, ARDS etiology, days of mechanical ventilation, intensive care unit outcomes, respiratory rate, Vt, PEEP, peak airway pressure, Pplat and arterial blood gases. Respiratory variables were recorded directly from the ventilator.

All patients were ventilated in volume control ventilation using the same ventilator model (Engström Carestation ICU ventilator, General Electric, Madison, WI, USA).

To avoid hypoxemia, defined as oxygen saturation ≤ 88% measured through pulse oximetry, we increased the $FiO_2$ to 0.8 1 h before starting the protocol.

### Measurements

Baseline ventilatory and hemodynamic parameters were collected before the protocol to measure lung volumes. The same procedures were carried out in SP and PP and are outlined below (see also Fig. 1):

1. Measurement of end-expiratory lung volume (EELV): EELV is the resting end-expiratory lung volume measured at baseline PEEP.
2. Removal of PEEP and continuation of mechanical ventilation at ZEEP. This derecruitment maneuver

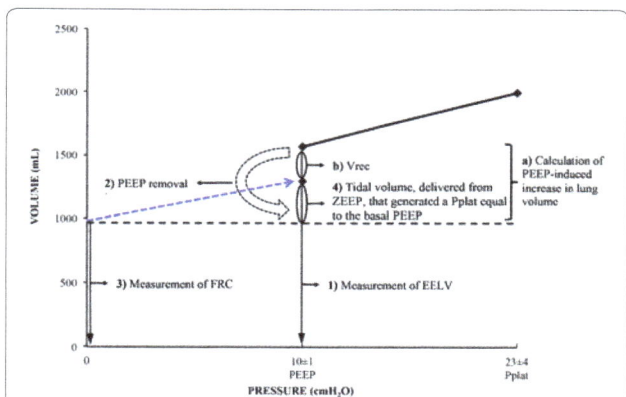

**Fig. 1** Lung volumes, measurements and calculations made in the study. The same procedures were carried out in supine and prone positions as follows: (1) measurement of end-expiratory lung volume (EELV): EELV is defined as the resting end-expiratory lung volume at PEEP. (2) Removal of PEEP and continuation of mechanical ventilation at zero end-expiratory pressure (ZEEP). (3) Measurement of functional residual capacity (FRC): FRC is defined as the resting lung volume at ZEEP. (4) Measurement of the tidal volume, delivered from ZEEP, that generated a Pplat equal to the basal PEEP. The same calculations were carried out in supine and prone positions as follows: (a) calculation of PEEP-induced increase in lung volume = EELV minus FRC. (b) Calculation of PEEP-induced lung volume recruitment (Vrec) = PEEP-induced increase in lung volume minus the Vt, delivered from ZEEP, that generated a Pplat equal to the basal PEEP. Blue line represents the compliance at ZEEP

is mandatory to conduct the following step 3, and it is the reason to increase the $FiO_2$ to 0.8 immediately before starting the protocol (i.e., to avoid hypoxemia).

3. Measurement of functional residual capacity (FRC): FRC is the resting lung volume measured at ZEEP.

4. Measurement of the Vt, delivered from ZEEP, that generated a Pplat equal to the basal PEEP. This step (see Fig. 1) is mandatory to allow a proper estimation of the PEEP-induced lung volume recruitment [19, 20, 23–25].

Once step 4 was completed, the same PEEP that was used at baseline was resumed.

Measurements at ZEEP (FRC and Vt delivered from ZEEP, that generated a Pplat equal to the basal PEEP) included a lung derecruitment maneuver (PEEP removal) that can produce hypoxemia. For the purpose of our investigation, we defined hypoxemia as oxygen saturation $\leq 88\%$ measured through pulse oximetry.

The safety limits and contraindications to remove PEEP were:

1. PEEP removal was contraindicated if $FiO_2 > 0.6$ and PEEP > 12 cm $H_2O$.

2. We increased the $FiO_2$ to 0.8 1 h before starting the protocol in order to avoid hypoxemia during PEEP removal.

3. If a patient presented with hypoxemia at any time during the protocol (saturation $\leq 88\%$ measured through pulse oximetry), the measurements were aborted and the patient was excluded.

Lung volumes (EELV and FRC) were measured twice using the nitrogen washout/washin technique available in Engström Carestation ICU ventilator as previously described [24, 26]. Washout/washin technique is a multiple breath maneuver that with a modification of 0.1 in $FiO_2$ calculates the residual nitrogen in the lung (assuming there is not exchange of nitrogen) by continuous measurements of oxygen and carbon dioxide. The ventilator was carefully calibrated before the measurements according to the manufacturer's specifications. We obtained four values for each lung volume. The mean of the four values was used. As previously suggested [27], patients were excluded if the differences between the four values were more than 20% (cutoff determined by the manufacturer).

After the procedures in SP, the patients were turned to PP and 1 h later the same procedures (from 1 to 4 above) were made in PP. This time span was based in previous data showing that after 1 h in PP gas exchange is stable in the majority of patients [28, 29]. If a patient presented with hypoxemia (oxygen saturation $\leq 88\%$) at any time

during the protocol, the measurements were aborted and the patient was excluded.

The normal reference values for FRC (liters) in the SP were calculated according to the equation described by Ibáñez and Raurich [30], as follows: 5.48 × height—7.05 for men and 1.39 × height—0.424 for women; height units are in meters. Compliance (ml/cm $H_2O$) was calculated as Vt/(Pplat minus total PEEP), being total PEEP the sum of PEEP plus intrinsic PEEP. Predicted body weight was calculated as follows: 50 + 0.91(height—152.4) for men and 45.5 + 0.91(height—152.4) for women; height units are in centimeters. Driving airway pressure was calculated as the difference between Pplat and total PEEP [31].

### Calculation of lung volumes and strain

(a) The PEEP-induced increase in lung volume was calculated as EELV minus FRC (see Fig. 1).

(b) PEEP-induced lung volume recruitment (Vrec) was calculated as PEEP-induced increase in lung volume minus the Vt, delivered from ZEEP, that generated a Pplat equal to the basal PEEP (see Fig. 1).

(c) Strain was calculated as previously described [24, 32, 33]:

1. Dynamic strain at ZEEP = Vt/FRC.
2. Dynamic strain at PEEP = Vt/(FRC + Vrec).
3. Static strain at PEEP = (EELV − FRC)/(FRC + Vrec).
4. Global strain at PEEP = (static strain at PEEP + dynamic strain at PEEP) = (EELV − FRC + Vt)/(FRC + Vrec).

### Statistical analysis

Data are expressed as mean ± SD. We used Wilcoxon test to compare variables between supine and prone positions and $U$ the Mann–Whiney test to compare early and non-early ARDS patients. A $p$ value < 0.05 was considered statistically significant. The SPSS® Statistics (version 20.0, Chicago, IL, USA) statistical software was used for statistical analysis.

### Results

The study was conducted from July 2010 to December 2013. Twenty-three patients were included in the study, and twenty were analyzed. One patient was excluded because of hypoxemia during the FRC measurement, and two were excluded because of a technical problem. (The differences between FRC measurements were > 20%.)

Table 1 summarizes the patients' main characteristics at baseline. The mean age of patients was 58 ± 18 years. The main causes of ARDS were pneumonia ($n = 11$) and septic shock ($n = 4$). The study was performed 4 ± 3 days

**Table 1** Patients' characteristics at study entry (with FiO$_2$ 0.8)

| Patient | Age (years) | Days on MV before study | SAPS III | Vt (ml/kg PBW) | RR (rpm) | PEEP (cm H$_2$O) | Pplat (cm H$_2$O) | Δ Paw (cm H$_2$O) | PaO$_2$/FiO$_2$ (mm Hg) | PaCO$_2$ (mm Hg) | Cause of ARDS | Outcome |
|---|---|---|---|---|---|---|---|---|---|---|---|---|
| 1 | 43 | 6 | 65 | 7.4 | 24 | 8 | 28 | 20 | 255 | 40 | Pneumonia | S |
| 2 | 66 | 1 | 52 | 6.1 | 22 | 10 | 20 | 10 | 254 | 60 | Pneumonia | S |
| 3 | 77 | 5 | 91 | 6.7 | 20 | 10 | 22 | 12 | 165 | 44 | Pneumonia | S |
| 4 | 68 | 4 | 69 | 8.4 | 24 | 12 | 21 | 9 | 255 | 44 | Pneumonia | S |
| 5 | 75 | 4 | 65 | 7.8 | 22 | 10 | 18 | 8 | 115 | 38 | Pneumonia | S |
| 6 | 65 | 7 | 94 | 9.2 | 30 | 10 | 21 | 11 | 240 | 53 | Pneumonia | S |
| 7 | 55 | 2 | 67 | 6.8 | 20 | 10 | 22 | 12 | 229 | 35 | Peritonitis | S |
| 8 | 43 | 2 | 77 | 8.1 | 20 | 8 | 26 | 18 | 151 | 48 | Peritonitis | D |
| 9 | 78 | 3 | 100 | 6.3 | 27 | 10 | 29 | 19 | 188 | 41 | Peritonitis | D |
| 10 | 74 | 2 | 82 | 11.0 | 25 | 10 | 28 | 18 | 198 | 43 | Pneumonia | D |
| 11 | 81 | 4 | 89 | 6.7 | 24 | 10 | 20 | 10 | 230 | 34 | Septic shock | S |
| 12 | 30 | 4 | 83 | 6.8 | 21 | 10 | 23 | 13 | 265 | 41 | Septic shock | D |
| 13 | 58 | 5 | 71 | 5.0 | 30 | 10 | 20 | 10 | 173 | 43 | Pneumonia | S |
| 14 | 69 | 1 | 101 | 5.9 | 28 | 10 | 28 | 18 | 300 | 44 | Septic shock | D |
| 15 | 50 | 14 | 95 | 6.0 | 30 | 10 | 25 | 15 | 206 | 42 | Septic shock | D |
| 16 | 55 | 3 | 68 | 7.0 | 20 | 8 | 19 | 11 | 129 | 37 | Thoracic Trauma | S |
| 17 | 30 | 4 | 64 | 6.2 | 24 | 12 | 22 | 10 | 104 | 41 | Pneumonia | S |
| 18 | 37 | 3 | 76 | 5.0 | 30 | 12 | 22 | 10 | 299 | 29 | Pneumonia | D |
| 19 | 80 | 2 | 82 | 6.1 | 17 | 12 | 19 | 7 | 230 | 35 | Pneumonia | S |
| 20 | 31 | 5 | 65 | 6.7 | 26 | 12 | 27 | 15 | 218 | 24 | Pancreatitis | D |
| Mean ± SD | 58 ± 18 | 4 ± 3 | 78 ± 14 | 6.9 ± 1.4 | 24 ± 4 | 10 ± 1 | 23 ± 4 | 13 ± 4 | 41 ± 8 | 41 ± 8 | | |

*ARDS* acute respiratory distress syndrome, *D* died, *PBW* predicted body weight, *MV* mechanical ventilation, *PEEP* positive end-expiratory pressure, *Pplat* end-inspiratory plateau airway pressure, *RR* respiratory rate, *S* survived, *SAPS III* simplified acute physiology score III, *Vt* tidal volume, *Δ Paw* driving airway pressure after starting mechanical ventilation. At baseline, mean Vt was $6.9 \pm 1.4$ ml/kg of predicted body weight and mean PEEP was $10 \pm 1$ cm $H_2O$.

After assuming the PP, the $PaO_2/FiO_2$ ratio increased significantly, from $210 \pm 57$ mm Hg in supine to $281 \pm 109$ mm Hg in prone ($p = 0.008$) (Table 2).

The mean FRC in SP was significantly lower than its reference value in healthy normal subjects ($965 \pm 397$ vs. $2424 \pm 459$ ml, $p \leq 0.001$). The change from SP to PP significantly increased both FRC (from $965 \pm 397$ to $1140 \pm 490$ ml, $p = 0.008$) and EELV (from $1566 \pm 476$ to $1832 \pm 719$ ml, $p = 0.008$) (Figs. 2, 3).

We did not calculate Vrec and derived parameters in four patients because the tidal volume delivered from ZEEP, that generated a Pplat equal to the basal PEEP, was not measured in accordance to the protocol. Vrec ($n = 16$) did not significantly vary with the change of position ($269 \pm 186$ ml in SP to $324 \pm 188$ ml in PP, $p = 0.263$) (Fig. 2).

We found a significant decrease in the dynamic strain at PEEP with the change from SP to PP from $0.38 \pm 0.14$ to $0.33 \pm 0.13$ ($p = 0.040$) (Fig. 4). The dynamic strain at ZEEP also decreased, from $0.52 \pm 0.23$ in SP to $0.44 \pm 0.18$ in PP ($p = 0.047$). The remaining variables did not change significantly between supine and prone positions (Table 2) (Additional file 2: Table S1).

In the whole population, the driving pressure in the non-survivor group ($n = 8$) was significantly higher than in the survivor group ($n = 12$) in both SP ($16 \pm 3$ cm $H_2O$ vs. $11 \pm 3$ cm $H_2O$, respectively, $p = 0.003$) and

in PP ($15 \pm 3$ cm $H_2O$ vs. $11 \pm 3$ cm $H_2O$, respectively, $p = 0.005$). Additional data are also shown (Additional file 2: Table S2).

## Discussion

The main findings in this study were that: (1) Prone position significantly increased lung volumes; (2) dynamic strain decreased significantly in prone position compared to supine position; and (3) the change of position from supine to prone did not modify the calculated PEEP-induced lung volume recruitment.

### Prone position, oxygenation and lung volumes

In ARDS patients, lung volumes at ZEEP (FRC) and at PEEP (EELV) are typically decreased [18]. Two previous studies have shown that PP significantly increases FRC in ARDS patients [15, 16]. Nevertheless, data about the changes in EELV with the change from SP to PP in ARDS patients are not consistent. Four previous studies have shown that PP increases EELV in ARDS patients as compared to SP [14–17], but another study [4] found that the change of EELV from SP to PP was not significant. These contradictory findings might be explained by differences in lung recruitability, distribution and extension of lung volume alterations, differences in chest wall compliance, the influence of abdominal weight and heart compression, the inclination from the horizontal plane and the use or not of ventral supports [3, 9, 34, 35].

In the present study, we found a 40% decrease in FRC as compared to its reference value in SP, confirming

**Table 2 Main characteristics of all patients in each position**

| Variable | Supine $n = 20$ | Prone $n = 20$ | p |
|---|---|---|---|
| $PaO_2/FiO_2$ (mm Hg) | $210 \pm 57$ | $281 \pm 109$ | 0.021 |
| $PaCO_2$ (mm Hg) | $41 \pm 8$ | $42 \pm 9$ | 0.400 |
| Peak airway pressure (cm $H_2O$) | $41 \pm 7$ | $41 \pm 6$ | 0.284 |
| Pplat (cm $H_2O$) | $23 \pm 4$ | $23 \pm 4$ | 0.446 |
| Compliance (ml/cm $H_2O$) | $36 \pm 11$ | $37 \pm 10$ | 0.594 |
| $\Delta$ Paw (cm $H_2O$) | $13 \pm 4$ | $12 \pm 4$ | 0.446 |
| FRC (ml) | $965 \pm 397$ | $1140 \pm 490$ | 0.021 |
| EELV (ml) | $1566 \pm 476$ | $1832 \pm 719$ | 0.009 |
| Vt delivered from ZEEP, that generated a Pplat equal to basal PEEP [ml ($n = 16$)] | $333 \pm 105$ | $360 \pm 127$ | 0.073 |
| Vrec [ml ($n = 16$)] | $269 \pm 186$ | $324 \pm 188$ | 0.501 |
| Dynamic strain at ZEEP | $0.52 \pm 0.23$ | $0.44 \pm 0.18$ | 0.040 |
| Dynamic strain at PEEP ($n = 16$) | $0.38 \pm 0.14$ | $0.33 \pm 0.13$ | 0.020 |
| Static strain at PEEP ($n = 16$) | $0.51 \pm 0.16$ | $0.48 \pm 0.13$ | 0.438 |
| Global strain at PEEP ($n = 16$) | $0.89 \pm 0.24$ | $0.81 \pm 0.18$ | 0.121 |

Data are presented as mean $\pm$ SD. Dynamic strain at ZEEP = Vt/FRC; dynamic strain at PEEP = Vt/(FRC + Vrec); static strain at PEEP = (EELV − FRC)/(FRC + Vrec); global strain at PEEP = (EELV − FRC + Vt)/(FRC + Vrec)

*EELV* end-expiratory lung volume, *FRC* functional residual capacity, *PEEP* positive end-expiratory pressure, *Pplat* end-inspiratory plateau airway pressure, *Vrec* PEEP-induced lung volume recruitment, *Vt* tidal volume, *$\Delta$ Paw* driving airway pressure

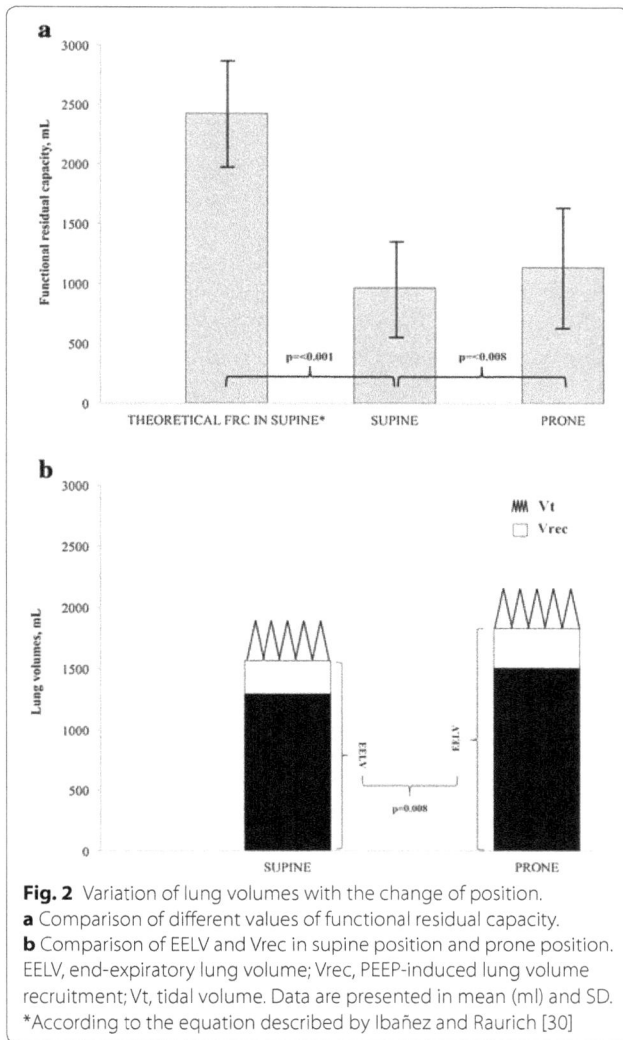

**Fig. 2** Variation of lung volumes with the change of position.
**a** Comparison of different values of functional residual capacity.
**b** Comparison of EELV and Vrec in supine position and prone position.
EELV, end-expiratory lung volume; Vrec, PEEP-induced lung volume
recruitment; Vt, tidal volume. Data are presented in mean (ml) and SD.
*According to the equation described by Ibañez and Raurich [30]

### Prone position and strain

During passive mechanical ventilation, the force applied by the ventilator generates an internal tension in the fibers of the lung skeleton, called "stress," and the elongation of these fibers from their resting position is called "strain" [2]. High values of dynamic lung strain (lung deformation caused by Vt) and static lung strain (lung deformation caused by PEEP) are associated with ventilator-induced lung injury [32, 37].

In an animal model, Protti et al. [33] showed that for the same global strain, a large static strain is less harmful than a large dynamic strain. On the same vein, González-López et al. [38] found that increased strain was associated with a proinflammatory lung response in patients with acute lung injury. Moreover, Bellani et al. [39] found in patients with acute lung injury that the intensity of metabolic activity (a surrogate of inflammation) detected by positron emission tomography was correlated with regional strain. Consequently, the significant decrease in dynamic strain in PP as compared to SP could be another mechanism of protection of PP against ventilator-induced lung injury. Therefore, the measurement of lung volumes at bedside may be an important tool to deliver a more physiologically based ventilation and encourage physicians to increase the use of PP in moderately to severe ARDS patients [40].

### Prone position and PEEP-induced lung volume recruitment

It is still unclear whether the PEEP-induced alveolar recruitment varies with the change from SP to PP. In an experimental study in animals with lung injury, Richard et al. [5] analyzed the variation of alveolar recruitment at PEEP 10 cm $H_2O$ in SP and PP by means of the positron emission tomography technique. They found that in PP, PEEP-induced alveolar recruitment was not higher than in SP. Interestingly, in this study, the authors observed a redistribution of densities in PP (recruitment in dorsal regions with derecruitment in ventral regions). Cornejo et al. [6] performed another study in ARDS patients to determine the effects of PEEP and PP on alveolar recruitment. Using the CT scan technique, they found that increasing PEEP from 5 cm $H_2O$ to 15 cm $H_2O$ significantly increased alveolar recruitment. However, the percentage of recruitment was similar in both positions (36% in SP and 33% in PP). Using a different methodology, the data from our study are consistent with these findings, indicating that the effects of PEEP on lung volume recruitment are similar in both positions (around 17% of EELV).

A previous study by Grasso et al. [41] found that alveolar recruitment was higher in the early phase ($1 \pm 0.3$ days of mechanical ventilation) than in the late phase of ARDS, but a subsequent study by Gattinoni

previous results [18]. We also observed that the FRC and EELV increased significantly with the change of position (18% in FRC and 17% in EELV). Santini et al. [7] performed a study in animals with normal lungs, and they found a significant increase in FRC with the change from SP to PP. The increase in resting lung volume was mainly related to a redistribution of aeration: a minor decrease in non-aerated lung tissue (3%), a major decrease in poorly aerated tissue (17%) and a major increase (20%) in well-aerated tissue. Since recruitment, as precisely measured by thoracic CT scan, refers to tissue recruitment (i.e., amount of non-inflated tissue that reinflates at a higher pressure), the decrease in poorly aerated tissue and the increase in well-aerated tissue (which contribute to the end-expiratory lung volume increase induced by PEEP) are thus considered as better gas distribution within the lung and not recruitment per se [36].

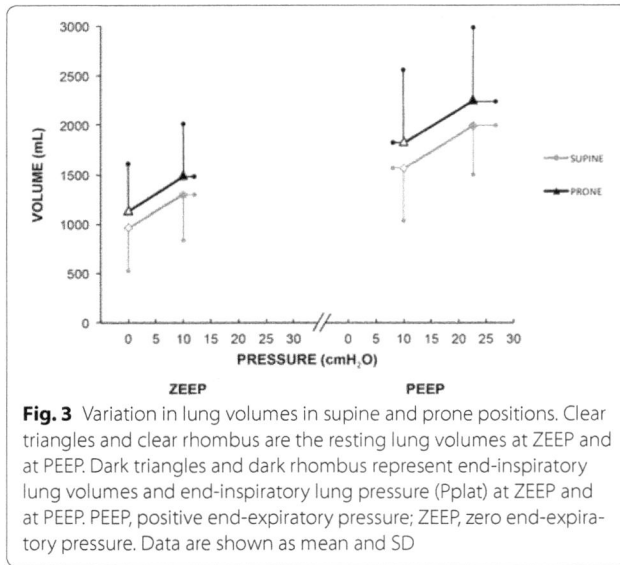

**Fig. 3** Variation in lung volumes in supine and prone positions. Clear triangles and clear rhombus are the resting lung volumes at ZEEP and at PEEP. Dark triangles and dark rhombus represent end-inspiratory lung volumes and end-inspiratory lung pressure (Pplat) at ZEEP and at PEEP. PEEP, positive end-expiratory pressure; ZEEP, zero end-expiratory pressure. Data are shown as mean and SD

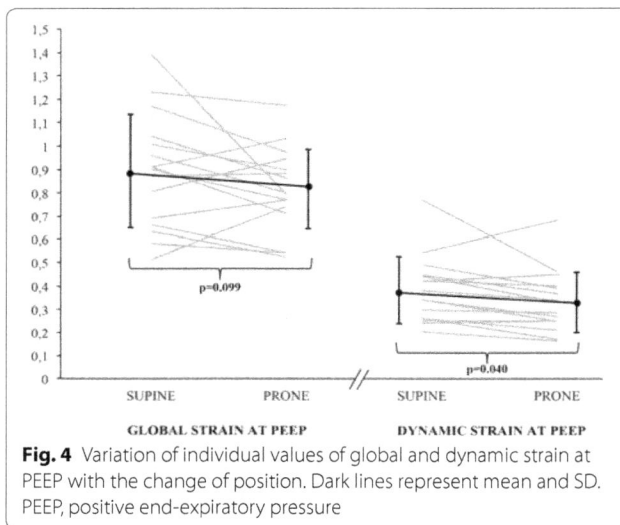

**Fig. 4** Variation of individual values of global and dynamic strain at PEEP with the change of position. Dark lines represent mean and SD. PEEP, positive end-expiratory pressure

et al. [42] did not find the same results. In the study of Gattinoni et al. [42], they found that the number of days of mechanical ventilation before the study was similar in patients with a lower percentage of potentially recruitable lung and those with a higher percentage ($5 \pm 6$ vs. $6 \pm 6$ days, respectively, $p = 0.50$). In our study when we classified ARDS patients in the early phase ($< 72$ h) and in late phase ($> 72$ h) (Additional file 2: Table S2), we observed results similar to those of Gattinoni et al. [42]: no statistical differences in lung volume recruitment between the early and late phase group were detected. In our study, however, in the early phase of

ARDS, lung volumes increased and strain decreased with the change from SP to PP, whereas in late phase ARDS we did not observe these findings (Additional file 2: Table S2). These differences could be related to the presence of some degree of hydrostatic pulmonary edema in the early phase of ARDS, and to the presence of fibrosis in the non-early phase of ARDS that predisposes to non-responsiveness to PP in terms of increasing in lung volumes and decreasing strain [43]. Our findings thus suggest that the survival benefit may, in part, be related to the early application of PP as it increases resting lung volumes and decreases lung strain compared to SP. It is also tempting to speculate that the lack of differences in Vrec between supine and prone, and the increase in overall lung volume in prone as compared to supine, can be explained by a decrease of poorly ventilated areas and an increase of well ventilated areas, which in turn might help to decrease lung inhomogeneity. It has been shown that the extent of lung inhomogeneities (as quantified by the amount of poorly ventilated tissue) is associated with worse outcomes in ARDS patients, possibly due to a mechanism of "stress raisers" [44].

### Limitations
Like many physiological studies [4, 6, 14–17, 34], our study has a relatively low number of patients. Another limitation is that the measurement of FRC could be subject to the tolerance to PEEP removal and the $FiO_2$ used. However, when the study was performed, all the patients met the criteria for mild–moderate ARDS according to the Berlin definition [22]. We did not perform a multi-slice spiral lung computed tomography to measure the quantitative changes in alveolar aeration induced by PEEP and PP. Other measurements of lung mechanics (i.e., esophageal pressure and derived variables) and lung biomarkers could help to further explain the effects of PEEP and positioning in ARDS patients, but we did not do these because of lack of adequate equipment at the time of the study. Finally, to confirm the changes, it might have been useful to return the patients from PP to SP and to repeat the same procedures and measurements; this was not done, however, because most patients remained in the PP as per clinical decision after the study had been completed.

### Conclusions
As compared to supine, prone position increases resting lung volumes without significantly changing the recruited volume kept by PEEP. Moreover, the change of position from supine to prone decreases dynamic lung strain. These findings help to better understand the beneficial effects of prone position in ARDS patients.

## Abbreviations

ARDS: acute respiratory distress syndrome; EELV: end-expiratory lung volume; FRC: functional residual capacity; PEEP: positive end-expiratory pressure; PP: prone position; Pplat: end-inspiratory plateau airway pressure; SP: supine position; Vrec: PEEP-induced lung volume recruitment; Vt: tidal volume; ZEEP: zero end-expiratory pressure.

## Authors' contributions

All authors participated in the study design, data collection and analysis, manuscript writing and final approval. All authors read and approved the final manuscript.

## Competing interests

General Electric provided the equipment (Engström Carestation ICU ventilator) to conduct this research.

## Acknowledgements

Not applicable.

## References

1. Ware LB, Matthay MA. The acute respiratory distress syndrome. N Engl J Med. 2000;342:1334–49.
2. Gattinoni L, Pesenti A. The concept of "baby lung". Intensive Care Med. 2005;31:776–84.
3. Gattinoni L, Taccone P, Carlesso E, Marini JJ. Prone position in acute respiratory distress syndrome. Rationale, indications, and limits. Am J Respir Crit Care Med. 2013;188:1286–93.
4. Pelosi P, Tubiolo D, Mascheroni D, Vicardi P, Crotti S, Valenza F, Gattinoni L. Effects of the prone position on respiratory mechanics and gas exchange during acute lung injury. Am J Respir Crit Care Med. 1998;157:387–93.
5. Richard JC, Bregeon F, Costes N, Bars DL, Tourvieille C, Lavenne F, Janier M, Bourdin G, Gimenez G, Guerin C. Effects of prone position and positive end-expiratory pressure on lung perfusion and ventilation. Crit Care Med. 2008;36:2373–80.
6. Cornejo RA, Diaz JC, Tobar EA, Bruhn AR, Ramos CA, Gonzalez RA, Repetto CA, Romero CM, Galvez LR, Llanos O, Arellano DH, Neira WR, Diaz GA, Zamorano AJ, Pereira GL. Effects of prone positioning on lung protection in patients with acute respiratory distress syndrome. Am J Respir Crit Care Med. 2013;188:440–8.
7. Santini A, Protti A, Langer T, Comini B, Monti M, Sparacino CC, Dondossola D, Gattinoni L. Prone position ameliorates lung elastance and increases functional residual capacity independently from lung recruitment. Intensive Care Med Exp. 2015;3:55.
8. Guerin C, Reignier J, Richard JC, Beuret P, Gacouin A, Boulain T, Mercier E, Badet M, Mercat A, Baudin O, Clavel M, Chatellier D, Jaber S, Rosselli S, Mancebo J, Sirodot M, Hilbert G, Bengler C, Richecoeur J, Gainnier M, Bayle F, Bourdin G, Leray V, Girard R, Baboi L, Ayzac L. Prone positioning in severe acute respiratory distress syndrome. N Engl J Med. 2013;368:2159–68.
9. Albert RK, Keniston A, Baboi L, Ayzac L, Guerin C. Prone position-induced improvement in gas exchange does not predict improved survival in the acute respiratory distress syndrome. Am J Respir Crit Care Med. 2014;189:494–6.
10. Guerin C, Baboi L, Richard JC. Mechanisms of the effects of prone positioning in acute respiratory distress syndrome. Intensive Care Med. 2014;40:1634–42.
11. Broccard A, Shapiro RS, Schmitz LL, Adams AB, Nahum A, Marini JJ. Prone positioning attenuates and redistributes ventilator-induced lung injury in dogs. Crit Care Med. 2000;28:295–303.
12. Valenza F, Guglielmi M, Maffioletti M, Tedesco C, Maccagni P, Fossali T, Aletti G, Porro GA, Irace M, Carlesso E, Carboni N, Lazzerini M, Gattinoni L. Prone position delays the progression of ventilator-induced lung injury in rats: does lung strain distribution play a role? Crit Care Med. 2005;33:361–7.
13. Mutoh T, Guest RJ, Lamm WJ, Albert RK. Prone position alters the effect of volume overload on regional pleural pressures and improves hypoxemia in pigs in vivo. Am Rev Respir Dis. 1992;146:300–6.
14. Pelosi P, Bottino N, Chiumello D, Caironi P, Panigada M, Gamberoni C, Colombo G, Bigatello LM, Gattinoni L. Sigh in supine and prone position during acute respiratory distress syndrome. Am J Respir Crit Care Med. 2003;167:521–7.
15. Mentzelopoulos SD, Roussos C, Zakynthinos SG. Static pressure volume curves and body posture in acute respiratory failure. Intensive Care Med. 2005;31:1683–92.
16. Mentzelopoulos SD, Roussos C, Zakynthinos SG. Prone position reduces lung stress and strain in severe acute respiratory distress syndrome. Eur Respir J. 2005;25:534–44.
17. Reutershan J, Schmitt A, Dietz K, Unertl K, Fretschner R. Alveolar recruitment during prone position: time matters. Clin Sci (Lond). 2006;110:655–63.
18. Chiumello D, Carlesso E, Cadringher P, Caironi P, Valenza F, Polli F, Tallarini F, Cozzi P, Cressoni M, Colombo A, Marini JJ, Gattinoni L. Lung stress and strain during mechanical ventilation for acute respiratory distress syndrome. Am J Respir Crit Care Med. 2008;178:346–55.
19. Jonson B, Richard JC, Straus C, Mancebo J, Lemaire F, Brochard L. Pressure-volume curves and compliance in acute lung injury: evidence of recruitment above the lower inflection point. Am J Respir Crit Care Med. 1999;159:1172–8.
20. Maggiore SM, Jonson B, Richard JC, Jaber S, Lemaire F, Brochard L. Alveolar derecruitment at decremental positive end-expiratory pressure levels in acute lung injury: comparison with the lower inflection point, oxygenation, and compliance. Am J Respir Crit Care Med. 2001;164:795–801.
21. Crotti S, Mascheroni D, Caironi P, Pelosi P, Ronzoni G, Mondino M, Marini JJ, Gattinoni L. Recruitment and derecruitment during acute respiratory failure: a clinical study. Am J Respir Crit Care Med. 2001;164:131–40.
22. Ranieri VM, Rubenfeld GD, Thompson BT, Ferguson ND, Caldwell E, Fan E, Camporota L, Slutsky AS. Acute respiratory distress syndrome: the Berlin Definition. JAMA. 2012;307:2526–33.
23. Ranieri VM, Giuliani R, Fiore T, Dambrosio M, Milic-Emili J. Volume-pressure curve of the respiratory system predicts effects of PEEP in ARDS: "occlusion" versus "constant flow" technique. Am J Respir Crit Care Med. 1994;149:19–27.
24. Dellamonica J, Lerolle N, Sargentini C, Beduneau G, Di Marco F, Mercat A, Richard JC, Diehl JL, Mancebo J, Rouby JJ, Lu Q, Bernardin G, Brochard L. PEEP-induced changes in lung volume in acute respiratory distress syndrome. Two methods to estimate alveolar recruitment. Intensive Care Med. 2011;37:1595–604.
25. Richard JC, Brochard L, Vandelet P, Breton L, Maggiore SM, Jonson B, Clabault K, Leroy J, Bonmarchand G. Respective effects of end-expiratory and end-inspiratory pressures on alveolar recruitment in acute lung injury. Crit Care Med. 2003;31:89–92.
26. Olegard C, Sondergaard S, Houltz E, Lundin S, Stenqvist O. Estimation of functional residual capacity at the bedside using standard monitoring equipment: a modified nitrogen washout/washin technique requiring a small change of the inspired oxygen fraction. Anesth Analg. 2005;101:206–12.
27. Dellamonica J, Lerolle N, Sargentini C, Beduneau G, Di Marco F, Mercat A, Richard JC, Diehl JL, Mancebo J, Rouby JJ, Lu Q, Bernardin G, Brochard L. Accuracy and precision of end-expiratory lung-volume measurements by automated nitrogen washout/washin technique in patients with acute respiratory distress syndrome. Crit Care. 2011;15:R294.
28. Chatte G, Sab JM, Dubois JM, Sirodot M, Gaussorgues P, Robert D. Prone position in mechanically ventilated patients with severe acute respiratory failure. Am J Respir Crit Care Med. 1997;155:473–8.
29. Mancebo J, Fernandez R, Blanch L, Rialp G, Gordo F, Ferrer M, Rodriguez F, Garro P, Ricart P, Vallverdu I, Gich I, Castano J, Saura P, Dominguez G, Bonet A, Albert RK. A multicenter trial of prolonged prone ventilation in severe acute respiratory distress syndrome. Am J Respir Crit Care Med. 2006;173:1233–9.
30. Ibanez J, Raurich JM. Normal values of functional residual capacity in the sitting and supine positions. Intensive Care Med. 1982;8:173–7.
31. Amato MB, Meade MO, Slutsky AS, Brochard L, Costa EL, Schoenfeld DA, Stewart TE, Briel M, Talmor D, Mercat A, Richard JC, Carvalho CR, Brower RG. Driving pressure and survival in the acute respiratory distress syndrome. N Engl J Med. 2015;372:747–55.

32.  Protti A, Cressoni M, Santini A, Langer T, Mietto C, Febres D, Chierichetti M, Coppola S, Conte G, Gatti S, Leopardi O, Masson S, Lombardi L, Lazzerini M, Rampoldi E, Cadringher P, Gattinoni L. Lung stress and strain during mechanical ventilation: any safe threshold? Am J Respir Crit Care Med. 2011;183:1354–62.

33.  Protti A, Andreis DT, Monti M, Santini A, Sparacino CC, Langer T, Votta E, Gatti S, Lombardi L, Leopardi O, Masson S, Cressoni M, Gattinoni L. Lung stress and strain during mechanical ventilation: any difference between statics and dynamics? Crit Care Med. 2013;41:1046–55.

34.  Galiatsou E, Kostanti E, Svarna E, Kitsakos A, Koulouras V, Efremidis SC, Nakos G. Prone position augments recruitment and prevents alveolar overinflation in acute lung injury. Am J Respir Crit Care Med. 2006;174:187–97.

35.  Nieszkowska A, Lu Q, Vieira S, Elman M, Fetita C, Rouby JJ. Incidence and regional distribution of lung overinflation during mechanical ventilation with positive end-expiratory pressure. Crit Care Med. 2004;32:1496–503.

36.  Chiumello D, Marino A, Brioni M, Cigada I, Menga F, Colombo A, Crimella F, Algieri I, Cressoni M, Carlesso E, Gattinoni L. Lung recruitment assessed by respiratory mechanics and computed tomography in patients with acute respiratory distress syndrome. What Is the relationship? Am J Respir Crit Care Med. 2016;193:1254–63.

37.  Dreyfuss D, Saumon G. Ventilator-induced lung injury: lessons from experimental studies. Am J Respir Crit Care Med. 1998;157:294–323.

38.  Gonzalez-Lopez A, Garcia-Prieto E, Batalla-Solis E, Amado-Rodriguez L, Avello N, Blanch L, Albaiceta GM. Lung strain and biological response in mechanically ventilated patients. Intensive Care Med. 2012;38:240–7.

39.  Bellani G, Guerra L, Musch G, Zanella A, Patroniti N, Mauri T, Messa C, Pesenti A. Lung regional metabolic activity and gas volume changes induced by tidal ventilation in patients with acute lung injury. Am J Respir Crit Care Med. 2011;183:1193–9.

40.  Guerin C, Beuret P, Constantin JM, Bellani G, Garcia-Olivares P, Roca O, Meertens JH, Maia PA, Becher T, Peterson J, Larsson A, Gurjar M, Hajjej Z, Kovari F, Assiri AH, Mainas E, Hasan MS, Morocho-Tutillo DR, Baboi L, Chretien JM, Francois G, Ayzac L, Chen L, Brochard L, Mercat A, investigators of the APRONET Study Group, the REVA Network, the Réseau recherche de la Société Française d'Anesthésie-Réanimation (SFAR-recherche), the ESICM Trials Group. A prospective international observational prevalence study on prone positioning of ARDS patients: the APRONET (ARDS Prone Position Network) study. Intensive Care Med. 2018;44:22–37. https://doi.org/10.1007/s00134-017-4996-5.

41.  Grasso S, Mascia L, Del Turco M, Malacarne P, Giunta F, Brochard L, Slutsky AS, Marco Ranieri V. Effects of recruiting maneuvers in patients with acute respiratory distress syndrome ventilated with protective ventilatory strategy. Anesthesiology. 2002;96:795–802.

42.  Gattinoni L, Caironi P, Cressoni M, Chiumello D, Ranieri VM, Quintel M, Russo S, Patroniti N, Cornejo R, Bugedo G. Lung recruitment in patients with the acute respiratory distress syndrome. N Engl J Med. 2006;354:1775–86.

43.  Nakos G, Tsangaris I, Kostanti E, Nathanail C, Lachana A, Koulouras V, Kastani D. Effect of the prone position on patients with hydrostatic pulmonary edema compared with patients with acute respiratory distress syndrome and pulmonary fibrosis. Am J Respir Crit Care Med. 2000;161:360–8.

44.  Cressoni M, Cadringher P, Chiurazzi C, Amini M, Gallazzi E, Marino A, Brioni M, Carlesso E, Chiumello D, Quintel M, Bugedo G, Gattinoni L. Lung inhomogeneity in patients with acute respiratory distress syndrome. Am J Respir Crit Care Med. 2014;189:149–58.

# 8

# Stool cultures at the ICU

Carolin F. Manthey[1]* , Darja Dranova[2], Martin Christner[3], Laura Berneking[3], Stefan Kluge[2], Ansgar W. Lohse[1] and Valentin Fuhrmann[2]

## Abstract

**Background:** Stool cultures for *Campylobacter*, *Salmonella* and *Shigella* and/or *Yersinia* spp. are frequently ordered in critically ill patients with diarrhea. The aim of this study is to analyze the diagnostic yield in a large cohort of critically ill patients. Therefore, we performed a cohort study at the Department of Intensive Care Medicine of a University Hospital (11 ICUs).

**Results:** From all patients who were admitted to the ICU between 2010 and 2015, stool cultures were taken from 2.189/36.477 (6%) patients due to diarrhea. Results of all stool cultures tested for *Campylobacter*, *Salmonella* and *Shigella* and/or *Yersinia* spp. were analyzed. Overall, 5.747 tests were performed; only six were positive (0.1%). In four of these, *Campylobacter* spp. were detected; diarrhea started within 48 h after ICU admission. Two patients with *Salmonella* spp. detection were chronic shedders. On the contrary, testing for *Clostridium difficile* via GDH- and toxin A/B-EIA yielded positive results in 179/2209 (8.1%) tests and revealed 144/2.189 (6.6%) patients with clinically relevant *C. difficile* infection.

**Conclusions:** Stool testing for enteric pathogens other than *C. difficile* should be avoided in ICU patients and is only reasonable when diarrhea commenced less than 48 h after hospital admission.

**Keywords:** Diarrhea, Stool culture, Critically ill, *Clostridium difficile*, *Campylobacter* spp., *Salmonella* spp.

## Background

Diarrhea is a common problem in critically ill patients. Reported prevalence varies from 2 to 95% [1] mostly owing to heterogeneous case definitions. The most common risk factors associated with diarrhea in this patient population are side effects of medications, dysbiosis due to antibiotic therapy, enteral feedings and enteric infections [2] as well as severe disease accompanying multiple organ dysfunction syndrome (MODS) [3]. *Clostridium difficile* infections (CDI) affect a significant amount of hospitalized patients [4], especially critically ill patients are at risk, whereas numbers for other enteric infections in this patient group remain elusive.

Current guidelines are recommending stool cultures for enteropathogenic bacteria for hospitalized patients with fever (> 101 °F/38.3 °C) and diarrhea that developed within 72 h after hospital admission [5]. However, this is not valid for critically ill patients as they have a significantly higher risk of complications (e.g., elderly, immunocompromised, certain comorbidities) [6]. Therefore, it is common practice to, even repeatedly, test for enteropathogenic bacteria in critically ill patients developing diarrhea [7]. This practice is cost-consuming, and in the case of *C. difficile* infections, repeated testing does not even increase diagnostic yield [7]. The aim of this study is to assess the clinical impact of diagnostic stool testing in critically ill patients.

## Methods

We performed a retrospective analysis of all stool samples collected during January 2010 and September 2015 in 11 ICUs (specialized for heart surgery, cardiology, internal medicine, neurosurgery, neurology and surgery, in addition to five interdisciplinary wards) of the Department of Intensive Care at the University Medical Center Hamburg. In addition to *C. difficile* toxin testing, cultures for enteropathogenic bacteria had consistently been requested for ICU patients with diarrhea during

*Correspondence: cmanthey@uke.de
[1] First Department of Internal Medicine and Gastroenterology, University Hospital Hamburg-Eppendorf, Martinistr. 52, 20246 Hamburg, Germany
Full list of author information is available at the end of the article

that time. Stool cultures for *Campylobacter* (modified Karmali agar), *Salmonella–Shigella* (MacConkey agar, Salmonella–Shigella agar, xylose lysine deoxycholate agar and selenite enrichment broth) and enteropathogenic *Yersinia* (CIN agar) had been performed by the Department of Medical Microbiology according to current practice guidelines by the German Society for Hygiene and Microbiology [8], while the C. diff Quik Chek Complete EIA (TechLab; Blacksburg, VA, USA) had been used for *C. difficile* glutamate dehydrogenase antigen (GDH) and toxin A/B testing of non-formed stool samples as recommended by the manufacturer. Only liquid stools were analyzed as a definition of diarrhea by C. diff Quik Chek, whereas culturing for other enteropathogenic bacteria was performed also from solid specimens. The number of stool passages per day for each patient was not available.

Anonymized data were extracted from our hospital and laboratory information systems.

The study was performed in accordance with the local regulations of the ethics committee (General Medical Council Hamburg, Ärztekammer Hamburg, reference number WF 11/16). Data analysis was performed anonymously, and informed consent was waived by the ethics committee for this retrospective study.

## Results

During the study period, 3188 stool samples from 2189 ICU patients were sent to the microbiology laboratory (Fig. 1). Patients tested represented 6.0% of all patients admitted (2010–2015: 41.415 admissions of 36.477 patients). Ninety-four samples (2.9%) were rejected by the laboratory due to several reasons (solid stool, scarcity of material).

Overall, 5.747 tests were performed; only six were positive (0.1%).

Only four out of 2500 *Campylobacter* cultures yielded a positive result (0.16% of all tests performed, 0.01% of all patients admitted); three samples were positive for *Campylobacter jejuni*, and one for *Campylobacter coli*. Symptoms in all four patients with *Campylobacter* infection had started less than 48 h after hospital admission implying that these patients had community acquired diarrhea. None of these patients received specific antibiotic therapy as symptoms had already resolved spontaneously. Length of ICU stay after diagnosis of *Campylobacter* enteritis was not increased, since all four patients were transferred to the normal ward the next day. None of the patients with *Campylobacter* enteritis died during their hospital stay.

Testing for *Salmonella* and *Shigella* (Salmonella–Shigella culture) was done for 2488 samples (1678 patients), two of these were positive for *Salmonella enterica* (0.08% of all tests performed, 0.005% of all patients), and none

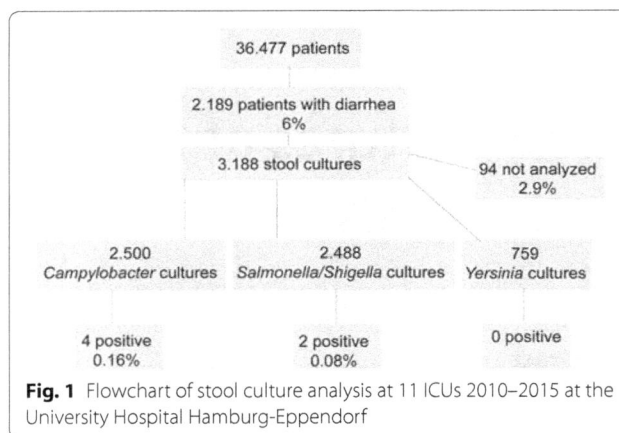

**Fig. 1** Flowchart of stool culture analysis at 11 ICUs 2010–2015 at the University Hospital Hamburg-Eppendorf

were positive for *Shigella*. *Salmonella enterica* was detected in the accidental submission of stool from two chronic shedders 20 and 23 days after hospital admission. The patients were not treated antimicrobially due to lack of symptoms. Detection of infection did not delay hospital dismissal or further transfer to another hospital. The main diagnoses in patients with *Campylobacter* enteritis were pneumonia (patient no. 1), postoperative due to thymectomy (patient no. 2) and vascular graft (patient no. 3), as well as epileptical attack (patient no. 4). Underlying comorbidities in these patients included Korsakov syndrome (patient no. 1), myasthenia gravis, arterial hypertension (patient no. 2), chronic obstructive pulmonary disease, reflux disease, sigma diverticulitis (patient no. 3), and cerebral infarction and arterial hypertension (patient no. 4). Patients with *Salmonella* detection were not on any immunosuppressive medication; however, one patient was suffering from head and neck cancer requiring multiple surgeries. The other patient with *Salmonella* infection was admitted due to subarachnoid hemorrhage.

None of the 759 samples tested for enteropathogenic *Yersinia* spp. yielded positive results (Fig. 1).

Regarding ICU characteristics, all six patients tested positive for *Salmonella* or *Campylobacter* required vasopressor support (mean 5.7 days ± 6.1) during their stay. Only one patient received vasopressor infusion on the day of the diagnosis, and the charts do not indicate that the dosage of vasopressor infusion was increased in patients due to diarrhea. Five out of six patients were in need of mechanical ventilation, although only one patient was on mechanical ventilation at the time of diagnosis. Length of mechanical ventilation was < 3 days in all three patients with *Campylobacter* enteritis. None of the patients required renal replacement therapy.

In contrast, *C. difficile* toxin testing yielded positive results in 242 (GDH antigen only) and 179 (GDH antigen and toxin A/B) of 2209 samples from 1654 patients (11.0

and 8.1% of all tests, 0.7 and 0.5% of all patients), the latter group fulfilling criteria for clinically relevant *C. difficile* infection in symptomatic patients [9]. 52/144 (36.1%) episodes of CDI occurred within 48 h of ICU admission, and 108/144 (75%) were antibiotic-associated.

Regarding stool tests in the overall hospital community, results between 2010 and 2015 in all departments of our hospital are illustrated in Fig. 2. Patients presenting to the emergency room (ER) with diarrhea showed the highest rates of infection with *Campylobacter* spp. (11.6% of all analyzed specimens) and *Salmonella* or *Shigella* spp. (2.4%). Also, patients presenting to the infectious diseases department showed higher infection rates with *Campylobacter* (4.6%) and *Salmonella* or *Shigella* spp. (2.9%). Infection rates with *Yersinia* were overall very low with a maximum rate of infection in general outpatients (0.2% of samples). The lowest rate of bacterial infection in patients presenting with diarrhea was observed in patients treated at the ICU and bone marrow transplant unit.

Economic impact was estimated based on national medical fee schedules in Germany. Considering usual local discounts, we conferred costs of 20 € for enteric bacteria stool culture and 10 € for *C. difficile* testing adding up to 50,000 € (enteric bacteria stool culture) and 22,090 € (*C. difficile*), total 72,090 €.

## Discussion

Our data from 5 years of extensive testing for enteric bacterial pathogens in adult critically ill patients show that *C. difficile* can be regarded as the only relevant bacterial cause of gastrointestinal infection in critically ill patients with diarrhea. The very low yield of stool cultures from patients at the ICU observed in our study confirms current guideline recommendations for non-critically ill

patients [5, 10] to limit testing in cases of suspected nosocomial gastrointestinal infection to *C. difficile*. Infections with *C. difficile* pose an important risk of increased mortality in patients at the ICU, and diagnostics regarding infection have to be conducted in case of suspected infection [8]. We can show that the highest rates of infections with enteric pathogens other than *C. difficile* are observed in patients presenting to the emergency room. *Campylobacter* spp. are the most important bacterial pathogen detected in outpatients; this reflects national reports by the Robert Koch Institute.

Simple stratification by time since hospital admission would have reduced the number of stool cultures at the ICU by more than 75% (72 h) or 80% (48 h) while still allowing for the detection of all four *Campylobacter* patients, which presented with diarrhea within a 48-h time frame. Application of more sophisticated rejection rules (considering patient age, comorbidities or non-diarrheal manifestations) would have decreased test numbers without significant effects on yield. Former reports have also demonstrated that stool cultures taken after the third day of hospitalization in non-critically ill adult patients only yielded positive results in 0.2% [11]–0.6% [12].

We present data applicable to management of diarrhea in critically ill patients at the ICU and hereby confirm previous findings [13]. Our findings undermine the fact that critically ill patients with diarrhea should be managed in exactly the same way as patients on the normal ward to reduce the number of unnecessary stool cultures. The comparably high costs of stool cultures do not seem justified given the low yield and limited consequences. Due to the retrospective study design of our single-center study, further studies are needed to confirm our findings.

## Conclusion

Our data indicate that diarrhea in patients at the ICU is seldom caused by enteropathogenic bacteria. Critically ill patients should be assessed for alternative reasons underlying diarrhea and be tested once to exclude infection with *C. difficile* and in cases of suspected outbreaks for viruses but not for other enteropathogenic bacteria as long as symptoms commenced > 48 h after admission.

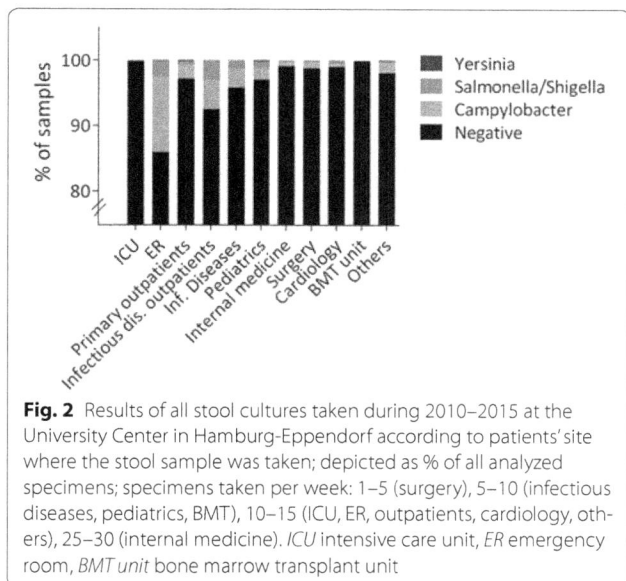

**Fig. 2** Results of all stool cultures taken during 2010–2015 at the University Center in Hamburg-Eppendorf according to patients' site where the stool sample was taken; depicted as % of all analyzed specimens; specimens taken per week: 1–5 (surgery), 5–10 (infectious diseases, pediatrics, BMT), 10–15 (ICU, ER, outpatients, cardiology, others), 25–30 (internal medicine). *ICU* intensive care unit, *ER* emergency room, *BMT unit* bone marrow transplant unit

**Authors' contributions**
All authors have done substantial contributions to conception and design. CFM helped in study design, data collection, data interpretation, data analysis and preparation of article. DD helped in data collection and data analysis. MC helped in data extraction, data interpretation and preparation of the manuscript. LB helped in data extraction and interpretation. SK helped in preparation of the manuscript. AWL helped in preparation of the manuscript. VF helped in study design, data analysis, data interpretation and preparation of the manuscript. All authors read and approved the final manuscript.

**Author details**
[1] First Department of Internal Medicine and Gastroenterology, University Hospital Hamburg-Eppendorf, Martinistr. 52, 20246 Hamburg, Germany. [2] Department of Intensive Care Medicine, University Hospital Hamburg-Eppendorf,

Hamburg, Germany. [3] Department of Microbiology, University Hospital Hamburg-Eppendorf, Hamburg, Germany.

**Acknowledgements**
None.

**Competing interests**
The authors declare that they have no competing interests.

## References

1. Thibault R, Graf S, Clerc A, Delieuvin N, Heidegger CP, Pichard C. Diarrhoea in the ICU: respective contribution of feeding and antibiotics. Crit Care. 2013;17:R153.
2. Wiesen P, Van Gossum A, Preiser JC. Diarrhoea in the critically ill. Curr Opin Crit Care. 2006;12:149–54.
3. Wei Y, Yang J, Wang J, et al. Successful treatment with fecal microbiota transplantation in patients with multiple organ dysfunction syndrome and diarrhea following severe sepsis. Crit Care. 2016;20:332.
4. Manthey CF, Eckmann L, Fuhrmann V. Therapy for *Clostridium difficile* infection—any news beyond Metronidazole and Vancomycin? Exp Rev Clin Pharmacol. 2017;10:1–12.
5. Riddle MS, DuPont HL, Connor BA. ACG clinical guideline: diagnosis, treatment, and prevention of acute diarrheal infections in adults. Am J Gastroenterol. 2016;111:602–22.
6. Bauer TM, Lalvani A, Fehrenbach J, et al. Derivation and validation of - guidelines for stool cultures for enteropathogenic bacteria other than *Clostridium difficile* in hospitalized adults. JAMA. 2001;285:313–9.
7. Deshpande A, Pasupuleti V, Patel P, et al. Repeat stool testing to diagnose *Clostridium difficile* infection using enzyme immunoassay does not increase diagnostic yield. Clin Gastroenterol Hepatol. 2011;9:665-9e1.
8. Mauch HPA, Herrmann M, Kniehl E, Kist M. MIQ 09: Gastrointestinale Infektionen Qualitätsstandards in der mikrobiologisch-infektiologischen Diagnostik. Amsterdam: Urban & Fischer Verlag/Elsevier GmbH; 2013.
9. Planche TD, Davies KA, Coen PG, et al. Differences in outcome according to *Clostridium difficile* testing method: a prospective multicentre diagnostic validation study of *C. difficile* infection. Lancet Infect Dis. 2013;13:936–45.
10. Hagel S, Epple HJ, Feurle GE, et al. S2k-guideline gastrointestinal infectious diseases and Whipple's disease. Z Gastroenterol. 2015;53:418–59.
11. Le Guern R, Loiez C, Grandbastien B, Courcol R, Wallet F. Performance of stool cultures before and after a 3-day hospitalization: fewer cultures, better for patients and for money. Diagn Microbiol Infect Dis. 2013;77:5–7.
12. Valenstein P, Pfaller M, Yungbluth M. The use and abuse of routine stool microbiology: a College of American Pathologists Q-probes study of 601 institutions. Arch Pathol Lab Med. 1996;120:206–11.
13. Tirlapur N, Puthucheary ZA, Cooper JA, et al. Diarrhoea in the critically ill is common, associated with poor outcome, and rarely due to *Clostridium difficile*. Sci Rep. 2016;6:24691.

# 9

# Use of speckle-tracking strain in preload-dependent patients, need for cautious interpretation!

C. Nafati[1,4*†] [ID], M. Gardette[1†], M. Leone[2,3], L. Reydellet[1], V. Blasco[1], A. Lannelongue[1], F. Sayagh[1], S. Wiramus[1], F. Antonini[2], J. Albanèse[1] and L. Zieleskiewicz[2]

## Abstract

**Background:** In critical patients, left ventricular ejection fraction and fractional shortening are used to reflect left ventricular systolic function. An emerging technique, two-dimensional-strain echocardiography, allows assessment of the left ventricle systolic longitudinal deformation (global longitudinal strain) and the speed at which this deformation occurs (systolic strain rate). This technique is of increasing use in critical patients in intensive care units and in the peri-operative period where preload constantly varies. Our objective, in this prospective single-center observational study, was to evaluate the effect of fluid resuscitation on two-dimensional-strain echocardiography measurements in preload-dependent critically ill patients. We included 49 patients with preload dependence attested by an increase of at least 10% in the left ventricular outflow track velocity–time integral measured by echocardiography during a passive leg raising maneuver. Echocardiography was performed before fluid resuscitation (echocardiography 1) and after preload independency achievement (echocardiography 2).

**Results:** Two-dimensional-strain echocardiography was feasible in 40 (82%) among the 49 patients. With preload dependence correction, the absolute value of global longitudinal strain and systolic strain rate was significantly increased from, respectively, $- 13.3 \pm 3.5$ to $- 18.4\% \pm 4.5$ ($p < 0.01$) and $- 1.11$ s$^{-1}$ $\pm 0.29$ to $- 1.55$ s$^{-1}$ $\pm 0.55$ ($p < 0.001$). The fluid resuscitation affects GLS and SSR in preload-dependent patients, with a shift, for GLS, from pathological to normal values.

**Conclusion:** In critically ill patients, the assessment of the systolic function by two-dimensional-strain echocardiography needs prior evaluation of preload dependency, in order to adequately interpret this variable. Future studies should assess the ability of global longitudinal strain to guide fluid management in the critically ill patients.

**Keywords:** Preload dependence, Fluid responsiveness, Passive leg raising, 2D-strain echocardiography, Speckle tracking

## Background

Systolic function assessment is crucial in the management of the critically ill patient. Using conventional echocardiography, left ventricular ejection fraction (LV EF) and fractional shortening are routinely used [1]. However, these variables depend on preload and afterload conditions [2]. They can be difficult to interpret in unstable patients such as those in septic shock [3].

Strain echocardiography (2D-strain) is a noninvasive ultrasound imaging technique that allows for an objective and quantitative evaluation of myocardial function. It measures the percentage of deformation of the left ventricle (LV) during systole (systolic strain) and the speed at which this deformation occurs (strain rate) [4, 5]. This technique has been validated after comparison with reference techniques: magnetic resonance imaging and sonomicrometry [5, 6]. The American Society

*Correspondence: Cyril.nafati@ap-hm.fr
†C. Nafati and M. Gardette are joint first authors and contributed equally
⁴ Service d'anesthésie et de réanimation, CHU de la Timone, 264 rue Saint Pierre, 13005 Marseille, France
Full list of author information is available at the end of the article

of Echocardiography and the European Association of Cardiovascular Imaging recommended measuring the Global Longitudinal Strain Systolic in apical 2-, 3- and 4-chamber views (GLS) using 2D-strain to evaluate the LV systolic function [7]. Normal values are below − 18% in healthy subjects [8, 9].

In critically ill patients, 2D-strain allows early diagnosis of cardiac injuries that are non-detectable with conventional examinations [10, 11]. Previous studies identified GLS as an independent factor of mortality [12, 13]. In the peri-operative setting, speckle tracking is an emerging tool for the early detection of right and left ventricular dysfunction [14]. Kovács et al. [15] found that 2D-strain reflects inotropism and correlates with elastance ($E_{max}$) and intraventricular pressure–volume curves in a rat model. In cardiology patients undergoing routine coronary angiography, fluid resuscitation did not affect GLS and systolic strain rate (SSR) [16]. Other studies [17, 18] in normal volunteers found diverging results. Conversely, animal studies suggest that fluid loading or acute unloading affects GLS and SSR [19, 20]. One clinical study in postcardiac surgery patients finds the same results, showing that the GLS and SSR are dependent on preload condition [21]. If for GLS, preload dependence is accepted, for the SSR this remains controversial. We hypothesized that this discrepancy was due to the position of the patient on the Frank and Starling curve. In the critically ill patient, preload and afterload constantly vary and preload dependency is an important parameter concerning up to 50% of these patients [22, 23]. The goal of our study was to evaluate for the first time in the ICU, the effect of fluid resuscitation on GLS and SSR in preload-dependent critically ill patients.

## Methods

Our study was a prospective observational study carried out in a single 12-bed polyvalent ICU at the University Hospital La Timone in Marseille, from August to December 2016. The protocol was approved by the Ethics Committee of the French Society of Anesthesiology and Intensive Care (IRB 00010254-2016-078) on August 18, 2016. Data collection was authorized by the CNIL (French Data Protection Authority, Receipt No. 1995927v0). Exclusion criteria were: patient under 18 years of age, absence of normal sinus rhythm, patient and/or person of trust's refusal to participate in the study.

We included all patients with preload dependence. Patients in acute circulatory failure were also included, if they were preload dependent. First, preload dependency was suspected according to at least one of the following criteria: hypotension or/and oligo-anuria or/and difficulty in weaning of catecholamine. Second, preload dependence was confirmed by an increase of at least 10% of the

left ventricular outflow track velocity–time integral (Δ LVOT VTI ≥ 10%) measured by echocardiography during a passive leg raising (PLR) [24]. If preload dependence was confirmed, the first echocardiogram was performed (echocardiography 1) with conventional and 2D-strain measurements. Then fluid resuscitation was started as follows: 500 mL of crystalloids administered over 30 min or 100 mL of 20% albumin administered over 60 min. The patient was considered as responsive if this fluid challenge was followed by a 15% increase in the LVOT VTI, and the patient was otherwise considered non-responsive [25]. The patient was considered as non-preload-dependent if the change in the (Δ) LVOT VTI during the PLR was below 10%. The fluid resuscitation could be repeated if needed, after checking the persistence of preload dependence criteria. When the patient was no longer preload dependent (Δ LVOT VTI PLR < 10%), a second echocardiogram was performed (echocardiography 2) with conventional and 2D-strain measurements. The choice of the resuscitation fluid (crystalloid or albumin 20%) was determined by the attending physician (Fig. 1).

Acute circulatory failure was defined as mean arterial pressure < 65 mmHg, urine output < 0.5 ml/kg/h, mottled skin or arterial blood lactate > 2 mmol/L [26].

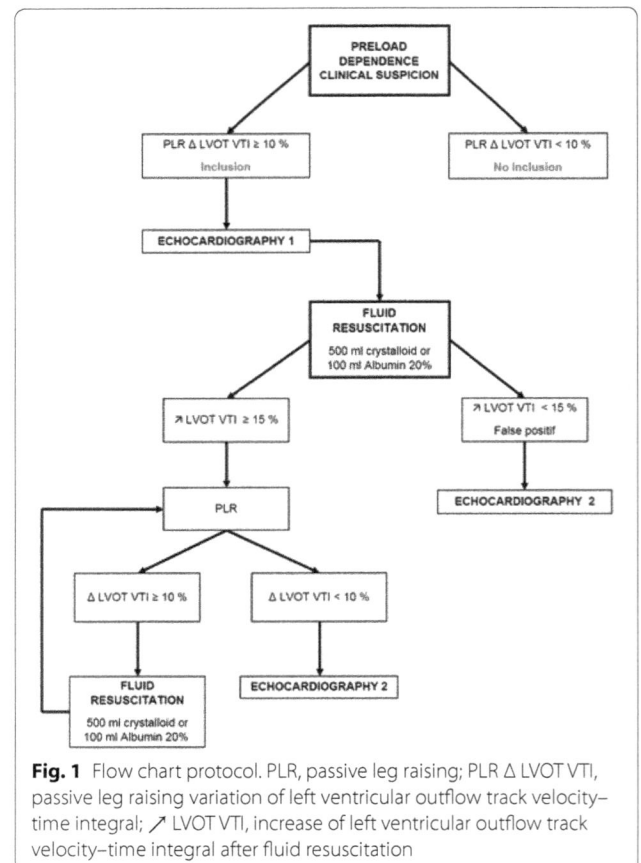

**Fig. 1** Flow chart protocol. PLR, passive leg raising; PLR Δ LVOT VTI, passive leg raising variation of left ventricular outflow track velocity–time integral; ↗ LVOT VTI, increase of left ventricular outflow track velocity–time integral after fluid resuscitation

The features (age, sex, weight, height, reason for admission), the cardiovascular comorbidities, SAPS II, SOFA and the arterial lactate levels were recorded for each patient included in the study. The arterial pressures (systolic, diastolic and mean) and heart rate were recorded before and after each fluid resuscitation. Mortality at 28 days was recorded by consulting the electronic patient files.

### Echocardiography protocol

Once the preload dependence was confirmed, two echocardiography studies were performed, the first one before fluid resuscitation (echocardiography 1) and the second one after, when the patient was no longer preload dependent (echocardiography 2). Both were performed by an expert certified physician (CN) and using a Philips CX 50 Compact Xtreme Ultrasound System (Philips Medical System. Andover. MA) and a 3.5-Hz probe. Conventional and 2D-strain echocardiography was used in each study.

The conventional evaluation was performed following the American Society of Echocardiography Recommendations [7]. The bi-dimensional measures were taken using a parasternal long-axis view with a motion ($M$)-mode to determine the right ventricle size, interventricular septal wall thickness, left ventricle size, ratio of right ventricle/left ventricle and the diameter of the LV outflow tract. The tricuspid annular plane systolic excursion (TAPSE) was measured from an apical 4-chamber view with M-mode. We visually verified using an apical 4-chamber view that the RV/LV ratio was < 1. The LVOT VTI was measured using pulse-wave Doppler from an apical 5-chamber view. Mitral flow was assessed using an apical 4-chamber view with pulse-wave Doppler allowing measurement of the $E$- and $A$-wave velocities, the $E/A$ ratio and the $E$-wave deceleration time.

Using tissue Doppler imaging from an apical 4-chamber view, the velocity of the septal and lateral mitral annulus $E'$ waves was measured ($E'_{lateral}$ and $E'_{medial}$), and $E'_{median}$ (average between $E'_{lateral}$ and $E'_{medial}$), $E/E'_{lateral}$, $E/E'_{medial}$ and $E/E'_{median}$ ratios were calculated. The ejection fraction was measured using the Simpson's biplane method in a 4- and 2-chamber view. All recorded values were averaged using three measurements.

With regard to the 2D-strain, a 2-s loop was recorded in DICOM format for each view with a frame rate above 50/s. The analysis and measures of strain and strain rate were performed off-line using the QLAB Philips software (Philips Medical System Andover, MA, USA) by a level 3 [27] operator (C.N.) fully trained in 2D-strain echocardiography. Particular attention was given to obtain an adequate grayscale image, allowing reliable delineation of myocardial tissue. The left ventricular myocardial contour was traced using the semiautomatized method of speckle tracking after identification of baso-septal, baso-lateral and apical points [28]. Adequate tracking can be verified in real time from the dynamic loop and manually adjusted if needed. The GLS was calculated as the average speckle-tracking systolic peak of strain from each of 18 LV segments from the apical 4-chamber view, 2-chamber view and 3-chamber view as recommended [7]. The SSR was the most negative value of the strain rate curve occurring after the opening of the aortic valve. The measure of GLS was considered successful if at least the 4-chamber systolic strain (S4C) and one or both strain among the 2 (S2C)- and 3-chamber view (S3C) were obtained [8]; otherwise, the LV was considered to have insufficient image quality. Segmental data were not analyzed. Strain and strain rate are negative values; the more negative the value is, the greater the deformation and LV function are. GLS and SSR were considered decreased when GLS > − 15% and SSR > − 1 s$^{-1}$ [29].

### Statistical analysis

All analyses were performed using R-Project for Statistical Computing 2.14 (The R Foundation, Vienna, Austria). Categorical variables were expressed as numbers and percentages (%). Continuous variables were expressed as mean ± SD or median and interquartile range (25th–75th) depending on their distribution. The Kruskal–Wallis test, the Fisher exact test and the ANOVA test $r^2$ were used to compare the distribution of variables. In univariate analysis, factors were considered significant when $p < 0.05$. We calculated that at least 38 patients would need to be enrolled to detect a 4% increase in GLS after fluid expansion with a 90% statistical power and a two-sided alpha value of 0.05. In order to exclude the patients in whom cardiac ultrasound was not technically feasible, we decided to include 49 patients. The correlation between the global longitudinal strain and the 4-chamber strain was performed using Spearman's method. From all patients, intraoperator variability of GLS was determined by the intraclass correlation coefficient.

### Results

Forty-nine patients were included over the period of August–December 2016.

### Clinical characteristics of study patients

The patients' clinical characteristics are presented in Table 1. Preload dependency was suspected because of hypotension in 29 (59%) patients, anuria in 8 (16%) patients and due to difficult catecholamine weaning in 12 (25%) patients.

**Table 1 Clinical characteristics of study patients**

| | |
|---|---|
| Total number of patient (*n*) | 49 |
| Sex ratio (m/w) | 29/20 |
| Age (years) | 64 ± 15 |
| *BMI* (kg/cm²) | 25 ± 5 |
| Mechanical ventilation [*n* (%)] | 18 (36) |
| Vasopressor [*n* (%)] | 22 (45) |
| Lactate | 2.9 ± 3.9 |
| SAPS II | 51 ± 17 |
| SOFA | 7.2 ± 3.5 |
| 28 Days mortality rate [*n* (%)] | 11 (22) |
| Cardiovascular comorbidities | |
|   Arterial hypertension | 18 (37) |
|   Coronary disease | 5 (10) |
|   Arrhythmia | 1 (2) |
|   Valvular disease | 1 (2) |
| Reason for admission in ICU [*n* (%)] | |
|   Septic shock | 16 (32) |
|   Hemorrhagic shock | 6 (12) |
|   Cardiogenic shock | 1 (2) |
|   Surgery | 15 (30) |
|   Cardiac arrest | 2 (4.10) |
|   Acute pancreatitis | 1 (2) |
|   Myasthenia | 1 (2) |
|   Hepatitis | 2 (4.1) |
|   Suicide | 2 (4.1) |
|   Liver transplantation | 3 (6.1) |

Data are expressed as number (%) or mean ± SD

*BMI* body mass index, *SAPS* Simplified Acute Physiology Score, *SOFA* Sequential Organ Failure Assessment, *ICU* intensive care unit

## Ultrasound data

Data are shown in Table 2. For 9 (18%) patients, the echocardiography quality was insufficient for strain measurement resulting in analysis of data in 40 patients. The average frame rate was 60/s ± 1.6.

## Effect of fluid resuscitation on standard clinical and echocardiographic values

Crystalloid, albumin or both were administered to 25 (51%) patients, 15 (30%) patients and 9 (19%) patients, respectively. The volume of crystalloid and albumin was 960 ± 310 and 256 ± 51 mL, respectively.

There was a significant increase in systolic arterial pressure (SAP), diastolic arterial pressure (DAP) and mean arterial pressure (MAP) after fluid resuscitation. There was also a nonsignificant decrease in heart rate (HR).

Out of the 49 preload-dependent patients, 48 patients increased their cardiac output after fluid resuscitation by at least 15%. The LVOT VTI increased from 15.6 cm ± 3.7 to 21.1 cm ± 4.5 before and after fluid

**Table 2 Echocardiography and clinical data before and after fluid resuscitation**

| | Before | After | *p* value |
|---|---|---|---|
| Heart rate (p/m) | 103 ± 20 | 97 ± 15 | 0.18 |
| SAP (mmHg) | 95 ± 17 | 119 ± 14 | < 0.001 |
| DAP (mmHg) | 50 ± 12 | 57 ± 10 | 0.01 |
| MAP (mmHg) | 65 ± 13 | 77 ± 10 | < 0.001 |
| E (cm/s) | 73 ± 23 | 91 ± 26 | 0.003 |
| E/A | 0.9 ± 0.3 | 1.0 ± 0.3 | 0.13 |
| DTE | 200 ± 16 | 200 ± 12 | 0.78 |
| $E'_{SEPT}$ (cm/s) | 13.6 ± 3.7 | 12.9 ± 3.4 | 0.36 |
| $E'_{LAT}$ (cm/s) | 14.2 ± 3.6 | 14.3 ± 3.5 | 0.79 |
| $E/E'_{SEPT}$ | 5.8 ± 2 | 7.3 ± 2.4 | 0.004 |
| $E/E'_{lat}$ | 5.4 ± 1.9 | 6.7 ± 2.4 | 0.001 |
| $E/E'_{moy}$ | 5.5 ± 1.9 | 6.9 ± 3.3 | 0.005 |
| LVOT VTI (cm) | 15.6 ± 3.7 | 21.1 ± 4.5 | < 0.001 |
| CO (L/min) | 4.4 ± 1.8 | 5.7 ± 5.7 | 0.007 |
| CI (L/min/m²) | 2.4 ± 0.9 | 3.1 ± 1.2 | 0.007 |
| LV EF (%) | 61.3 ± 15.9 | 60.7 ± 15 | 0.78 |
| LVOT diameter (cm) | 1.8 ± 0.1 | 1.8 ± 0.1 | 0.89 |
| LVTDV (mL) | 104.5 ± 29 | 131 ± 34 | < 0.001 |
| RV/LV | 0.6 ± 0.1 | 0.6 ± 0.1 | 0.62 |
| TAPSE (mm) | 22 ± 7 | 23 ± 5 | 0.87 |
| SSR (s⁻¹⁾ | − 1.1 ± 0.29 | − 1.55 ± 0.55 | < 0.001 |
| GLS | − 13.3 ± 3.5 | − 18.4 ± − 4.5 | < 0.001 |
| S4C (%) | − 13.5 ± 4.1 | − 18.7 ± 4.9 | < 0.001 |
| S2C (%) | − 13.4 ± 3 | − 18.4 ± 4.8 | < 0.001 |
| S3C (%) | − 12.6 ± 3.7 | − 18.4 ± 4.8 | < 0.001 |

Data are expressed as mean ± SD

*SAP* systolic arterial pressure, *DAP* diastolic arterial pressure, *MAP* mean arterial pressure, *E* peak early diastolic transmittal flow velocity, *E/A* ratio of e to a, *TDE* E-wave deceleration time, *E'ₗ* peak early diastolic lateral mitral annulus velocity, *E'ₛ* peak early diastolic septal mitral annulus velocity, *E/E'* ratio of E to E', *LVTO VTI* left ventricular outflow tract velocity–time integral, *CO* cardiac output, *LV EF* left ventricle ejection fraction, *TAPSE* tricuspid annular systolic excursion, *LVDV* left ventricular tele-diastolic volume, *SSR* systolic strain rate, *GLS* global longitudinal strain, *S4C* 4-chamber systolic strain, *S2C* two-chamber systolic strain, *S3C* three-chamber systolic strain

resuscitation ($p < 0.01$). After fluid resuscitation ($p < 0.01$), cardiac index increased from 2.4 ± 0.9 to 3.1 ± 1.2 L/min/m² ($p < 0.01$) (Fig. 2). We observed a significant increase in left ventricular end-diastolic volume (LVEDV): 104.5 ± 29–131 ± 34 mL ($p < 0.001$). We did not find a significant change in the LV EF after fluid resuscitation. In our study, no patients had right heart failure.

After fluid resuscitation, *E*-wave significantly increased from 73 ± 23 to 91 ± 27 cm/s ($p < 0.01$). $E/E'_{lateral}$, $E/E'_{medial}$ and $E/E'_{median}$ increased from 5.4 ± 1.9 to 6.7 ± 2.4 ($p < 0\ 0.01$), 5.8 ± 2 to 7.3 ± 2.4 ($p < 0.01$) and 5.5 ± 1.9 to 6.9 ± 2.3 ($p < 0.01$).

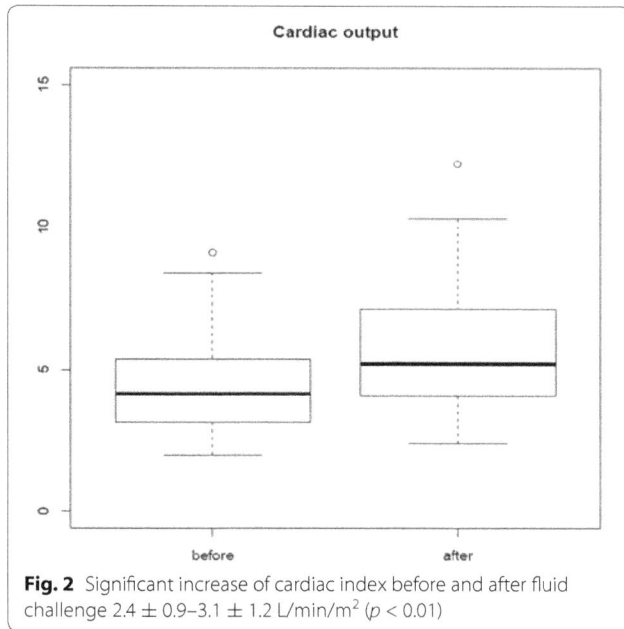

**Fig. 2** Significant increase of cardiac index before and after fluid challenge $2.4 \pm 0.9$–$3.1 \pm 1.2$ L/min/m$^2$ ($p < 0.01$)

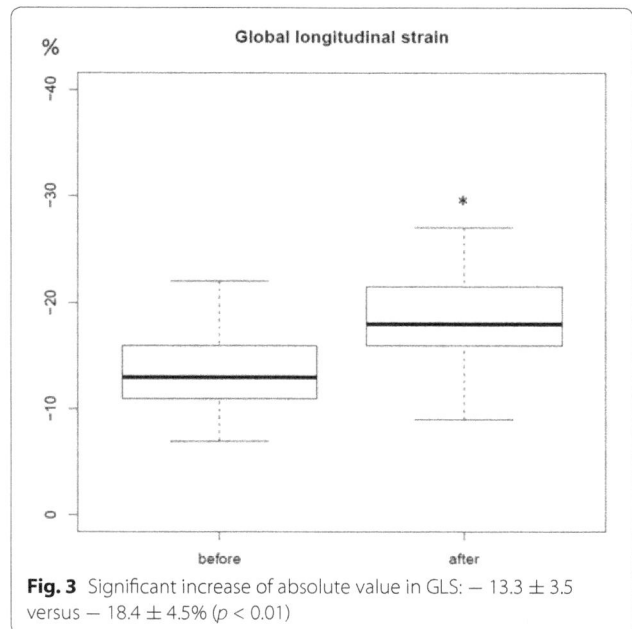

**Fig. 3** Significant increase of absolute value in GLS: $-13.3 \pm 3.5$ versus $-18.4 \pm 4.5\%$ ($p < 0.01$)

### Effect of fluid resuscitation on strain and strain rate values

After fluid resuscitation, the absolute value of GLS significantly changed from $-13.3\% \pm 3.5$ to $-18.4\% \pm 4.5$ ($p < 0.01$) (Fig. 3). This variation was confirmed by the absolute strain values measured in the four-chamber ($14\% \pm 4.1$ vs. $19\% \pm 4.9$), three-chamber ($13\% \pm 3.5$ vs. $18\% \pm 4.3$) and two-chamber ($13\% \pm 3.7$ vs. $18\% \pm 4.8$) views ($p < 0.01$). The GLS and the 4-chamber view strain values had good correlation ($r = 0.81$, $p < 0.01$) (Fig. 4). Regarding the SSR, the absolute value of SSR significantly changed from $-1.11$ s$^{-1}$ $\pm 0.29$ to $-1.55$ s$^{-1}$ $\pm 0.55$ ($p < 0.001$).

The intraclass correlation coefficient of the intraoperator variability of GLS was 0.92 ($p < 0.001$).

### Discussion

The main result of our study was to show that fluid resuscitation affects GLS and SSR in preload-dependent patients, with a shift, for GLS, from pathological to normal values.

Hence, in the critically ill patient, pathological values of GLS should be interpreted with prudence.

Recently, Boissier et al. [30] showed that GLS was inversely correlated with afterload. They did not find a correlation between preload and GLS values. However, based on the low collapsibility index of the superior vena cava reported in their patients, preload dependency was unlikely. Certain studies do not find modification of the SSR [17, 31] and/or of the GLS [18, 31] following preload variations. In these studies, this can be explained by the population consisting of healthy conscious volunteers

(Abali et al. and Anderson et al.), the preload variation being smaller than that observed in the ICU patient and that the patients were not necessarily in a preload dependency state (Mendes et al.). Furthermore, these variations would activate baroreceptor-mediated counter-regulatory changes in the sympathetic outflow to the heart in such a population. This physiologic response was probably insufficient in our population of preload-dependent patients. Recently, Fredholm et al. [21] in a clinical study of postoperative cardiac surgery found similar results. They conclude that GLS and SSR were preload dependent. We explain the significant increase in the GLS and SSR, after preload correction, by the increased end-diastolic stretch of the left ventricle fibers (a significant increase in LVEDV $104.5 \pm 29$ mL to $131 \pm 34$, $p < 0.001$). The patients being in the preload-dependent zone are on the steep portion of the Franck–Starling curve. The preload increase then leads to an increase in the contraction force and velocity, as shown by Sonnenblick et al. in an experimental study in 1962 [32]. This does not occur in non-preload-dependent patients. In our false-negative patient, GLS or SSR did not change after fluid resuscitation.

More specifically for the SSR, in our study, there was a significant increase with preload correction; however, in contrast with the GLS, its value in hypovolemic patients is not pathological ($-1.11 \pm 0.29$ s$^{-1}$). We explain this by the fact that not only is SSR influenced by preload, but it is also influenced by the heart rate. These results are aligned with those of Fredholm et al., who found in their

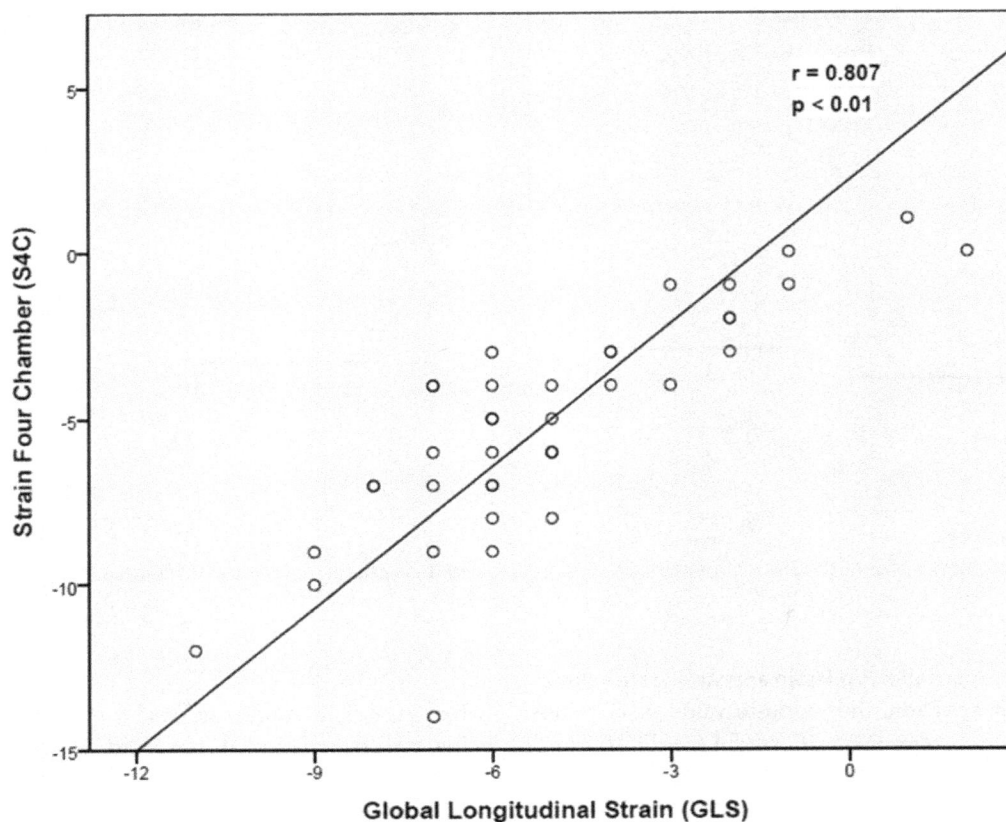

**Fig. 4** Correlation of global longitudinal strain and strain 4 chamber $r = 0.81$ ($p < 0.01$)

study that the SSR is both preload and pace dependent. We believe that the SSR staying in a physiologic zone is due to the tachycardia provoked by the hypovolemia (HR: $103 \pm 20$ in our study). This is, in our opinion, a physiologically adaptive mechanism to maintain a certain intrinsic contractility in hypovolemic patients. This phenomenon is known as the force–frequency relationship [33].

We are not surprised that the LV EF is around 60% in our preload-dependent cohort. Indeed, in these hypovolemic patients, the preload is lowered and the cardiac chambers are reduced in size. The LVESV is decreased and tends toward zero (kissing heart) which leads to an LV EF increase tending toward 100% (LV EF = LVEDV − LVESV/LVEDV × 100). Thus, in our hypovolemic patients, the LV EF is mathematically elevated. Furthermore, we had a high proportion of septic shock patients in our population (32%), and because of the vasoplegia intrinsic to this pathology, there were numerous hyperkinetic patients with a LV EF > 60%. Boissier et al. found, in their cohort of septic shock patients, 103 patients with normal or hyperkinetic LV EF out of 130 [30].

We did not find a significant increase in LV EF after preload correction, whereas we did find a significant increase in LVEDV and GLS. We explain this because the LV EF and GLS are not comparable. The GLS formula $L - L_o/L_o$ ($L$: the length of contracted myocardial fibers, $L_o$: the length of stretched myocardial fibers) refers to deformation of myocardial fibers, whereas LV EF refers to volumes and is therefore also dependent on ventriculo-arterial coupling [2]. Consequently, the fluid expansion induces changes in arterial elastance which may have more impact on EF than on GLS. Moreover, in the case of acute hypovolemia, as previously discussed, falsely elevated LV EF may be encountered due to a end-systolic collapse of the left ventricular. Therefore, after fluid loading and correction of left ventricular collapse the LV EF may not systematically increase even in the case of fluid responsiveness and increased inotropy. Finally, the LV EF was measured by Simpson's biplane method, and even if this is the reference technique, it is associated with a non-negligible inter- and intraobserver variability which could have masked the LV EF modification.

Based on our study, the influence of preload on the strain values measured is critical to consider. Indeed, for preload-dependent patients, a low absolute value of GLS can lead to erroneous diagnoses of systolic dysfunction. As compared with previous studies evaluating strain in septic shock, our study sheds a new light on this technology [34–37]. Pathological strain values detect early myocardial dysfunction. However, it may not be relevant to assess systolic function in patients with unstable hemodynamic conditions. Therefore, in these patients, a low GLS value should push the clinician to question first a preload dependency and then a myocardial dysfunction. Before any strict evaluation of LV systolic function and before starting any inotropic treatment, hypovolemia should be ruled out.

In line with our previous study [13], the success rate of strain measurement was 82%, matching with cardiology studies [38]. However, in the critically ill patient, the success rate can drop to 50% [30]. In this regard, the use of a single apical 4-chamber view could facilitate the diffusion of speckle-tracking use in critically ill patients. Indeed, in our cohort, GLS (the average of the two, three and four apical views) and longitudinal strain of the apical four-chamber view only were strongly correlated.

Our study has several limitations of which we are aware. It is a single-center study. A single operator performed all of the measurements. Therefore, we could not assess the interoperator variability. Our resuscitation protocol left the choice of fluid solution to the prescribing physician. The albumin was administered over 30 min and the crystalloid over 60 min. These are indeed longer durations than recommended. Future studies should consider the association of this value and GLS.

## Conclusion

Our study showed that GLS was influenced by fluid resuscitation in preload-dependent patients. Interestingly, values shifted from pathological to normal after fluid resuscitation. In the critically ill patients, the assessment of systolic function by 2D-strain needs prior evaluation of preload dependency, in order to adequately interpret this variable. GLS variations after an increase in venous return could be a marker of the patient position in the Frank–Starling curve. Future studies evaluating the interest of GLS for guiding fluid resuscitation are required.

### Abbreviations
LV EF: left ventricular ejection fraction; LV: left ventricle; LVTDV: left ventricular tele-diastolic volume; LVSTV: left ventricular tele-systolic volume; LVOT VTI: left ventricular outflow track velocity–time integral; Δ LVOT VTI: variation of left ventricular outflow track velocity; PLR: passive leg raising; GLS: global longitudinal systolic strain; S4C: four-chamber systolic strain; S3C: three-chamber systolic strain; S2C: two-chamber systolic strain.

### Authors' contributions
CN helped in conception and design of the study, analysis and interpretation of the data and final approval of the article; MG analyzed and interpreted the data, drafted the article, collected and assembled the data; CN and MG contributed equally and are joint first authors; ML and LZ critically revised the article for important intellectual content; LR and FA contributed to statistical expertise; VB collected and assembled the data; AL, FS and SW contributed to provision of study materials or patients; and JA helped in administrative, technical or logistical support. All authors read and approved the final manuscript.

### Author details
[1] Department of Anesthesia and Intensive Care Medicine, University Hospital of Marseille, la Timone Hospital, Marseille, France. [2] Department of Anaesthesia and Intensive Care Medicine, University Hospital of Marseille, North Hospital, Marseille, France. [3] Centre d'Investigation Clinique, Aix-Marseille University, AP-HM, 14901 Marseille, France. [4] Service d'anesthésie et de réanimation, CHU de la Timone, 264 rue Saint Pierre, 13005 Marseille, France.

### Acknowledgements
None.

### Competing interests
The authors declare that they have no competing interests.

### Funding
None.

### References
1. McLean AS. Echocardiography in shock management. Crit Care Lond Engl. 2016;20:275.
2. Robotham JL, Takata M, Berman M, Harasawa Y. Ejection fraction revisited. Anesthesiology. 1991;74(1):172–83.
3. Jardin F, et al. Persistent preload defect in severe sepsis despite fluid loading: a longitudinal echocardiographic study in patients with septic shock. Chest. 1999;116(5):1354–9.
4. D'hooge J, et al. Regional strain and strain rate measurements by cardiac ultrasound: principles, implementation and limitations. Eur J Echocardiogr J Work Group Echocardiogr Eur Soc Cardiol. 2000;1(3):154–70.
5. Pellerin D, Sharma R, Elliott P, Veyrat C. Tissue Doppler, strain, and strain rate echocardiography for the assessment of left and right systolic ventricular function. Heart. 2003;89(Suppl 3):iii9–17.
6. Amundsen BH, et al. Noninvasive myocardial strain measurement by speckle tracking echocardiography: validation against sonomicrometry and tagged magnetic resonance imaging. J Am Coll Cardiol. 2006;47(4):789–93.
7. Lang RM, et al. Recommendations for cardiac chamber quantification by echocardiography in adults: an update from the American Society of Echocardiography and the European Association of Cardiovascular Imaging. J Am Soc Echocardiogr Off Publ Am Soc Echocardiogr. 2015;28(1):1. e14–39.e14.
8. Muraru D, et al. Left ventricular myocardial strain by three-dimensional speckle-tracking echocardiography in healthy subjects: reference values and analysis of their physiologic and technical determinants. J Am Soc Echocardiogr Off Publ Am Soc Echocardiogr. 2014;27(8):858.e1–871.e1.
9. Smiseth OA, Torp H, Opdahl A, Haugaa KH, Urheim S. Myocardial strain imaging: how useful is it in clinical decision making? Eur Heart J. 2016;37(15):1196–207.
10. Shahul S, et al. Detection of myocardial dysfunction in septic shock: a speckle-tracking echocardiography study. Anesth Analg. 2015;121(6):1547–54.
11. Dalla K, Hallman C, Bech-Hanssen O, Haney M, Ricksten S-E. Strain echocardiography identifies impaired longitudinal systolic function in patients with septic shock and preserved ejection fraction. Cardiovasc Ultrasound. 2015;13:30.
12. Orde SR, et al. Outcome prediction in sepsis: speckle tracking echocardiography based assessment of myocardial function. Crit Care Lond Engl. 2014;18(4):R149.
13. Nafati C, et al. Two-dimensional-strain echocardiography in intensive care unit patients: a prospective, observational study. J Clin Ultrasound JCU. 2016;44(6):368–74.

14. Kumar A, Puri GD, Bahl A. Transesophageal echocardiography, 3-dimensional and speckle tracking together as sensitive markers for early outcome in patients with left ventricular dysfunction undergoing cardiac surgery. J Cardiothorac Vasc Anesth. 2017;31(5):1695–701.

15. Kovács A, et al. Strain and strain rate by speckle-tracking echocardiography correlate with pressure-volume loop-derived contractility indices in a rat model of athlete's heart. Am J Physiol Heart Circ Physiol. 2015;308(7):H743–8.

16. Burns AT, La Gerche A, D'hooge J, MacIsaac AI, Prior DL. Left ventricular strain and strain rate: characterization of the effect of load in human subjects. Eur J Echocardiogr J Work Group Echocardiogr Eur Soc Cardiol. 2010;11(3):283–9.

17. Abali G, Tokgözoğlu L, Ozcebe OI, Aytemir K, Nazli N. Which Doppler parameters are load independent? A study in normal volunteers after blood donation. J Am Soc Echocardiogr Off Publ Am Soc Echocardiogr. 2005;18(12):1260–5.

18. Andersen NH, Terkelsen CJ, Sloth E, Poulsen SH. Influence of preload alterations on parameters of systolic left ventricular long-axis function: a Doppler tissue study. J Am Soc Echocardiogr Off Publ Am Soc Echocardiogr. 2004;17(9):941–7.

19. Rösner A, et al. Left ventricular size determines tissue Doppler-derived longitudinal strain and strain rate. Eur J Echocardiogr J Work Group Echocardiogr Eur Soc Cardiol. 2009;10(2):271–7.

20. Dahle GO, et al. The influence of acute unloading on left ventricular strain and strain rate by speckle tracking echocardiography in a porcine model. Am J Physiol Heart Circ Physiol. 2016;310(10):H1330–9.

21. Fredholm M, Jörgensen K, Houltz E, Ricksten S-E. Load-dependence of myocardial deformation variables—a clinical strain-echocardiographic study. Acta Anaesthesiol Scand. 2017;61(9):1155–65.

22. Monnet X, Marik PE, Teboul J-L. Prediction of fluid responsiveness: an update. Ann Intensive Care. 2016;6(1):111.

23. Michard F, Teboul J-L. Predicting fluid responsiveness in ICU patients: a critical analysis of the evidence. Chest. 2002;121(6):2000–8.

24. Monnet X, Marik P, Teboul J-L. Passive leg raising for predicting fluid responsiveness: a systematic review and meta-analysis. Intensive Care Med. 2016;42:1935–47.

25. Marik PE, Monnet X, Teboul J-L. Hemodynamic parameters to guide fluid therapy. Ann. Intensive Care. 2011;1(1):1.

26. Muller L, et al. An increase in aortic blood flow after an infusion of 100 mL colloid over 1 min can predict fluid responsiveness: the mini-fluid challenge study. Anesthesiology. 2011;115(3):541–7.

27. Mayo PH, et al. American College of Chest Physicians/La Société de Réanimation de Langue Française statement on competence in critical care ultrasonography. Chest. 2009;135(4):1050–60.

28. Mondillo S, et al. Speckle-tracking echocardiography: a new technique for assessing myocardial function. J Ultrasound Med Off J Am Inst Ultrasound Med. 2011;30(1):71–83.

29. Dalen H, et al. Segmental and global longitudinal strain and strain rate based on echocardiography of 1266 healthy individuals: the HUNT study in Norway. Eur J Echocardiogr J Work Group Echocardiogr Eur Soc Cardiol. 2010;11(2):176–83.

30. Boissier F, et al. Left ventricular systolic dysfunction during septic shock: the role of loading conditions. Intensive Care Med. 2017;43(5):633–42.

31. Mendes L, et al. Load-independent parameters of diastolic and systolic function by speckle tracking and tissue doppler in hemodialysis patients. Rev Port Cardiol Orgao Of Soc Port Cardiol Port J Cardiol Off J Port Soc Cardiol. 2008;27(9):1011–25.

32. Sonnenblick EH. Force–velocity relations in mammalian heart muscle. Am J Physiol. 1962;202:931–9.

33. Bombardini T, Correia MJ, Cicerone C, Agricola E, Ripoli A, Picano E. Force–frequency relationship in the echocardiography laboratory: a noninvasive assessment of Bowditch treppe? J Am Soc Echocardiogr Off Publ Am Soc Echocardiogr. 2003;16(6):646–55.

34. Basu S, Frank LH, Fenton KE, Sable CA, Levy RJ, Berger JT. Two-dimensional speckle tracking imaging detects impaired myocardial performance in children with septic shock, not recognized by conventional echocardiography. Pediatr Crit Care Med J Soc Crit Care Med World Fed Pediatr Intensive Crit Care Soc. 2012;13(3):259–64.

35. De Geer L, Engvall J, Oscarsson A. Strain echocardiography in septic shock—a comparison with systolic and diastolic function parameters, cardiac biomarkers and outcome. Crit Care Lond Engl. 2015;19:122.

36. Ng PY, Sin WC, Ng AK-Y, Chan WM. Speckle tracking echocardiography in patients with septic shock: a case control study (SPECKSS). Crit Care Lond Engl. 2016;20(1):145.

37. Yang F, et al. Two-dimensional speckle tracking imaging in assessing the left ventricular systolic function and its dynamic changes of patients with septic shock. Zhonghua Wei Zhong Bing Ji Jiu Yi Xue. 2017;29(8):721–5.

38. Yingchoncharoen T, Agarwal S, Popović ZB, Marwick TH. Normal ranges of left ventricular strain: a meta-analysis. J Am Soc Echocardiogr Off Publ Am Soc Echocardiogr. 2013;26(2):185–91.

# 10

# Nutrition delivery of a model-based ICU glycaemic control system

Kent W. Stewart[1]*[iD], J. Geoffrey Chase[1], Christopher G. Pretty[1] and Geoffrey M. Shaw[2]

## Abstract

**Background:** Hyperglycaemia is commonplace in the adult intensive care unit (ICU), associated with increased morbidity and mortality. Effective glycaemic control (GC) can reduce morbidity and mortality, but has proven difficult. STAR is a proven, effective model-based ICU GC protocol that uniquely maintains normo-glycaemia by changing both insulin and nutrition interventions to maximise nutrition in the context of GC in the 4.4–8.0 mmol/L range. Hence, the level of nutrition it provides is a time-varying estimate of the patient-specific ability to take up glucose.

**Methods:** First, the clinical provision of nutrition by STAR in Christchurch Hospital, New Zealand ($N = 221$ Patients) is evaluated versus other ICUs, based on the Cahill et al. survey of 158 ICUs. Second, the inter- and intra- patient variation of nutrition delivery with STAR is analysed. Nutrition rates are in terms of percentage of caloric goal achieved.

**Results:** Mean nutrition rates clinically achieved by STAR were significantly higher than the mean and best ICU surveyed, for the first 3 days of ICU stay. There was large inter-patient variation in nutrition rates achieved per day, which reduced overtime as patient-specific metabolic state stabilised. Median intra-patient variation was 12.9%; however, the interquartile range of the mean per-patient nutrition rates achieved was 74.3–98.2%, suggesting patients do not deviate much from their mean patient-specific nutrition rate. Thus, the ability to tolerate glucose intake varies significantly between, rather than within, patients.

**Conclusions:** Overall, STAR's protocol-driven changes in nutrition rate provide higher nutrition rates to hyperglycaemic patients than those of 158 ICUs from 20 countries. There is significant inter-patient variability between patients to tolerate and uptake glucose, where intra-patient variability over stay is much lower. Thus, a best nutrition rate is likely patient specific for patients requiring GC. More importantly, these overall outcomes show high nutrition delivery and safe, effective GC are not exclusive and that restricting nutrition for GC does not limit overall nutritional intake compared to other ICUs.

**Keywords:** Glycaemic control, Nutrition delivery, Clinical workload, Intensive care unit, Critical care, Hyperglycaemia, Hypoglycaemia, Model-based, Targeted

## Background

The ICU patient is under considerable physiological stress, resulting in 20–40% of patients experiencing dysregulation of blood glucose (BG) levels [1] and hyperglycaemia [2, 3], which is associated with increased morbidity and mortality [4–6]. Glycaemic variability due to poor control [7] has also been independently associated with mortality [7–10]. Effective glycaemic control (GC) can reduce mortality and morbidity [11–14], organ failure [15] and cost of care [16, 17]. However, due to inter- and intra- patient variability [18–21], GC has proven difficult, and many protocols have increased hypoglycaemia, also associated with increased mortality [22–25], due to the inability to provide consistent, safe and effective GC [25–31].

The model-based STAR (Stochastic TARgeted) protocol has proven to be safe, consistent and effective [32, 33]. The tablet-based STAR protocol uses a clinically evaluated [34, 35] physiological insulin–glucose model [36, 37]

*Correspondence: kent.stewart@pg.canterbury.ac.nz
[1] Department of Mechanical Engineering, Centre for Bio-Engineering, University of Canterbury, Private Bag 4800, Christchurch 8140, New Zealand
Full list of author information is available at the end of the article

in conjunction with a stochastic model of metabolic variability [38, 39], to estimate a patient-specific current metabolic state and its potential future variability [40, 41]. Thus, treatments are selected by forward simulation with a clinically specified desired risk of light hypoglycaemia (5% BG < 4.4 mmol/L) due to these possible future variations. STAR has proven to be safe, effective and replicable across ICUs [32].

Uniquely, STAR maintains normal BG levels by changing both insulin and nutrition interventions [33]. Changing nutrition interventions differentiates STAR from other ICU GC protocols [42], as most only change insulin interventions (e.g. [43–47]). STAR maximises nutrition in the context of GC in the 4.4–8.0 mmol/L range [33, 40]. Hence, the level of nutrition it provides is a patient-specific, time-varying estimate of the ability to take up glucose and is reduced in the face of significant insulin resistance.

Currently, there is also significant debate over the appropriate amount to feed an ICU patient. Many studies have shown mixed results in reviewing caloric intake, route, and timing and their relation to outcome [48–58]. Cahill et al. [59] surveyed the overall nutrition performance of 158 ICUs, from 20 countries, finding significant variation in nutrition delivery. This study also found an ideal relation to mortality at 85% of the caloric goal nutrition rate set by the respective ICU [51], based on a model fit to the large collection of retrospective survey data obtained from 158 ICUs in 20 countries. This 'Heyland ideal' value and the best performing unit surveyed are used in this study as a guideline for assessing the clinical performance of STAR nutrition delivery.

This paper first evaluates the clinical provision of nutrition by STAR, to a cohort of hyperglycaemic ICU patients, versus all ICU patients in other ICUs based on the survey results of Cahill et al. [59] to assess if safe, effective GC precludes or limits high nutrition delivery, as well as determining if nutrition restriction to obtain GC limits total nutritional intake. Second, the inter- and intra- patient variation of nutritional delivery, while maintaining normo-glycaemia, is assessed to evaluate a range of glucose/nutrition tolerance in ICU patients on GC. The main outcomes assess clinically provided nutrition using STAR at the cohort level in an international context and then show a best nutrition rate is likely patient specific, particularly for patients requiring GC.

## Methods
### STAR GC protocol
#### GC protocol overview
Starting criteria for STAR is two successive BG measurements over 8.0 mmol/L within a 4-h period. After two measurements are taken, integral-based parameter fitting

[60] is used to identify a clinically evaluated model-based insulin sensitivity [34–36]. This value is used with a stochastic model, based on historical data, [33, 38, 39, 61] to find the 5th and 95th percentile potential future insulin sensitivity values. These 5th and 95th percentile insulin sensitivity values and a potential insulin and nutrition intervention are then used to forward-simulate the likely resulting 5th and 95th percentile BG values for that intervention to find the intervention with 5% risk of BG < 4.4–4.6 mmol/L [33, 40]. Full details can be found in [33].

STAR modifies nutrition rate depending on the bounds of predicted potential behaviour, with a preference to increase insulin before reducing nutrition, and to raise nutrition whenever possible [33, 40]. STAR modulates this nutrition rate between 30 and 100% of the caloric goal, with a maximum step change of ± 30% caloric goal per hour [33]. ACCP guidelines are used to determine patient-specific daily caloric goal intake of 25 kcal/kg/day [62].

Overall, STAR attempts to provide the maximum nutrition rate a patient can tolerate while safely keeping BG in the 4.4–8.0 mmol/L range. However, insulin saturation limits the impact of insulin to lower BG levels on its own [63–65], requiring nutrition restriction in some patients or time periods. Hence, based on STAR's control predictions, providing excess carbohydrates to a patient above this limit would result in excess BG. Therefore, the nutrition rate achieved by STAR represents a 'STAR ideal' patient-specific nutrition rate that maximises their likelihood of falling within the targeted 4.4–8.0 mmol/L BG band, based on their current ability to tolerate glucose.

#### Christchurch clinical implementation
Clinical data from 221 hyperglycaemic ICU patients treated with STAR (2011–2015) [32] in the Christchurch Hospital ICU (mixed medical surgical) were used to assess the performance of its variable nutrition delivery. BG, insulin and nutrition data were collected from STAR tablets and thus only exists when patients are on GC. STAR has proven to provide excellent GC in this cohort spending over 88% time, per patient, in the targeted 4.4–8.0 mmol/L range, as shown in Table 1. STAR patients in Christchurch are typically fed enterally with the low carbohydrate Glucerna™ Select (74.6 g/L Carbohydrate, 50 g/L Protein, 21.1 g/L Fibre, Abbott Labs, Illinois, USA), where carbohydrate concentrations exclude indigestible fibre. Parenteral nutrition (PN) is used occasionally, at clinician discretion, to supplement enteral nutrition. While STAR knows of the PN value, it does not regulate it and will still try to provide 100% of the caloric goal through enteral nutrition (EN). Thus, enabling the possibility of nutrition delivery over 100% of goal. Cohort demographics are given in Table 1.

**Table 1 STAR cohort patient demographics and GC performance statistics**

| | |
|---|---|
| *Patient demographics* | |
| Number of patients | 221 |
| Number hours of GC | 21,769 |
| Age | 64.0 [54.0–72.0] |
| Sex (% Male) | 66.1 |
| ICU length of stay | 8.4 [3.1–15.3] |
| Days on GC | 2.2 [1.2–3.9] |
| Admission to GC start (h) | 17.5 [7.3–53.8] |
| Operative (%) | 29.0 |
| APACHE II score | 21.0 [16.0–27.0] |
| ICU mortality (%) | 28.0 |
| *GC performance statistics* | |
| BG mean per patient | 6.66 [6.36–7.21] |
| BG SD per patient | 1.17 [0.85–1.65] |
| % Time in targeted band (4.4–8.0 mmol/L) per patient | 88.42 [77.42–94.44] |
| % Time in targeted band (4.4–8.0 mmol/L) cohort | 83.2 |
| % Time < 4.4 mmol/L cohort | 1.35 |
| # Patients < 2.2 mmol/L | 4 |
| Patients fed PN (%) | 46.8 |
| Mean days on PN | 2.0 [1.0–5.8] |
| Mean PN per day (% caloric goal) | 6.4 [1.5–14.5] |

Data presented as median [IQR] where appropriate

Patients are not weighed in the Christchurch ICU, so ACCP caloric goal feed is approximated by estimating the patient weight. This estimation first assumes an 80 kg individual and then modifies this value based on frame size (subjective assessment; small, medium, large), age and sex, using Table 2 and Eq. 1 [66].

$$A * F * G * 80 * 25 = \text{kcal Goal/Day} \quad (1)$$

Equation 1 modifies the goal feed rate of 25 kcal/kg/day into a maximum range of 1152–2420 kcal/day. In this cohort, the median interquartile range (IQR) goal feed rate was 1800 [1608–1992] kcal/day. Due to clinical circumstances, such as planned surgery requiring a fasted state, medical imaging, and/or gastric tolerances, a patient's

**Table 2 Coefficients used to determine an ICU patients daily caloric goal in Christchurch ICU Hospital**

| Frame size (F) | Small | Medium | | Large |
|---|---|---|---|---|
| | 0.9 | 1.0 | | 1.1 |
| Age (A) | ≤39 | 40–59 | 60–79 | ≥80 |
| | 1.1 | 1.0 | 0.9 | 0.8 |
| Gender (G) | Male | | Female | |
| | 1.0 | | 0.8 | |

nutrition may be stopped or reduced significantly, for short periods, not reflective of the STAR feeding algorithm. In this analysis, all occurrences of feeding less than 30% caloric goal are ignored (3,135 h, 14.4% of the time).

### Ethics, consent and permissions
STAR is the standard of care in Christchurch Hospital, New Zealand; therefore, no consent was required from patients to be placed on the STAR GC protocol. The Upper South Regional Ethics Committee, New Zealand, granted approval for the audit, analysis and publication of the retrospective data.

### Analysis
#### Overall clinical performance of current STAR variable nutrition protocol
The mean cohort caloric goal achieved per day in the ICU by STAR, with hyperglycaemic ICU patients, is calculated and compared to the entire ICU patient cohorts reviewed by Cahill et al. [59]. For STAR, information only exists for periods of GC, which are aligned to the appropriate day of ICU stay so comparisons to Cahill et al. [59] are valid. The percentage of caloric goal achieved represents the total caloric intake (including protein calories) from both EN and PN, in regard to the ACCP caloric goal. This analysis helps answer whether caloric restriction for GC, or safe, effective GC in general, preclude or limit nutrition delivery when compared to that achieved by the entire ICU patient cohort.

#### Per-patient nutrition delivery
The distribution per patient (median, IQR, 5th–95th range) of caloric goal achieved per day on STAR is calculated. The per-day distribution is compared to the best performing ICU surveyed in [59] and the 85% 'Heyland ideal' caloric goal presented in [51] to evaluate the percentage of patients who can tolerate more, or less, nutrition than these results. This comparison delineates the range and distribution of glucose and nutrition tolerance for these medical ICU patients.

The mean and variation of caloric goal achieved over a patient's entire stay is assessed in terms of median IQR between patients and to the overall variation seen per day across the entire cohort. This assesses if the overall variability seen per day is due to variable patients or different patient-specific tolerances of nutritional uptake.

### Results
#### Overall clinical performance of current STAR variable nutrition protocol
The percentage caloric goal clinically achieved by STAR, each day in ICU, was compared to the survey results in Cahill et al. [59]. Figure 1 shows mean nutrition delivered

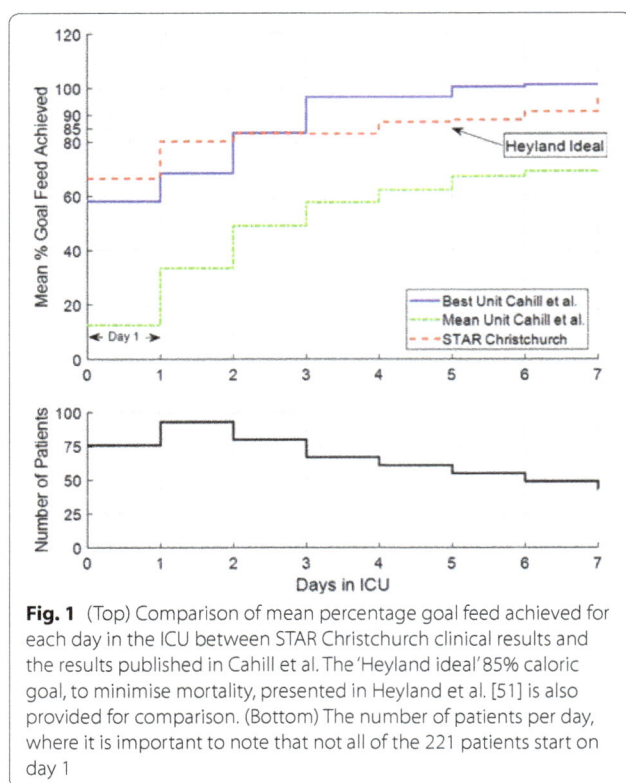

**Fig. 1** (Top) Comparison of mean percentage goal feed achieved for each day in the ICU between STAR Christchurch clinical results and the results published in Cahill et al. The 'Heyland ideal' 85% caloric goal, to minimise mortality, presented in Heyland et al. [51] is also provided for comparison. (Bottom) The number of patients per day, where it is important to note that not all of the 221 patients start on day 1

[51] after day 2, reaching 73.5% on day 7. The percentage of patients over the mean ICU result in [59] are also shown in Table 3 to be ranging from 100% on day 1 to 85.7% on day 7. Overall, in comparison with Fig. 1, the per-patient results clearly show some patients cannot achieve this cohort mean rate or the ideal 100% caloric goal. As noted, the rates in Fig. 2 are an estimate of the 'STAR ideal' time-varying patient-specific nutrition uptake in the context of GC to the 4.4-8.0 mmol/L BG range.

Table 4 shows the median of the mean feed rate achieved over a patient's stay, per patient, is relatively high at 89.8% caloric goal, but has a large IQR of 23.9%. However, the relatively small median standard deviation of feed rate achieved over a patient's stay, per patient, of 12.9% shows that individual patients are less variable than the cohort and thus that the overall ability to tolerate glucose is patient specific. Thus, it is clear the ability to take up, and thus to deliver, nutrition varies significantly between GC patients.

## Discussion
### Overall clinical performance of current STAR variable nutrition protocol
Figure 1 shows STAR's nutrition protocol, on hyperglycaemic ICU patients, performs equal to or better than the average of all the ICU patients in the best ICU surveyed by Cahill et al. [59] over the first 3 days of ICU stay. After day 3, the best ICU performs slightly better. However, the number of patients on GC is shown to diminish after day 3. This outcome makes the relevance of nutrition performance less significant after this time. Overall, these outcomes show the current STAR nutrition protocol delivers clinical nutrition results for hyperglycaemic patients, which are equal to, or better than, those reported in the Cahill et al. survey for all ICU patients in 158 ICUs in 20 countries. It is clear that high nutritional delivery and safe, effective GC are not mutually exclusive and that variable nutrition to achieve GC does not reduce total nutritional intake when compared to an entire ICU cohort.

### Per-patient nutrition delivery
Figure 2 shows a large variation in nutrition rates achieved per day, per patient, narrowing and rising as

to hyperglycaemic ICU patients by the variable nutrition protocol in STAR performs very well compared to all ICU patients in the best ICU reviewed in Cahill et al., only slightly underperforming after day 3. It is well above the mean ICU surveyed on all days, as shown in Table 3. In addition, the mean percentage caloric goal nutrition, per day in ICU, exceeds the 'Heyland ideal' 85% caloric goal [51] from day 4 onwards.

### Per-patient nutrition delivery
Figure 2 shows the distribution of per-patient mean nutrition rates delivered per day by STAR, including IQR and 5th–95th percentile values. It clearly shows large variation in patient-specific nutrition rates on the first day of ICU stay, which narrows as patient-specific metabolic state stabilises [21]. Table 3 shows over 56.2% of patients reach or exceed the 'Heyland ideal' 85% caloric goal in

**Table 3  Percentage of patients above the Mean ICU reviewed by Cahill et al. [59] and 'Heyland ideal' rate of 85% [51]**

| Day in ICU | Day 1 | Day 2 | Day 3 | Day 4 | Day 5 | Day 6 | Day 7 |
|---|---|---|---|---|---|---|---|
| % Patients > Mean Unit Cahill et al. | 100.0 | 96.8 | 92.5 | 86.6 | 85.3 | 90.9 | 85.7 |
| % Patients > 'Heyland ideal' (85%). | 25.0 | 41.9 | 56.2 | 58.2 | 63.9 | 60.0 | 73.5 |

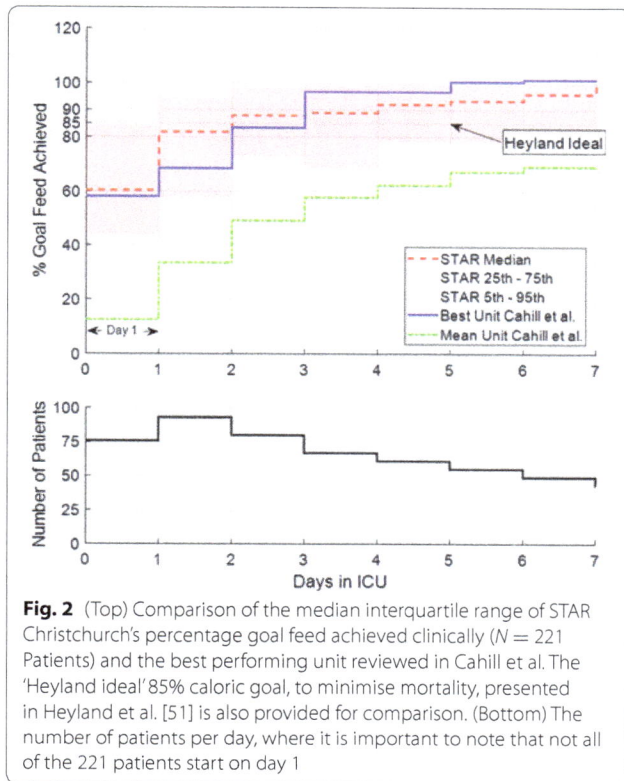

**Fig. 2** (Top) Comparison of the median interquartile range of STAR Christchurch's percentage goal feed achieved clinically (*N* = 221 Patients) and the best performing unit reviewed in Cahill et al. The 'Heyland ideal' 85% caloric goal, to minimise mortality, presented in Heyland et al. [51] is also provided for comparison. (Bottom) The number of patients per day, where it is important to note that not all of the 221 patients start on day 1

the patient-specific metabolic state stabilises [21], similar to that seen in Heyland et al. [67]. However, the median variation per patient was only 12.9 [4.6–20.4] % (Table 4), suggesting patients do not deviate significantly from their mean nutrition rate. This result and the large IQR of the mean feed rates achieved (74.3–98.2%, Table 4) suggest the lower nutritional delivery to the 5th and 25th percentile are a result of a few patients who had a lower ability to tolerate glucose intake.

It is very uncommon for patients not on GC in Christchurch ICU to have their feed rates changed due to the strong clinical culture of patients achieving their caloric goal. In addition, prior to STAR's predecessor, SPRINT, being implemented (2005) [14], feed rates were fixed at 100% caloric goal during GC for all patients. Hence, if they are not on GC, they are likely to have a fixed 100% caloric goal nutrition rate and have a BG within 4.4–8.0 mmol/L, having a relatively constant glucose tolerance

**Table 4  Per-patient feed rate characteristics**

| Number of patients | 221 |
|---|---|
| Mean of a patient's feed rate over entire stay, per patient (%) | 89.8 [74.3–98.2] |
| SD of a patient's feed rate over entire stay, per patient (%) | 12.9 [4.6–20.4] |

Data presented as median [IQR] where appropriate

and reduced insulin sensitivity variability [21, 68]. Therefore, if all patient data were considered, the intra-patient variability seen in Table 4 would likely go down.

Considering STAR feeds the maximum possible nutrition, while safely maintaining normo-glycaemia, the nutrition rates achieved give a good indication of the patient-specific ability to tolerate glucose and thus of their 'STAR ideal' nutrition rate. In essence, every patient is fed the maximum they can achieve with added insulin, within the bounds of the future predicted variability. Therefore, the spread of nutrition rates per patient in the results infer this 'STAR ideal' nutrition rate is very patient specific and evolves with time.

The 'STAR ideal' nutrition rate achieved by STAR was less than the 100% caloric goal for more than 50% of patients, over all days. However, the best unit surveyed in Cahill et al. [59] was still considerably lower than this predetermined caloric goal suggesting these generalised approximations do not represent all ICU patients well, as seen in the results for STAR in Christchurch. In addition, over 56% of patients exceeded the lower 85% 'Heyland ideal' of [51] by day 3, as shown in Table 3.

### Limitations

Cahill et al. [59] provides the percentage caloric goal nutrition achieved by each ICU. However, caloric goals may vary across ICUs. Additionally, the estimation of patient body weight in Christchurch ICU [69], as shown in Table 2, may also bias the caloric goal feed estimate which outlines the need for patients to be weighed on the day of ICU admission in Christchurch Hospital. As a result, some ICUs may thus achieve caloric goal nutrition targets 'more easily' than others, making comparison difficult. However, the 25 kcal/kg/day ACCP guideline [62] used in the Christchurch ICU, or a similar value guideline (25–30 kcal/kg/day SCCM/ASPEN [70], and 20–25 kcal/kgBW/day initial phase and recovery phase 25–30 kcal/kgBW/day ESPEN [71]), is commonly used and these cover the range used with STAR patients.

In addition, Cahill et al. review nutrition achieved during the first day of ICU stay, which is not necessarily when GC starts for all patients. Although GC commonly starts at the beginning of ICU stay, it may not always be the case. However, as an ICU patient is under the most amount of stress immediately post-surgery or insult [72], they are most likely to require GC at or near the beginning of their ICU stay [1–3]. In this study, 59.3% of patients started GC within 24 h of being admitted to the ICU (Median 15.5 h, Table 1).

Moreover, Cahill et al. survey the nutrition given to all ICU patients. However, this study only considered patients who required GC. The 25–35% of patients who require GC in the ICU [28] are the most metabolically stressed and, as a result, have a reduced glucose uptake capacity. They are thus often harder to deliver the target nutrition rates [20, 52, 57, 58]. In addition, given that 158 ICUs over 20 countries were surveyed by Cahill et al. [59], and this ICU was 1 of the 22 surveyed in Australia, and New Zealand the mixed medical surgical ICU in Christchurch Hospital would likely have patients with similar parameters. Therefore, achieving nutrition rates with high performance GC similar to that achieved for all ICU patients, normoglycaemic and hyperglycaemic, in the best ICU reviewed by Cahill et al. [59] is a significant outcome. More importantly, this outcome and the inter-patient variability in the results indicate high nutrition delivery and safe, effective GC are not exclusive, an equally, that nutrition restriction to obtain GC does not necessarily reduce total nutrition in an international context.

The insulin–glucose model used by STAR has been shown to be effective in predicting a patient's response [35, 36, 73]. However, as STAR doses based on the 5th and 95th percentile future metabolic variability [38], ensuring only a 5% risk of hypoglycaemia [74], the majority of patient's future BG will fall within the targeted band. Hence, many patients could possibly remain within the targeted BG range (4.4–8.0 mmol/L) if given a higher than recommended nutrition rate. As a result, some patients may be able to receive higher nutrition rates than reported here and still be able to be provided effective GC. However, this choice would also increase the likelihood of hyperglycaemia, reducing the safety of GC provided by STAR.

The 85% caloric goal presented in Heyland et al. is calculated by a model fit to retrospective data from 158 ICUs and clinical practices, and while it represents a significant body of multi-centre data, it may not be causative. Many prospective trials have found improved outcomes for even lower hypo-caloric feeding [50, 75–77]. Therefore, this 'Heyland ideal' value may overestimate the caloric goal required for improved outcomes and may be reflective of 'less sick' patients tolerating higher nutrition. This study is designed to show that STAR can provide high nutrition rates while still providing safe and effective GC. In addition, STAR is designed to be flexible to different nutrition goals while still providing effective GC.

Other factors, such as mechanical ventilation, neurologic injury, gastric emptying and paresis patients, are well known to influence the nutritional requirements of ICU patients. This is another strong limitation of this retrospective analysis, as this detailed information was not available. However, the cohort was typical of medical ICU in Christchurch.

The STAR GC protocol uses model-based patient-specific control in conjunction with a stochastic model to predict the best treatment for a patient. As shown in Table 1 and [32], STAR is able to achieve very good GC with a compliance of over 96.8% in all interventions and near identical results across multiple ICUs [32]. However, in many clinical practices, the idea of protocol-driven changes in the nutrition given to a patient for GC is foreign and thus clinically unacceptable. Thus, the main focus of this study is to show that protocol-driven changes in nutrition rate do not preclude in achieving better nutrition delivery rates than those of 158 ICUs from 20 countries. In addition, the concept of nutritional tolerances in relation to glucose tolerances provides a potentially new method of calculating patient-specific feed rates and should be investigated further in future studies.

## Conclusions

The STAR GC protocol clinical provision of nutrition to hyperglycaemic patients was compared to nutrition rates of entire ICU cohorts surveyed in 158 ICUs in Cahill et al. [59]. Mean nutrition rates clinically achieved by the STAR variable nutrition protocol were significantly higher than the mean and best ICU surveyed, for the first 3 days of ICU stay. Overall, STAR's protocol-driven changes in nutrition rate provide on average nutrition rates for hyperglycaemic patients which are equal to, or better than the mean of all ICU patients in 158 ICUs from 20 countries. More importantly, these outcomes show high nutrition delivery and safe, effective GC are not exclusive and that restricting nutrition for GC does not limit overall nutritional intake compared to other ICUs.

The inter- and intra- patient variation of nutritional delivery was assessed in the STAR cohort There was large inter-patient variation in nutrition rates achieved per day, which reduced overtime as patient-specific metabolic state stabilised. Median intra-patient variation was 12.9%; however, the IQR of the mean per-patient nutrition rates achieved was 74.3–98.2%, suggesting patients do not deviate much from their mean patient-specific nutrition rate and thus that the ability to tolerate glucose intake varies significantly between, rather than within, patients. There is significant inter-patient variability between patients to tolerate and uptake glucose, where intra-patient variability over stay is much lower. Thus, a best nutrition rate is likely patient specific for patients requiring GC.

**Abbreviations**
STAR: stochastic TARgeted; GC: glycaemic control; BG: blood glucose; IQR: interquartile range; ICU: intensive care unit; ACCP: American College of Chest Physicians; PN: parenteral nutrition.

**Author's contributions**
JGC, GS and CP conceived and developed the STAR protocol. GS assisted implementing the protocol in the Christchurch ICU, New Zealand. KS assisted in the data collection. KS undertook all of the analysis, interpretation of the clinical data. KS, CP and JGC drafted the manuscript. All authors approved the final manuscript.

## Author details
[1] Department of Mechanical Engineering, Centre for Bio-Engineering, University of Canterbury, Private Bag 4800, Christchurch 8140, New Zealand. [2] Department of Intensive Care, Christchurch Hospital, Christchurch, New Zealand.

## Acknowledgements
None.

## Competing interests
The authors declare that they have no competing interests.

## Funding
We acknowledge the support of UC Doctoral Scholarships for Kent Stewart, as well as funding from EU FP7, RSNZ IRSES mobility grants and the HRC of NZ.

## References

1. Clutter WE, Bier DM, Shah SD, Cryer PE. Epinephrine plasma metabolic clearance rates and physiologic thresholds for metabolic and hemodynamic actions in man. J Clin Investig. 1980;66:94–101.
2. McCowen KC, Malhotra A, Bistrian BR. Stress-induced hyperglycemia. Crit Care Clin. 2001;17:107–24.
3. Shamoon H, Hendler R, Sherwin RS. Synergistic interactions among anti-insulin hormones in the pathogenesis of stress hyperglycemia in humans. J Clin Endocrinol Metab. 1981;52:1235–41.
4. Capes SE, Hunt D, Malmberg K, Gerstein HC. Stress hyperglycaemia and increased risk of death after myocardial infarction in patients with and without diabetes: a systematic overview. Lancet. 2000;355:773–8.
5. Krinsley JS. Association between hyperglycemia and increased hospital mortality in a heterogeneous population of critically ill patients. Mayo Clin Proc. 2003;78:1471–8.
6. Mizock BA. Alterations in fuel metabolism in critical illness: hyperglycaemia. Best Pract Res Clin Endocrinol Metab. 2001;15:533–51.
7. Uyttendaele V, Dickson JL, Shaw GM, Desaive T, Chase JG. Untangling glycaemia and mortality in critical care. Crit Care. 2017;21:152.
8. Egi M, Bellomo R, Stachowski E, French CJ, Hart G. Variability of blood glucose concentration and short-term mortality in critically ill patients. Anesthesiology. 2006;105:244–52.
9. Krinsley JS. Glycemic variability: a strong independent predictor of mortality in critically ill patients. Crit Care Med. 2008;36:3008–13.
10. Lanspa MJ, Dickerson J, Morris AH, Orme JF, Holmen J, Hirshberg EL. Coefficient of glucose variation is independently associated with mortality in critically ill patients receiving intravenous insulin. Crit Care. 2014;18:R86.
11. Finney SJ, Zekveld C, Elia A, Evans TW. Glucose control and mortality in critically ill patients. JAMA. 2003;290:2041–7.
12. Van den Berghe G, Wouters P, Weekers F, Verwaest C, Bruyninckx F, Schetz M, et al. Intensive insulin therapy in the critically ill patients. N Engl J Med. 2001;345:1359–67.
13. Krinsley JS. Effect of an intensive glucose management protocol on the mortality of critically ill adult patients. Mayo Clin Proc. 2004;79:992–1000.
14. Chase JG, Shaw G, Le Compte A, Lonergan T, Willacy M, Wong XW, et al. Implementation and evaluation of the SPRINT protocol for tight glycaemic control in critically ill patients: a clinical practice change. Crit Care. 2008;12:R49.
15. Chase JG, Pretty CG, Pfeifer L, Shaw GM, Preiser JC, Le Compte AJ, et al. Organ failure and tight glycemic control in the SPRINT study. Crit Care. 2010;14:R154.
16. Krinsley JS, Jones RL. Cost analysis of intensive glycemic control in critically ill adult patients. Chest. 2006;129:644–50.
17. Van den Berghe G, Wouters PJ, Kesteloot K, Hilleman DE. Analysis of healthcare resource utilization with intensive insulin therapy in critically ill patients. Crit Care Med. 2006;34:612–6.
18. Dickson JL, Gunn CA, Chase JG. Humans are horribly variable. Int J Clin Med Imaging. 2014; 1.
19. Chase JG, Le Compte AJ, Suhaimi F, Shaw GM, Lynn A, Lin J, et al. Tight glycemic control in critical care—the leading role of insulin sensitivity and patient variability: a review and model-based analysis. Comput Methods Programs Biomed. Elsevier Ireland Ltd; 2011;102:156–71.
20. Suhaimi F, Le Compte A, Preiser JC, Shaw GM, Massion P, Radermecker R, et al. What makes tight glycemic control (TGC) Tight? The impact of variability and nutrition in 2 clinical studies. J Diabetes Sci Technol. 2010;4:284–98.
21. Pretty CG, Le Compte AJ, Chase JG, Shaw GM, Preiser JC, Penning S, et al. Variability of insulin sensitivity during the first 4 days of critical illness: implications for tight glycemic control. Ann Intensive Care. 2012;2:17.
22. Egi M, Bellomo R, Stachowski E, French CJ, Hart GK, Taori G, et al. Hypoglycemia and outcome in critically ill patients. Mayo Clin Proc. 2010;85:217–24.
23. Bagshaw SM, Bellomo R, Jacka MJ, Egi M, Hart GK, George C. The impact of early hypoglycemia and blood glucose variability on outcome in critical illness. Crit Care. 2009;13:R91.
24. Finfer S, Liu B, Chittock DR, Norton R, Myburgh JA, McArthur C, et al. Hypoglycemia and risk of death in critically ill patients. N Engl J Med. 2012;367:1108–18.
25. Griesdale DEG, de Souza RJ, van Dam RM, Heyland DK, Cook DJ, Malhotra A, et al. Intensive insulin therapy and mortality among critically ill patients: a meta-analysis including NICE-SUGAR study data. Can Med Assoc J. 2009;180:821–7.
26. Finfer S, Delaney A. Tight glycemic control in critically ill adults. JAMA. 2008;300:963–5.
27. Brunkhorst FM, Engel C, Bloos F, Meier-Hellmann A, Ragaller M, Weiler N, et al. Intensive insulin therapy and pentastarch resuscitation in severe sepsis. N Engl J Med. 2008;358:125–39.
28. Treggiari MM, Karir V, Yanez ND, Weiss NS, Daniel S, Deem SA. Intensive insulin therapy and mortality in critically ill patients. Crit Care. 2008;12:R29.
29. Kalfon P, Giraudeau B, Ichai C, Guerrini A, Brechot N, Cinotti R, et al. Tight computerized versus conventional glucose control in the ICU: a randomized controlled trial. Intensive Care Med. 2014;40:171–81.
30. Hamimy W, Khedr H, Rushdi T, Zaghloul A, Hosni M, Aal AA. Application of conventional blood glucose control strategy in surgical ICU in developing countries: is it beneficial? Egypt J Anaesth. 2015;32:123–9.
31. Van den Berghe G, Wilmer A, Hermans G, Meersseman W, Wouters PJ, Milants I, et al. Intensive insulin therapy in the medical ICU. N Engl J Med. 2006;354:449–61.
32. Stewart KW, Pretty CG, Tomlinson H, Thomas FL, Homlok J, Noémi SN, et al. Safety, efficacy and clinical generalization of the STAR protocol: a retrospective analysis. Ann Intensive Care. 2016;6:24.
33. Fisk L, Lecompte A, Penning S, Desaive T, Shaw G, Chase G. STAR development and protocol comparison. IEEE Trans Biomed Eng. 2012;59:3357–64.
34. Dickson JL, Stewart KW, Pretty CG, Flechet M, Desaive T, Penning S, et al. Generalisability of a virtual trials method for glycaemic control in intensive care. IEEE Trans Biomed Eng. 2017;1–1.
35. Chase JG, Suhaimi F, Penning S, Preiser JC, Le Compte AJ, Lin J, et al. Validation of a model-based virtual trials method for tight glycemic control in intensive care. Biomed Eng Online. 2010;9:84.
36. Lin J, Razak NN, Pretty CG, Le Compte A, Docherty P, Parente JD, et al. A physiological Intensive Control Insulin-Nutrition-Glucose (ICING) model validated in critically ill patients. Comput Methods Programs Biomed. 2011;102:192–205.
37. Stewart KW, Pretty CG, Tomlinson H, Fisk L, Shaw GM, Chase JG. Stochastic Model Predictive (STOMP) glycaemic control for the intensive care unit: development and virtual trial validation. Biomed Signal Process Control. 2015;16:61–7.
38. Lin J, Lee D, Chase JG, Shaw GM, Hann CE, Lotz T, et al. Stochastic modelling of insulin sensitivity variability in critical care. Biomed Signal Process Control. 2006;1:229–42.
39. Lin J, Lee D, Chase JG, Shaw GM, Le Compte A, Lotz T, et al. Stochastic modelling of insulin sensitivity and adaptive glycemic control for critical care. Comput Methods Programs Biomed. 2008;89:141–52.
40. Evans A, Le Compte A, Tan CS, Ward L, Steel J, Pretty CG, et al. Stochastic targeted (STAR) glycemic control: design, safety, and performance. J Diabetes Sci Technol. 2012;6:102–15.
41. Evans A, Shaw GM, Le Compte A, Tan CS, Ward L, Steel J, et al. Pilot proof of concept clinical trials of Stochastic Targeted (STAR) glycemic control. Ann Intensive Care. 2011;1:38.
42. Kalfon P, Preiser JC. Tight glucose control: should we move from intensive

insulin therapy alone to modulation of insulin and nutritional inputs? Crit Care. 2008;12:156.

43. Amrein K, Ellmerer M, Hovorka R, Kachel N, Fries H, von Lewinski D, et al. Efficacy and safety of glucose control with Space GlucoseControl in the medical intensive care unit: an open clinical investigation. Diabetes Technol Ther. 2012;14:690–5.

44. Van Herpe T, Mesotten D, Wouters PJ, Herbots J, Voets E, Buyens J, et al. LOGIC-insulin algorithm-guided versus nurse-directed blood glucose control during critical illness: the LOGIC-1 single-center, randomized, controlled clinical trial. Diabetes Care. 2013;36:188–94.

45. Pachler C, Plank J, Weinhandl H, Chassin LJ, Wilinska ME, Kulnik R, et al. Tight glycaemic control by an automated algorithm with time-variant sampling in medical ICU patients. Intensive Care Med. 2008;34:1224–30.

46. Finfer S, Chittock DR, Su SY-S, Blair D, Foster D, Dhingra V, et al. Intensive versus conventional glucose control in critically ill patients. N Engl J Med. 2009;360:1283–97.

47. Preiser JC, Devos P, Ruiz-Santana S, Melot C, Annane D, Groeneveld J, et al. A prospective randomised multi-centre controlled trial on tight glucose control by intensive insulin therapy in adult intensive care units: the Glucontrol study. Intensive Care Med. 2009;35:1738–48.

48. Doig GS, Simpson F, Finfer S, Delaney A, Davies AR, Mitchell I, et al. Effect of evidence-based feeding guidelines on mortality of critically ill adults: a cluster randomized controlled trial. JAMA. 2008;300:2731–41.

49. Villet S, Chiolero RL, Bollmann MD, Revelly JP, Cayeux RNM, Delarue J, et al. Negative impact of hypocaloric feeding and energy balance on clinical outcome in ICU patients. Clin Nutr. 2005;24:502–9.

50. Krishnan JA, Parce PB, Martinez A, Diette GB, Brower RG. Caloric intake in medical ICU patients: consistency of care with guidelines and relationship to clinical outcomes. Chest. 2003;124:297–305.

51. Heyland DK, Cahill N, Day AG. Optimal amount of calories for critically ill patients: depends on how you slice the cake! Crit Care Med. 2011;39:1.

52. Arabi YM, Aldawood AS, Haddad SH, Al-Dorzi HM, Tamim HM, Jones G, et al. Permissive underfeeding or standard enteral feeding in critically ill adults. N Engl J Med. 2015;372:2398–408.

53. Preiser J-C, van Zanten AR, Berger MM, Biolo G, Casaer MP, Doig GS, et al. Metabolic and nutritional support of critically ill patients: consensus and controversies. Crit Care. 2015;19:1–11.

54. Rice TW. Gluttony in the intensive care unit. Am J Respir Crit Care Med. 2013;187:223–4.

55. Weijs PJM, Stapel SN, de Groot SDW, Driessen RH, de Jong E, Girbes ARJ, et al. Optimal protein and energy nutrition decreases mortality in mechanically ventilated, critically ill patients: a prospective observational cohort study. JPEN J Parenter Enteral Nutr. 2012;36:60–8.

56. Singer P, Anbar R, Cohen J, Shapiro H, Shalita-Chesner M, Lev S, et al. The tight calorie control study (TICACOS): a prospective, randomized, controlled pilot study of nutritional support in critically ill patients. Intensive Care Med. 2011;37:601–9.

57. Casaer MP, Mesotten D, Hermans G, Wouters PJ, Schetz M, Meyfroidt G, et al. Early versus late parenteral nutrition in critically ill adults. N Engl J Med. 2011.

58. Rice TW, Wheeler AP, Thompson BT, Steingrub J, Hite RD, Moss M, et al. Initial trophic vs full enteral feeding in patients with acute lung injury: the EDEN randomized trial. JAMA. 2012;307:795–803.

59. Cahill NE, Dhaliwal R, Day AG, Jiang X, Heyland DK. Nutrition therapy in the critical care setting: what is "best achievable" practice? An international multicenter observational study*. Crit Care Med. 2010;38:395–401.

60. Hann CE, Chase JG, Lin J, Lotz T, Doran CV, Shaw GM. Integral-based parameter identification for long-term dynamic verification of a glucose–insulin system model. Comput Methods Programs Biomed. 2005;77:259–70.

61. Haidar A, Elleri D, Allen JM, Harris J, Kumareswaran K, Nodale M, et al. Validity of triple- and dual-tracer techniques to estimate glucose appearance. AJP Endocrinol Metab. 2012;302:E1493–501.

62. Cerra FB, Benitez MR, Blackburn GL, Irwin RS, Jeejeebhoy K, Katz DP, et al. Applied nutrition in ICU patients: a consensus statement of the American College of Chest Physicians. Chest. 1997;111:769–78.

63. Fugleberg S, Kolendorf K, Thorsteinsson B, Bliddal H, Lund B, Bojsen F. The relationship between plasma concentration and plasma disappearance rate of immunoreactive insulin in normal subjects. Diabetologia. 1982;22:437–40.

64. Thorsteinsson B. Kinetic models for insulin disappearance from plasma in man. Dan Med Bull. 1990;37:143–53.

65. Natali A, Gastaldelli A, Camastra S, Sironi AM, Toschi E, Masoni A, et al. Dose-response characteristics of insulin action on glucose metabolism: a non-steady-state approach. Am J Physiol Endocrinol Metab. 2000;278:E794–801.

66. Chase JG, Shaw GM, Lotz T, LeCompte A, Wong J, Lin J, et al. Model-based insulin and nutrition administration for tight glycaemic control in critical care. Curr Drug Deliv. 2007;4:283–96.

67. Heyland DK, Schroter-Noppe D, Drover JW, Jain M, Keefe L, Dhaliwal R, et al. Nutrition support in the critical care setting: current practice in canadian ICUs—opportunities for improvement? JPEN J Parenter Enteral Nutr. 2003;27:74–83.

68. Thomas F, Pretty CG, Fisk L, Shaw GM, Chase JG, Desaive T. Reducing the impact of insulin sensitivity variability on glycaemic outcomes using separate stochastic models within the STAR glycaemic protocol. Biomed Eng Online. 2014;13:43.

69. Chase JG, Shaw GM, Lotz T, LeCompte A, Wong J, Lin J, et al. Model-based insulin and nutrition administration for tight glycaemic control in critical care. Curr Drug Deliv. 2007;4:283–96.

70. Taylor BE, McClave SA, Martindale RG, Warren MM, Johnson DR, Braunschweig C, et al. Guidelines for the provision and assessment of nutrition support therapy in the adult critically ill patient. Crit Care Med. 2016;44:390–438.

71. Kreymann KG, Berger MM, Deutz NEP, Hiesmayr M, Jolliet P, Kazandjiev G, et al. ESPEN guidelines on enteral nutrition: intensive care. Clin Nutr. 2006;25:210–23.

72. Cuthbertson DP. Post-shock metabolic response. Lancet. 1942;239:433–7.

73. Stewart KW, Chase JG, Dickson J, Pretty C, Shaw G. Can we fix it? Yes we can! Simplifying nutrition in STAR Glycemic Control. 16th annual diabetes technology meet. 2016.

74. Fisk LM, Le Compte AJ, Shaw GM, Penning S, Desaive T, Chase JG. STAR development and protocol comparison. IEEE Trans Biomed Eng. 2012;59:3357–64.

75. Patino JF, de Pimiento SE, Vergara A, Savino P, Rodriguez M, Escallon J. Hypocaloric support in the critically ill. World J Surg. 1999;23:553–9.

76. Dickerson RN, Boschert KJ, Kudsk KA, Brown RO. Hypocaloric enteral tube feeding in critically ill obese patients. Nutrition. 2002;18:241–6.

77. Arabi YM, Tamim HM, Dhar GS, Al-Dawood A, Al-Sultan M, Sakkijha MH, et al. Permissive underfeeding and intensive insulin therapy in critically ill patients: a randomized controlled trial. Am J Clin Nutr. 2011;93:569–77.

# 11

# Outcome of in- and out-of-hospital cardiac arrest survivors with liver cirrhosis

Kevin Roedl[1,3†], Christian Wallmüller[2†], Andreas Drolz[1,3], Thomas Horvatits[1,3], Karoline Rutter[1,3], Alexander Spiel[1,2], Julia Ortbauer[3], Peter Stratil[2], Pia Hubner[2], Christoph Weiser[2], Jasmin Katrin Motaabbed[3], Dominik Jarczak[1], Harald Herkner[2], Fritz Sterz[2] and Valentin Fuhrmann[1,3*]

## Abstract

**Background:** Organ failure increases mortality in patients with liver cirrhosis. Data about resuscitated cardiac arrest patients with liver cirrhosis are missing. This study aims to assess aetiology, survival and functional outcome in patients after successful cardiopulmonary resuscitation (CPR) with and without liver cirrhosis.

**Methods:** Analysis of prospectively collected cardiac arrest registry data of consecutively hospital-admitted patients following successful CPR was performed. Patient's characteristics, admission diagnosis, severity of disease, course of disease, short- and long-term mortality as well as functional outcome were assessed and compared between patients with and without cirrhosis.

**Results:** Out of 1068 patients with successful CPR, 47 (4%) had liver cirrhosis. Acute-on-chronic liver failure (ACLF) was present in 33 (70%) of these patients on admission, and four patients developed ACLF during follow-up. Mortality at 1 year was more than threefold increased in patients with liver cirrhosis (OR 3.25; 95% CI 1.33–7.96). Liver cirrhosis was associated with impaired neurological outcome (OR for a favourable cerebral performance category: 0.13; 95% CI 0.04–0.36). None of the patients with Child–Turcotte–Pugh (CTP) C cirrhosis survived 28 days with good neurological outcome. Overall nine (19%) patients with cirrhosis survived 28 days with good neurological outcome. All patients with ACLF grade 3 died within 28 days.

**Conclusion:** Cardiac arrest survivors with cirrhosis have worse outcome than those without. Although one quarter of patients with liver cirrhosis survived longer than 28 days after successful CPR, patients with CTP C as well as advanced ACLF did not survive 28 days with good neurological outcome.

**Keywords:** Cardiac arrest, Cirrhosis, Acute-on-chronic liver failure, Multiple organ failure, Intensive care unit

## Background

Patients with liver cirrhosis [1] and organ failure admitted to intensive care units (ICU) have high morbidity and mortality [2, 3]. Mortality rates of up to 80% are reported in critically ill cirrhotic patients, progressively increasing with the number of organs failing [4–6]. Recently, chronic liver failure-SOFA (CLIF-SOFA) score [3] was developed as a tool for risk stratification in patients with cirrhosis and acute-on-chronic liver failure (ACLF) [2, 3].

Cardiac arrest (CA) can be the consequence of or lead to multiple organ failure. It is one of the leading causes of death in many parts of the world. Every year estimated 375,000–700,000 citizens are suffering CA in Europe and the USA [7, 8] and receive cardiopulmonary resuscitation (CPR). Patients who achieve return of spontaneous circulation (ROSC) following CA have high morbidity and mortality mainly due to cerebral and cardiac dysfunction that accompany whole-body ischaemia and reperfusion [9]. These disabilities can lead to the post-CA syndrome, which is defined as multiple organ failure after CA. Despite advances in critical and emergency care, survival

*Correspondence: v.fuhrmann@uke.de
†Kevin Roedl and Christian Wallmüller have contributed equally to this work
[1] Department of Intensive Care Medicine, University Medical Center Hamburg-Eppendorf, Martinistraße 52, 20246 Hamburg, Germany
Full list of author information is available at the end of the article

rates after in-hospital cardiac arrest (IHCA) and out-of-hospital cardiac arrest (OHCA) are generally poor and varying greatly for OHCA between 8–16% [10, 11] and for IHCA 14–23% [12–14].

Data on occurrence and outcome of CA in patients with liver cirrhosis are not available. Therefore, the aim of the study was to investigate cause and outcome in patients with liver cirrhosis after CA and ROSC compared to a large cohort of patients with CA and ROSC without liver cirrhosis.

## Methods

This study was based on a prospectively maintained registry at the Emergency Department of the Medical University of Vienna. This registry was approved by the ethics committee of the Medical University of Vienna. Due to the observational character of the study, informed consent was waived. The study was performed between January 2005 and January 2012. All consecutive patients admitted to the Emergency Department of the Medical University Vienna after CA and ROSC were included in the analysis. CPR and post-CA care were performed in accordance with the European Resuscitation Council guidelines [15, 16]. The data were collected prospectively according to Utstein-style guidelines [17, 18]. Patients suffering from OHCA were treated by the Viennese two-tier EMS system, featured by an EMS physician and paramedics; the EMS system was described previously in detail [19, 20]. No-flow time was defined as the time period from onset of CA to the start of resuscitation efforts. Low-flow time was defined as the time period from the start of resuscitation efforts until ROSC. Time to ROSC was defined as time from onset of CA until ROSC. CA survivors were followed prospectively for at least 1 year after admission to the emergency department for assessment of survival and neurological outcome. Rates of 28-day mortality, 6-month mortality and 1-year mortality were assessed on site or by contacting the patients or their attending physicians. Cerebral function and overall performance were assessed on admission and after 28 days, 6 months and 1 year, by clinical visits, by physicians on site or contacting the attending physician, the patients or the family of the patient directly by telephone. Cerebral performance categories (CPC) [21] and overall performance categories (OPC) scales were used to assess neurological and overall outcome. A CPC/OPC score of 1–2 was defined as favourable neurological/overall outcome, such as 3–5 as unfavourable. The primary outcome was good neurological survival (CPC 1/2) after 6 months; our secondary outcome was overall mortality after 1 year.

Routine laboratory assessment including coagulation and liver function parameters was performed on daily basis. Furthermore, aetiology of CA (cardiac and non-cardiac origin like pulmonary, traumatic, cerebral, septic, intoxication, drowning, hypothermia, unclear and others) and underlying diseases were assessed and documented.

Severity of illness was evaluated in all patients using Sequential Organ Failure Assessment (SOFA) score [22] and Simplified Acute Physiology Score (SAPS II) [23]. Charlson comorbidity index (CCI) [24] was calculated in all patients. For patients with liver cirrhosis, model of end-stage liver disease score (MELD) [25], Child–Turcotte–Pugh (CTP) score [26] and CLIF-SOFA score [3] were calculated on admission, and CLIF-SOFA was additionally calculated 24 and 48 h after ROSC.

All patients were screened for signs of liver cirrhosis. Presence of liver cirrhosis was defined via histology, if available, otherwise by a combination of clinical characteristics (ascites, spider angiomata, caput medusa), laboratory and radiological findings (typical morphological changes of the liver, sings of portal hypertension, etc. in ultrasonography or computed tomography scanning).

## Statistical analysis

Data are presented as count and relative frequency or median and 25–75% interquartile range (IQR). We tabulated clinical variables according to liver cirrhosis status and used Chi-squared, Fisher exact or Mann–Whitney $U$ test for hypothesis testing as appropriate. The prognostic factor of interest was liver cirrhosis, and we used logistic regression to estimate the effect on neurological intact survival. The dependent variable was favourable neurological survival (best CPC 1 or 2; yes vs. no). In a multivariable logistic regression model, we entered liver cirrhosis as main covariable and age, sex, OHCA, witnessed CA, time to ROSC, presence of shockable rhythm, cardiac cause of CA, mechanical ventilation, SOFA on admission, initiation of MTH, CCI and cumulative adrenaline dose as other covariates to the model. To allow for potentially non-random missing data for time to ROSC caused by unwitnessed cardiac arrest, we categorised this variable for 0–4, 5–12, 13–24, 25–44, 45 + minutes as well as 'missing' as the sixth category. We used a similar model to estimate the associations with mortality at one year as the outcome. In all models, we tested for linear effects, first-order interactions and model fit using the likelihood ratio test. Survival function estimates were calculated using Kaplan–Meier method and were compared by the log-rank test. Statistical analysis was conducted using Stata 14 (StataCorp, College Station, TX) and IBM SPSS Statistics version 23.0 (IBM Corp., Armonk, NY). Generally, a $p$ value < 0.05 was considered statistically significant.

# Results

## Study population

In total, 1068 patients (72% male, median age 61 years) after CA and ROSC were included in this study. Forty-seven (4%) of these patients had liver cirrhosis. Main cause of CA was cardiac in 678 (63%) patients of the total cohort. A total of 798 (75%) patients suffered CA out of hospital. Patients with liver cirrhosis had a significantly higher underlying non-cardiac cause compared to patients without cirrhosis. Median SOFA, SAPS II and CCI on admission were significantly higher in patients with liver cirrhosis. Sex, age, height and weight were distributed equally between both groups. Detailed characteristics of the study population are given in Table 1. Liver function and coagulation parameters were significantly different between patients with and without cirrhosis on hospital admission as illustrated in Additional file 1: Table S1.

## Characteristics of patients with liver cirrhosis

Main underlying aetiology of liver cirrhosis was alcoholic liver disease ($n = 35$, 74%) followed by viral hepatitis ($n = 6$, 13%) and others ($n = 6$, 13%). Child–Turcotte–Pugh (CTP) class prior to admission was A in 17 (36%), B in 17 (36%) and C in 13 (28%) patients. Hepatocellular carcinoma (HCC) was present in three patients. Three patients had transjugular intrahepatic portosystemic shunt (TIPS), and one patient was listed for liver transplantation prior to occurrence of CA. No patient had liver transplantation during follow-up. Aetiology of CA was cardiac ($n = 21$, 45%), variceal bleeding ($n = 6$, 13%), sepsis ($n = 5$, 11%), respiratory insufficiency ($n = 5$, 11%), electrolyte disturbances ($n = 4$, 9%) and other causes ($n = 6$, 13%). Detailed data are illustrated in Table 2.

CLIF-SOFA on admission, 24 and 48 h following hospital admission, and MELD, SOFA and SAPS II on admission and CTP score prior to CA were significantly higher in patients with unfavourable neurological outcome or mortality within 28 days.

Thirty-three patients (70%) had ACLF on admission. Four (29%) out of 14 patients without ACLF on admission developed ACLF within 48 h after ROSC. Two (4%) of the patients had ACLF prior to admission. ACLF

**Table 1 Patients' characteristics of the study population at admission stratified according to the presence of cirrhosis**

| Parameters | All patients ($n = 1068$) | Cirrhosis ($n = 47$) | No cirrhosis ($n = 1021$) | p value |
|---|---|---|---|---|
| Age, years median; IQR | 61 (50–72) | 62 (51–67) | 61 (50–72) | 0.92 |
| Male, n % | 765 (72) | 35 (74) | 730 (72) | 0.66 |
| Weight, kg median; IQR | 80 (70–90) | 80 (69.5–93) | 80 (70–90) | 0.72 |
| Height, cm median; IQR | 175 (168–180) | 175 (165–180) | 175 (168–180) | 0.59 |
| SOFA admission, pts median; IQR | 9 (6–12) | 11 (7.5–13) | 9 (6–12) | < 0.05 |
| SAPS II admission, pts median; IQR | 80 (74–88) | 87 (77.5–100) | 80 (73–87) | < 0.001 |
| Charlson comorbidity index, pts. median; IQR | 1 (0–3) | 4 (2.5–6) | 1 (0–2) | < 0.001 |
| Cause of arrest, n % | | | | |
|   Cardiac | 678 (63) | 21 (45) | 657 (64) | < 0.05 |
| Out of hospital, n % | 798 (75) | 31 (66) | 767 (75) | 0.16 |
| Invasive mechanical ventilation, n % | 850 (80) | 35 (74) | 815 (80) | 0.37 |
| Before cardiac arrest—normal CPC, n % | 1043 (98) | 45 (96) | 998 (98) | 0.45 |
| Before cardiac arrest—normal OPC, n % | 973 (91) | 39 (83) | 934 (91) | 0.09 |
| Ischaemic time, min median; IQR* | | | | |
|   No flow | 0 (0–3) | 0 (0–3.5) | 0 (0–3) | 0.49 |
|   Low flow | 13 (4–25) | 11 (3–23) | 13 (4–25) | 0.51 |
|   Time to ROSC | 16 (5–30) | 15 (3–27) | 16 (5–30) | 0.42 |
| Epinephrine cumulative (mg) median; IQR | 3 (1–4) | 3 (1–5.5) | 3 (1–4) | < 0.001 |
| Witnessed cardiac arrest, n % | 921 (86) | 42 (89) | 879 (86) | 0.56 |
| Initial rhythm, n % | | | | |
|   VT/VF | 550 (51) | 10 (21) | 540 (53) | < 0.001 |
|   PEA/asystole | 465 (44) | 35 (75) | 430 (42) | |
|   Other/unknown | 53 (5) | 2 (4) | 51 (5) | 0.82 |
| Defibrillation, n % | 646 (60) | 14 (30) | 632 (62) | < 0.001 |
| Therapeutic hypothermia, n % | 666 (62) | 18 (38) | 648 (63) | < 0.001 |

*SOFA* Sequential Organ Failure Assessment, *SAPS* Simplified Acute Physiology Score, *CPC* cerebral performance categories, *OPC* overall performance categories, *ROSC* return of spontaneous circulation, *VT* ventricular tachycardia, *VF* ventricular fibrillation, *PEA* pulseless electrical activity

* Overall ($n = 926$), cirrhosis ($n = 41$), no cirrhosis ($n = 1021$)

**Table 2 Characteristics of patients with cirrhosis stratified according to good 28-day outcome and bad 28-day outcome**

| Parameters | Overall (n = 47) | Good 28-day outcome (n = 9) | Bad 28-day outcome (n = 38) | p value* |
|---|---|---|---|---|
| Aetiology of cirrhosis, n % | | | | 0.33 |
| Alcoholic | 35 (74) | 7 (78) | 28 (74) | |
| Viral | 6 (13) | 2 (22) | 4 (10) | |
| Other (cryptogenic, cardiac, etc.) | 6 (13) | 0 (0) | 6 (16) | |
| Hepatocellular carcinoma, n % | 3 (6) | 0 (0) | 3 (8) | 0.38 |
| Liver TX during follow-up, n % | 0 (0) | 0 (0) | 0 (0) | |
| TIPS, n % | 3 (6) | 0 (0) | 3 (8) | 0.38 |
| CLIF-SOFA—admission median; IQR | 10 (6–12.5) | 4 (3–4) | 11 (9–13) | < 0.001 |
| CLIF-SOFA—24 h median; IQR | 10 (4.5–14) | 4 (2–7) | 12 (8.25–15.5) | 0.01 |
| CLIF-SOFA—48 h median; IQR | 7 (2–12.5) | 1 (1–7) | 11 (6–13.75) | 0.01 |
| CTP—before admission, n % | | | | 0.05 |
| A | 17 (36) | 6 (67) | 11 (29) | |
| B | 17 (36) | 3 (33) | 14 (37) | |
| C | 13 (28) | 0 (0) | 13 (34) | |
| CTP points—before admission median; IQR | 7 (5.5–10) | 6 (5–7) | 8 (6–11) | 0.03 |
| MELD—admission median; IQR | 19 (10.5–24) | 10 (9–10) | 21 (14–24) | < 0.001 |
| SOFA—admission median; IQR | 11 (7.5–13) | 4 (3–7) | 12 (10–13.75) | < 0.001 |
| SAPS II—admission median; IQR | 87 (77.5–100) | 66 (66–75) | 92 (85–102.75) | < 0.001 |
| Ascites—before admission, n % | | | | 0.33 |
| None | 15 (32) | 4 (44) | 11 (29) | |
| Mild | 25 (53) | 5 (56) | 20 (53) | |
| Severe | 7 (15) | 0 (0) | 7 (18) | |
| HE—before admission, n % | | | | 0.22 |
| None | 25 (53) | 7 (78) | 18 (47) | |
| I–II | 17 (36) | 2 (22) | 15 (40) | |
| III–IV | 5 (11) | 0 (0) | 5 (13) | |
| ACLF—on admission, n % | | | | < 0.001 |
| Grade 1 | 11 (23) | 1 (11) | 10 (26) | |
| Grade 2 | 11 (23) | 0 (0) | 11 (30) | |
| Grade 3 | 11 (23) | 0 (0) | 11 (30) | |
| No ACLF | 14 (30) | 8 (89) | 6 (16) | |
| ACLF—during follow-up, n % | | | | < 0.001 |
| Grade 1 | 1 (2) | 1 (11) | 0 (0) | |
| Grade 2 | 3 (6) | 1 (11) | 2 (5) | |
| Grade 3 | 0 (0) | 0 (0) | 0 (0) | |
| No ACLF | 10 (21) | 6 (67) | 4 (11) | |
| Ischaemic time, min median; IQR | | | | |
| No flow | 0 (0–3.5) | 0 (0–0) | 0 (0–5) | < 0.01 |
| Low flow | 11 (3–23) | 1 (1–3) | 16 (8–23.5) | 0.06 |
| Time to ROSC | 15 (3–27) | 1 (1–3) | 19.5 (11–28) | < 0.05 |
| Initial rhythm, n % | | | | |
| VT/VF | 10 (21) | 3 (33) | 7 (18) | 0.569 |
| PEA/Asystole | 35 (75) | 4 (45) | 31 (82) | < 0.05 |
| Other/unknown | 2 (4) | 2 (22) | 0 (0) | 0.305 |
| Witnessed cardiac arrest, n % | 42 (89) | 9 (100) | 33 (87) | 0.118 |
| Defibrillation, n % | 14 (30) | 3 (33) | 11 (29) | 0.569 |
| Therapeutic hypothermia, n % | 18 (38) | 1 (11) | 17 (45) | < 0.01 |

*CPC* cerebral performance categories, *TX* transplantation, *TIPS* transjugular intrahepatic portosystemic shunt, *CLIF-SOFA* chronic liver failure-Sequential Organ Failure Assessment, *CTP* Child–Turcotte–Pugh, *MELD* model for end-stage liver disease, *SOFA* Sequential Organ Failure Assessment, *SAPS* Simplified Acute Physiology Score, *HE* hepatic encephalopathy, *ACLF* acute-on-chronic liver failure

* CPC 1/2 versus CPC 3/4 or mortality

grades 1, 2 and 3 were present in 12 (32%), 14 (38%) and 11 (30%) patients, respectively.

## CPR-specific data

The majority of patients of the total cohort (75%) suffered OHCA. This rate did not differ significantly in patients with and without cirrhosis. Cardiac arrest was witnessed in 921 (86%) patients. No-flow time was median 0 (IQR 0–3) minutes, low-flow 13 (IQR 4–25) minutes and time to ROSC 16 (IQR 5–30) minutes, which did not differ significantly between patients with and without cirrhosis. Initial shockable rhythm (VT/VF) was significantly more frequent present in patients without cirrhosis. Accordingly, frequency of defibrillation during CPR was significantly lower in patients with liver cirrhosis. Furthermore, cumulative epinephrine dosage during CPR was significantly higher in patients with cirrhosis. First measured lactate levels were significantly higher in patients with liver cirrhosis. Table 1 and Additional file 1: Table S3 illustrate the detailed CPR data.

## Functional outcome and survival after CA

Almost all patients both with and without cirrhosis showed a normal CPC and OPC score prior to occurrence of CA as given in Table 1. Rate of favourable neurological outcome was 19% after 28 days, 6 months and 1 year in patients with cirrhosis, compared to 47% after 28 days and 6 months and 43% after 1 year in patients without cirrhosis, respectively. Rate of favourable neurological outcome in CA survivors after 6 months was significantly lower in patients with liver cirrhosis (19 vs. 47%, crude OR 0.26; 95% CI 0.13–0.53). This association continued to be statistically significant after adjustment for covariables (multivariable-adjusted OR 0.13; 95% CI 0.04–0.36, see Table 3). Mortality in patients with cirrhosis was significantly higher compared to patients without cirrhosis (74, 77 and 79% versus 41, 48 and 50% after 28 days, 6 months and 1 year, respectively; OR for 1-year mortality 3.69; 95% CI 1.82–7.51). Figure 1 demonstrates the survival of patients with and without cirrhosis. Cirrhosis was an independent risk factor for 1-year mortality in multivariate regression analysis (multivariable-adjusted OR 3.25; 95% CI 1.33–7.96, see Table 4).

No patient with liver cirrhosis CTP C as well as no patient with HCC or pre-existing TIPS survived longer than 28 days following ROSC with good neurological outcome. Figure 2 demonstrates the survival of patients with favourable neurological outcome in cirrhosis CTP A + B versus CTP C.

Forty per cent ($n = 4$) of patients with cirrhosis without ACLF died within 28 days following ROSC or had unfavourable neurological outcome compared to 92% ($n = 34$) of patients with ACLF ($p < 0.001$). In detail, 83%

**Table 3 Logistic regression model for factors associated with good neurological outcome (CPC 1/2 vs. > 2 or deceased)**

| Parameter | OR (95% CI) | p value |
|---|---|---|
| Cirrhosis (yes vs. no) | 0.13 (0.04–0.36) | < 0.001 |
| Age (years) | 0.96 (0.96–0.98) | < 0.001 |
| Time to ROSC (per category)* | 0.56 (0.47–0.67) | < 0.001 |
| Shockable rhythm (yes vs. no) | 2.16 (1.45–3.23) | < 0.001 |
| Intubated on admission (yes vs. no) | 0.17 (0.09–0.34) | < 0.001 |
| SOFA admission (per category)* | 0.73 (0.64–0.82) | < 0.001 |
| Cardiac cause (yes vs. no) | 1.73 (1.17–2.58) | 0.01 |
| Epinephrine cumulative dose (per mg) | 0.91 (0.85–0.98) | 0.01 |
| Witnessed cardiac arrest (yes vs. no) | 0.62 (0.32–1.23) | 0.17 |
| Mild therapeutic hypothermia (yes vs. no) | 1.23 (0.80–1.90) | 0.36 |
| Out-of-hospital cardiac arrest (yes vs. no) | 0.89 (0.58–1.38) | 0.61 |
| Male (vs. female) | 0.92 (0.65–1.31) | 0.65 |
| Charlson comorbidity index (per category)* | 0.97 (0.84–1.12) | 0.67 |

*OR* multivariable-adjusted odds ratio, *CI* confidence interval, *ROSC* return of spontaneous circulation, *SOFA* Sequential Organ Failure Assessment, *mg* milligram

* Time to ROSC categories: 0–4, 5–12, 13–24, 25–44, 45 + min, or missing; SOFA categories (score): 5, 6–8, 9–10, 11–12, 12 +, or missing; Carlson comorbidity categories: 0, 1, 2 + 3, 4 +, or missing

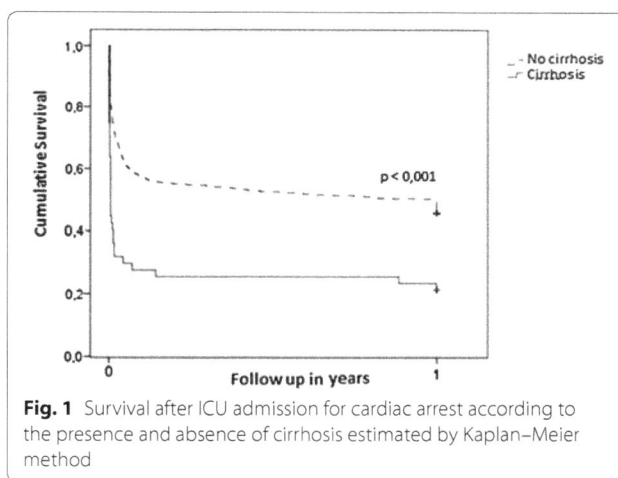

**Fig. 1** Survival after ICU admission for cardiac arrest according to the presence and absence of cirrhosis estimated by Kaplan–Meier method

($n = 10$) of patients with ACLF grade 1, 93% ($n = 13$) with ACLF grade 2 and 100% ($n = 11$) with ACLF grade 3 had unfavourable neurological outcome or died within 28 days. Multiple organ failure as cause of death was observed in 30 patients with cirrhosis, one patient had cerebral herniation following hypoxic brain injury, and four patients died with palliative care following irreversible hypoxic brain damage.

Mild therapeutic hypothermia (MTH) was applied in 666 (62%) patients of the total cohort [18 (38%) patients with cirrhosis and 648 (63%) without cirrhosis ($p < 0.001$)]. Furthermore, MTH was significantly

**Table 4 Logistic regression model for factors associated with 1-year mortality**

| 1-year mortality | OR | (95% CI) | p value |
|---|---|---|---|
| Age | 1.05 | (1.03–1.06) | < 0.001 |
| Time to ROSC* | 1.57 | (1.32–1.87) | < 0.001 |
| Shockable rhythm | 0.45 | (0.31–0.67) | < 0.001 |
| Tube admission | 2.33 | (1.35–4.03) | < 0.001 |
| SOFA admission* | 1.36 | (1.20–1.54) | < 0.001 |
| Cirrhosis | 3.25 | (1.33–7.96) | 0.01 |
| Charlson comorbidity index* | 1.19 | (1.03–1.37) | 0.02 |
| Epinephrine cumulative | 1.07 | (1.01–1.15) | 0.03 |
| Male | 1.41 | (1.00–1.98) | 0.05 |
| Cardiac cause of CA | 0.68 | (0.46–1.00) | 0.05 |
| Mild therapeutic hypothermia | 0.68 | (0.45–1.05) | 0.09 |
| OHCA | 0.99 | (0.66–1.50) | 0.98 |
| Witnessed CA | 1.00 | (0.51–1.94) | 0.99 |

*OR* multivariable-adjusted odds ratio, *CI* confidence interval, *OHCA* out-of-hospital cardiac arrest, *CA* cardiac arrest, *ROSC* return of spontaneous circulation, *SOFA* Sequential Organ Failure Assessment

* Time to ROSC categories: 0–4, 5–12, 13–24, 25–44, 45 + min, or missing; SOFA categories (score): 5, 6–8, 9–10, 11–12, 12 +, or missing; Charlson comorbidity categories: 0, 1, 2 + 3, 4 +, or missing

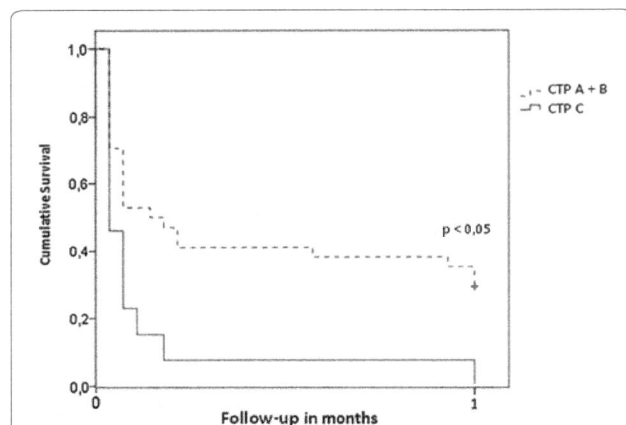

**Fig. 2** Probability of having a good neurological outcome after a cardiac arrest among cirrhotic patients according to Child–Turcotte–Pugh score estimated by Kaplan–Meier method

less frequent applied in patients with liver cirrhosis. In the cirrhosis population, patients with MTH were older, had lower SOFA, SAPS II, CLIF-SOFA and MELD score on admission and had significantly longer time to ROSC compared to patients without MTH. We could not observe bleeding or any other complication related to MTH. Twenty-eight-day mortality did not differ significantly between patients with cirrhosis and MTH versus no MTH (78 vs. 72%). Additional file 1: Table S2 illustrates the detailed data on MTH in patients with cirrhosis.

## Discussion

In our study, we analysed 1068 critically ill patients following CA and ROSC. Forty-seven of these patients suffered from liver cirrhosis. Presence of cirrhosis was associated with low rates of favourable neurological outcome and increased mortality. Highest rates of unfavourable functional outcome were found in advanced stages of cirrhosis and ACLF.

Cardiac arrest was witnessed in 921 (86%) patients of our cohort, and this is comparable to a previous publication [27]. Seventy-five per cent of the total cohort had OHCA. The first recorded rhythm was shockable in 52% of these patients which is comparable to the reported prevalence of 20–60% in the literature [10, 11, 28]. In contrast, shockable rhythms (35%) were found less frequent in IHCA in accordance with the literature (21–39%) [13, 14, 29]. In the total cohort, 1-year mortality was 50% and favourable functional outcome was observed in 43% of patients following CA. This high rate of favourable outcome may be the consequence of several circumstances. First, we included only patients following ROSC after CA. Accordingly, the rate of good functional outcome was comparable to other studies including only patients with ROSC [27, 30]. Second, we observed in average a short no-flow period in our cohort, which may contribute to the high rate of favourable functional outcome. Third, the vast majority (86%) of CAs was witnessed and we observed a shockable rhythm in about half of the patients.

We identified 47 (4%) patients with cirrhosis in our cohort. This finding is comparable to publications of critical illness, where prevalence of cirrhosis was about 4–7% in the general intensive care setting [31, 32]. These patients had significantly higher SOFA, SAPS II and CCI on hospital admission. Time to ROSC was comparable between patients with and without cirrhosis. However, we observed several significant differences in CA in patients with and without cirrhosis. First, a cardiac aetiology was less frequent and patients with cirrhosis were more likely to have a non-shockable initial ECG rhythm. Second, cumulative epinephrine dosage was higher during CPR and third defibrillations were less frequently performed in patients with cirrhosis. These differences seem to be mainly a consequence of the fact that patients with cirrhosis frequently developed CA following complications of cirrhosis like variceal haemorrhage, severe infection or severe electrolyte disturbances.

Rates of unfavourable functional outcome and mortality were significantly higher in patients with cirrhosis despite no-flow times that were comparable to patients without cirrhosis. This can be explained by the higher comorbidity rate, higher rate of non-cardiac cause and higher rate of non-shockable rhythm in patients with cirrhosis. Furthermore, multivariate regression analysis identified presence of cirrhosis *per se* as an independent predictor of unfavourable outcome.

Overall 38 (81%) patients with cirrhosis had unfavourable neurological outcome or died within 28 days following CA. These patients had a significant higher severity of liver disease and organ failure represented by CTP class, CLIF-SOFA, MELD and ACLF grade as illustrated in Table 2. ACLF was present in 33 (70%) cirrhotic patients at ICU admission following ROSC, and four patients developed ACLF within 48 h after admission. These patients had dramatically worse functional outcome: out of 37 patients with ACLF, 34 (92%) had unfavourable neurology or died within 28 days. Moreover, we observed significant differences in CA characteristics. Patients with cirrhosis and favourable 28-day outcome had a significantly lower no-flow time and time to ROSC and a significantly lower rate of non-shockable rhythm compared to patients with unfavourable neurological outcome or mortality. Furthermore, CA was witnessed in all cases in patients with favourable 28-day outcome. Ischaemic times, especially no flow, seem to be crucial for development of organ failure and unfavourable outcome in patients with cirrhosis. The higher rate of unfavourable 28-day outcome in patients with cirrhosis following CA and ROSC compared to critically ill patients with liver cirrhosis [3, 4, 33] may be explained mainly by the higher severity of illness at baseline in our cohort [4].

The post-CA phase is frequently complicated by the post-CA syndrome, a unique pathophysiological process involving multiple organs [9]. For instance, post-CA brain injury frequently complicates the post-CA phase and accounts for high morbidity and mortality [9, 33]. Factors like hyperglycaemia, impaired cerebral autoregulation as well as pre-existing cerebral impairment in the sense of hepatic encephalopathy could lead to further cerebral injury in patients with cirrhosis. Additionally, post-CA myocardial dysfunction and systemic ischaemia and reperfusion response are frequent findings and account for high morbidity and mortality after CA [15]. The severity of the post-CA syndrome varies according to duration and cause of CA [15]. In our cohort of patients with cirrhosis, death was mainly related to multiple organ failure (86%). Post-anoxic encephalopathy as solitaire cause of death was observed in a minority of patients with cirrhosis, only. Patients with cirrhosis seem to be more prone to organ impairment following CA. This seems to be a consequence of a higher vulnerability for new onset of organ failure and higher severity of illness during CA as discussed previously.

Mild therapeutic hypothermia, i.e. targeted temperature 32–36 °C for 24 h [15], is frequently used despite recent controversial findings as standardised post-CA

care [27, 30, 34]. MTH was performed in 666 (62%) patients of our total cohort and in 18 (38%) patients with cirrhosis. Main reason for withholding MTH in cirrhosis was severely abnormal coagulation. A recent study of patients with cirrhosis demonstrated that abnormal coagulation parameters, especially fibrinogen and platelet counts, predict new onset of major bleeding in patients with cirrhosis at the ICU [33]. Data on bleeding complications due to MTH in patients with liver diseases are scarce. Two small case series [35, 36], a randomised controlled trial [37] and a retrospective study [38] of MTH in patients with acute liver failure did not observe an association of MTH and increased rate of bleeding complications. We could not observe new onset of bleeding or any other complication related to MTH in our cohort of critically ill patients with cirrhosis. Twenty-eight-day mortality did not differ significantly in patients with cirrhosis and MTH compared to patients with cirrhosis without MTH. This may be a consequence of the rather small number of patients with cirrhosis, the higher rate of OHCA and a significantly longer time to ROSC in the MTH group. In addition, this study was not powered to analyse the effect of MTH on prognosis in cirrhotic patients. Additional file 1: Table S2 illustrates the detailed data.

Multiple organ failure is associated with high mortality in patients with liver cirrhosis. ACLF is a dynamic condition, which can improve or worsen in a short period of time [39]. Early and repeated risk stratification may help and guide clinical decision making in this extremely sick population [40, 41]. Although our study is able to identify the population that is at highest risk of worst outcome (patients with advanced stages of ACLF and patients with cirrhosis CTP C), we do not believe that current knowledge is already sufficient to provide (i.e. score-based) cut-offs in regard to the decision whether to continue or to stop treatment due to futility. Rather, we are convinced that further therapeutic decisions, especially for withdrawal of care, must take individual patient based factors (i.e. severity of acute and chronic illness, patient's wishes, etc.) into account. Furthermore, remaining treatment options (e.g. liver transplantation), course of the disease and severity of acute illness should be taken into account for further decisions by the attending physician. Future studies are warranted for end-of-life decisions in critically ill patients with cirrhosis [41, 42].

Our study has some limitations. The number of patients with cirrhosis is rather small. However, this is the first study investigating CA in patients with cirrhosis. Furthermore, this study was conducted in a medical intensive care setting. Thus, our data may not be transferable to surgical ICUs. Residual confounding arising from unmeasured covariates cannot be entirely excluded.

In conclusion, CA survivors with cirrhosis have worse outcome than those without pre-existent chronic liver disease. Although one quarter of patients with liver cirrhosis survived longer than 28 days after successful CPR, patients with CTP C as well as advanced ACLF did not survive 28 days with good neurological outcome.

## Abbreviations

CA: cardiac arrest; ROSC: return of spontaneous circulation; ICU: intensive care unit; OHCA: out-of-hospital cardiac arrest; IHCA: in-hospital cardiac arrest; MTH: mild therapeutic hypothermia; CPC: cerebral performance categories; OPC: overall performance categories; SOFA: Sequential Organ Failure Assessment; SAPS: Simplified Acute Physiology Score; CCI: Charlson comorbidity index; MELD: model of end-stage liver disease; CTP: Child–Turcotte–Pugh; TIPS: transjugular intrahepatic portosystemic shunt; HCC: hepatocellular carcinoma; PCI: percutaneous coronary intervention.

## Authors' contributions

KRo, CWa, FS and VF participated in study conception and design. AD, TH, KRu, AS, JO, PH, CWe, JKM, DJ, CWa, VF and KRo were involved in acquisition of data. KRo, VF, FS, CWa and HH contributed to analysis and interpretation of data. KRo and CWa drafted the manuscript. VF, FS and HH were involved in critical revision of the manuscript for important intellectual content. VF and FS participated in supervision. All authors read and approved the final manuscript.

## Author details

[1] Department of Intensive Care Medicine, University Medical Center Hamburg-Eppendorf, Martinistraße 52, 20246 Hamburg, Germany. [2] Department of Emergency Medicine, Medical University of Vienna, Vienna, Austria. [3] Division of Gastroenterology and Hepatology, Department of Internal Medicine 3, Medical University of Vienna, Vienna, Austria.

## Acknowledgements

The authors would like to thank the staff of the Emergency Department and ICUs of the Medical University of Vienna and appreciate their work.

## Competing interests

The authors declare that they have no competing interests.

## Funding

No financial support has been received conducting this study.

## References

1. Shellman RG, Fulkerson WJ, DeLong E, Piantadosi CA. Prognosis of patients with cirrhosis and chronic liver disease admitted to the medical intensive care unit. Crit Care Med. 1988;16:671–8.
2. Jalan R, Gines P, Olson JC, Mookerjee RP, Moreau R, Garcia-Tsao G, et al. Acute-on chronic liver failure. J Hepatol. 2012;57:1336–48.
3. Moreau R, Jalan R, Gines P, Pavesi M, Angeli P, Cordoba J, et al. Acute-on-chronic liver failure is a distinct syndrome that develops in patients with acute decompensation of cirrhosis. Gastroenterology. 2013;144:1426–37 **(1437.e1421–1429)**.
4. McPhail MJW, Shawcross DL, Abeles RD, Chang A, Patel V, Lee G-H, et al. Increased survival for patients with cirrhosis and organ failure in liver intensive care and validation of the chronic liver failure-sequential organ failure scoring system. Clin Gastroenterol Hepatol. 2015;13(1353–1360):e1358.
5. Arabi Y, Ahmed QA, Haddad S, Aljumah A, Al-Shimemeri A. Outcome predictors of cirrhosis patients admitted to the intensive care unit. Eur J Gastroenterol Hepatol. 2004;16:333–9.
6. Cholongitas E, Senzolo M, Patch D, Kwong K, Nikolopoulou V, Leandro G, et al. Risk factors, sequential organ failure assessment and model for end-stage liver disease scores for predicting short term mortality in cirrhotic patients admitted to intensive care unit. Aliment Pharmacol Ther. 2006;23:883–93.
7. Berdowski J, Berg RA, Tijssen JGP, Koster RW. Global incidences of out-of-hospital cardiac arrest and survival rates: systematic review of 67 prospective studies. Resuscitation. 2010;81:1479–87.
8. Mozaffarian D, Benjamin EJ, Go AS, Arnett DK, Blaha MJ, Cushman M, et al. Heart disease and stroke statistics-2016 update: a report from the American Heart Association. Circ. 2016;133(4):e38–360.
9. Neumar RW, Nolan JP, Adrie C, Aibiki M, Berg RA, Böttiger BW, et al. Post-cardiac arrest syndrome: epidemiology, pathophysiology, treatment, and prognostication. A consensus statement from the International Liaison Committee on Resuscitation (American Heart Association, Australian and New Zealand Council on Resuscitation, European Resuscitation Council, Heart and Stroke Foundation of Canada, InterAmerican Heart Foundation, Resuscitation Council of Asia, and the Resuscitation Council of Southern Africa); the American Heart Association Emergency Cardiovascular Care Committee; the Council on Cardiovascular Surgery and Anesthesia; the Council on Cardiopulmonary, Perioperative, and Critical Care; the Council on Clinical Cardiology; and the Stroke Council. Circulation. 2008;118:2452–83.
10. Atwood C, Eisenberg MS, Herlitz J, Rea TD. Incidence of EMS-treated out-of-hospital cardiac arrest in Europe. Resuscitation. 2005;67:75–80.
11. Nichol G, Thomas E, Callaway CW, Hedges J, Powell JL, Aufderheide TP, et al. Regional variation in out-of-hospital cardiac arrest incidence and outcome. JAMA. 2008;300:1423–31.
12. Peberdy MA, Kaye W, Ornato JP, Larkin GL, Nadkarni V, Mancini ME, et al. Cardiopulmonary resuscitation of adults in the hospital: a report of 14720 cardiac arrests from the National Registry of Cardiopulmonary Resuscitation. Resuscitation. 2003;58:297–308.
13. Meaney PA, Nadkarni VM, Kern KB, Indik JH, Halperin HR, Berg RA. Rhythms and outcomes of adult in-hospital cardiac arrest. Crit Care Med. 2010;38:101–8.
14. Girotra S, Nallamothu BK, Spertus JA, Li Y, Krumholz HM, Chan PS. Trends in survival after in-hospital cardiac arrest. N Engl J Med. 2012;367:1912–20.
15. Nolan JP, Soar J, Cariou A, Cronberg T, Moulaert VRM, Deakin CD, et al. European Resuscitation Council and European Society of Intensive Care Medicine Guidelines for Post-resuscitation Care 2015: Section 5 of the European Resuscitation Council Guidelines for Resuscitation 2015. Resuscitation. 2015;95:202-22.
16. Soar J, Nolan JP, Böttiger BW, Perkins GD, Lott C, Carli P, et al. Section 3. Adult advanced life support: European Resuscitation Council guidelines for resuscitation 2015. Resuscitation. 2015;95:100-47.
17. Cummins RO, Chamberlain D, Hazinski MF, Nadkarni V, Kloeck W, Kramer E, et al. Recommended guidelines for reviewing, reporting, and conducting research on in-hospital resuscitation: the in-hospital 'Utstein style'. A statement for healthcare professionals from the American Heart Association, the European Resuscitation Council, the Heart and Stroke Foundation of Canada, the Australian Resuscitation Council, and the Resuscitation Councils of Southern Africa. Resuscitation. 1997;34:151–83.
18. Cummins RO, Chamberlain DA, Abramson NS, Allen M, Baskett PJ, Becker L, et al. Recommended guidelines for uniform reporting of data from out-of-hospital cardiac arrest: the Utstein Style. A statement for health professionals from a task force of the American Heart Association, the European Resuscitation Council, the Heart and Stroke Foundation of Canada, and the Australian Resuscitation Council. Circulation. 1991;84:960–75.
19. Schober A, Sterz F, Laggner AN, Poppe M, Sulzgruber P, Lobmeyr E, et al. Admission of out-of-hospital cardiac arrest victims to a high volume cardiac arrest center is linked to improved outcome. Resuscitation. 2016;106:42–8.
20. Nurnberger A, Sterz F, Malzer R, Warenits A, Girsa M, Stockl M, et al. Out of hospital cardiac arrest in Vienna: incidence and outcome. Resuscitation. 2013;84:42–7.

21. Jennett B, Bond M. Assessment of outcome after severe brain damage. Lancet. 1975;1:480–4.
22. Vincent JL, Moreno R, Takala J, Willatts S, De Mendonça A, Bruining H, et al. The SOFA (Sepsis-related Organ Failure Assessment) score to describe organ dysfunction/failure. On behalf of the Working Group on Sepsis-Related Problems of the European Society of Intensive Care Medicine. Intensive Care Med. 1996;22:707–10.
23. Le Gall JR, Lemeshow S, Saulnier F. A new Simplified Acute Physiology Score (SAPS II) based on a European/North American multicenter study. JAMA. 1993;270:2957–63.
24. Charlson ME, Pompei P, Ales KL, MacKenzie CR. A new method of classifying prognostic comorbidity in longitudinal studies: development and validation. J Chronic Dis. 1987;40:373–83.
25. Kamath PS, Wiesner RH, Malinchoc M, Kremers W, Therneau TM, Kosberg CL, et al. A model to predict survival in patients with end-stage liver disease. Hepatology. 2001;33:464–70.
26. Cholongitas E, Papatheodoridis GV, Vangeli M, Terreni N, Patch D, Burroughs AK. Systematic review: the model for end-stage liver disease—should it replace Child-Pugh's classification for assessing prognosis in cirrhosis? Aliment Pharmacol Ther. 2005;22:1079–89.
27. Nielsen N, Wetterslev J, Cronberg T, Erlinge D, Gasche Y, Hassager C, et al. Targeted temperature management at 33 °C versus 36 °C after cardiac arrest. N Engl J Med. 2013;369:2197–206.
28. Schober A, Sterz F, Herkner H, Locker GJ, Heinz G, Fuhrmann V, et al. Post-resuscitation care at the emergency department with critical care facilities—a length-of-stay analysis. Resuscitation. 2011;82:853–8.
29. Wallmuller C, Meron G, Kurkciyan I, Schober A, Stratil P, Sterz F. Causes of in-hospital cardiac arrest and influence on outcome. Resuscitation. 2012;83:1206–11.
30. Group HaCAS. Mild therapeutic hypothermia to improve the neurologic outcome after cardiac arrest. N Engl J Med. 2002;346:549–56.
31. Piton G, Chaignat C, Giabicani M, Cervoni JP, Tamion F, Weiss E, et al. Prognosis of cirrhotic patients admitted to the general ICU. Ann Intensive Care. 2016;6:94.
32. Fuhrmann V, Kneidinger N, Herkner H, Heinz G, Nikfardjam M, Bojic A, et al. Impact of hypoxic hepatitis on mortality in the intensive care unit. Intensive Care Med. 2011;37:1302–10.
33. Drolz A, Horvatits T, Roedl K, Rutter K, Staufer K, Kneidinger N, et al. Coagulation parameters and major bleeding in critically ill patients with cirrhosis. Hepatology. 2016;64:556–68.
34. Bernard SA, Gray TW, Buist MD, Jones BM, Silvester W, Gutteridge G, et al. Treatment of comatose survivors of out-of-hospital cardiac arrest with induced hypothermia. N Engl J Med. 2002;346:557–63.
35. Jalan R, Olde Damink SWM, Deutz NEP, Hayes PC, Lee A. Moderate hypothermia in patients with acute liver failure and uncontrolled intracranial hypertension. Gastroenterology. 2004;127:1338–46.
36. Jalan R, ODamink SW, Deutz NE, Lee A, Hayes PC. Moderate hypothermia for uncontrolled intracranial hypertension in acute liver failure. Lancet. 1999;354:1164–8.
37. Bernal W, Murphy N, Brown S, Whitehouse T, Bjerring PN, Hauerberg J, et al. A multicentre randomized controlled trial of moderate hypothermia to prevent intracranial hypertension in acute liver failure. J Hepatol 2016;65(2):273-9.
38. Karvellas CJ, Todd Stravitz R, Battenhouse H, Lee WM, Schilsky ML, Group UALFS. Therapeutic hypothermia in acute liver failure: a multicenter retrospective cohort analysis. Liver Transpl. 2015;21:4–12.
39. Arroyo V, Moreau R, Jalan R, Gines P. Acute-on-chronic liver failure: a new syndrome that will re-classify cirrhosis. J Hepatol. 2015;62:S131–43.
40. Saliba F, Ichai P, Levesque E, Samuel D. Cirrhotic patients in the ICU: prognostic markers and outcome. Curr Opin Crit Care. 2013;19:154–60.
41. Gustot T, Fernandez J, Garcia E, Morando F, Caraceni P, Alessandria C, et al. Clinical course of acute-on-chronic liver failure syndrome and effects on prognosis. Hepatology. 2015;62:243–52.
42. McPhail MJ, Auzinger G, Bernal W, Wendon JA. Decisions on futility in patients with cirrhosis and organ failure. Hepatology. 2016;64:986.

# 12

# The 2014 updated version of the Confusion Assessment Method for the Intensive Care Unit compared to the 5th version of the Diagnostic and Statistical Manual of Mental Disorders and other current methods used by intensivists

Gérald Chanques[1,2*†], E. Wesley Ely[3,4†], Océane Garnier[1], Fanny Perrigault[5], Anaïs Eloi[5], Julie Carr[1], Christine M. Rowan[3], Albert Prades[1], Audrey de Jong[1,2], Sylvie Moritz-Gasser[5,6], Nicolas Molinari[7] and Samir Jaber[1,2]

## Abstract

**Background:** One third of patients admitted to an intensive care unit (ICU) will develop delirium. However, delirium is under-recognized by bedside clinicians without the use of delirium screening tools, such as the Intensive Care Delirium Screening Checklist (ICDSC) or the Confusion Assessment Method for the ICU (CAM-ICU). The CAM-ICU was updated in 2014 to improve its use by clinicians throughout the world. It has never been validated compared to the new reference standard, the Diagnostic and Statistical Manual of Mental Disorders 5th version (DSM-5).

**Methods:** We made a prospective psychometric study in a 16-bed medical–surgical ICU of a French academic hospital, to measure the diagnostic performance of the 2014 updated CAM-ICU compared to the DSM-5 as the reference standard. We included consecutive adult patients with a Richmond Agitation Sedation Scale (RASS) $\geq -3$, without preexisting cognitive disorders, psychosis or cerebral injury. Delirium was independently assessed by neuropsychological experts using an operationalized approach to DSM-5, by investigators using the CAM-ICU and the ICDSC, by bedside clinicians and by ICU patients. The sensitivity, specificity, positive and negative predictive values were calculated considering neuropsychologist DSM-5 assessments as the reference standard (primary endpoint). CAM-ICU inter-observer agreement, as well as that between delirium diagnosis methods and the reference standard, was summarized using $\kappa$ coefficients, which were subsequently compared using the $Z$-test.

**Results:** Delirium was diagnosed by experts in 38% of the 108 patients included for analysis. The CAM-ICU had a sensitivity of 83%, a specificity of 100%, a positive predictive value of 100% and a negative predictive value of 91%. Compared to the reference standard, the CAM-ICU had a significantly ($p < 0.05$) higher agreement ($\kappa = 0.86 \pm 0.05$) than the physicians', residents' and nurses' diagnoses ($\kappa = 0.65 \pm 0.09$; $0.63 \pm 0.09$; $0.61 \pm 0.09$, respectively), as well as the patient's own impression of feeling delirious ($\kappa = 0.02 \pm 0.11$). Differences between the ICDSC ($\kappa = 0.69 \pm 0.07$)

*Correspondence: g-chanques@chu-montpellier.fr
†Gérald Chanques and E. Wesley Ely contributed equally to this study
[1] Department of Anaesthesia and Critical Care Medicine, University of Montpellier Saint Eloi Hospital, 80, avenue Augustin Fliche, 34295 Montpellier Cedex 5, France
Full list of author information is available at the end of the article

and CAM-ICU were not significant ($p = 0.054$). The CAM-ICU demonstrated a high reliability for inter-observer agreement ($\kappa = 0.87 \pm 0.06$).

**Conclusions:** The 2014 updated version of the CAM-ICU is valid according to DSM-5 criteria and reliable regarding inter-observer agreement in a research setting. Delirium remains under-recognized by bedside clinicians.

**Keywords:** Delirium, Intensive care unit, Critical care

## Background

Nearly one third of patients admitted to an intensive care unit (ICU) will develop delirium [1], which is subsequently associated with sedation–analgesia management issues [2–4], an increased duration of mechanical ventilation, length of stay in the ICU and hospital, risk of death, as well as of having long-term neurocognitive dysfunction [1, 5]. Guidelines recommend the routine use of validated clinical tools for the early recognition and treatment of delirium by medical and nursing ICU teams, even if they are not expert neuropsychologists [6].

Among the delirium diagnosis tools that can be used by ICU clinicians in routine practice, the Confusion Assessment Method for the ICU (CAM-ICU) [7, 8] and the Intensive Care Delirium Screening Checklist (ICDSC) [9] have been extensively studied for more than 15 years, demonstrating good psychometric properties in a research setting [6]. In 2014, the CAM-ICU and its training manual were updated to avoid any misinterpretation by users (Table 1). Also, the original version of the CAM-ICU [7, 8] was validated against the American Psychiatric Association's fourth edition of the Diagnostic and Statistical Manual of Mental Disorders (DSM-IV). Differences between the 4th and the new 5th versions (DSM-5) regarding delirium assessment are still under debate [10, 11].

The primary objective of this study was to measure the ability of the 2014 updated version of the CAM-ICU to diagnose delirium according to the most updated neuropsychological reference standard, i.e., the DSM-5 method. Secondary objectives were (1) to measure inter-observer agreement for the CAM-ICU, and (2) within the context of a comprehensive investigation of delirium assessment in a real-life intensive care setting, to compare the diagnostic accuracy of the CAM-ICU to the ICDSC and to physician, resident and nurse recognition of delirium, as well as to common orientation questions and to the patient's own impression of feeling delirious.

## Methods

### Ethics and consent

The protocol was approved by an independent ethics committee [*Comité de Protection des Personnes (CPP) Sud Méditerranée.IV* (N°ID-RCB: 2015-A01084-45; Protocol version 1: 06/23/2015)] and was conducted in accordance with the Declaration of Helsinki (clinicaltrials.gov: NCT02760446). Written consent was required from the patient or the legally authorized representative or a proxy/surrogate decision maker (patient's next of kin) who gave consent on the patient's behalf, followed by the patient's consent as soon they could communicate.

**Table 1 Principal changes made in the 2014 updated version of the CAM-ICU training manual**

| Features | Changes in the 2014 updated version |
|---|---|
| Feature 1 = *Acute onset or fluctuating course of mental status* | The term "sedation level" was intertwined with the "level of consciousness" throughout the method because some clinicians used these two terms interchangeably, but others were confused by the fact that patients could not receive sedatives. Note that RASS can be used in patients sedated or non-sedated |
| Feature 2 = *Inattention* | Another new 10-letter set (C–A–S–A–B–L–A–N–C–A) is now provided to allow for international understanding |
| Feature 3 = *Altered level of consciousness* | Following many institutions, the former feature #3 (disorganized thinking) was switched with former feature #4 (altered level of consciousness). The new feature #3 (level of consciousness) is often sufficient to rate a CAM-ICU as positive, while the new feature #4 (disorganized thinking) is less often necessary to perform in the end |
| Feature 4 = *Disorganized thinking* | This feature was rewritten to avoid any confusion in the total number of errors required among the 4 questions and 1 command: > 1 error = feature #4 present |
| Supporting materials | The updated method was associated with a 32-page complete training manual (available at www.icudelirium.org), including an extensive Frequently Asked Questions section, new case studies and links to the ICUDelirium.org Web site that was completely remodeled |

*CAM-ICU* Confusion Assessment Method for the Intensive Care Unit, *RASS* Richmond Agitation Sedation Scale

## Population

The study took place in the 16-bed medical–surgical ICU of the University of Montpellier Saint Eloi Hospital, an academic tertiary-care hospital, from November 2015 to April 2016. All consecutive French-speaking patients $\geq$ 18-year old were eligible for enrollment if they had a Richmond Agitation Sedation Scale (RASS) $\geq$ −3 [12–14]. Exclusion criteria were preexisting cognitive disorder/psychosis (baseline cognitive status is often unknown early in the ICU stay, precluding accurate evaluation of change in mental status, a key feature of delirium), visual/hearing loss without helpers, pregnancy (according to French law), patients under tutelage, withdrawal of consent or change in clinical status that would preclude a complete cognitive testing.

## Study conduct

All consecutive patients admitted to our ICU were screened by the ICU research team every morning including weekends, until they reached the inclusion criteria during a period of 5 months (November 2015–March 2016). After having obtained consent and enrolling the patient, the ICU research team contacted one of two neuropsychological experts participating in the study to independently perform a neuropsychological assessment of delirium. Figure 1 summarizes the timing of delirium assessments by the neuropsychological experts and the ICU research team.

## Data collection

### Delirium

Delirium was assessed once, the same day, in five ways that occurred as close together as possible in time, but strictly independent of each other. Separate clinical research forms were used to assure independence between observers.

*1. ICU delirium tools: CAM-ICU and ICDSC* The ICU research team used the French versions of the 2014 updated CAM-ICU training manual and the ICDSC [9, 15]. The CAM-ICU was assessed by two independent investigators to estimate inter-observer agreement.

*2. Expert neuropsychological assessment of delirium (the reference standard)* The neuropsychological experts were members of the speech and language therapy team, usually in charge of neuropsychological testing in the neurology/neurosurgery/neuro-ICU departments of the Neurosciences University Hospital of Montpellier. A standardized method for diagnosing delirium was used based on the DSM-5 [16] using the Montreal Cognitive Assessment (MOCA) [17], Dubois' 5-word test [18], Language Screening Test (LAST) [19], with helpers for intubated ICU patients (see Additional file 1: Supplemental Digital Content).

*3. Bedside–clinician assessment of delirium* When immediately available, the patient's bedside ICU team

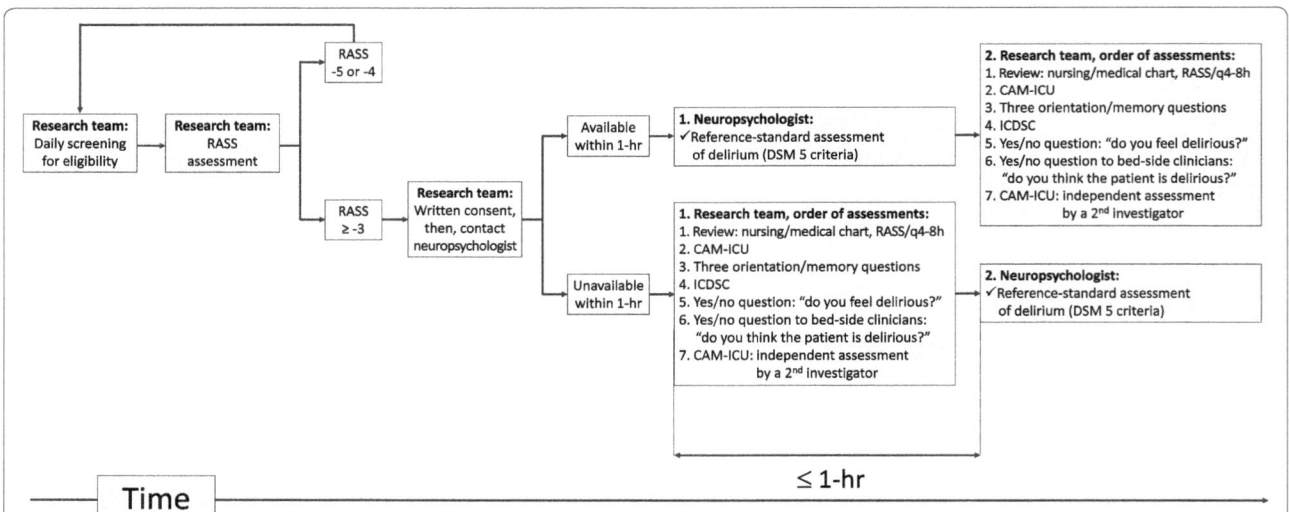

**Fig. 1** Study design. The order of assessments by the research team was determined to check both the patient's eligibility and the presence of some CAM-ICU and ICDSC features (i.e., fluctuating course of mental status assessed by RASS ratings). ICDSC was assessed after CAM-ICU because ICDSC included some CAM-ICU features (i.e., inattention). *RASS* Richmond Agitation Sedation Scale, *CAM-ICU* Confusion Assessment Method for the Intensive Care Unit, *ICDSC* Intensive Care Delirium Screening Checklist, *DSM-5* 5th version of the Diagnostic and Statistical Manual of Mental Disorders

(i.e., the patient's nurse, resident and attending physician) were contacted by the ICU research team to get their personal feeling about the presence or absence of delirium.

*4. The 3 simple orientation/memory questions for the assessment of delirium* The ICU research team also assessed delirium by asking three simple questions commonly used to assess delirium at our institution: Where are you? What day is it today? Who is the president? (because long-term memory is frequently altered in delirium) [20]. The number of incorrect and absent response(s) was recorded.

*5. The patient's own feeling* At the end of testing, the patients were asked by the ICU research team if they had the impression they were confused.

### Demographic and medical data

Age, gender, comorbidities and the reason for ICU admission were recorded. The Simplified Acute Physiological Score II (SAPS-II) score [21] and the Sequential Organ Failure Assessment (SOFA) score [22] were calculated within 24 h after ICU admission and upon enrollment. In case enrollment occurred before 24 h, the SAPS-II score took into account the worst value available during the 24 h preceding enrollment. Therapeutics such as sedation, mechanical ventilation and the use of vasopressors were collected upon enrollment.

### Data presentation and statistical analysis
### Psychometric properties of the CAM-ICU

*Validity (primary endpoint)* The performance of the CAM-ICU for diagnosing delirium was assessed by measuring the sensitivity, specificity, positive predictive value (PPV) and negative predictive value (NPV) according to standardized definitions [23, 24]. Expert assessments were used as the reference standard.

*Reliability* The kappa coefficient was calculated between the two ICU research investigators. Kappa coefficients above 0.80, 0.60 and 0.40 are considered as measuring 'near perfect', 'strong' and 'moderate' levels of agreement [25], respectively.

### The diagnostic performance of other methods commonly used to assess delirium (ICSDC, bedside clinician assessments, 3-question test), as well as patients' impressions)

The sensitivity, specificity, PPV and NPV were also calculated using the expert assessments as the reference standard. To compare all five methods for diagnosing delirium, kappa coefficients were calculated between the expert assessments and the other methods. Kappa coefficient comparisons between methods were made using

the Z-test [26]. A $p$ value of $< 0.05$ was considered statistically significant.

*Power analysis* The study sample size was determined in relation to the primary endpoint. For expected values [8] of sensitivity and specificity at 85 and 75%, respectively, a desired level of precision set at 10% and the prevalence of delirium set at 50%, the number of patient inclusions required for achieving appropriate power would be 95. Taking into account possible post-enrollment exclusions, 115 patients needed to be enrolled in the study. The prevalence of delirium ranged from 30 to 90% in the literature [1]. Thus, we set the prevalence of delirium at 50% which is conservative regarding the number of patients needed to be analyzed, in order to maximize the power.

*Data presentation* Quantitative data are shown as medians and 25th–75th percentiles. Data were analyzed using SAS version 9.2 (SAS Institute, Cary, NC).

### Results

A total of 108 patients were included for analysis among the 115 patients enrolled in the study. A Standards for Reporting of Diagnostic Accuracy (STARD) diagram for patient enrollment is shown in Additional file 1: Supplemental Digital Content. Table 2 summarizes patient demographic and medical characteristics. Delirium was diagnosed by the neuropsychological experts for 41 of the 108 patients (38%).

### Validation of the 2014 updated CAM-ICU

A positive CAM-ICU was found for 34 (31%) patients. Compared to expert assessments, there were 7 misclassified CAM-ICU ratings among the 108 ratings, of which there were 7 false negatives and no false positives. Compared to expert assessments, the CAM-ICU had a sensitivity of 83% [95% confidence interval 71–94], a specificity of 100% [100–100], a PPV of 100% [100–100] and a NPV of 91% [84–97].

To measure the inter-observer reliability of the CAM-ICU, 98 patients were assessed by a second investigator. For the ten remaining patients, a second assessment was impossible because of changes in vigilance status or clinical condition. The kappa coefficient for inter-observer reliability was 0.87 (SD $\pm$ 0.06) demonstrating strong agreement. There were no significant differences between the 5 ICU investigators and the 2 neuropsychological experts (kappa coefficients ranging from 0.82 $\pm$ 0.1 to 0.88 $\pm$ 0.2). First and second CAM-ICU investigators obtained similar agreement with experts' assessments (kappa coefficients = 0.86 $\pm$ 0.1 and 0.85 $\pm$ 0.1, respectively).

**Table 2 Demographic and medical characteristics of the 108 patients included for analysis**

| Characteristics | Median [IQR] or n (%) |
| --- | --- |
| Upon ICU admission | |
| Age (years) | 62 [54–68] |
| Sex [n (%)] | |
| Male | 64 (59%) |
| Female | 44 (41%) |
| Body mass index (kg/m$^{-2}$) | 25 [23–29] |
| Type of admission | |
| Unplanned surgical (from operating room) [n (%)] | 26 (24%) |
| Planned surgical (from operating room) [n (%)] | 15 (14%) |
| Surgical (from ward) [n (%)] | 5 (05%) |
| Medical [n (%)] | 62 (57%) |
| SAPS II score | 39 [31–49] |
| SOFA score | 7 [4–9] |
| Sepsis at admission [n (%)] | 47 (44%) |
| Intubation at admission [n (%)] | 70 (65%) |
| Upon study enrollment | |
| Time between ICU admission and enrollment (days) | 3 [2–5] |
| SAPS II score | 29 [23–38] |
| SOFA score | 4 [2–7] |
| Vigilance status | |
| Median RASS level | 0 [0–0] |
| RASS level = +2 [n (%)] | 2 (2%) |
| RASS level = +1 [n (%)] | 8 (7%) |
| RASS level = 0 [n (%)] | 76 (70%) |
| RASS level = −1 [n (%)] | 13 (12%) |
| RASS level = −2 [n (%)] | 4 (4%) |
| RASS level = −3 [n (%)] | 5 (5%) |
| Therapeutics | |
| Invasive mechanical ventilation [n (%)] | 23 (21%) |
| Noninvasive mechanical ventilation [n (%)] | 8 (07%) |
| Vasopressors [n (%)] | 18 (17%) |
| Sedation (propofol) [n (%)] | 12 (11%) |
| At ICU discharge | |
| Total duration of mechanical ventilation (days) | 1.6 [0.3–5.5] |
| ICU length of stay (days) | 6.5 [3.0–12.4] |

*BMI* body mass index, *ICU* Intensive Care Unit, *IQR* inter-quartile range, *RASS* Richmond Agitation Sedation Scale, *SAPS II* Simplified Acute Physiological Score II, *SOFA* Sequential Organ Failure Assessment score

## Diagnostic performance of commonly used methods for assessing delirium

Table 3 presents the statistical measurement of performance regarding delirium recognition via the CAM-ICU, and the ICDSC, by nurses, residents and physicians, as well as via three simple questions. The CAM-ICU demonstrated good performance, while the 3 simple questions demonstrated poor performance. The 3 simple questions demonstrated the highest sensitivity for a false or absent response, but with the lowest specificity and PPV. The ICDSC and clinicians' diagnosis demonstrated similar performances.

Figure 2 shows the graphic representation of kappa coefficients for each of the methods used to assess delirium. The kappa coefficient measured the agreement between each of the methods and the assessment by the neuropsychological experts using DSM-5 criteria (reference standard). There was a significant difference between the level of agreement found for the CAM-ICU (kappa $0.86 \pm 0.05$) and that found for other methods ($p < 0.047$), except the ICDSC ($0.69 \pm 0.07$, $p = 0.054$, Z-test). Detailed data regarding CAM-ICU/ICDSC procedures are provided in Additional file 1: Supplemental Digital Content.

The 3 simple questions and the patient's own impression had the lowest agreements with experts and demonstrated significant differences with other methods.

### Patient's own impression of feeling delirious

Among the 108 patients, 77 (71%) were able to answer the question as to whether they felt delirious or not (all had a RASS level $\geq -1$). Among these patients, 27 (35%) answered that they were. The patient's sensitivity for recognizing delirium compared to expert assessments was 38%, with a specificity of 66%, a PPV of 22% and a NPV of 80%.

## Discussion

The main finding of this study is that the 2014 updated version of the CAM-ICU was valid compared to the DSM-5 reference standard, with strong inter-observer agreement. CAM-ICU and ICDSC agreed with experts' opinion without significant difference. The CAM-ICU had superior performance for diagnosing delirium compared to the bedside–clinicians' opinion, as well as compared to simple questions that are commonly used to assess delirium. Patient impressions of feeling delirious are not accurate, with a false-positive rate at 78%.

Delirium is multifactorial and frequent in critically ill ICU patients [6, 27–35]. It is diagnosed in 10–90% of ICU patients, depending on the diagnosis tool, the timing of assessment (during or after interrupting sedation), as well as the frequency of assessment (one-point assessment for validation studies or throughout the ICU stay) [6, 36]. A recent review of 42 studies estimated the prevalence of delirium at 5280 (31.8%) out of 16,595 critically ill patients [1]. The prevalence of delirium in the present study is close to this result: 38% according to neuropsychological assessment and 31% according to the CAM-ICU. Although frequent, delirium is under-recognized

**Table 3** Patients' clinical diagnosis and simple orientation questions

| Measure-ment | ICU delirium tools | | Patients' clinician diagnosis[a] | | | 3 Simple orientation questions | | | |
|---|---|---|---|---|---|---|---|---|---|
| | CAM-ICU | ICDSC | Physician | Resident | Nurse | 1 false or absent response | 2 false or absent responses | 1 false response[b] | 2 false responses[b] |
| Sensitivity | 83% [71–94] | 83% [71–94] | 79% [65–94] | 68% [52–83] | 70% [54–86] | 90% [81–99] | 68% [54–83] | 78% [59–97] | 28% [7–48] |
| Specificity | 100% [100–100] | 87% [78–95] | 85% [75–96] | 93% [86–100] | 89% [82–97] | 66% [54–77] | 82% [73–91] | 73% [62–85] | 92% [85–99] |
| PPV | 100% [100–100] | 79% [67–91] | 79% [65–94] | 85% [72–99] | 78% [62–93] | 62% [49–74] | 70% [56–84] | 47% [29–65] | 50% [19–81] |
| NPV | 91% [84–97] | 89% [82–97] | 85% [75–96] | 82% [72–92] | 85% [76–94] | 92% [84–99] | 81% [72–90] | 92% [84–99] | 81% [72–90] |
| Delirium diagnosis by non experts | 31% | 40% | 41% | 31% | 31% | 56% | 37% | 38% | 13% |
| by experts | 38% | 38% | 41% | 39% | 34% | 38% | 38% | 21% | 21% |
| Agreement with experts ($\kappa \pm SD$)[c] | 0.86 ± 0.05 | 0.69 ± 0.07 | 0.65 ± 0.09 | 0.63 ± 0.09 | 0.61 ± 0.09 | 0.51 ± 0.08 | 0.51 ± 0.09 | 0.41 ± 0.10 | 0.23 ± 0.13 |

The statistical measurement of performance is expressed as the percentage and its 95% confidence interval. *CAM-ICU* Confusion Assessment Method for the Intensive Care Unit, *ICDSC* Intensive Care Delirium Screening Checklist, *PPV* positive predictive value, *NPV* negative predictive value

[a] Among the 108 patients included for analysis, patients' clinicians were available upon study completion for 91 patient nurses (84%), 89 patient residents (82%) and 71 patient physicians (66%). Among the clinicians participating in the study, the 4 nurses, 1 resident and 1 physician who could not answer the question whether the patient was or was not delirious were not taken into account for the analysis

[b] Analysis was performed among the 78 patients (72%) who were able to answer all three simple questions

[c] The agreement between each method of delirium diagnosis and the assessment by the neuropsychological experts using DSM-5 criteria (reference standard) was measured using kappa coefficients

by both physicians and nurses [37]. Compared to the CAM-ICU, clinician sensitivity for diagnosing delirium is about 30% [38, 39]. The recognition of delirium by physicians and nurses in the present study was better, with a sensitivity of nearly 70%, suggesting that there might have been an increase in clinician awareness regarding delirium in the ICU over the past decade [40]. However, with PPVs under 80% and NPVs under 90% in the present study, clinicians should still use an ICU delirium tool to improve their diagnostic performance, according to current guidelines [6]. In the present study, agreement with expert diagnosis was not significantly different between the CAM-ICU and the ICDSC. In previous studies, the pooled sensitivity and specificity were 76 and 96%, respectively, for the CAM-ICU, and 80 and 75% for the ICDSC [41]. Sensitivity and specificity were slightly higher for both tools in the present study. This could be due to the study setting where a research team with experience in conducting research in the area of sedation–analgesia was available to conduct this psychometric study. Indeed, performance measurements for ICU delirium tools are higher in research settings than in real life [41]. However, the original study validating the CAM-ICU reported higher sensitivity and specificity than in the present study, with a sensitivity ranging from 93 to 100% and a specificity ranging from 98 to 100% [8]. This

could be due to differences in the studied populations. In the original study [8], patients had a median Glasgow score of 7 at enrollment, while in the present study, 80% of patients had a RASS level ≥ 0, suggesting they were more alert. It has been reported that the CAM-ICU could have a lower sensitivity in alert patients, possibly because of better cognitive function [42, 43]. Because delirium prevalence and recognition may depend on the level of consciousness, some authors recommend stratifying delirium assessments for sedation score using a cutoff of RASS − 2 [44]. In the present study also, when taking into account only the 99 patients who had a RASS level of > −2 for a sensitivity analysis, the delirium prevalence was lower than in the overall population (32% instead of 38% according to the experts, 25% instead of 31%, according to the CAM-ICU). The CAM-ICU had a slightly lower sensitivity (78%, instead of 83%), while conserving the same specificity, positive and negative predictive values. Similar findings were obtained when excluding from the analysis the 12 patients who were sedated (8 of them having a RASS level of > −2).

Our study has several limitations. For example, all the methods for diagnosing delirium were assessed within a short time. This may have tired patients and decreased their cognitive functions. The research team planned the assessments within the space of an hour to increase

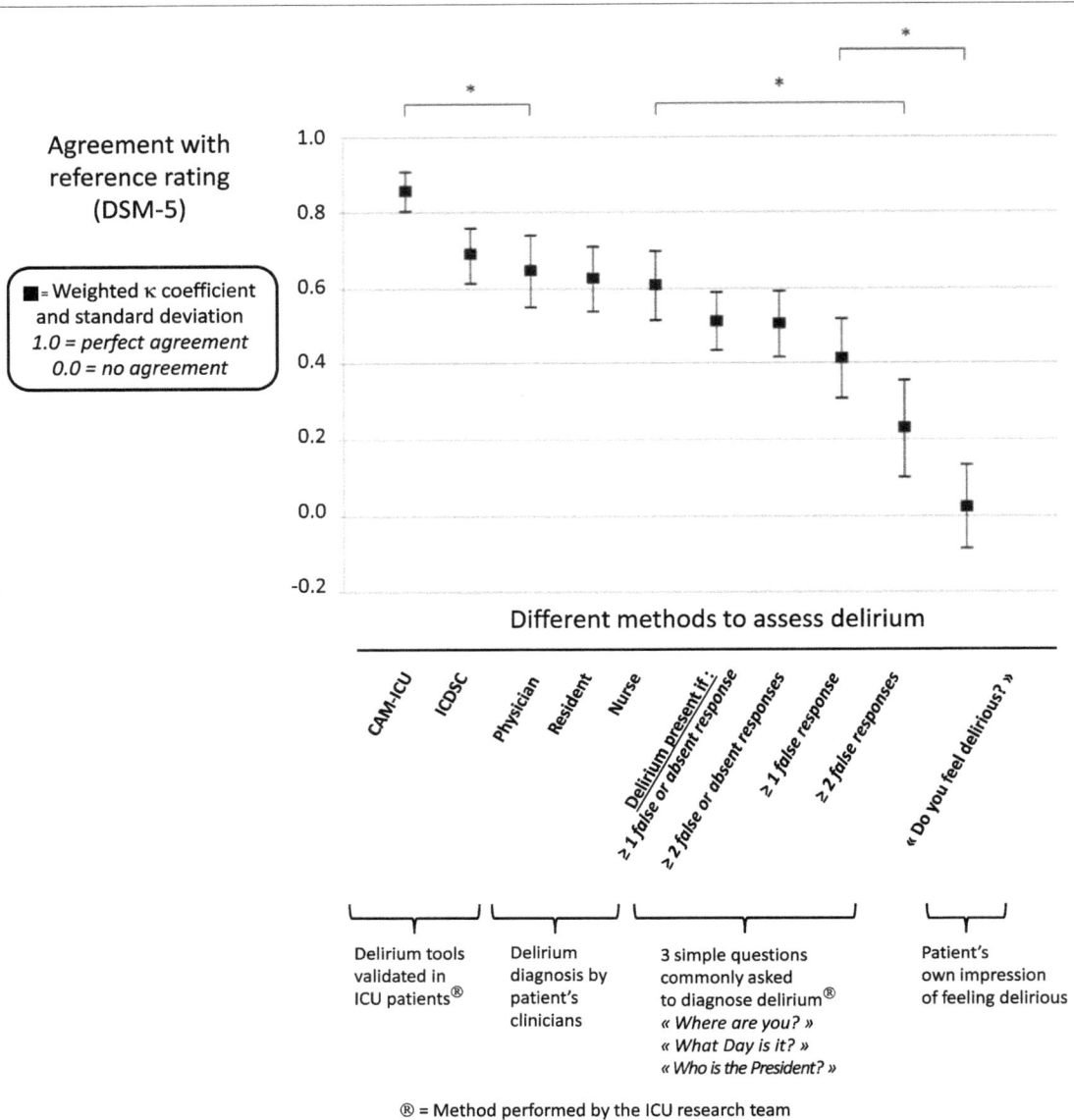

**Fig. 2** Agreement between different delirium assessment methods and the neurological experts' reference rating using the DSM-5 criteria. This figure shows the graphic representation of kappa coefficients and their standard deviations for each of the methods used to assess delirium. The kappa coefficient measured the agreement between each of the methods and the assessment by the neuropsychologist experts using DSM-5 criteria (reference standard). For simple questions, we did not decide a priori how to analyze the answers. Because some patients answered some questions but did not answer other ones, we decided a posteriori to analyze these data following two approaches: including all patients and including only the patients able to answer all the questions. Several thresholds were tested, i.e., delirium was defined in all patients if they gave at least 1 or 2 false or no response(s), or, among the patients who were able to answer all simple questions, if the patients gave at least 1 or 2 false response(s). There was a significant difference ($p < 0.047$) between the CAM-ICU and each of the other methods, except the ICDSC ($p = 0.054$). There were significant differences between "all methods from CAM-ICU to $\geq$ 1 false response to simple questions" and "patient's own impression of feeling delirious," as well as between "all methods from CAM-ICU to nurse diagnosis" and "$\geq$ 2 false responses to simple questions" or "patient's own impression of feeling delirious." *: Significant difference ($p < 0.05$); *CAM-ICU* Confusion Assessment Method for the Intensive Care Unit, *ICDSC* Intensive Care Delirium Screening Checklist

the chance of measuring delirium at the same time for a given patient (Fig. 1). The agreement between the neuropsychological expert and the CAM-ICU was not significantly different whether the expert performed the assessment before or after the research team (kappa coefficient $0.86 \pm 0.1$ vs $0.85 \pm 0.1$, respectively). Secondly, except ICDSC, many other validated delirium tools [42] were not performed in order to make the duration of assessment feasible. In the same way, the ICDSC could have demonstrated higher sensitivity and specificity if it had been performed in more alert patients, and by the patient's clinicians rather than by the research team. To perform the ICDSC, the research team took into account all nursing/medical charts (Fig. 1) but performed only "punctual" cognitive evaluations instead of evaluations over a nursing shift. The ICDSC was not performed by the patient's clinicians to avoid any bias regarding their raw opinion about the presence or the absence of delirium. In other words, clinicians did not use a validated delirium tool which is to take into account for the interpretation of the data. The primary goal of the present study was to validate the 2014 updated version of the CAM-ICU. Measuring the psychometric properties of the ICDSC was only informative because it is a second recommended tool for assessing delirium and therefore frequently used throughout the world [6]. Moreover, the present study demonstrated no significant difference between the ICDSC and CAM-ICU regarding the agreement between the ICU research team and the neuropsychological experts (Fig. 2). However, this study was not calibrated to measure this difference. A longer period of evaluation could have resulted in a higher sensitivity for ICDS. Similarly, repeated measurements of delirium on a longer period of time could have lead to a higher sensitivity. Regarding the expert's assessment, DSM-5 interpretations and use as a reference standard for delirium are a source of debate and thus may vary according to assessor [10, 11]. Finally, all the causes of delirium were not investigated because this was out of the scope of this psychometric study. Sepsis was present in 44% of patients at admission, and 11% of patients received sedatives at enrollment. Thus, a few intubated patients were included, due to a strategy of "early-sedation-interruption." This study should be further performed in different settings/ICU populations.

Study strengths include the reference standard method used by experts to diagnose delirium, which was provided for the first time in detail to facilitate study reproducibility (see Additional file 1: Supplemental Digital Content). Aside from the expert assessment, a pragmatic approach for diagnosing delirium was also evaluated in order to reflect real-life situations in intensive care. This included nurse, resident and physician diagnoses, as well as commonly used simple orientation/memory questions. These questions are not appropriate for diagnosing delirium. This might be due to patient disorientation, which can be related to environment (absence of windows). The recommendation to use a validated delirium tool is reinforced by the fact that the ICU team is used

to conducting clinical research and quality improvement projects in the area of agitation, sedation and analgesia [45–47]. Even in such an "a priori" favorable setting for the early recognition of delirium, bedside–clinicians still need to use a validated tool during their routine practice, repeatedly during the day and throughout the ICU stay. This is paramount for treating the factors associated with delirium [6, 27–35] as soon as possible, especially when taking into account the negative outcomes associated with delirium [5, 6]. A comprehensive approach [48] integrating delirium management with analgesia, sedation, mechanical ventilation, mobility/exercise and family engagement/empowerment has shown a positive impact on increasing ventilatory-free days [49, 50], decreasing delirium incidence [49–51] and improving hospital mortality [51].

Finally, the study investigated the patient's ability to recognize delirium. Though delusional memories are frequent in ICU survivors, they have not been investigated during hospitalization in the ICU setting [52–54]. Recent studies found no significant association between delirium in the ICU and mental disorders in survivors [55–57]. However, memories of being delirious in the ICU are associated with anxiety [56]. The link between delirium recollection, feelings of being delirious while in the ICU (which is possibly theoretically wrong or too abstract for some patients) and long-term psychological outcomes thus requires further exploration.

## Conclusions

The 2014 updated version of the CAM-ICU is a valid tool for delirium diagnosis in a research setting in critically ill patients according to the DSM-5 criteria used by neuropsychological experts. It demonstrated important inter-observer reliability, and better performance for diagnosing delirium in ICU patients than physicians, residents and nurses, despite increased awareness regarding delirium in the ICU for many years. Future studies should investigate the discrepancies between validated methods to diagnose delirium (DSM-5, CAM-ICU, ICDSC) and the ICU team. Moreover, the patient's own ability to report delirium might be inaccurate. Ethics committees should pay attention to delirium assessment when checking for patient's ability to consent to participate in ICU studies [58]. This suggests also that delusional memories reported by survivors should be investigated in regard to a valid assessment of delirium during the ICU stay. In the ICU, patients should be asked about feeling delirious, comforted if they are not, but be taken care of regarding what could make them feel so.

## Abbreviations

CAM-ICU: Confusion Assessment Method for the Intensive Care Unit; DSM-5: 5th version of the Diagnostic and Statistical Manual of Mental Disorders; ICDSC: Intensive Care Delirium Screening Checklist; ICU: Intensive care unit; NPV: negative predictive value; PPV: positive predictive value; RASS: Richmond Agitation Sedation Scale; SAPS II: Simplified Acute Physiological Score II score; SOFA: Sequential Organ Failure Assessment.

## Authors' contributions

GC, EWE, CMR, SMG and SJ contributed to study concept and design; OG, FP, AE and AP contributed to data acquisition; GC, EWE, SMG and SJ contributed to data analysis and interpretation; GC, ADJ and NM contributed to statistical methods and statistical data analysis; GC, EWE and JC contributed to manuscript preparation and drafting; CMR, ADJ, SMG and SJ contributed to manuscript critique and review. All authors read and approved the final manuscript.

## Author details

[1] Department of Anaesthesia and Critical Care Medicine, University of Montpellier Saint Eloi Hospital, 80, avenue Augustin Fliche, 34295 Montpellier Cedex 5, France. [2] PhyMedExp, INSERM U1046, CNRS, UMR 9214, University of Montpellier, Montpellier, France. [3] Department of Medicine, Division of Allergy, Pulmonary, and Critical Care Medicine and the Center for Health Services Research, Vanderbilt University School of Medicine, Nashville, TN, USA. [4] Geriatric Research Education Clinical Center (GRECC), Department of Veterans Affairs, Tennessee Valley Healthcare System, Nashville, TN, USA. [5] Department of Speech and Language Therapy, School of Medicine, University of Montpellier, Montpellier, France. [6] Institute of Neurosciences of Montpellier, INSERM U105, University of Montpellier, Montpellier, France. [7] Department of Statistics, University of Montpellier Hospitals, Montpellier, France.

## Acknowledgements

We would like to thank all patients who participated in the study and the families who gave their consent for participation, as well as the clinical and research staff. We also thank Dr. Carey M. Suehs for her help with English corrections.

## Competing interests

In contexts unrelated to the present work, Pr Jaber has consulted for and received honorarium from the following companies: Dräger, Hamilton, Maquet and Fisher Paykel. No other conflicts of interest related to this article exist for the other authors.

## Funding

Support for this study was provided solely via institutional and/or departmental sources (Montpellier University Hospitals; 34000, France).

## References

1. Salluh JI, Wang H, Schneider EB, Nagaraja N, Yenokyan G, Damluji A, et al. Outcome of delirium in critically ill patients: systematic review and meta-analysis. BMJ. 2015;350:h2538.
2. Chanques G, Tarri T, Ride A, Prades A, De Jong A, Carr J, et al. Analgesia nociception index for the assessment of pain in critically ill patients: a diagnostic accuracy study. Br J Anaesth. 2017;119:812–20.
3. Chanques G, Payen JF, Mercier G, de Lattre S, Viel E, Jung B, et al. Assessing pain in non-intubated critically ill patients unable to self report: an adaptation of the Behavioral Pain Scale. Intensive Care Med. 2009;35:2060–7.
4. Wang PP, Huang E, Feng X, Bray CA, Perreault MM, Rico P, et al. Opioid-associated iatrogenic withdrawal in critically ill patients: a multicenter prospective observational study. Ann Intensive Care. 2017;7:88.
5. Pandharipande PP, Girard TD, Jackson JC, Morandi A, Thompson JL, Pun BT, et al. Long-term cognitive impairment after critical illness. N Engl J Med. 2013;369:1306–16.
6. Barr J, Fraser GL, Puntillo K, Ely EW, Gelinas C, Dasta JF, et al. Clinical practice guidelines for the management of pain, agitation, and delirium in adult patients in the intensive care unit. Crit Care Med. 2013;41:278–80.
7. Ely EW, Margolin R, Francis J, May L, Truman B, Dittus R, et al. Evaluation of delirium in critically ill patients: validation of the Confusion Assessment Method for the Intensive Care Unit (CAM-ICU). Crit Care Med. 2001;29:1370–9.
8. Ely EW, Inouye SK, Bernard GR, Gordon S, Francis J, May L, et al. Delirium in mechanically ventilated patients: validity and reliability of the confusion assessment method for the intensive care unit (CAM-ICU). JAMA. 2001;286:2703–10.
9. Bergeron N, Dubois MJ, Dumont M, Dial S, Skrobik Y. Intensive Care Delirium Screening Checklist: evaluation of a new screening tool. Intensive Care Med. 2001;27:859–64.
10. Adamis D, Rooney S, Meagher D, Mulligan O, McCarthy G. A comparison of delirium diagnosis in elderly medical inpatients using the CAM, DRS-R98, DSM-IV and DSM-5 criteria. Int Psychogeriatr. 2015;27:883–9.
11. Meagher DJ, Morandi A, Inouye SK, Ely W, Adamis D, Maclullich AJ, et al. Concordance between DSM-IV and DSM-5 criteria for delirium diagnosis in a pooled database of 768 prospectively evaluated patients using the delirium rating scale-revised-98. BMC Med. 2014;12:164.
12. Sessler CN, Gosnell MS, Grap MJ, Brophy GM, O'Neal PV, Keane KA, et al. The Richmond Agitation–Sedation Scale: validity and reliability in adult intensive care unit patients. Am J Respir Crit Care Med. 2002;166:1338–44.
13. Ely EW, Truman B, Shintani A, Thomason JW, Wheeler AP, Gordon S, et al. Monitoring sedation status over time in ICU patients: reliability and validity of the Richmond Agitation–Sedation Scale (RASS). JAMA. 2003;289:2983–91.
14. Chanques G, Jaber S, Barbotte E, Verdier R, Henriette K, Lefrant J, et al. Validation of the French translated Richmond vigilance-agitation scale. Ann Fr Anesth Reanim. 2006;25:696–701.
15. Chanques G, Garnier O, Carr J, Conseil M, de Jong A, Rowan CM, et al. The CAM-ICU has now a French "official" version. The translation process of the 2014 updated Complete Training Manual of the Confusion Assessment Method for the Intensive Care Unit in French (CAM-ICU.fr). Anaesth Crit Care. Pain Med. 2017;36:297–300.
16. American Psychiatric Association: Diagnostic and Statistical Manual of Mental Disorders. 5th edition. Arlington, VA; 2013.
17. Nasreddine ZS, Phillips NA, Bedirian V, Charbonneau S, Whitehead V, Collin I, et al. The Montreal Cognitive Assessment, MoCA: a brief screening tool for mild cognitive impairment. J Am Geriatr Soc. 2005;53:695–9.
18. Dubois B, Touchon J, Portet F, Ousset PJ, Vellas B, Michel B. "The 5 words": a simple and sensitive test for the diagnosis of Alzheimer's disease. Presse Med. 2002;31:1696–9.
19. Flamand-Roze C, Falissard B, Roze E, Maintigneux L, Beziz J, Chacon A, et al. Validation of a new language screening tool for patients with acute stroke: the Language Screening Test (LAST). Stroke. 2011;42:1224–9.
20. Meagher D, Adamis D, Trzepacz P, Leonard M. Features of subsyndromal and persistent delirium. Br J Psychiatry. 2012;200:37–44.
21. Legall J-R, Lemeshow S, Saulnier F. New Simplified Acute Physiology Score (SAPS II) based on a European/North American Multicenter Study. JAMA. 1993;270:2957–63.
22. Vincent J, de Mendonça A, Cantraine F, Moreno R, Takala J, Suter P, et al. Use of the SOFA score to assess the incidence of organ dysfunction/failure in intensive care units: results of a multicenter, prospective study. Working group on "sepsis-related problems" of the European Society of Intensive Care Medicine. Crit Care Med. 1998;26:1793–800.
23. Altman DG, Bland JM. Diagnostic tests 2: predictive values. BMJ. 1994;309:102.
24. Altman DG, Bland JM. Diagnostic tests. 1: sensitivity and specificity. BMJ. 1994;308:1552.
25. Landis J, Koch G. The measurement of observer agreement for categorical data. Biometrics. 1977;33:159–74.
26. Altman DG, editor. Practical statistics for medical research. London: Chapman and Hall; 1991.
27. Page VJ, Davis D, Zhao XB, Norton S, Casarin A, Brown T, et al. Statin use and risk of delirium in the critically ill. Am J Respir Crit Care Med. 2014;189:666–73.
28. Van Rompaey B, Elseviers MM, Van Drom W, Fromont V, Jorens PG. The effect of earplugs during the night on the onset of delirium and sleep

perception: a randomized controlled trial in intensive care patients. Crit Care. 2012;16:R73.

29. Kamdar BB, Niessen T, Colantuoni E, King LM, Neufeld KJ, Bienvenu OJ, et al. Delirium transitions in the medical ICU: exploring the role of sleep quality and other factors. Crit Care Med. 2015;43:135–41.

30. Serafim RB, Dutra MF, Saddy F, Tura B, de Castro JE, Villarinho LC, et al. Delirium in postoperative nonventilated intensive care patients: risk factors and outcomes. Ann Intensive Care. 2012;2:51.

31. Rafat C, Flamant M, Gaudry S, Vidal-Petiot E, Ricard JD, Dreyfuss D. Hyponatremia in the intensive care unit: How to avoid a Zugzwang situation? Ann Intensive Care. 2015;5:39.

32. Delaney LJ, Van Haren F, Lopez V. Sleeping on a problem: the impact of sleep disturbance on intensive care patients—a clinical review. Ann Intensive Care. 2015;5:3.

33. Dittrich T, Tschudin-Sutter S, Widmer AF, Ruegg S, Marsch S, Sutter R. Risk factors for new-onset delirium in patients with bloodstream infections: independent and quantitative effect of catheters and drainages—a four-year cohort study. Ann Intensive Care. 2016;6:104.

34. van Ewijk CE, Jacobs GE, Girbes ARJ. Unsuspected serotonin toxicity in the ICU. Ann Intensive Care. 2016;6:85.

35. Neuville M, El-Helali N, Magalhaes E, Radjou A, Smonig R, Soubirou JF, et al. Systematic overdosing of oxa- and cloxacillin in severe infections treated in ICU: risk factors and side effects. Ann Intensive Care. 2017;7:34.

36. Patel SB, Poston JT, Pohlman A, Hall JB, Kress JP. Rapidly reversible, sedation-related delirium versus persistent delirium in the intensive care unit. Am J Respir Crit Care Med. 2014;189:658–65.

37. SRLF Trial Group. Sedation in French intensive care units: a survey of clinical practice. Ann Intensive Care. 2013;3:24.

38. Spronk PE, Riekerk B, Hofhuis J, Rommes JH. Occurrence of delirium is severely underestimated in the ICU during daily care. Intensive Care Med. 2009;35:1276–80.

39. van Eijk MM, van Marum RJ, Klijn IA, de Wit N, Kesecioglu J, Slooter AJ. Comparison of delirium assessment tools in a mixed intensive care unit. Crit Care Med. 2009;37:1881–5.

40. Patel RP, Gambrell M, Speroff T, Scott TA, Pun BT, Okahashi J, et al. Delirium and sedation in the intensive care unit: survey of behaviors and attitudes of 1384 healthcare professionals. Crit Care Med. 2009;37:825–32.

41. Neto AS, Nassar AP Jr, Cardoso SO, Manetta JA, Pereira VG, Esposito DC, et al. Delirium screening in critically ill patients: a systematic review and meta-analysis. Crit Care Med. 2012;40:1946–51.

42. Luetz A, Heymann A, Radtke FM, Chenitir C, Neuhaus U, Nachtigall I, et al. Different assessment tools for intensive care unit delirium: which score to use? Crit Care Med. 2010;38:409–18.

43. Mitasova A, Kostalova M, Bednarik J, Michalcakova R, Kasparek T, Balabanova P, et al. Poststroke delirium incidence and outcomes: validation of the Confusion Assessment Method for the Intensive Care Unit (CAM-ICU). Crit Care Med. 2012;40:484–90.

44. Haenggi M, Blum S, Brechbuehl R, Brunello A, Jakob SM, Takala J. Effect of sedation level on the prevalence of delirium when assessed with CAM-ICU and ICDSC. Intensive Care Med. 2013;39:2171–9.

45. Chanques G, Jaber S, Barbotte E, Violet S, Sebbane M, Perrigault P, et al. Impact of systematic evaluation of pain and agitation in an intensive care unit. Crit Care Med. 2006;34:1691–9.

46. de Jong A, Molinari N, de Lattre S, Gniadek C, Carr J, Conseil M, et al. Decreasing severe pain and serious adverse events while moving intensive care unit patients: a prospective interventional study (the NURSE-DO project). Crit Care. 2013;17:R74.

47. Dodek P, Chanques G, Brown G, Norena M, Grubisic M, Wong H, et al. Role of organisational structure in implementation of sedation protocols: a comparison of Canadian and French ICUs. BMJ Qual Saf. 2012;21:715–21.

48. Ely EW. The ABCDEF bundle: science and philosophy of how ICU liberation serves patients and families. Crit Care Med. 2017;45:321–30.

49. Balas MC, Vasilevskis EE, Olsen KM, Schmid KK, Shostrom V, Cohen MZ, et al. Effectiveness and safety of the awakening and breathing coordination, delirium monitoring/management, and early exercise/mobility bundle. Crit Care Med. 2014;42:1024–36.

50. Chanques G, Conseil M, Roger C, Constantin JM, Prades A, Carr J, et al. Immediate interruption of sedation compared with usual sedation care in critically ill postoperative patients (SOS-Ventilation): a randomised, parallel-group clinical trial. Lancet Respir Med. 2017;5:795–805.

51. Barnes-Daly MA, Phillips G, Ely EW. Improving hospital survival and reducing brain dysfunction at seven California community hospitals: implementing PAD guidelines via the ABCDEF bundle in 6,064 patients. Crit Care Med. 2017;45:171–8.

52. Jones C, Bäckman C, Capuzzo M, Flaatten H, Rylander C, Griffiths RD. Precipitants of post-traumatic stress disorder following intensive care: a hypothesis generating study of diversity in care. Intensive Care Med. 2007;33:978–85.

53. Jones C, Griffiths RD, Humphris G, Skirrow PM. Memory, delusions, and the development of acute posttraumatic stress disorder-related symptoms after intensive care. Crit Care Med. 2001;29:573–80.

54. Parker AM, Sricharoenchai T, Raparla S, Schneck KW, Bienvenu OJ, Needham DM. Posttraumatic stress disorder in critical illness survivors: a metaanalysis. Crit Care Med. 2015;43:1121–9.

55. Wolters AE, Peelen LM, Welling MC, Kok L, de Lange DW, Cremer OL, et al. Long-term mental health problems after delirium in the ICU. Crit Care Med. 2016;44:1808–13.

56. Svenningsen H, Egerod I, Christensen D, Tonnesen EK, Frydenberg M, Videbech P. Symptoms of posttraumatic stress after intensive care delirium. Biomed Res Int. 2015;2015:876947.

57. Jackson JC, Pandharipande PP, Girard TD, Brummel NE, Thompson JL, Hughes CG, et al. Depression, post-traumatic stress disorder, and functional disability in survivors of critical illness in the BRAIN-ICU study: a longitudinal cohort study. Lancet Respir Med. 2014;2:369–79.

58. Fan E, Shahid S, Kondreddi VP, Bienvenu OJ, Mendez-Tellez PA, Pronovost PJ, et al. Informed consent in the critically ill: a two-step approach incorporating delirium screening. Crit Care Med. 2008;36:94–9.

# 13

# Response to different furosemide doses predicts AKI progression in ICU patients with elevated plasma NGAL levels

Ryo Matsuura[1], Yohei Komaru[1], Yoshihisa Miyamoto[3], Teruhiko Yoshida[1], Kohei Yoshimoto[2], Rei Isshiki[1], Kengo Mayumi[1], Tetsushi Yamashita[1], Yoshifumi Hamasaki[3], Masaomi Nangaku[1,3], Eisei Noiri[1], Naoto Morimura[2] and Kent Doi[2]*

## Abstract

**Background:** Furosemide responsiveness (FR) is determined by urine output after furosemide administration and has recently been evaluated as a furosemide stress test (FST) for predicting severe acute kidney injury (AKI) progression. Although a standardized furosemide dose is required for FST, variable dosing is typically employed based on illness severity, including renal dysfunction in the clinical setting. This study aimed to evaluate whether FR with different furosemide doses can predict AKI progression. We further evaluated the combination of an AKI biomarker, plasma neutrophil gelatinase-associated lipocalin (NGAL), and FR for predicting AKI progression.

**Results:** We retrospectively analyzed 95 patients who were treated with bolus furosemide in our medical–surgical intensive care unit. Patients who had already developed AKI stage 3 were excluded. A total of 18 patients developed AKI stage 3 within 1 week. Receiver operating curve analysis revealed that the area under the curve (AUC) values of FR and plasma NGAL were 0.87 (0.73–0.94) and 0.80 (0.67–0.88) for AKI progression, respectively. When plasma NGAL level was < 142 ng/mL, only one patient developed stage 3 AKI, indicating that plasma NGAL measurements were sufficient to predict AKI progression. We further evaluated the performance of FR in 51 patients with plasma NGAL levels > 142 ng/mL. FR was associated with AUC of 0.84 (0.67–0.94) for AKI progression in this population with high NGAL levels.

**Conclusions:** Although different variable doses of furosemide were administered, FR revealed favorable efficacy for predicting AKI progression even in patients with high plasma NGAL levels. This suggests that a combination of FR and biomarkers can stratify the risk of AKI progression in a clinical setting.

**Keywords:** Acute kidney injury, Biomarkers, Intensive care unit, Progression, Diuretics

## Background

Acute kidney injury (AKI) is highly prevalent in an intensive care unit (ICU) and is associated with significant morbidity and mortality [1–3]. Severe AKI has an unacceptably high mortality, especially when renal replacement therapy (RRT) is required [4–6]. Prediction of AKI progression from a mild to severe form is clinically important for several reasons. First, the early initiation of RRT can be supported for highly possible AKI progression, although there is currently no consensus regarding the timing of initiating RRT [7, 8]. Second, AKI diagnosis is based on the changes of serum creatinine concentration, but it is well known that changes in serum creatinine levels are delayed. Although the Kidney Disease: Improving Global Outcomes (KDIGO) Clinical Practice Guideline for Acute Kidney Injury suggests considering an invasive diagnostic workup (stage 1) along with ICU admission (stage 2) for AKI management based on AKI severity determined by serum creatinine [9], establishing

*Correspondence: kdoi-tky@umin.ac.jp
[2] Department of Emergency and Critical Care Medicine, The University of Tokyo Hospital, 7-3-1 Hongo, Bunkyo-ku, Tokyo 113-8655, Japan
Full list of author information is available at the end of the article

a triage decision for management and prevention of AKI progression is difficult with a late marker of serum creatinine. Finally, identifying possible AKI progressors may contribute to the development of novel drugs for AKI by reducing inappropriate enrollment of patients with mild AKI who recover spontaneously.

To date, multiple biomarkers, such as plasma neutrophil gelatinase-associated lipocalin (NGAL), L-type fatty acid binding protein (L-FABP), interleukin (IL)-18, and tissue inhibitor of metalloproteinases (TIMP-2)/insulin-like growth factor-binding protein 7 (IGFBP7), have been developed [10–14]. Moreover, urinary NGAL and L-FABP can reportedly discriminate between prerenal and renal AKI [15–17] and TIMP-2/IGFBP7 can predict AKI progression [18, 19].

Furosemide is excreted from the blood into the urine through the proximal tubules by the human organic anion transporter and inhibits luminal sodium transporters in the loop of Henle from the urinal lumen [20]. If furosemide administration increases the urine output, it could be assumed that the tubules are functional. Koyner et al. [21] recently demonstrated that the 2-h urine output after a standardized high-dose intravenous furosemide injection (furosemide stress test; FST) was sensitive in predicting AKI progression to stage 3 in patients with early AKI.

To better stratify the risk of AKI progression, a combination of renal functional and damage biomarkers is recommended [22]. However, there are no reports in the literature that have examined the combination of functional and damage biomarkers for predicting AKI progression. In this study, we retrospectively evaluated the combination of AKI biomarkers and urine output in response to the administration of bolus furosemide for stratifying the risk of AKI progression in critically ill patients.

## Methods

### Definition

Furosemide responsiveness (FR) is newly defined as total urine output in 2 h (mL) divided by the dose of bolus furosemide (mg) administered. A previous study reported that the urine output within the first 2 h after a standardized dose of furosemide administration provided the highest prediction of the development of severe AKI [23]. We reviewed furosemide dose and hourly urine output using ICU medical charts and determined FR of each patient. The timing and dose of furosemide administration were determined by the physician involved. In our regular clinical practice, furosemide dose was decided based on body weight, volume status, cardiac function, serum creatinine concentration at the time of furosemide administration, and presence of complications of chronic

kidney disease (CKD). All patients finally enrolled in this study had an indwelling catheter, and hourly urine output could be accurately measured.

### Study design

This study is a subanalysis of our prospective observational studies [24–26]. The cohort in this study was selected from these previous prospective observational studies conducted in the medical–surgical mixed ICU at the University of Tokyo Hospital. In previous studies, we measured the AKI biomarkers of plasma NGAL, urinary L-FABP, and urinary N-acetyl-β-D-glucosaminidase (NAG) and evaluated the association with AKI biomarkers and AKI progression within 1 week. Among 523 adult critically ill patients enrolled, 153 were retrospectively identified to have received furosemide on the same day that the above-mentioned AKI biomarkers were measured. Finally, 95 patients were eligible for analysis after excluding 33 patients who were administered continuous intravenous furosemide infusion instead of a bolus and 25 patients who had already progressed to AKI stage 3 at the time of ICU admission (Fig. 1). Volume depletion was evaluated by the clinical context, physical signs, and findings on cardiac ultrasound examination in all 95 patients.

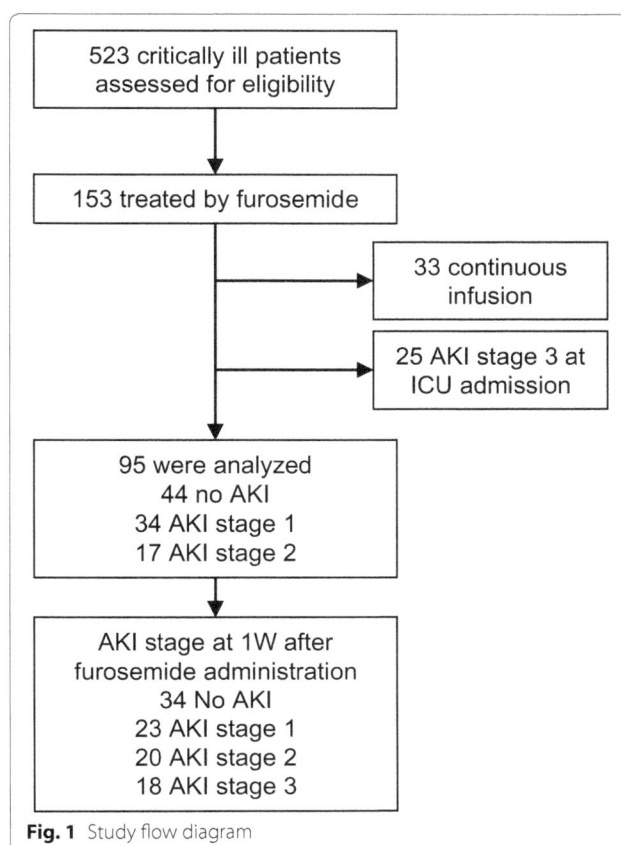

**Fig. 1** Study flow diagram

The study protocol was approved by the institutional review board of the University of Tokyo and adhered to the Declaration of Helsinki. Patient informed consent was obtained at the time of ICU admission. The following clinical variables during the ICU and hospital stay were evaluated: age, sex, weight, causes of ICU admission, acute physiology and chronic health evaluation II score [27], and the length of ICU and hospital stay.

### Assessment of kidney function
Baseline serum creatinine level was defined as the last outpatient value within 6 months prior to ICU admission. If the creatinine level prior to admission was not known, the baseline value was defined as the lowest among creatinine values in hospital but prior to ICU admission, the last level before hospital discharge, and the estimated value using the Modification of Diet in Renal Disease equation at the lower end of the normal range [28]. The definition and classification of AKI were made according to the KDIGO Clinical Practice Guideline for Acute Kidney Injury [29].

### Measurement of AKI biomarkers
Urine and plasma samples were collected at the time of ICU admission and were frozen at − 80 °C within 1 h of collection. As urine output was measured hourly by an indwelling catheter, we could obtain a fresh urine sample that was collected within 1 h previously. The plasma NGAL level was determined using the Triage NGAL Device (AlereMedical, San Diego, CA, USA). Urinary L-FABP level was measured using commercially available enzyme-linked immunosorbent assay kits (Human L-FABP Assay Kit; CMIC Co. Ltd., Tokyo, Japan). Urinary NAG level was measured at the University of Tokyo Hospital Clinical Laboratory using the 4-HP-NAG substrate method (L-Type NAG; Wako Pure Chemical Industries Ltd., Osaka, Japan). Urinary L-FABP and NAG level measurements were evaluated by adjusting with urine creatinine concentration [11, 30].

### Statistical analyses
Data are presented as median (interquartile range). Continuous variables were compared using Wilcoxon rank-sum tests if they were non-normally distributed. Categorical variables were compared using the Pearson Chi-square or Fisher exact test. The urinary and plasma biomarker performance was ascertained using a receiver operating characteristic (ROC) curve analysis. The optimal cutoff values were acquired using the Youden index (sensitivity + specificity − 1), which is a common summary measure of the ROC curve representing the maximum potential effectiveness of a marker [31]. Comparisons of the ROC curves were performed as

previously reported [30, 32]. All analyses were performed using a statistical analysis software (JMP ver. 11.2; SAS Institute Inc., Cary, NC). A conventional criterion of an $\alpha$ level of 0.05 was used to assess statistical significance.

## Results
### Patient characteristics and AKI progression to AKI stage 3
Characteristics of all 95 patients studied are presented in Table 1. Among these, 51 patients (54%) were diagnosed with AKI at the time of furosemide administration;

**Table 1  Characteristics of the 95 enrolled patients**

| | |
|---|---|
| Age | 67 (57–77) |
| Male/female | 58/37 |
| Body weight (kg) | 59.7 (48.7–66.6) |
| APACHE II score | 17 (14–22) |
| Chronic heart failure | 13 |
| Furosemide use before ICU | 25 |
| Doses of furosemide before ICU (mg) | 30 (20–55) |
| Indication for ICU admission | |
| Cardiovascular | 11 |
| Cerebrovascular | 12 |
| Pulmonary | 17 |
| Sepsis | 17 |
| Others | 38 |
| Baseline serum creatinine (mg/dl) | 0.8 (0.51–0.98) |
| Serum creatinine at hospitalization (mg/dl) | 0.89 (0.64–1.30) |
| Serum creatinine at ICU admission (mg/dl) | 0.97 (0.60–1.37) |
| Serum creatinine at furosemide administration (mg/dl) | 1.09 (0.68–1.40) |
| Serum albumin at furosemide administration (g/dL) | 2.9 (2.5–3.2) |
| AKI stage at ICU admission | |
| No AKI | 55 |
| Stage 1 | 29 |
| Stage 2 | 11 |
| AKI stage at furosemide administration | |
| No AKI | 44 |
| Stage 1 | 34 |
| Stage 2 | 17 |
| AKI stage at 1 week | |
| No AKI | 34 |
| Stage 1 | 23 |
| Stage 2 | 20 |
| Stage 3 | 18 |
| Length of hospitalization (days) | 50 (25–93) |
| Length of ICU stay (days) | 6 (3–11) |
| Plasma NGAL at furosemide administration (ng/mL) | 147 (78–309) |
| Urinary L-FABP at furosemide administration (µg/gCr) | 39.9 (15.1–208) |
| Urinary NAG at furosemide administration (U/gCr) | 3.5 (2.0–6.4) |
| Dose of furosemide (mg) | 10 (10–20) |

*AKI* acute kidney injury, *APACHE* acute physiology and chronic health evaluation, *ICU* intensive care units, *L-FABP* L-type fatty acid binding protein, *NAG* N-acetyl-β-D-glucosaminidase, *NGAL* neutrophil gelatinase-associated lipocalin

34 were diagnosed with AKI stage 1 (36%) and 17 with AKI stage 2 (18%). Within 1 week following furosemide administration, 18 patients progressed to AKI stage 3 (Fig. 1). Among this, 10 patients had progressed from AKI stage 1 and four patients from stage 2. Four patients did not have AKI at the time of furosemide administration.

## Biomarkers, FR, and AKI stages at 1 week

First, the association between progression to AKI stage 3 after 1 week with FR and AKI biomarkers was evaluated. FR and plasma NGAL level showed significant differences between the AKI progression group (from any stage to stage 3) and the non-progression group (Fig. 2). When

weight-adjusted FR is defined as the total urine output in 2 h divided by furosemide dose per kilogram body weight (mg/kg), weight-adjusted FR showed a significant difference between the groups (Additional file 1: Figure S1). Measurement of urinary L-FABP and NAG levels could not significantly differentiate AKI progression to stage 3. The ROC analysis demonstrated that FR, weight-adjusted FR, and plasma NGAL could significantly predict AKI progression to stage 3; in contrast, urinary L-FABP and NAG levels could not predict AKI progression (Table 2). Similar results were obtained when a composite outcome of AKI stage 3 or death within 1 week after furosemide administration was used (Table 2; Figs. 2, 3; Additional file 1: Figure S2).

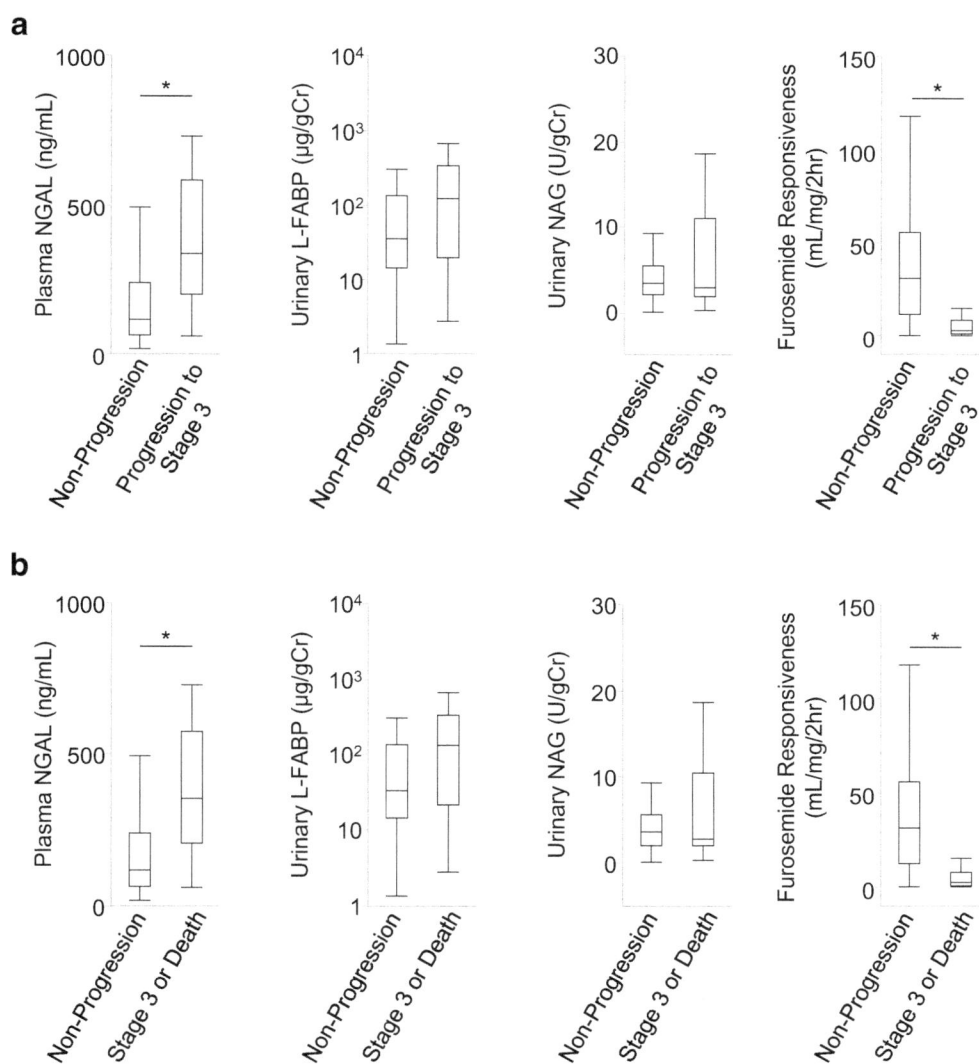

**Fig. 2** Biomarkers and furosemide responsiveness (FR) in AKI progression. The boxplots show the differences in the AKI biomarkers and FR between patients **a** without and with the progression to AKI stage 3 and **b** without and with the progression to AKI stage 3 or death within 1 week. *p < 0.01

**Table 2  ROC analysis for the progression to AKI stage 3 or death within 1 week**

|  | AUC (95% CI) | Cutoff |
|---|---|---|
| Progression to AKI stage 3 | | |
| FR | 0.87 (0.73–0.94) | 3.9 mL/mg/2 h |
| Plasma NGAL | 0.80 (0.67–0.88) | 199 ng/mL |
| Urinary L-FABP | 0.61 (0.45–0.75) | 83.0 mg/μCr |
| Urinary NAG | 0.54 (0.37–0.71) | 9.3 U/gCr |
| Progression to AKI stage 3 or death within 1 week | | |
| FR | 0.88 (0.75–0.95) | 3.9 mL/mg/2 h |
| Plasma NGAL | 0.81 (0.68–0.89) | 199 ng/mL |
| Urinary L-FABP | 0.62 (0.47–0.76) | 83.0 mg/μCr |
| Urinary NAG | 0.53 (0.37–0.69) | 9.3 U/gCr |

*AKI* acute kidney injury, *FR* furosemide responsiveness, *L-FABP* L-type fatty acid binding protein, *NAG* N-acetyl-β-ᴅ-glucosaminidase, *NGAL* neutrophil gelatinase-associated lipocalin

### FR for the prediction of AKI progression in the population with high NGAL levels

Among the 95 enrolled patients, 51 were diagnosed with AKI of different stages at the time of furosemide administration. For predicting AKI progression to stage 3, the plasma NGAL level measured at the time of furosemide administration showed a good AUC in the ROC analysis, 0.79 (0.68–0.86) with a cutoff value of 142 ng/mL, as determined by the Youden index (sensitivity, 72.1%; specificity, 79.4%). When the plasma NGAL level was < 142 ng/mL, only one patient progressed to AKI stage 3, indicating that plasma NGAL level alone was sufficient to predict AKI progression to stage 3. Therefore, we further evaluated the efficacy of FR in predicting AKI progression in patients with plasma NGAL levels > 142 ng/

mL. Among the 51 patients with plasma NGAL levels > 142 ng/mL at the time of furosemide administration, 17 progressed to AKI stage 3 (eight patients required RRT) and four died (Fig. 4). FR was associated with AUCs of 0.84 (0.67–0.94) and 0.88 (0.70–0.96) to predict the development of AKI stage 3 and the composite outcome of AKI stage 3 progression or death. Cutoff values of FR for both AKI progression to stage 3 and the composite outcome as determined by Youden index were 3.9 mL/mg/2 h.

The characteristics of the population with higher NGAL levels divided by FR positive ($n = 36$) or FR negative ($n = 15$) with the cutoff value of 3.9 mL/mg/2 h described above are shown in Table 3. The serum creatinine levels at the time of hospitalization and furosemide administration were higher in the FR-positive patients compared with the FR-negative patients. The proportion of patients at each stage of AKI at the time of ICU admission and furosemide administration, as well as the plasma NGAL level measured at the time of furosemide administration, were not significantly different. A higher dose of furosemide was administered to patients who were FR negative than to those who were FR positive. Among the 15 patients who were FR negative, 13 (86.7%) progressed to AKI stage 3, while six (40%) required RRT. On the other hand, among 36 patients who were FR positive, only four (11%) progressed to AKI stage 3 and two (5.6%) required RRT (Table 4).

### Discussion

AKI progression frequently occurs in ICU in the context of multiple organ failure [33] and is significantly associated with high mortality in different cohorts of ICU and

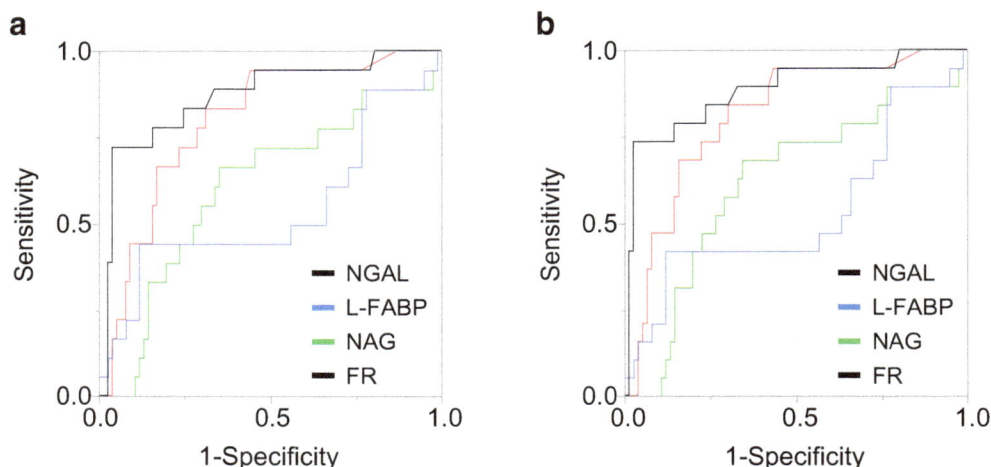

**Fig. 3** Prediction of AKI progression by biomarkers and furosemide responsiveness (FR). Receiver operating characteristic curves (ROC) in **a** progression to AKI stage 3 and **b** progression to AKI stage 3 or death at 1 week. NGAL, neutrophil gelatinase-associated lipocalin; L-FABP, L-type fatty acid binding protein; NAG, N-acetyl-β-ᴅ-glucosaminidase; FR, furosemide responsiveness

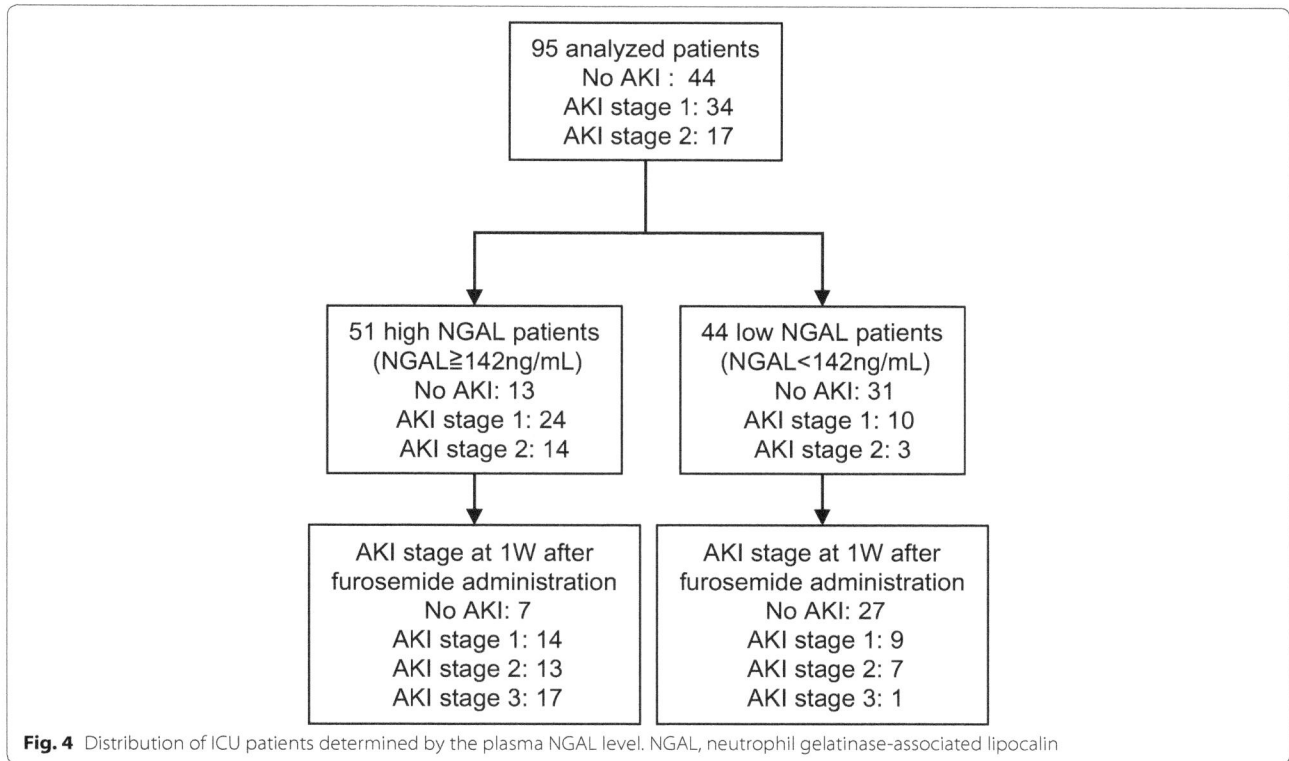

**Fig. 4** Distribution of ICU patients determined by the plasma NGAL level. NGAL, neutrophil gelatinase-associated lipocalin

in patients who have undergone cardiac surgery and those with cardiorenal syndrome [10, 34, 35]. The identification of the potential AKI progression may allow us to initiate early interventions (e.g., more invasive monitoring and RRT) before the development of life-threatening complications. In addition, with the likely development of novel therapies for AKI, an accurate prediction of AKI progression may help to determine patients at the highest risk and those most likely to benefit from such treatment. Several emerging AKI biomarkers, including TIMP-2/IGFBP-7, IL-18, and plasma NGAL, have been demonstrated to predict AKI progression [10, 34]. In particular, TIMP-2/IGFBP-7 was validated for early AKI risk stratification in critically ill patients in multicenter studies [18, 36, 37]. These cell-cycle arrest biomarkers are expected to help in the early detection of patients at risk of AKI in various clinical settings. Recently, FST was suggested to be a significant predictor of progression to AKI stage 3 in patients with AKI stage 1 or 2 [23]. Moreover, Koyner et al. [21] reported a superior efficacy of FST than urinary AKI biomarkers for the prediction of AKI progression. This study demonstrates that both FR and plasma NGAL levels could successfully predict AKI progression as shown by previous studies described above. The novel findings of this study are as follows: (1) FST, as described originally, requires a standardized intravenous

furosemide dose of 1 mg/kg. However, this study demonstrated that response to a variable dose of frusemide could also predict AKI progression under actual clinical conditions, when different doses of furosemide were chosen based on patient condition; (2) FR could predict AKI progression in patients with high plasma NGAL levels, while few patients with low plasma NGAL levels exhibited AKI progression. These results indicate that both functional (furosemide response) and structural evaluations (plasma NGAL level) in AKI may be helpful for the prediction of AKI progression.

As described above, FR (mL/mg/2 h) in this study was determined by the 2-h total urine output (mL) following furosemide administration divided by the dose of furosemide (mg). It is well known that the effect of loop diuretics is dose dependent [38]. The delivery of furosemide to the thick ascending limb of the loop of Henle depends on the secretion from the proximal tubular epithelial cells. Because the rate of delivery to the site of action is the most important determining factor for natriuresis induced by furosemide administration, FR in this study might reflect the proximal tubule function even with variable furosemide doses. In the studies involving normal healthy subjects, 10 mg furosemide produced diuresis and 40 mg intravenously administered was associated with the maximal effect. In oliguric AKI, the dose with

**Table 3  Characteristics of patients with high plasma NGAL levels**

|  | All (*N* = 51) | FR positive (*N* = 36) | FR negative (*N* = 15) | P value |
|---|---|---|---|---|
| Age | 65 (55–76) | 63.5 (49–73) | 73 (61–78) | 0.08 |
| Male/female | 34/17 | 24/12 | 10/5 | 1.00 |
| APACHE II score | 20 (14–22) | 19.5 (15–22) | 20 (14–28) | 0.56 |
| Chronic heart failure | 10 | 5 | 5 | 0.12 |
| Furosemide use before ICU | 18 | 10 | 8 | 0.08 |
| Dose of furosemide before ICU (mg) | 20 (15–40) | 40 (15–60) | 20 (12.5–40) | 0.52 |
| Serum creatinine (mg/dl) |  |  |  |  |
| Baseline | 0.83 (0.51–1.36) | 0.81 (0.49–1.13) | 1.24 (0.8–2.59) | 0.07 |
| At hospitalization | 1.1 (0.78–1.92) | 0.97 (0.69–1.7) | 1.81 (0.96–3.64) | 0.04 |
| At ICU admission | 1.26 (0.92–1.94) | 1.13 (0.78–1.48) | 1.56 (1.01–2.14) | 0.08 |
| At furosemide administration | 1.33 (0.99–1.94) | 1.17 (0.98–1.67) | 1.77 (1.26–2.77) | 0.03 |
| Serum albumin (g/dL) | 2.8 (2.3–3.1) | 2.8 (2.3–3.1) | 2.7 (2.3–3.2) | 0.79 |
| AKI stage at ICU admission |  |  |  | 0.92 |
| No AKI | 20 | 15 | 5 |  |
| Stage 1 | 21 | 14 | 7 |  |
| Stage 2 | 10 | 7 | 3 |  |
| AKI stage at furosemide administration |  |  |  | 0.80 |
| No AKI | 13 | 10 | 3 |  |
| Stage 1 | 24 | 16 | 8 |  |
| Stage 2 | 14 | 10 | 4 |  |
| Length of hospitalization (days) | 42 (25–85) | 45 (26–90) | 33 (17–77) | 0.23 |
| Length of ICU stays (days) | 6 (3–13) | 5 (3–9) | 12 (4–16) | 0.04 |
| Plasma NGAL at furosemide administration (ng/ml) | 303 (199–495) | 274 (190–399) | 354 (260–576) | 0.26 |
| Dose of furosemide (mg) | 20 (10–20) | 10 (10–20) | 40 (20–45) | < 0.01 |

*AKI* acute kidney injury, *APACHE* acute physiology and chronic health evaluation, *ICU* intensive care units, *NGAL* neutrophil gelatinase-associated lipocalin

**Table 4  Odds ratio by FR in the high NGAL population**

|  | FR positive | FR negative | Odds ratio (95% CI) |
|---|---|---|---|
| AKI stage 3 at 1 week | 4/36 (11%) | 13/15 (86.7%) | 52 (8.5–319.5) |
| RRT | 2/36 (5.6%) | 6/15 (40%) | 11.3 (2.0–65.9) |
| AKI stage 3 or death at 1 week | 4/36 (11%) | 14/15 (93.3%) | 112 (11.5–1094.4) |

*AKI* acute kidney injury, *FR* furosemide responsiveness

the maximum effect of furosemide is assumed to be as high as 500 mg [39]. In this study, the furosemide dose ranged from 10 to 340 mg. Our findings provide useful information to clinicians as FR calculated with different doses of furosemide can be used to predict AKI progression. This is because furosemide dosing should be individually determined based on patient condition in a clinical setting.

Another important issue regarding the physiology of furosemide is serum albumin concentration. Hypoalbuminemia results in lower oncotic pressure and fluid shift to the interstitial compartment, which may depress fluid

excretion by the kidneys. Previously, colloid infusion with loop diuretics was shown to increase urine output and lower net fluid balance in critically ill patients with hypoalbuminemia and fluid overload [40, 41]. In contrast, despite a possible role of albumin in furosemide-induced diuresis, serum albumin levels were not different between the FR-positive and FR-negative patients in the population with high NGAL levels. Thus, serum albumin levels seemed to have little impact on the response to furosemide.

An ideal AKI biomarker should aid in determining the degree of damage and functional changes in the kidney and help to adequately manage AKI and initiate RRT when needed [22]. Emerging AKI biomarkers, including NGAL, L-FABP, IL-18, and TIMP-2/IGFBP7, are reported to be useful for the early detection of AKI and prediction of progression because AKI impacts the metabolism and excretion of these biomarkers that are produced, excreted, or reabsorbed in the renal tubules [14, 18, 37, 42–47]. However, these biomarkers may be insufficient for the measurement of residual function of the kidney because they monitor damage but not severity of impairment of kidney function [48]. Therefore, we suggest a two-step approach for the prediction of AKI progression: (1) the evaluation of structural damage by plasma NGAL and (2) the subsequent functional assessment by FR (Fig. 5).

This study has several limitations. First, this was a retrospective observational study and the number of patients included in this single-center study was small. Among 523 patients, only 153 were analyzed because furosemide administration was determined based on the clinical situation. In addition, plasma NGAL levels had to be measured on the same day as furosemide administration for study enrollment. Although we showed the significance of FR for predicting severe AKI progression, unmeasured factors could have biased our results. Therefore, inherent bias should be carefully considered while interpreting this study. However, it should be stated that the preliminary findings of this study may suggest that a novel approach combining structural damage makers and functional evaluation may be useful for predicting AKI progression. Future multicenter prospective studies with larger cohorts should be conducted to validate our strategy and findings. Second, the plasma NGAL cutoff level in this study was retrospectively determined and could not be extrapolated in other cohorts. A prospective cohort analysis is required to confirm our results. Third, furosemide was administered based on clinician judgment and criteria for administration depended on clinicians' decision and the criteria to administer furosemide were vague. Although 1 mg/kg furosemide was used in the original paper for FST [21, 23], furosemide dose administered in our study was different in each patient and was determined by the physician based on the patient's condition. Again, a prospective study with a predefined furosemide administration protocol is necessary.

Finally, we did not evaluate the long-term outcomes in this study. Recent clinical reports demonstrate that AKI has a significant impact on mortality and the progression of kidney disease (e.g., chronic kidney disease or end-stage kidney disease) [49–51]. Further investigation is necessary to determine whether the combination of FR and AKI biomarkers is significant for predicting long-term AKI-related outcomes.

## Conclusions

This retrospective study demonstrated that FR and plasma NGAL may be significant predictors of severe AKI progression in general ICU patients. In addition, FR could predict AKI progression even in patients with high NGAL values, indicating that the sequential evaluation with FR and plasma NGAL could identify patients at a high risk for the development of severe AKI. Of note, identifying high-risk patients may enable to decrease potential adverse effects of furosemide. Finally, careful consideration is necessary before applying the findings of this small retrospective study to clinical practice.

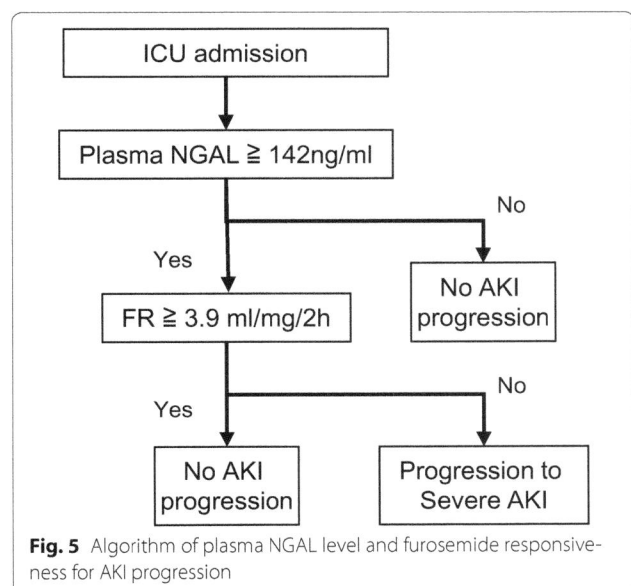

**Fig. 5** Algorithm of plasma NGAL level and furosemide responsiveness for AKI progression

**Abbreviations**
AKI: acute kidney injury; AUC: area under the curve; FR: furosemide responsiveness; FST: furosemide stress test; ICU: intensive care unit; IGFBP7: insulin-like growth factor-binding protein 7; IL-18: interleukin 18; KDIGO: Kidney Disease: Improving Global Outcomes; L-FABP: L-type fatty acid binding protein; NAG: N-acetyl-β-D-glucosaminidase; NGAL: neutrophil gelatinase-associated lipocalin; ROC: receiver operating characteristic; RRT: renal replacement therapy; TIMP-2: tissue inhibitor of metalloproteinases.

**Authors' contributions**
RM and KD conceived the study, participated in its design and coordination, conducted sample collection, measured biomarkers, analyzed the data, and drafted the manuscript. YK, YM, TY, KY, RI, KM, and TY participated in the study design and coordination, analyzed the data, and drafted the manuscript. MN, EN, and NM conceived the study, participated in its design and coordination, analyzed the data, and drafted the manuscript. All authors read and approved the final manuscript.

**Author details**
[1] Department of Nephrology and Endocrinology, The University of Tokyo Hospital, 7-3-1 Hongo, Bunkyo-ku, Tokyo 113-8655, Japan. [2] Department of Emergency and Critical Care Medicine, The University of Tokyo Hospital, 7-3-1 Hongo, Bunkyo-ku, Tokyo 113-8655, Japan. [3] Department of Dialysis and Apheresis, The University of Tokyo Hospital, 7-3-1 Hongo, Bunkyo-ku, Tokyo 113-8655, Japan.

**Acknowledgements**
This study was partly supported by grants from the Tokyo Society of Medical Sciences (KD). Alere Medical Co Ltd. (Tokyo, Japan) partly supported blood

sample collection and testing but did not contribute to the study design, data analysis, or preparation of the manuscript.

## Competing interests
The authors declare that they have no competing interests.

## Funding
This work was supported by a grant by the Tokyo Society of Medical Sciences.

## References

1. Bellomo R, Kellum JA, Ronco C. Acute kidney injury. Lancet. 2012;380:756–66.
2. Rewa O, Bagshaw SM. Acute kidney injury-epidemiology, outcomes and economics. Nat Rev Nephrol. 2014;10:193–207.
3. Singbartl K, Kellum JA. AKI in the ICU: definition, epidemiology, risk stratification, and outcomes. Kidney Int. 2012;81:819–25.
4. Iwagami M, Yasunaga H, Noiri E, Horiguchi H, Fushimi K, Matsubara T, et al. Current state of continuous renal replacement therapy for acute kidney injury in Japanese intensive care units in 2011: analysis of a national administrative database. Nephrol Dial Transplant. 2015;30:988–95.
5. Vesconi S, Cruz DN, Fumagalli R, Kindgen-Milles D, Monti G, Marinho A, et al. Delivered dose of renal replacement therapy and mortality in critically ill patients with acute kidney injury. Crit Care. 2009;13:R57.
6. RENAL Replacement Therapy Study Investigators, Bellomo R, Cass A, Cole L, Finfer S, Gallagher M, et al. Intensity of continuous renal-replacement therapy in critically ill patients. N Engl J Med. 2009;361:1627–38.
7. Gibney N, Hoste E, Burdmann EA, Bunchman T, Kher V, Viswanathan R, et al. Timing of initiation and discontinuation of renal replacement therapy in AKI: unanswered key questions. Clin J Am Soc Nephrol. 2008;3:876–80.
8. Vaara ST, Reinikainen M, Wald R, Bagshaw SM, Pettila V. Timing of RRT based on the presence of conventional indications. Clin J Am Soc Nephrol. 2014;9:1577–85.
9. Kidney Disease: Improving Global Outcomes (KDIGO) Work Group. KDIGO clinical practice guideline for acute kidney injury. Dialysis interventions for treatment of AKI. Section 3. Prevention and treatment of AKI. Kidney Int Suppl. 2012;2:37–68.
10. Koyner JL, Garg AX, Coca SG, Sint K, Thiessen-Philbrook H, Patel UD, et al. Biomarkers predict progression of acute kidney injury after cardiac surgery. J Am Soc Nephrol. 2012;23:905–14.
11. Koyner JL, Parikh CR. Clinical utility of biomarkers of AKI in cardiac surgery and critical illness. Clin J Am Soc Nephrol. 2013;8:1034–42.
12. Arthur JM, Hill EG, Alge JL, Lewis EC, Neely BA, Janech MG, et al. Evaluation of 32 urine biomarkers to predict the progression of acute kidney injury after cardiac surgery. Kidney Int. 2014;85:431–8.
13. Parikh CR, Thiessen-Philbrook H, Garg AX, Kadiyala D, Shlipak MG, Koyner JL, et al. Performance of kidney injury molecule-1 and liver fatty acid-binding protein and combined biomarkers of AKI after cardiac surgery. Clin J Am Soc Nephrol. 2013;8:1079–88.
14. Charlton JR, Portilla D, Okusa MD. A basic science view of acute kidney injury biomarkers. Nephrol Dial Transplant. 2014;29:1301–11.
15. Doi K, Katagiri D, Negishi K, Hasegawa S, Hamasaki Y, Fujita T, et al. Mild elevation of urinary biomarkers in prerenal acute kidney injury. Kidney Int. 2012;82:1114–20.
16. Singer E, Elger A, Elitok S, Kettritz R, Nickolas TL, Barasch J, et al. Urinary neutrophil gelatinase-associated lipocalin distinguishes pre-renal from intrinsic renal failure and predicts outcomes. Kidney Int. 2011;80:405–14.
17. Nejat M, Pickering JW, Devarajan P, Bonventre JV, Edelstein CL, Walker RJ, et al. Some biomarkers of acute kidney injury are increased in pre-renal acute injury. Kidney Int. 2012;81:1254–62.
18. Kashani K, Al-Khafaji A, Ardiles T, Artigas A, Bagshaw SM, Bell M, et al. Discovery and validation of cell cycle arrest biomarkers in human acute kidney injury. Crit Care. 2013;17:R25.
19. Vijayan A, Faubel S, Askenazi DJ, Cerda J, Fissell WH, Heung M, et al. Clinical use of the urine biomarker [TIMP-2] × [IGFBP7] for acute kidney injury risk assessment. Am J Kidney Dis. 2016;68:19–28.
20. Huang X, Dorhout Mees EJ, Vos PF, Hamza S, Braam B. Everything we always wanted to know about furosemide but were afraid to ask. Am J Physiol Renal Physiol. 2016. https://doi.org/10.1152/ajprenal.00476.2015.
21. Koyner JL, Davison DL, Brasha-Mitchell E, Chalikonda DM, Arthur JM, Shaw AD, et al. Furosemide stress test and biomarkers for the prediction of AKI severity. J Am Soc Nephrol. 2015;26:2023–31.
22. Murray PT, Mehta RL, Shaw A, Ronco C, Endre Z, Kellum JA, et al. Potential use of biomarkers in acute kidney injury: report and summary of recommendations from the 10th Acute Dialysis Quality Initiative consensus conference. Kidney Int. 2014;85:513–21.
23. Chawla LS, Davison DL, Brasha-Mitchell E, Koyner JL, Arthur JM, Shaw AD, et al. Development and standardization of a furosemide stress test to predict the severity of acute kidney injury. Crit Care. 2013;17:R207.
24. Isshiki R, Asada T, Sato D, Sumida M, Hamasaki Y, Inokuchi R, et al. Association of urinary neutrophil gelatinase-associated lipocalin with long-term renal outcomes in ICU survivors: a retrospective observational cohort study. Shock. 2016;46:44–51.
25. Hayase N, Yamamoto M, Asada T, Isshiki R, Yahagi N, Doi K. Association of heart rate with N-terminal pro-B-type natriuretic peptide in septic patients: a prospective observational cohort study. Shock. 2016;46:642–8.
26. Asada T, Aoki Y, Sugiyama T, Yamamoto M, Ishii T, Kitsuta Y, et al. Organ system network disruption in nonsurvivors of critically ill patients. Crit Care Med. 2016;44:83–90.
27. Knaus WA, Draper EA, Wagner DP, Zimmerman JE. APACHE II: a severity of disease classification system. Crit Care Med. 1985;13:818–29.
28. Matsuo S, Imai E, Horio M, Yasuda Y, Tomita K, Nitta K, et al. Revised equations for estimated GFR from serum creatinine in Japan. Am J Kidney Dis. 2009;53:982–92.
29. The Kidney Disease: Improving Global Outcomes (KDIGO) Work Group. KDIGO clinical practice guideline for acute kidney injury. Dialysis interventions for treatment of AKI. Section 2. AKI Definition. Kidney Int Supple. 2012;2:19–36.
30. DeLong ER, DeLong DM, Clarke-Pearson DL. Comparing the areas under two or more correlated receiver operating characteristic curves: a nonparametric approach. Biometrics. 1988;44:837–45.
31. Ruopp MD, Perkins NJ, Whitcomb BW, Schisterman EF. Youden Index and optimal cut-point estimated from observations affected by a lower limit of detection. Biom J. 2008;50:419–30.
32. Hanley JA, McNeil BJ. A method of comparing the areas under receiver operating characteristic curves derived from the same cases. Radiology. 1983;148:839–43.
33. Russell JA, Singer J, Bernard GR, Wheeler A, Fulkerson W, Hudson L, et al. Changing pattern of organ dysfunction in early human sepsis is related to mortality. Crit Care Med. 2000;28:3405–11.
34. Doi K, Noiri E, Nangaku M, Yahagi N, Jayakumar C, Ramesh G. Repulsive guidance cue semaphorin 3A in urine predicts the progression of acute kidney injury in adult patients from a mixed intensive care unit. Nephrol Dial Transplant. 2014;29:73–80.
35. Chen C, Yang X, Lei Y, Zha Y, Liu H, Ma C, et al. Urinary biomarkers at the time of AKI diagnosis as predictors of progression of AKI among patients with acute cardiorenal syndrome. Clin J Am Soc Nephrol. 2016;11:1536–44.
36. Hoste EA, McCullough PA, Kashani K, Chawla LS, Joannidis M, Shaw AD, et al. Derivation and validation of cutoffs for clinical use of cell cycle arrest biomarkers. Nephrol Dial Transplant. 2014;29:2054–61.
37. Bihorac A, Chawla LS, Shaw AD, Al-Khafaji A, Davison DL, Demuth GE, et al. Validation of cell-cycle arrest biomarkers for acute kidney injury using clinical adjudication. Am J Respir Crit Care Med. 2014;189:932–9.
38. Brater DC, Day B, Burdette A, Anderson S. Bumetanide and furosemide in heart failure. Kidney Int. 1984;26:183–9.
39. Brater D, Voelker J. Use of diuretics in patients with renal disease. New York: Churchill Livingstone; 1987.
40. Martin GS, Moss M, Wheeler AP, Mealer M, Morris JA, Bernard GR. A randomized, controlled trial of furosemide with or without albumin in hypoproteinemic patients with acute lung injury. Crit Care Med. 2005;33:1681–7.
41. Cordemans C, De Laet I, Van Regenmortel N, Schoonheydt K, Dits H, Martin G, et al. Aiming for a negative fluid balance in patients with acute

lung injury and increased intra-abdominal pressure: a pilot study looking at the effects of PAL-treatment. Ann Intensive Care. 2012;2:S15.

42. Waring WS, Moonie A. Earlier recognition of nephrotoxicity using novel biomarkers of acute kidney injury. Clin Toxicol. 2011;49:720–8.

43. Goetz DH, Willie ST, Armen RS, Bratt T, Borregaard N, Strong RK. Ligand preference inferred from the structure of neutrophil gelatinase associated lipocalin. Biochemistry. 2000;39:1935–41.

44. Cai L, Rubin J, Han W, Venge P, Xu S. The origin of multiple molecular forms in urine of HNL/NGAL. Clin J Am Soc Nephrol. 2010;5:2229–35.

45. Yamamoto T, Noiri E, Ono Y, Doi K, Negishi K, Kamijo A, et al. Renal L-type fatty acid-binding protein in acute ischemic injury. J Am Soc Nephrol. 2007;18:2894–902.

46. Doi K, Noiri E, Maeda-Mamiya R, Ishii T, Negishi K, Hamasaki Y, et al. Urinary L-type fatty acid-binding protein as a new biomarker of sepsis complicated with acute kidney injury. Crit Care Med. 2010;38:2037–42.

47. Kuwabara T, Mori K, Mukoyama M, Kasahara M, Yokoi H, Saito Y, et al. Urinary neutrophil gelatinase-associated lipocalin levels reflect damage to glomeruli, proximal tubules, and distal nephrons. Kidney Int. 2009;75:285–94.

48. Mehta RL. Biomarker explorations in acute kidney injury: the journey continues. Kidney Int. 2011;80:332–4.

49. Cohen SD, Kimmel PL. Long-term sequelae of acute kidney injury in the ICU. Curr Opin Crit Care. 2012;18:623–8.

50. Lo LJ, Go AS, Chertow GM, McCulloch CE, Fan D, Ordonez JD, et al. Dialysis-requiring acute renal failure increases the risk of progressive chronic kidney disease. Kidney Int. 2009;76:893–9.

51. Bucaloiu ID, Kirchner HL, Norfolk ER, Hartle JE, Perkins RM. Increased risk of death and de novo chronic kidney disease following reversible acute kidney injury. Kidney Int. 2012;81:477–85.

# 14

# Admission of tetanus patients to the ICU: a retrospective multicentre study

Rafael Mahieu[1] [ID], Thomas Reydel[1], Adel Maamar[2], Jean-Marc Tadié[2], Angeline Jamet[3], Arnaud W. Thille[3], Nicolas Chudeau[4], Julien Huntzinger[5], Steven Grangé[6], Gaetan Beduneau[6], Anne Courte[7], Stephane Ehrmann[8], Jérémie Lemarié[9], Sébastien Gibot[9], Michael Darmon[10], Christophe Guitton[11], Julia Champey[12], Carole Schwebel[12], Jean Dellamonica[13], Thibaut Wipf[14], Ferhat Meziani[14], Damien Du Cheyron[15], Achille Kouatchet[1] and Nicolas Lerolle[1*]

## Abstract

**Background:** An extended course of tetanus (up to 6 weeks) requiring ICU admission and protracted mechanical ventilation (MV) may have a significant impact on short- and long-term survival. The subject is noteworthy and deserves to be discussed.

**Methods:** Twenty-two ICUs in France performed tetanus screenings on patients admitted between January 2000 and December 2014. Retrospective data were collected from hospital databases and through the registers of the town hall of the patients.

**Results:** Seventy patients were included in 15 different ICUs. Sixty-three patients suffered from severe or very severe tetanus according to the Ablett classification. The median age was 80 years [interquartile range 73–84], and 86% of patients were women. Ninety per cent of patients ($n = 63$) required MV for a median of 36 days [26–46], and 66% required administration of a neuromuscular-blocking agent for 23 days [14–29]. A nosocomial infection occurred in 43 patients (61%). ICU and 1-year mortality rates were 14% ($n = 10$) and 16% ($n = 11$), respectively. Forty-five per cent of deaths occurred during the first week. Advanced age, a higher SAPS II, any infection, and the use of vasopressors were significantly associated with a lower number of days alive without ventilator support by day 90. Age was the only factor that significantly differed between deceased and survivors at 1 year (83 [81–85] vs. 79 [73–84] years, respectively; $p = 0.03$). Sixty-one per cent of survivors suffered no impairment to their functional status.

**Conclusion:** In a high-income country, tetanus mainly occurs in healthy elderly women. Despite prolonged MV and extended ICU length of stay, we observed a low 1-year mortality rate and good long-term functional status.

**Keywords:** Tetanus, Intensive care unit, Outcome, Mechanical ventilation, Elderly patient, Prognosis, Ventilators, Mechanical, Aged, Comorbidity

## Background

Tetanus is caused by the neurological effects of the toxin produced by *Clostridium tetani*. Although it is a completely preventable disease, tetanus remains responsible for around 60,000 deaths per year worldwide [1]. The blockage of neuromuscular transmission by the toxin causes painful muscle spasms and respiratory distress requiring ICU admission and mechanical ventilation (MV) in about 80% of patients [2]. Considering the long-lasting effect of the toxin, prolonged ventilation combined with sedation and neuromuscular blockade up to 6 weeks may be required [2, 3]. In developing countries, where access to high intensity care may be a challenge, the mortality rate of tetanus has risen to 50% for a mean age of 50 years with little improvement over time [4, 5, 6, 7].

*Correspondence: nicolas.lerolle@univ-angers.fr
[1] Département de réanimation médicale et médecine hyperbare, CHU Angers et faculté de santé Angers, 49933 Angers, France
Full list of author information is available at the end of the article

Data about severe tetanus are scarce in high-income countries. In Australia, a net decrease in tetanus-related mortality was observed between 1957 and 1985 (from 44 to 5%), which likely reflects the implementation of intensive care medicine over these years [8]. In developed countries, the enduring incidence of tetanus is mainly due to a lack of vaccination coverage of the elderly [9, 10]. In the USA and France, people over 65 years old have a twice to ten times greater risk of becoming infected with tetanus compared to younger patients [11, 12]. Elderly patients admitted to the ICU may be faced with a particularly high risk of poor outcome. Indeed, in elderly patients admitted to the ICU for medical reasons and requiring prolonged length of stay and/or MV, ICU- and 1-year mortality rates up to 50 and 70% have been reported, respectively [13, 14].

Treating tetanus in developed countries undoubtedly carries the challenge of prolonged ICU care for a particularly at-risk population. This may have a major impact on short- and long-term survival, which has not been described in recent years. We therefore conducted a multicentre retrospective study on such patients in France, reporting both short-term and 1-year mortality and long-term functional status.

## Patients and methods

### Study design

A retrospective cohort of adult tetanus patients was created. The study was conducted in 22 French ICUs. Patients were identified using hospital-based medical and administrative as well as ICU databases in each centre. All adult patients admitted to the ICU for tetanus from 1 January 2000 to 31 December 2014 were included.

### Data collection

Data on patient hospitalisations were retrieved from local ICU databases and medical files. Demographic data were collected, including age, sex, body mass index, Charlson Comorbidity Index, and Knaus' classification of functional limitation (ratings are A for no limitation, B for slight functional limitation, C for severe functional limitation, and D for bed-ridden patients) [15]. Severity of acute illness was recorded according the Sequential Organ Failure Assessment (SOFA) [16], the Simplified Acute Physiology Score (SAPS) II [17], and the Ablett classification of tetanus severity (mild for mild trismus, no dysphagia, and no respiratory involvement; moderate for moderate trismus, dysphagia, and moderate respiratory involvement; severe for generalised spasticity, severe respiratory involvement; and very severe when associated with autonomic disturbance involving the cardiovascular system) [18]. Data on the clinical presentation of tetanus included the presence of a wound, incubation time, time from symptom to admission to the ICU, status of vaccination protection, severity and extent of spasms (isolated trismus, localised spasm outside the jaw, dysphagia, generalised tetanus), and presence of an autonomic dysfunction. Autonomic dysfunction was defined by the report of labile blood pressure or heart rate, or ventricular arrhythmia in medical files [19]. Length of stay in ICU, mortality in ICU, duration of MV, use of vasopressors, renal replacement therapy (RRT), and nosocomial infections were recorded. Durations of the administration of neuromuscular-blocking agents and sedatives were registered. The use of magnesium and verapamil was recorded. Surgical treatment of the wound, antimicrobial therapy, and the use and dosage of human tetanus immunoglobulin (HTIg) were recorded.

### Long-term outcome

Long-term survival outcome was obtained by consulting hospital databases and by consulting patient's town hall registries. (The latter are used to record births and deaths, which is mandatory in France.) Last follow-up was determined depending on the date of inspecting town hall records and the day of admission into the ICU. Long-term functional status was defined using Knaus' functional classification and the number of patients who required long-term care facilities. The functional status was retrieved from hospital medical records and general practitioners.

### Statistical analysis

We performed analyses using the SPSS v15.0 statistical software package (IBM, New York, USA). Continuous variables were reported as medians with 25–75% percentiles (IQR). Categorical variables were reported as n and percentage. All parameters were tested for 1-year survival and for the number of days alive without ventilator support by day 90. Continuous data were compared using Student's $t$ test or the Mann–Whitney test, as appropriate. Categorical variables were compared using Pearson's Chi-squared test or Fisher's exact test, as appropriate. Kaplan–Meier survival curves were used to evaluate mortality.

## Results

Fifteen ICUs identified 70 patients with tetanus over the study period. Baseline characteristics and clinical presentations of patients are provided in Table 1. Characteristics of tetanus are detailed in Table 2. Fifty-seven patients (81%) received antibiotic treatment (benzyl penicillin for 51 patients, metronidazole for 13, both antibiotics for 4, other regimen for 23) for a median duration of 7 days (IQR 7–10). Human tetanus immunoglobulin (HTIg) was used in the case of 57 patients (81%) after a median

**Table 1  Baseline characteristics of patients**

| Parameters | Median [IQ] (min–max) or number (%) |
|---|---|
| Age | 80 [73–84] (22–91) |
| Male sex | 10 (14.3%) |
| Body mass index | 24 [21–29] |
| Coexisting conditions | |
|   Chronic heart failure | 16 (23%) |
|   Chronic respiratory failure | 4 (6%) |
|   Liver disease | 0 |
|   Chronic kidney disease | 4 (6%) |
|   Diabetes | 10 (14%) |
|   Dementia | 2 (3%) |
|   Active cancer | 2 (3%) |
| Charlson Comorbidity Index | 4 [3–5] |
| Knaus' classification | |
|   Knaus A | 35 (50%) |
|   Knaus B | 35 (50%) |
|   Knaus C or D | 0 |
| SAPS II upon ICU admission | 33 [26–41] |
| SOFA upon ICU admission | 1 [0–3] |

**Table 2  Characteristics of tetanus and specific management**

| Parameters | Median [IQ] or number (%) |
|---|---|
| Status of protection | |
|   No vaccination | 26 (37%) |
|   Vaccination > 10 years | 18 (26%) |
|   No information | 26 (37%) |
| Wound | 67 (96%) |
|   Gardening wound | 31 (44%) |
| Incubation time | 10 [8–14] |
| Time from symptoms to admission | 2 [1–3] |
| Ablett classification | |
|   Mild | 2 (3%) |
|   Moderate | 5 (7%) |
|   Severe | 29 (41%) |
|   Very severe | 34 (49%) |
| Trismus | 70 (100%) |
| Localised spasm | 34 (49%) |
| Dysphagia | 46 (66%) |
| Generalised tetanus | 39 (56%) |
| Autonomic dysfunction | 40 (57%) |
|   Blood pressure instability | 29 (41%) |
|   Heart rate instability | 17 (24%) |
|   Ventricular arrhythmia | 4 (6%) |

delay of 1 day after ICU admission, with a dose ranging from 250 to 5000 IU. None of the patients received verapamil to improve control of dysautonomia symptoms.

Magnesium intravenous infusion was used in 23 patients for a median duration of 6 (IQR 2–14) days. Baclofen was used in 12 patients (17%), by intrathecal route in the case of 7 patients, for a median duration of 10 (IQR 4–12) days; all of them required MV. MV was performed in 63 patients (90%) for a median duration of 36 days (IQR 26–46; range 1–131). Continuous administration of a neuromuscular-blocking agent (NMBA) was used in 50 (71%) patients for a median duration of 23 days (IQR 14–29; range 1–39). Ninety-eight per cent ($n = 61$) of patients with severe or very severe tetanus were administered a continuous infusion of benzodiazepines for a median duration of 28 (IQR 19–34) days. Twenty-four patients (34%) required vasopressor support (only norepinephrine was used) for a median duration of 9 days (IQR 4–20; range 1–34). Two-thirds of patients underwent a tracheotomy ($n = 46$) after a median duration of 7 days (IQR 1–9; range 0–48) in the ICU. Median length of stay in the ICU and hospital was 41 days (IQR 24–53; range 1–117) and 51 days (IQR 32–69; range 1–178), respectively. Only one patient required RRT. Sixty-one per cent of patients ($n = 43$) developed a nosocomial infection with 12 bloodstream infections (4 central venous catheter-associated bloodstream infections, 2 cases of ventilator acquired pneumonia (VAP) with bacteraemia, 1 sinusitis, 2 pyelonephritis, 3 primitive blood stream infection), 32 (51% of ventilated patients) VAPs (including the two with associated bloodstream infection), and 1 *Clostridium difficile* infection. The VAP rate was 15 episodes per 1000 ventilator days.

ICU, 90-day, and 1-year mortality rates were 14% ($n = 10$), 13% ($n = 9$), and 16% ($n = 11$), respectively (see Fig. 1). The ICU mortality rate was higher than the 90-day survival rate due to one late death in the ICU

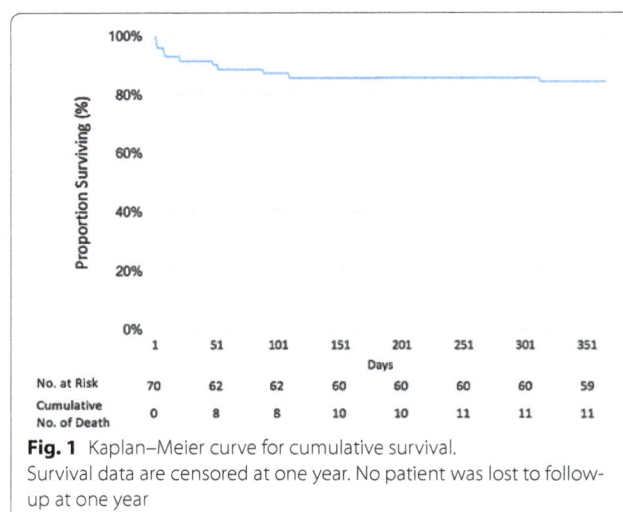

**Fig. 1** Kaplan–Meier curve for cumulative survival.
Survival data are censored at one year. No patient was lost to follow-up at one year

| | 1 | 51 | 101 | 151 | 201 | 251 | 301 | 351 |
|---|---|---|---|---|---|---|---|---|
| No. at Risk | 70 | 62 | 62 | 60 | 60 | 60 | 60 | 59 |
| Cumulative No. of Death | 0 | 8 | 8 | 10 | 10 | 11 | 11 | 11 |

of a patient at day 109. It is noteworthy that patients who did not receive MV had a mortality rate of 0% with a median length of stay in the ICU of 5 days (IQR 3–9; range 1–15), with all of them suffering from isolated cephalic tetanus. (Two patients had mild and five had moderate tetanus according to the Ablett classification.) Mortality status at 5 years was known for 57 patients (81%), among whom 36 (61% of the 57) were alive. Nearly half of the deaths that occurred during the first year occurred within the first week ($n = 5$). Four of these early deaths were caused by ventricular arrhythmia, possibly as a manifestation of autonomic dysfunction. Three patients died during the first 90 days in the ICU following the withdrawal of life-sustaining therapies, two patients died due to nosocomial infections, and one patient died after being discharged. None of the deaths could be attributed to delayed intubation resulting in hypoxic cardiac arrest. Among the survivors at last follow-up ($n = 38$), the health status according to Knaus' classification was known for 95% of them, after a median duration of 1385 [302–3096] days. Sixty-one per cent of these survivors had no impairment of their functional status. Seventeen per cent ($n = 6$) of patients initially classified as Knaus A before ICU admission evolved to Knaus B (the same number was observed for Knaus B patients evolving to Knaus C) and 5% ($n = 2$) of Knaus A patients evolved to Knaus C. Only six patients (17% of survivors with a known functional status) required admission to a long-term care facility.

Age was the only factor that significantly differed between deceased and survivors at 1 year (83 [81–85] vs. 79 [73–84] years, respectively; $p = 0.03$). Advanced age, higher SAPS II (above the median of 33), any infection, bloodstream infection, VAP, and the use of vasopressors were significantly associated with a lower number of days alive without ventilator support by day 90 (see Table 3).

## Discussion

### Epidemiology of tetanus in developed countries

In this study, tetanus mainly occurred in elderly patients (75% of patients were older than 73, median age 80 years), which is consistent with previous Italian and French studies reporting a median age of 76 years or 86% of patients being 70 years old or over, respectively [12, 20]. This is in contrast with US reports, which involved younger patients (median age of 49 years) [11]. The description of tetanus in injection drug users in the US [11] may explain part of these differences given that in our study a gardening wound was the main portal of entry in our patients. Women are a particular at-risk population (86% of tetanus patients in this study and 68% in Italy). It may be hypothesised that mandatory vaccination during

**Table 3 Factors significantly associated with the number of days alive without ventilator support by day 90**

| Parameters | Number of days alive without ventilator support by day 90. Median [interquartile range] | p value |
|---|---|---|
| Age (years) | | |
| ≥ 80 | 43 [0–57] | 0.03 |
| < 80 | 53 [45–59] | |
| SAPS II[a] | | |
| ≥ 34 | 44 [22–54] | 0.04 |
| < 34 | 57 [43–63] | |
| Any infection | | |
| Yes | 45 [27–57] | 0.01 |
| No | 60 [48–71] | |
| Bloodstream infection | | |
| Yes | 42 [6–51] | 0.04 |
| No | 54 [36–52] | |
| Ventilator acquired pneumonia | | |
| Yes | 42 [19–57] | 0.01 |
| No | 55 [47–63] | |
| Vasopressor use | | |
| Yes | 43 [0–57] | < 0.05 |
| No | 53 [42–62] | |

[a] Parameter dichotomised at median value

compulsory military service for men provides them with long-lasting immunisation [20].

### Controlling muscle spasms and autonomic dysfunction

Several treatments have been tested to control autonomic instability and muscle spasm and to hasten recovery. Despite little evidence, benzodiazepines remain the main treatment regimen for tetanus spasms [21]. Benzodiazepines in continuous infusion were used in all severe or very severe tetanus patients except one, while NMBAs were required in the majority of cases. Baclofen was used only marginally. Baclofen has the potential to relieve muscle spasms and may reduce the need for ventilation; however, evidence in favour of baclofen use is limited to case studies with conflicting results [22]. Severe autonomic dysfunction, and in particular early-onset ventricular arrhythmia, was responsible for 36% of deaths is this study; this percentage is commonly reported in tetanus studies [4, 23, 24]. The pathophysiological link between ventricular arrhythmia and tetanus toxin is still unclear. Verapamil and magnesium have been suggested as a prevention method. None of our patients received verapamil, while one-third of patients received magnesium treatment. We did not observe any association between magnesium use and outcome; however, this study was not designed to draw conclusions on this hypothesis. As shown by Thwaites et al. [2], magnesium may reduce autonomic dysfunction thanks to its calcium-antagonist properties [25]; however, no benefits for mortality were observed in our study, which is consistent with a recent meta-analysis [25].

### Neutralisation of toxin, antibiotic, and wound management

HTIg was used in more than 80% of patients, with no difference in outcome between the patients who received HTIg treatment and those who did not (data not shown). HTIg is conventionally recommended in tetanus to bind the unbound toxin in serum, which has been demonstrated in 10% of serum samples [26]. Notably, none of the patients in this study received HTIg by intrathecal route, while previous uncontrolled studies showed an association between this route of administration and reduced mortality [27]. More recently, the benefits of intrathecal route combined with intramuscular HTIg were assessed in a randomised study and only a reduction in hospital stay was observed [28]. Antimicrobial therapy probably plays a minor role in tetanus but is conventionally recommended to halt the toxin's production [21, 29]. No difference was observed in this study between patients treated with penicillin, metronidazole, or other regimens (data not shown). The first study that compared penicillin to metronidazole found a greater reduction in mortality in the metronidazole group [30]; however, more recent studies, including a randomised study, did not show any difference between these treatments [4, 31]. Penicillin and metronidazole are therefore equally recommended. Wound debridement, which can eradicate persistent spores of *C. tetani*, was only performed in 16% of cases. It is likely that in a context of a rare disease with severe symptoms, the portal of entry (sometimes a very small one) did not appear as a priority. However, persistence of *C. tetani* in the wound has been described despite antimicrobial therapy, and wound debridement therefore seems essential to haste the eradication of the bacteria [32].

### Prolonged mechanical ventilation and elderly patients

Most patients in our study required prolonged mechanical ventilation. Most of them were elderly (median age 80 years), but all had no or only slight functional limitation and a low burden of comorbidities as measured by Knaus' classification and the Charlson Comorbidity Index. Indeed, a gardening wound was identified in about half of the cases, thereby selecting a population of "healthy elderly". Despite a strikingly high duration of MV with frequent requirement for tracheotomy and a long ICU length of stay, ICU and 1-year survival were excellent, at 86 and 84%, respectively. The increasing number of elderly patients in the ICU, combined with concerns regarding their high mortality rate and uncertainty regarding the functional outcome, fuelled a continuous debate about the benefits of their admission [13, 33–38]. A recent study by Moitra showed that higher duration of MV and length of stay in the ICU were almost linearly correlated with outcome [13]. In sharp contrast with this late study, the very low rate of comorbidities in our population combined with a completely reversible disease may explain the very low ICU and 1-year mortality rate in our study [13, 14]. Finally, our study confirms and builds on a study performed in Italy that showed a 16.5% hospital mortality rate for tetanus patients in a population with a median age of 76 years [20]. Further comparison with this study is limited by the lack of any ICU data and a known outcome for only 43.9% of patients.

### Outcome of tetanus in high-income countries

The low mortality rate observed in our patients (16% 1-year mortality) in comparison with low-income countries likely reflects the availability of high-cost ICU facilities [8]. These are essential for managing prolonged MV, paralysing agents, autonomic dysfunction, and the high rate of infectious complications. Indeed, the mortality rate of severe tetanus patients remains between 30 and 50% in low-income countries [4, 5, 6], which is consistent with the mortality rate of tetanus before the implementation of ICUs [39] in Europe. A study in the 1970s reported a mortality rate of only 11% in England [40].

### Limitations

Our study presents certain limitations. The main concern is the lack of detailed information regarding the long-term functional status of survivors. Indeed, we could not assess it precisely due to the study's design. However, the functionality score according to Knaus' classification was known for 95% of survivors, with 61% of them suffering no loss of autonomy. Moreover, only six patients required admission to a long-term care facility. Another limitation is that we could not include tetanus patients subject to a Do-Not-Resuscitate order that would have prevented ICU admission, or patients who suffered hypoxic cardiac arrest before ICU admission. Finally, due to the incompleteness of most medical reports, we could not establish accurately the processes or indications that lead the physicians to intubate, start NMBA treatment or perform a tracheotomy.

### Conclusion

Tetanus in France occurs mainly in healthy elderly patients, especially women. In this population, despite prolonged MV with frequent NMBA use as well as extended ICU length of stay, we observed a low mortality rate and a good long-term functional status.

## Abbreviations

HTIg: human tetanus immunoglobulin; ICU: intensive care unit; MV: mechanical ventilation; NMBA: neuromuscular-blocking agent; RRT: renal replacement therapy; SAPS II: Simplified Acute Physiology Score II; SOFA: Sequential Organ Failure Assessment; VAP: ventilator-associated pneumonia.

## Authors' contributions

RM, TR, and NL drafted the manuscript. All authors participated in collecting data for the study and then read and approved the final manuscript.

## Author details

[1] Département de réanimation médicale et médecine hyperbare, CHU Angers et faculté de santé Angers, 49933 Angers, France. [2] Service des Maladies Infectieuses et Réanimation Médicale, Maladies Infectieuses et Réanimation Médicale, CHU Rennes, 35033 Rennes, France. [3] Service de Réanimation Médicale, CHU de Poitiers, 2, rue de la Milétrie, 86021 Poitiers, France. [4] Département d'anesthésie-réanimation, LUNAM université, université d'Angers, CHU d'Angers, 49933 Angers, France. [5] Service de réanimation, Centre hospitalier Bretagne Atlantique, 56017 Vannes Cedex, France. [6] Medical Intensive Care Unit, Rouen University Hospital, Rouen, France. [7] Medical-surgical ICU, Hospital of Saint-Brieuc, 10 rue Marcel Proust, 22000 Saint-Brieuc, France. [8] Médecine Intensive Réanimation, Centre Hospitalier Régional et Universitaire de Tours, 37044 Tours, France. [9] Service de Réanimation Médicale, CHRU Nancy, Hôpital Central, Nancy, France. [10] Medical-Surgical ICU, Saint-Etienne University Hospital, Saint-Priest-en-Jarez, France. [11] Medical intensive care unit, Nantes academic hospital, Nantes university, Nantes, France. [12] Intensive Care Medicine, CHU de Grenoble, BP 218, 38043 Grenoble Cedex 9, France. [13] Service de Réanimation, Centre Hospitalier-Universitaire, Nice, France. [14] Service de Réanimation Médicale, Nouvel Hôpital Civil, Centre Hospitalo-Universitaire, Strasbourg, France. [15] Intensive Care Unit, University Hospital of Caen, Caen, France.

## Competing interests

The authors declare that they have no competing interests.

## Funding

None.

## References

1. GBD 2015 Mortality and Causes of Death Collaborators. Global, regional, and national life expectancy, all-cause mortality, and cause-specific mortality for 249 causes of death, 1980–2015: a systematic analysis for the Global Burden of Disease Study 2015. Lancet. 2016;388:1459–544.
2. Thwaites CL, Yen LM, Loan HT, Thuy TTD, Thwaites GE, Stepniewska K, et al. Magnesium sulphate for treatment of severe tetanus: a randomised controlled trial. Lancet. 2006;368:1436–43.
3. da Nóbrega MVD, Reis RC, Aguiar ICV, Queiroz TV, Lima ACF, Pereira EDB, et al. Patients with severe accidental tetanus admitted to an intensive care unit in Northeastern Brazil: clinical–epidemiological profile and risk factors for mortality. Braz J Infect Dis. 2016;20:457–61.
4. Saltoglu N, Tasova Y, Midikli D, Burgut R, Dündar IH. Prognostic factors affecting deaths from adult tetanus. Clin Microbiol Infect. 2004;10:229–33.
5. Chalya PL, Mabula JB, Dass RM, Mbelenge N, Mshana SE, Gilyoma JM. Ten-year experiences with Tetanus at a Tertiary hospital in Northwestern Tanzania: a retrospective review of 102 cases. World J Emerg Surg WJES. 2011;6:20.
6. Tosun S, Batirel A, Oluk AI, Aksoy F, Puca E, Bénézit F, et al. Tetanus in adults: results of the multicenter ID-IRI study. Eur. J. Clin. Microbiol. Infect. 2017;36:1455–62.
7. Brauner JS, Vieira SRR, Bleck TP. Changes in severe accidental tetanus mortality in the ICU during two decades in Brazil. Intensive Care Med. 2002;28:930–5.
8. Gilligan JEF, Lawrence JR, Clayton D, Rowland R. Tetanus and the evolution of intensive care in Australia. Crit Care Resusc J Australas Acad Crit Care Med. 2012;14:316–23.
9. Centers for Disease Control and Prevention (CDC). Tetanus and pertussis vaccination coverage rates among adults aged > 18 years—United States, 1999 and 2008. MMWR. 2010;59:1302–6.
10. La Gergely A. couverture vaccinale contre le tétanos, la poliomyélite et la diphtérie en 2006 dans une population âgée francilienne. Bull Epidémiol Hebd. 2008;9:61–4.
11. Centers for Disease Control and Prevention (CDC). Tetanus surveillance—United States, 2001–2008. MMWR Morb Mortal Wkly Rep. 2011;60:365–9.
12. Antona D. Le tétanos en France en 2008–2011. Saint-Maurice: Institut de veille sanitaire. Bull Epidemiol Hebd. 2012;26:303–6.
13. Moitra VK, Guerra C, Linde-Zwirble WT, Wunsch H. Relationship between ICU length of stay and long-term mortality for elderly ICU survivors. Crit Care Med. 2016;44:655–62.
14. Roch A, Wiramus S, Pauly V, Forel J-M, Guervilly C, Gainnier M, et al. Long-term outcome in medical patients aged 80 or over following admission to an intensive care unit. Crit Care. 2011;15:R36.
15. Knaus WA, Zimmerman JE, Wagner DP, Draper EA, Lawrence DE. APACHE-acute physiology and chronic health evaluation: a physiologically based classification system. Crit Care Med. 1981;9:591–7.
16. Vincent JL, Moreno R, Takala J, Willatts S, De Mendonça A, Bruining H, et al. The SOFA (Sepsis-related Organ Failure Assessment) score to describe organ dysfunction/failure. On behalf of the Working Group on Sepsis-Related Problems of the European Society of Intensive Care Medicine. Intensive Care Med. 1996;22:707–10.
17. Le Gall JR, Lemeshow S, Saulnier F. A new Simplified Acute Physiology Score (SAPS II) based on a European/North American multicenter study. JAMA. 1993;270:2957–63.
18. Ablett J. Analysis and main experiences in 82 patients treated in the Leeds Tetanus Unit. In: Ellis M, editors, Symposium on Tetanus in Great Britain. Leeds General Infirmary; 1967. p. 1–10.
19. Kerr JH, Corbett JL, Spalding JM. Sympathetic overactivity in severe tetanus. Proc R Soc Med. 1969;62:659–62.
20. Filia A, Bella A, von Hunolstein C, Pinto A, Alfarone G, Declich S, et al. Tetanus in Italy 2001–2010: a continuing threat in older adults. Vaccine. 2014;32:639–44.
21. Rodrigo C, Fernando D, Rajapakse S. Pharmacological management of tetanus: an evidence-based review. Crit Care. 2014;18:217.
22. Müller H, Börner U, Zierski J, Hempelmann G. Intrathecal baclofen for treatment of tetanus-induced spasticity. Anesthesiology. 1987;66:76–9.
23. Thwaites CL, Yen LM, Glover C, Tuan PQ, Nga NTN, Parry J, et al. Predicting the clinical outcome of tetanus: the tetanus severity score. Trop Med Int Health TM IH. 2006;11:279–87.
24. Phillips LA. A classification of tetanus. Lancet. 1967;1:1216–7.
25. Rodrigo C, Samarakoon L, Fernando SD, Rajapakse S. A meta-analysis of magnesium for tetanus. Anaesthesia. 2012;67:1370–4.
26. Veronose R. Tetanus: important new concepts. Excerpta Medica. 1981; p. 183.
27. Sun KO, Chan YW, Cheung RT, So PC, Yu YL, Li PC. Management of tetanus: a review of 18 cases. J R Soc Med. 1994;87:135–7.
28. de Miranda-Filho D, De Alencar Ximenes RA, Barone AA, Vaz VL, Vieira AG, Albuquerque VMG. Randomised controlled trial of tetanus treatment with antitetanus immunoglobulin by the intrathecal or intramuscular route. BMJ. 2004;328:615.
29. Afshar M, Raju M, Ansell D, Bleck TP. Narrative review: tetanus-a health threat after natural disasters in developing countries. Ann Intern Med. 2011;154:329–35.
30. Ahmadsyah I, Salim A. Treatment of tetanus: an open study to compare the efficacy of procaine penicillin and metronidazole. Br Med J Clin Res Ed. 1985;291:648–50.
31. Ganesh Kumar AV, Kothari VM, Krishnan A, Karnad DR. Benzathine penicillin, metronidazole and benzyl penicillin in the treatment of tetanus: a randomized, controlled trial. Ann Trop Med Parasitol. 2004;98:59–63.
32. Campbell JI, Lam TMY, Huynh TL, To SD, Tran TTN, Nguyen VMH, et al. Microbiologic characterization and antimicrobial susceptibility of Clostrid-

*ium tetani* isolated from wounds of patients with clinically diagnosed tetanus. Am J Trop Med Hyg. 2009;80:827–31.

33. Heyland D, Cook D, Bagshaw SM, Garland A, Stelfox HT, Mehta S, et al. The very elderly admitted to ICU: a quality finish? Crit Care Med. 2015;43:1352–60.

34. Ely EW, Wheeler AP, Thompson BT, Ancukiewicz M, Steinberg KP, Bernard GR. Recovery rate and prognosis in older persons who develop acute lung injury and the acute respiratory distress syndrome. Ann Intern Med. 2002;136:25–36.

35. Martin GS, Mannino DM, Moss M. The effect of age on the development and outcome of adult sepsis. Crit Care Med. 2006;34:15–21.

36. Orwelius L, Nordlund A, Nordlund P, Simonsson E, Bäckman C, Samuelsson A, et al. Pre-existing disease: the most important factor for health related quality of life long-term after critical illness: a prospective, longitudinal, multicentre trial. Crit Care. 2010;14:R67.

37. Zivot JB. Elderly patients in the ICU: worth it or not? Crit Care Med. 2016;44:842–3.

38. Sjoding MW, Prescott HC, Wunsch H, Iwashyna TJ, Cooke CR. Longitudinal changes in ICU admissions among elderly patients in the United States. Crit Care Med. 2016;44:1353–60.

39. Trujillo MH, Castillo A, España J, Manzo A, Zerpa R. Impact of intensive care management on the prognosis of tetanus. Analysis of 641 cases. Chest. 1987;92:63–5.

40. Edmondson RS, Flowers MW. Intensive care in tetanus: management, complications, and mortality in 100 cases. Br Med J. 1979;1:1401–4.

# 15

# Fluid therapy and outcome: a prospective observational study in 65 German intensive care units between 2010 and 2011

Christian Ertmer[1], Bernhard Zwißler[2], Hugo Van Aken[1], Michael Christ[3], Fabian Spöhr[4,5], Axel Schneider[6], Robert Deisz[7] and Matthias Jacob[2,8]*

## Abstract

**Background:** Outcome data on fluid therapy in critically ill patients from randomised controlled trials may be different from data obtained by observational studies under "real-life" conditions. We conducted this prospective, observational study to investigate current practice of fluid therapy (crystalloids and colloids) and associated outcomes in 65 German intensive care units (ICUs). In total, 4545 adult patients who underwent intravenous fluid therapy were included. The main outcome measures were 90-day mortality, ICU mortality and acute kidney injury (AKI). Data were analysed using logistic and Cox regression models, as appropriate.

**Results:** In the predominantly post-operative overall cohort, unadjusted 90-day mortality was 20.1%. Patients who *also* received colloids (54.6%) had a higher median Simplified Acute Physiology Score II [25 (interquartile range 11; 41) vs. 17 (7; 31)] and incidence of severe sepsis (10.2 vs. 7.4%) on admission compared to patients who received *exclusively* crystalloids (45.4%). 6% hydroxyethyl starch (HES 130/0.4) was the most common colloid (57.0%). Crude rates of 90-day mortality were higher for patients who received colloids (OR 1.845 [1.560; 2.181]). After adjustment for baseline variables, the HR was 1.666 [1.405; 1.976] and further decreased to indicate no associated risk (HR 1.003 [0.980; 1.027]) when it was adjusted for vasopressor use, severity of disease and transfusions. Similarly, the crude risk of AKI was higher in the colloid group (crude OR 3.056 [2.528; 3.694]), after adjustment for baseline variables OR 1.941 [1.573; 2.397], and after full adjustment OR 0.696 [0.629; 0.770]), the risk of AKI turned out to be reduced. The same was true for the subgroup of patients treated with 6% HES 130/0.4 (crude OR 1.931 [1.541; 2.419], adjusted for baseline variables OR 2.260 [1.730; 2.953] and fully adjusted OR 0.800 [0.704; 0.910]) as compared to crystalloids only.

**Conclusions:** The present analysis of mostly post-operative patients in routine clinical care did not reveal an independent negative effect of colloids (mostly 6% HES 130/0.4) on renal function or survival after multivariable adjustment. Signals towards a reduced risk in subgroup analyses deserve further study.

**Keywords:** Fluid therapy, Critical illness, Colloids, Crystalloids, Hydroxyethyl starch, Acute kidney injury

## Background

Fluid therapy in critically ill patients is an important issue especially in initial stabilisation [1, 2]. The optimal fluid during the first "golden" hours remains controversial [3,

*Correspondence: Matthias.Jacob@klinikum-straubing.de
[8] Department of Anaesthesiology, Surgical Intensive Care and Pain Medicine, St. Elisabeth Hospital, St.-Elisabeth-Str. 23, 94315 Straubing, Germany
Full list of author information is available at the end of the article

4]. Comparing different fluids prospectively regarding survival and organ failure of hypovolemic patients is difficult, since transfer to the participating intensive care units (ICUs), obtaining consent, randomisation and preparing study fluids take time. Recent trials relating the use of hydroxyethyl starch (HES) in critically ill patients to negative outcomes [5–8] largely suffered from this problem: identifying participants to first infusion of study fluid took up to 24 h. Therefore, due to sufficient initial (pre-study) resuscitation [9], most patients were already stabilised at inclusion [10]. Thus, these studies did not compare crystalloids versus colloids for resuscitation, but for maintenance [5, 7, 8, 11]. Moreover, results in sepsis have been extrapolated to all patients with fluid depletion [12], suspecting harm in, for example, perioperative patients, although this is not supported by current evidence. In contrast, timing and indication for fluid therapy in early resuscitation appear to be decisive for harm or benefit. This may have contributed to the decision of the European Medicines Agency (EMA) to differentiate between specific disease entities.

The present prospective, non-interventional multicentre registry aimed at gaining data on the practice of fluid therapy and associated outcomes. The goals were to assess the impact of colloids per se, but also specific colloids on 90-day survival, ICU mortality and acute kidney injury (AKI). Notably, all data were obtained prior to the EMA decision on HES solutions in 2013.

## Methods
### Aim
The aim of this study is to gather data on the practice of fluid therapy and associated outcomes in order to assess the impact of specific colloids and colloids in general on 90-day survival, ICU mortality and acute kidney injury (AKI).

### Study design
RaFTinG (Rational Fluid Therapy in Germany) is a prospective, observational, multicentre database. It assessed the characteristics of unselected ICU patients, focusing on fluid therapy and related outcomes. For recruitment, all German ICUs received an invitation letter and a notification in "Deutsches Ärzteblatt".

### Setting
Sixty-five German ICUs participated in this registry.

### Study population
Patients with an indication for fluid therapy (judged by the attending physician) and presumed length of ICU stay > 24 h were included. Exclusion criteria were age < 18 years, psychological disorders, reasonable doubt regarding the patient's discernment and institutionalisation upon court or other official order. Inclusion started 01.06.2010 and ended 31.05.2011. Centres were offered four inclusion schemes to avoid selective inclusion: 1. all patients, 2. all patients admitted on a specific weekday, 3. all patients admitted in one week per month and 4. first 10 consecutive patients per month.

### Study protocol and collected data
No specifications regarding diagnostics, medication or procedures were made. All relevant decisions were performed as part of usual care. Only routine records were documented for the study starting at admission to the ICU. Basic biometrical data, admission diagnoses, haemodynamic and laboratory parameters and severity scores (Acute Physiology And Chronic Health Evaluation, APACHE II; Simplified Acute Physiology Score, SAPS II; Sequential Organ Failure Assessment score, SOFA) were documented. On each ICU day, new diagnoses, haemodynamic and laboratory variables, fluid balance and therapeutic interventions were assessed. Documentation was completed by the medical condition at discharge.

ICU survivors were contacted by postal mail to retrieve survival status 90 days after ICU admission. If no reply was returned, survival status was attempted to be retraced via telephone calls and the residents' registration offices.

Data entries were possible in electronic or paper forms (Additional file 1: Supplemental digital content 1) as preferred by the centres. Automatic enquiries for values outside of pre-specified limits ensured data validity. All data were continuously checked for formal and content-related errors. Missing and inconsistent information was reassessed.

### Outcome parameters and pre-defined subcohorts
Main outcome parameters were 90-day mortality (death within 90 days after first ICU admission), ICU mortality and AKI (RIFLE [13] "failure"). Renal replacement therapy (RRT) was analysed for completeness, despite the fact that, without protocol, it is an inaccurate parameter.

Patients were a priori stratified as having received crystalloids *and* colloids or exclusively crystalloids. Patients having received crystalloids *and* colloids were further substratified a priori as having received gelatine, HES 130/0.4, HES 130/0.42), HES 200/0.5 or human albumin. Patients who were treated with more than one type of colloid were excluded from subcohort analyses.

Data were also a priori stratified for surgical or medical patients and patients with or without severe sepsis on admission.

### Statistical analysis
Data are presented as median (25th; 75th percentiles) for numeric variables or percentages for categorical variables, if not otherwise specified. Crude results cover the whole study population. Univariate data comprise only patients eligible for multivariable analysis. The predicted individual risk of mortality on admission was calculated from SAPS II and APACHE II scores [14, 15]. We used the highest calculated risk for further analyses because

a relevant subset of patients only had entries for one of these scores. In order to assess the maximum mortality risk for each patient, the score that predicted a higher risk was used for the regression analyses. Comparison of predicted vs. actual mortality shows that both are well correlated (Additional file 1: Supplemental digital content 2).

For all multivariable tests, covariables with a clear clinical relevance on the investigated outcome were chosen as cofactors and restricted to those with a $p < 0.10$ in univariate analysis in the model. Colloid dose is entered as a continuous variable in mL into the statistical models.

For AKI, RRT and ICU mortality, a multiple logistic regression model was fitted with adjustment for the predicted mortality risk in percentile steps of 10% (resulting in an ordinal covariable stratifying the predicted risk from 0–10 up to 90–100%), gender, chronic kidney disease (CKD, according to KDOQI [16]) and severe sepsis (according to ACCP/SCCM [17]) on admission as categorical cofactors (model referred to as "baseline adjustment" in the tables).

To enhance structural equality of the cohorts, the covariables obtained at ICU admission and variables derived during ICU stay (AUC of SOFA score until event or end of stay, cumulative volume of red blood cell products, cumulative volume of other blood products, cumulative fluid balance, application of vasopressor equivalent > 0.6 mg/h and daily crystalloid infusion) were included as covariables in a second analysis (referred to as "full model").

Association of covariates was tested for significance and removed when not significant to reduce the number of model parameters to be estimated.

Norepinephrine equivalent was defined as 1 mg norepinephrine being equivalent to 1 mg epinephrine or 100 mg of dopamine [18].

90-day survival was analysed by Cox regression with the cofactors and covariables given above. To account for missing follow-up data, the following approaches were chosen: (1) include only patients with complete follow-up data; (2) assume that all patients with unknown status die 1 day after discharge ("worst case"); (3) assume that 10% of all patients die after discharge (unknown status is extrapolated based on post-ICU mortality); (4) assume that 28% of all patients die after discharge (unknown status is extrapolated based on mortality in the cohort without 90-d follow-up); (5) assume that all patients with unknown status survive until 90 days post-discharge ("best case").

For the multivariable analyses, hazard ratios (HRs) were used to describe point estimates of the instantaneous risk ratio between cohorts in Cox regression analysis.

Odds ratios (ORs) were used to quantify the cumulative risk estimate presented derived from logistic regression.

Factors with an exploratory p value of less than 0.05 in the regression equation were considered relevant for the event under investigation. The impact of specific fluids in each analysis is shown as the adjusted odds ratio or hazard ratio and the respective 95% confidence intervals [19], keeping all other covariables constant.

All statistical analyses were done with SAS version 9.3.

## Results

### Participating centres and patient recruitment

Sixty-five study centres documented 4545 patients. 70.9% (3223) of patients were admitted from the operating theatre. In total, 3902 (85.9%) had records for each adjustment variable and were valid for multivariable analysis (Fig. 1). Baseline characteristics are presented in Table 1. Patients with higher severity of illness (SAPS II and APACHE II scores) or with severe sepsis on admission were more likely to have received colloids later on. An overview about primary diagnoses of the patient populations is presented in Additional file 1: Supplemental digital content 3.

### Fluid therapy

During ICU stay, 54.6% (2482) of patients received *exclusively* crystalloids, whereas 45.4% (2063) received crystalloids *and* colloids. 57.0% (1175) of the latter collective received 6% HES 130/0.4 (Table 1). Considerably less patients were treated with other colloids (6% HES 130/0.42, gelatine and human albumin) and were therefore excluded from subgroup analyses (Additional file 1: Supplemental digital content 4). Sixteen centres used exclusively crystalloids in all documented patients (207).

Fluid balances are presented in Additional file 1: Supplemental digital content 5 and 6. Colloid dose is given in Additional file 1: Supplemental digital content 7. Cumulative fluid balance and fluid balance on day 1 were more positive for patients receiving crystalloids *and* colloids as compared to sole crystalloid therapy (Additional file 1: Supplemental digital content 6). Among patients treated with colloids, 77.2% (1555 patients) received colloids on day 1 (Fig. 2), with a median amount of one unit of 500 mL [500; 1000]. Amounts of infused blood products significantly differed between cohorts, but absolute differences were very small (Additional file 1: Supplemental digital content 6).

### 90-day survival

77.5% of patients had 90-day follow-up data (3115 plus 408 who died on ICU). 55.0% (1713) of patients with follow-up data received only crystalloids and 45.0% (1402)

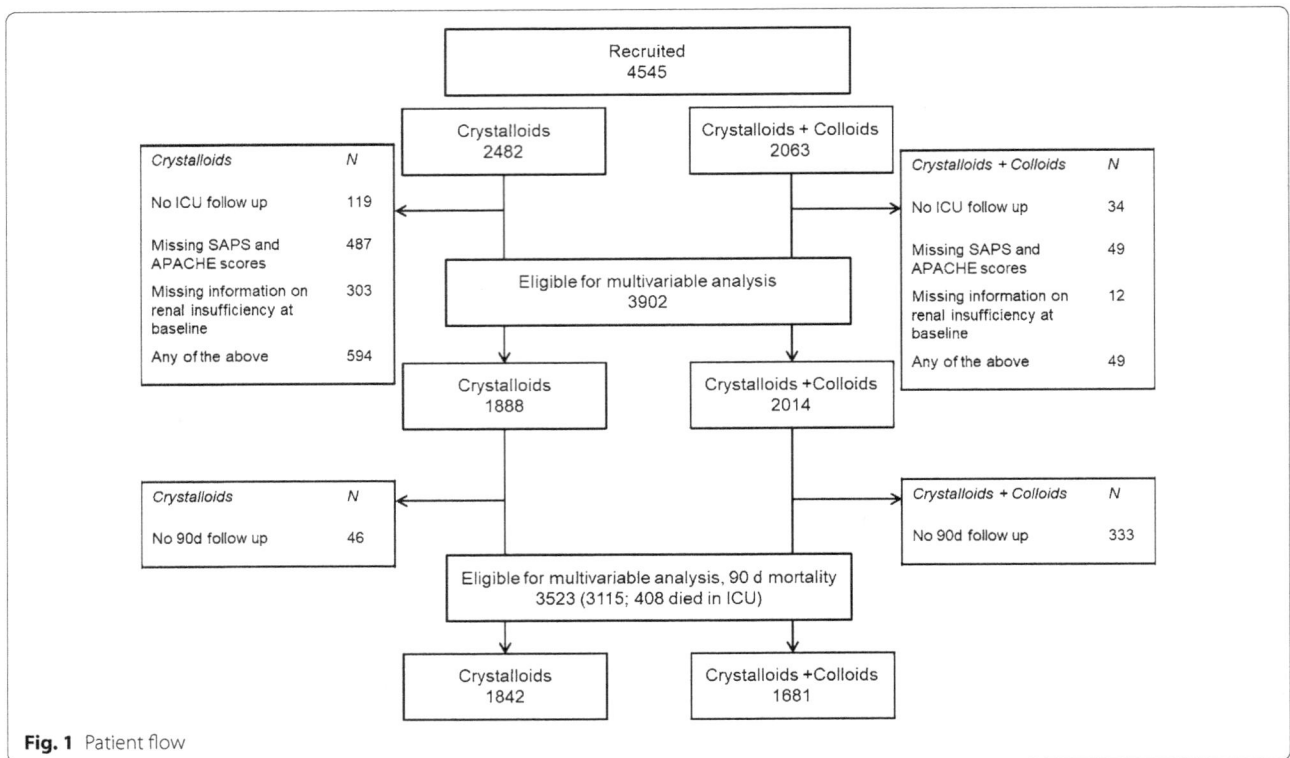

**Fig. 1** Patient flow

received colloids, a ratio that is similar to the total database (54.6 vs. 45.4%).

Unknown status for 90-day follow-up was associated with lower SAPS II and APACHE II scores on admission (SAPS II median 13 [6, 26] vs. 24 [11, 38], $p < 0.001$; APACHE II median 19 [13, 24] vs. 20 [15, 26], $p < 0.001$), as well as significantly lower cumulative crystalloid infusion and red blood cell transfusions. In contrast, there was no significant association of loss to 90-day follow-up with length of ICU stay, CKD or sepsis on admission.

Overall 90-day mortality was 20.1% (707 of 3523). Crude 90-day mortality of patients who received colloids was higher than in patients treated exclusively with crystalloids (25.5% (423 of 1681) vs. 15.4% (284 of 1842) (crude OR in the overall population 1.845 [1.560; 2.181]). After adjustment for baseline covariables only and adjustment for baseline and progress variables, the adjusted risk associated with colloids decreased stepwise by multivariable Cox regression and was no longer statistically significant (Table 2). Independent risk factors were predicted mortality, female gender, severe sepsis and CKD on admission, vasopressor use, SOFA score (AUC) and cumulative fluid balance. These findings were similar in patients who received HES 130/0.4 (Additional file 1: Supplemental digital content 8). In addition, results were homogenous among the subcohorts of septic and non-septic (colloid use 0.923 [0.874; 0.974]; 1.002 [0.908;

1.106]) as well as surgical and medical patients (colloid use 0.980 [0.912; 1.053], 0.945 [0.891; 1.001]). Sensitivity analysis did not suggest that data were influenced by missing follow-up data (Additional file 1: Supplemental digital content 9).

### ICU mortality
Overall ICU mortality was 9.3% (408 of 4392, 153 missing data). Treatment with colloids was associated with higher crude ICU mortality compared to crystalloids only (13.8% (279 of 2029) versus 5.5% (129 of 2363), crude OR in the overall population 2.761 [2.221; 3.433]). The risk of ICU mortality associated with colloids or 6% HES 130/0.4 decreased progressively after multiple logistic regression analysis using baseline and progress covariables (Additional file 1: Supplemental digital content 10 and 11). Independent risk factors were predicted mortality, female gender, vasopressor use, severe sepsis and CKD on admission, as well as cumulative fluid balance. Notably, for patients in the subcohort without severe sepsis on admission, the adjusted risk of ICU mortality was lower for patients treated with colloids in general (crude OR 2.367 [1.539; 3.643]; multivariable adjusted OR 0.923 [0.874; 0.974]) or 6% HES 130/0.4 (crude OR 2.179 [1.223; 3.882]; multivariable adjusted OR 0.905 [0.833; 0.983]) compared to crystalloids only.

**Table 1  Baseline characteristics of study patients and subcohorts**

| | All patients entered into database | | | | Only patients eligible for multivariable analysis | | | | p value |
|---|---|---|---|---|---|---|---|---|---|
| | All fluids | Crystalloids only | Crystalloids + colloids | Crystalloids + HES 130/0.4 | All Fluids | Crystalloids only | Crystalloids + colloids | Crystalloids + HES 130/0.4 | Crystalloids vs. colloids (all/eligible for multivariable analysis) |
| N (n [%]) | 4545 [100] | 2482 [54.6] | 2063 [45.4] | 1175 [25.9] | 3902 [100] | 1888 [48.4] | 2014 [51.6] | 1128 [28.9] | |
| Age (years) | 68 [55; 76] | 68 [55; 76] | 68 [56; 75] | 68 [55; 76] | 68 [55; 76] | 68 [55; 76] | 68 [56; 75] | 68 [55;76] | 0.784/0.641[b] |
| Gender, male (n [%]) | 2788 [61.3] | 1491 [60.1] | 1297 [62.9] | 761 [64.8] | 2392 [61.3] | 1123 [59.5] | 1269 [67.2] | 730 [64.7] | 0.058/0.026[c] |
| Admission type: surgical (n [%]) | 3223 [70.9] | 1714 [69.1] | 1509 [73.1] | 986 [83.9] | 2782 [71.3] | 1316 [69.7] | 1466 [72.8] | 955 [84.7] | 0.003/0.036[c] |
| Cardiac surgery (n [%]) | 686 [15.1] | 310 [12.5] | 376 [18.2] | 351 [29.9] | 659 [16.9] | 290 [15.4] | 369 [18.3] | 348 [30.9] | <0.001/0.015[c] |
| Severe sepsis on admission (n [%]) | 394 [8.7] | 184 [7.4] | 210 [10.2] | 71 [6.0] | 370 [9.5] | 163 [8.6] | 207 [10.3] | 71 [6.3] | 0.001/0.090[c] |
| History of CKD (n [%]) | 828 [18.2] | 449 [18.1] | 379 [18.4] | 161 [13.7] | 622 [15.9] | 312 [16.5] | 310 [16.4] | 144 [12.4] | 0.837/0.356[c] |
| APACHE II | 20 [14, 25] | 18 [13, 23] | 22 [17, 27] | 24 [19, 30] | 20 [14, 25] | 18 [13, 23] | 22 [17, 27] | 24 [19, 30] | <0.001/< 0.001[b] |
| SAPS II | 21 [9; 36] | 17 [7, 31] | 25 [11; 41] | 34 [18; 52] | 21 [9; 36] | 17 [8, 31] | 25 [11; 41] | 34 [18; 52] | <0.001/< 0.001[b] |
| Probability of mortality [%][a] | 39.0 | 33.3 | 44.7 | 50.7 | 39.1 | 33.1 | 44.7 | 51.0 | <0.001/< 0.001[b] |
| AKI (RIFLE "failure") (n [%]) | 560 [12.3] | 174 [7.0] | 386 [18.7] | 179 [15.2] | 549 [14.1] | 167 [8.8] | 382 [19] | 178 [15.8] | <0.001/< 0.001[c] |
| Renal replacement therapy in ICU (n [%]) | 361 [7.9] | 78 [3.1] | 283 [13.7] | 133 [11.3] | 358 [9.2] | 76 [4] | 282 [14] | 133 [11.8] | <0.001/< 0.001[c] |
| ICU mortality (n [%]) | 408 [9.3] | 129 [5.5] | 279 [13.8] | 119 [10.2] | 367 [9.4] | 92 [4.9] | 275 [13.7] | 118 [10.5] | <0.001/< 0.001[c] |
| Length of ICU stay (days) | 3 [1, 9] | 2 [1, 5] | 6 [3, 12] | 5 [2, 11] | 4 [2, 8] | 2 [1, 5] | 6 [3, 13] | 5 [3, 11] | <0.001/< 0.001[b] |
| 90-day mortality (n [%]) | 707 [20.1] | 284 [15.4] | 423 [25.2] | 191 [18.8] | 613 [22.4] | 198 [14.6] | 415 [30.1] | 187 [21.9] | <0.001/< 0.001[c] |

Data are given as absolute number and percentage or median [25th; 75th percentiles], as appropriate

AKI acute kidney injury, APACHE acute physiology and chronic health evaluation score, CKD chronic kidney disease, ICU intensive care unit, SAPS simplified acute physiology score

[a] Probability of mortality was calculated from APACHE II and SAPS II scores as given in methods

[b] Wilcoxon–Mann–Whitney test

[c] Chi-squared contingency table test

## Acute kidney injury

The overall incidence of AKI was 12.3% (560 of 4545). The crude incidence of AKI was higher in patients treated with colloids compared to crystalloids only (18.7% (386 of 2063) vs. 7.0% (174 of 2484), crude OR 3.056 [2.528; 3.694]). With multivariable logistic regression analysis, the risk associated with colloids or 6% HES 130/0.4 decreased after adjustment for baseline covariables. In the full model adjusted for baseline and progress covariables, colloids and 6% HES 130/0.4 were associated with a reduced risk of AKI (Table 3 and Additional file 1: Supplemental digital content 12). Independent risk factors were predicted mortality, severe sepsis and CKD on admission as well as SOFA score (AUC).

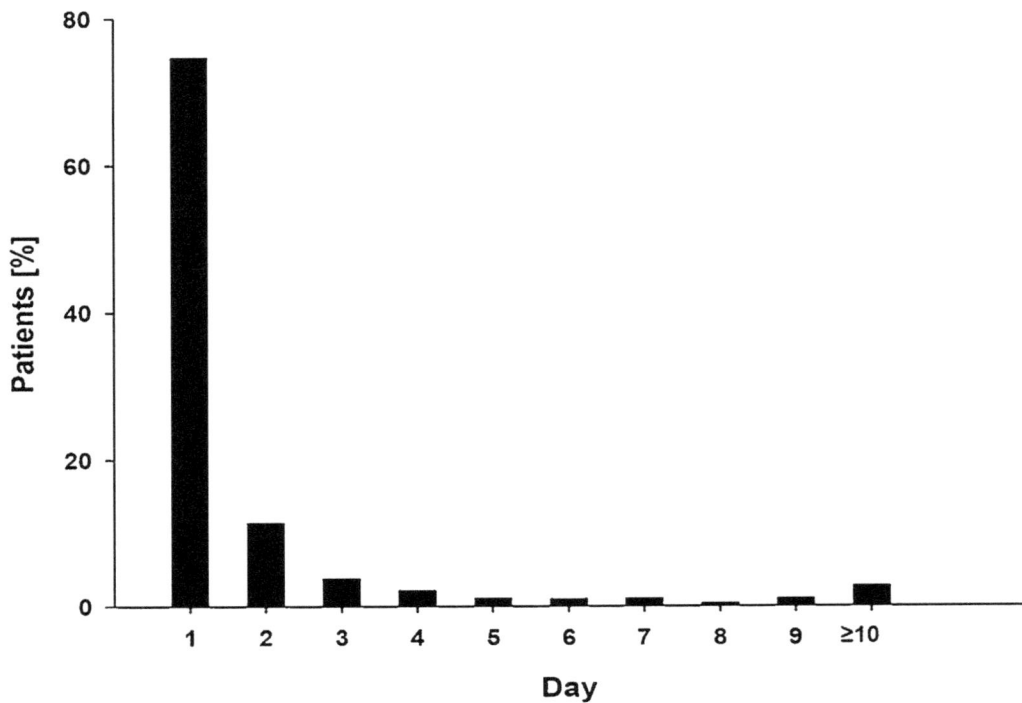

**Fig. 2** Day of first colloid infusion in study patients receiving colloids. This figure depicts the day of ICU stay on which the patients receiving colloids were infused the first dose of colloids

Further information about renal function and failure (incidences of AKI and RRT in patients with and without underlying CKD on admission; creatinine and diuresis) is given in Additional file 1: Supplemental digital content 13 and 14.

### Renal replacement therapy

During ICU stay, 7.9% (361) of the patients received RRT (see also Table 1). The crude incidence of RRT was considerably higher in patients treated with colloids compared to those without (13.7% (283 of 2063) vs. 3.1% (78 of 2484), crude OR for the overall population 4.904 [3.789; 6.348]). With multivariable logistic regression analysis, the risk associated with colloids or 6% HES 130/0.4 decreased after adjustment for baseline covariables. In the full model adjusted for baseline and progress covariables, colloids and 6% HES 130/0.4 were associated with a reduced risk of RRT (Additional file 1: Supplemental digital content 15). Independent risk factors for RRT included predicted risk of death, severe sepsis and CKD, AUC of the SOFA score and cumulative fluid balance. In contrast, vasopressor use was negatively associated with RRT.

### Discussion

In the present analysis of fluid therapy in roughly 4500 German ICU patients with predominantly post-operative admission, about half the patients were *exclusively* treated with crystalloids, whereas the remaining patients *also* received colloids (mainly 6% HES 130/0.4).

Whereas crude and unadjusted analyses suggested an association of colloids with adverse outcome, a stepwise adjustment for baseline and progress covariables indicates that the use of colloids per se did not affect the risk of mortality. Moreover, the association of colloids with AKI disappeared after multivariable adjustment. In subgroup analyses, the adjusted risk of AKI was lower in patients treated with colloids per se or HES 130/0.4. In the subcohort of patients admitted without severe sepsis, there was also a trend towards reduced ICU mortality with colloids per se or HES 130/0.4. The most important finding of the present study is that the effects of colloids turned from seemingly adverse in the raw data to neutral or potentially beneficial after multivariable analyses. This contradicts findings from randomised controlled trials (RCTs). One main reason for this may be the timing and dose of colloid use being different from the RCTs as detailed below.

RaFTinG is the largest database comparing crystalloids versus colloids in clinical routine for renal and overall

**Table 2** Effects of colloid infusion on 90-day mortality in Cox regression analysis

| Odds/hazard ratio estimates | Unadjusted/crude mortality (population eligible for multi-variable analysis)[a] | | | Adjustment for baseline variables | | | Full model, adjusted for evolution variables | | |
|---|---|---|---|---|---|---|---|---|---|
| Effect | OR | 95% CI | | HR | 95% CI | | HR | 95% CI | |
| Colloid infusion | 2.027 | 1.697 | 2.422 | 1.666 | 1.405 | 1.976 | 1.003 | 0.980 | 1.027 |
| Gender, male | | | | 1.141 | 0.974 | 1.337 | 0.798 | 0.679 | 0.936 |
| Predicted risk of death 90–99% | | | | 6.003 | 3.773 | 9.551 | 4.505 | 2.781 | 7.298 |
| Predicted risk of death 80–89% | | | | 3.266 | 2.046 | 5.212 | 2.630 | 1.637 | 4.226 |
| Predicted risk of death 70–79% | | | | 3.018 | 1.905 | 4.780 | 2.250 | 1.412 | 3.586 |
| Predicted risk of death 60–69% | | | | 2.893 | 1.870 | 4.474 | 2.184 | 1.403 | 3.401 |
| Predicted risk of death 50–59% | | | | 2.171 | 1.365 | 3.453 | 1.718 | 1.070 | 2.757 |
| Predicted risk of death 40–49% | | | | 2.073 | 1.353 | 3.176 | 1.732 | 1.128 | 2.660 |
| Predicted risk of death 30–39% | | | | 1.648 | 1.064 | 2.552 | 1.484 | 0.957 | 2.303 |
| Predicted risk of death 20–29% | | | | 1.777 | 1.154 | 2.736 | 1.611 | 1.045 | 2.482 |
| Predicted risk of death 10–19% | | | | 1.833 | 1.189 | 2.826 | 1.759 | 1.140 | 2.712 |
| Chronic kidney disease | | | | 2.149 | 1.812 | 2.549 | 1.960 | 1.645 | 2.336 |
| Severe sepsis on admission | | | | 2.017 | 1.648 | 2.469 | 1.284 | 1.025 | 1.608 |
| Vasopressor equivalent > 0.6 mg/h | | | | | | | 1.019 | 1.002 | 1.035 |
| SOFA score AUC | | | | | | | 1.030 | 1.024 | 1.036 |
| Cumulative red blood cell products (per litre) | | | | | | | 0.977 | 0.958 | 0.997 |
| Cumulative other blood products (per litre) | | | | | | | 1.002 | 0.968 | 1.037 |
| Cumulative fluid balance (per litre) | | | | | | | 1.014 | 1.008 | 1.020 |
| Daily crystalloid infusion (per litre) | | | | | | | 1.121 | 1.067 | 1.178 |

Risk of mortality was estimated from severity scores as detailed in the methods section. Gender, risk of mortality categories, vasopressor requirement, chronic kidney disease and severe sepsis on admission were used as binary variables (yes/no), whereas the hazard ratios (HRs) for fluid-based variables and Sequential Organ Failure Assessment (SOFA) score describe the excess risk per litre of fluid and per SOFA area under the curve (AUC), respectively

*CI* confidence interval

[a] To show the effect of the modelling, we showed the unadjusted odds ratio for the population that was eligible for the multivariable analysis. Crude OR for all patients in the registry is shown in the text

outcome. Demographic characteristics indicate its population to be representative for German and international ICUs [20, 21]. Incidence and mortality of severe sepsis were comparable to that observed in a German epidemiological trial [20] but lower than in the Sepsis Occurrence in Acutely Ill Patients (SOAP) study [22].

The present data demonstrated colloids to be reserved for more severely ill patients with risk factors for mortality or AKI beyond the type of i.v. fluids. It is not surprising that the crude incidences of AKI and mortality were higher in "colloid" patients, since the present study was no RCT. Therefore, the observational design of RaFTinG required adjustment for confounders with impact on patient outcome.

Our approach for adjustment included the baseline variables gender, severity of disease (based on risk of mortality derived from SAPS II and APACHE II scores), chronic kidney disease and severe sepsis on admission, which affect outcome in the ICU. However, these variables do not reflect the disease progression on the ICU. Patients with the same baseline risk may develop in opposed

directions, with some patients recovering without fluid resuscitation and others deteriorating and require crystalloids and/or colloids for haemodynamic support. Thus, we also included the following variables for adjustment in our final model: SOFA score to reflect the overall severity of organ failure over the course of the ICU stay, indicating a general deterioration of patient status, high-dose vasopressor infusion to reflect haemodynamic instability related to the vasculature as well as transfusions [23], which carry an independent risk of negative outcome. We consider the addition of these factors to the multivariate analysis as mandatory to approach the net effects of colloids on outcome. Nevertheless, it needs to be acknowledged, that the current approach also bears the risk of overadjustment, since some of the adjustment variables may also be affected by colloid infusion itself (e.g. transfusions). To make the data more transparent, we present crude data, baseline adjustment and full adjustment.

After multivariable adjustment for baseline covariables and progress variables, treatment with colloids in general practice did not appear to negatively affect survival.

**Table 3 Effects of colloid infusion in logistic regression analysis of RIFLE "failure"**

| Odds ratio estimates | Unadjusted/crude mortality (population eligible for multivariable analysis)[a] | | | Adjustment for baseline variables | | | Full model, adjusted for evolution variables | | |
|---|---|---|---|---|---|---|---|---|---|
| Effect | OR | 95% CI | | OR | 95% CI | | OR | 95% CI | |
| Colloid infusion | 2.412 | 1.987 | 2.929 | 1.941 | 1.573 | 2.397 | 0.696 | 0.629 | 0.770 |
| Gender, male | | | | 1.008 | 0.824 | 1.233 | 0.943 | 0.763 | 1.167 |
| Predicted risk of death 90–99% | | | | 20.787 | 11.773 | 36.700 | 12.490 | 6.724 | 23.201 |
| Predicted risk of death 80–89% | | | | 5.754 | 3.349 | 9.885 | 4.823 | 2.731 | 8.516 |
| Predicted risk of death 70–99% | | | | 3.934 | 2.326 | 6.653 | 3.061 | 1.769 | 5.297 |
| Predicted risk of death 60–69% | | | | 2.756 | 1.677 | 4.532 | 1.940 | 1.154 | 3.262 |
| Predicted risk of death 50–59% | | | | 2.461 | 1.470 | 4.121 | 1.921 | 1.129 | 3.268 |
| Predicted risk of death 40–49% | | | | 1.705 | 1.061 | 2.738 | 1.336 | 0.822 | 2.173 |
| Predicted risk of death 30–39% | | | | 1.331 | 0.819 | 2.163 | 1.100 | 0.672 | 1.800 |
| Predicted risk of death 20–29% | | | | 1.043 | 0.642 | 1.694 | 0.773 | 0.471 | 1.271 |
| Predicted risk of death 10–19% | | | | 1.237 | 0.763 | 2.005 | 1.041 | 0.639 | 1.696 |
| Chronic kidney disease | | | | 11.089 | 9.008 | 13.652 | 10.445 | 8.409 | 12.975 |
| Severe sepsis on admission | | | | 8.415 | 6.841 | 10.353 | 11.618 | 9.062 | 14.894 |
| Vasopressor equivalent > 0.6 mg/h | | | | | | | 0.957 | 0.891 | 1.029 |
| SOFA score AUC | | | | | | | 1.046 | 1.039 | 1.053 |
| Cumulative red blood cell products (per litre) | | | | | | | 0.976 | 0.923 | 1.032 |
| Cumulative other blood products (per litre) | | | | | | | 1.208 | 0.988 | 1.476 |
| Cumulative fluid balance (per litre) | | | | | | | 1.011 | 0.994 | 1.029 |
| Daily crystalloid infusion (per litre) | | | | | | | 0.843 | 0.792 | 0.896 |

Risk of mortality was estimated from severity scores as detailed in the methods section. Gender, risk of mortality categories, vasopressor requirement, chronic kidney disease and severe sepsis on admission were used as binary variables (yes/no), whereas the odds ratios (ORs) for fluid-based variables and Sequential Organ Failure Assessment (SOFA) score describe the excess risk per litre of fluid and per SOFA area under the curve (AUC), respectively

CI confidence interval

[a] To show the effect of the modelling, we showed the unadjusted OR for the population that was eligible for the multivariable analysis. Crude OR for all patients in the registry are shown in the text

Colloids being still associated with adverse outcomes after adjustment for baseline variables may be explained by evolution of patients' disease state after ICU admission with some patients improving and others deteriorating further. Since the latter patients are more likely to receive colloids, we also adjusted for variables of disease progress after ICU admission. Notably, the SOAP study used a very similar approach to adjustment in a very similar setting [24]. Surprisingly, our fully adjusted analysis suggests that, in low doses as used in the present cohort, colloids and specifically HES 130/0.4 are neutral in terms of 90-day mortality and might even be associated with reduced risks of AKI and ICU mortality in critically ill patients without severe sepsis. These adjusted results are in strong contrast to the unadjusted results and should therefore be judged with appropriate caution. Nevertheless, they are in agreement with the CRISTAL trial [25], which showed that in untreated shock from any reason initial treatment with crystalloids alone may limit survival. Furthermore, the present results indicate that trials

conducted in septic patients may not be extrapolated to non-septic patients [12, 26].

The advantage of the RaFTinG registry compared to previous RCTs [5, 7, 8, 25] is that colloids or crystalloids infusion was based exclusively on the clinical scenario, without being influenced by study protocols. The latter do often not reflect "real-life" fluid therapy, as has been demonstrated previously [5, 7, 8]. However, this also represents a major weakness, since the study cohorts are markedly different and the statistical analysis is sophisticated. Nevertheless, the present data give an estimate of the current use and dosing of fluid therapy and its changes throughout the ICU stay. This is important, as most positive and negative effects seen with colloids and fluids per se depend on timing and dosage [1, 9]. Therefore, RaFTinG not only adds relevant data but also helps to separate clinically relevant from artificial effects and allows the design of appropriate control groups for future RCTs. In this study, colloid use was completely different from that in VISEP [5], 6S [8] or CHEST [7]. Colloids were mainly given during the first day of ICU stay, with a consistent decline thereafter. When the interventional period of recent trials began, less than 60% of the RaFTinG population still received colloids. Furthermore, patients received median volumes of only 500 mL daily, which is considerably less than the amount that patients received on average per day in previous trials, e.g. 6S (1000–1500 mL) [8]. Neither physiology nor clinical practice randomises patients for several days into "colloid" and "crystalloid receivers". Rather, the decision to infuse the drug "fluid" should be the result of a careful and permanently re-evaluated individual assessment of the expected benefit versus the potential risk.

The current discussion about colloids, especially on the safety of HES, might have caused significant indication bias by some investigators. For example, severely ill patients may be prone to receive more colloids as their cardiac preload is thought to be more compromised. Additionally, in patients with renal impairment, some physicians might prefer gelatine, according to the results of mainly one clinical trial [27], or sole crystalloids instead of HES. Indeed, CKD at baseline was highest in patients who received gelatine in RaFTinG.

Most patients in our study were post-operative without severe sepsis on admission (Table 1). Many patients in the RCTs suggesting negative effects of HES solutions, by contrast, were admitted to the ICU due to severe sepsis [5, 7, 8]. For patients in the perioperative setting, there is no evidence for harm with the use of 6% HES 130/0.4 [28, 29] or HES solutions in general [30] from the recent literature.

The results of the present multivariable analysis are in accordance with the previous literature on 6% HES 130/0.4 in non-septic and perioperative patients, which does not suggest an adverse effect on kidney function or survival.

## Limitations of the present study

Our study has several limitations. Since it is observational, unblinded outcome assessment is unavoidable. Patients were not randomised and the cohorts are heterogeneous, with significant imbalances at baseline (e.g. severity scores, prevalence of sepsis) and many potential confounders on outcome. Even though we are confident that we were able to identify most of them and perform an appropriate adjustment, several approaches to adjusting the data are possible. It appears virtually impossible to account for the different severity of illness in the colloid cohort versus the crystalloid cohort without using adjustment parameters that are also influenced by disease progress. Thus, both risks of residual confounding and overadjustment exist. As a consequence, the adjusted results should be interpreted with caution. However, the small adjusted confidence intervals around or below 1

strongly suggest neutrality of the investigated colloids in terms of mortality and AKI. Unfortunately, although the analysis plan for the major endpoints (AKI, 90-day and ICU mortality) was designed a priori, no statistical analysis plan has been pre-published, which would have further strengthened the present results.

The present study did not investigate pre-admission fluid therapy or haemodynamics and can therefore not provide an estimate of the indication and effectiveness, which would have required a different study design [31]. Nevertheless, the timing of colloid infusion suggests colloids were used predominantly for initial or post-operative resuscitation (with pre-ICU fluid therapy, e.g. in the OR, being a blind spot).

Subcohorts having received other colloids than HES 130/0.4 were small compared to HES 130/0.4 or crystalloids. Any comparison between these subgroups must be done with caution, if at all.

Furthermore, the incidence of RRT may be a unreliable outcome measure, since most centres had no clear protocol for it. Any conclusion based on RRT should therefore be drawn with great caution.

It also needs to be acknowledged that an estimated mortality risk calculation by combining APACHE II and SAPS II (as available) may be less accurate than having a full set of both scores.

Finally, the follow-up might be considered incomplete. Besides that, missing information was not evenly distributed between both analysed groups with more incomplete baseline data with crystalloids only and more incomplete 90-day follow-up with colloids. The reason for this imbalance in missing data remains unknown, although we found that patients lost to follow-up were less severely ill on ICU admission. It is unclear how this finding may have led to a lower follow-up rate in the colloid cohort. Therefore, it is possible that unknown confounders influenced follow-up rates in the two cohorts. Nevertheless, a 90-day follow-up rate of 77.5% appears to be reasonably high when compared to 50–80% in other epidemiological cohort studies [32].

We also checked the effect of missing data on our full multivariable analysis with a best-/worst-case scenario. As expected, all risks were "diluted" by the assumption that all patients without follow-up had died. However, the risk associated with colloid use did not increase by this approach although colloid use was associated with greater loss to 90-day follow-up. Thus, the best-case/worst-case analysis suggests that missing follow-up data did not substantially affect the overall result.

## Conclusions

The present analysis of mostly post-operative patients in routine clinical care did not reveal an independent negative effect of colloids (mostly HES 130/0.4) on AKI or survival after multivariable adjustment. Contrasting results compared to published RCTs may be explained by differences in dose and duration of colloid infusion. Signals towards a reduced risk in non-septic, perioperative patients deserve further study.

### Abbreviations

AKI: acute kidney injury; AUC: area under the curve; HES: hydroxyethyl starch; ICU: intensive care unit; OR: odds ratio; RCT: randomised controlled trial; CKD: chronic kidney disease.

### Authors' contributions

CE and MJ were involved in study conception and design, data acquisition and drafting of the manuscript. They performed the statistical analysis. HVA and BZ conceived of the study, participated in its design and coordination and helped to draft the manuscript. MC, FS, AS and RD were responsible for data acquisition and revision of the manuscript. All authors read an approved the final manuscript and confirm that they meet the requirements for authorship. All authors believe that the paper represents honest work and are able to verify the validity of the results. All authors read and approved the final manuscript.

### Author details

[1] Department of Anaesthesiology, Intensive Care and Pain Medicine, University Hospital Münster, 48149 Münster, Germany. [2] Department of Anaesthesiology, University Hospital, LMU Munich, 80337 Munich, Germany. [3] Department of Emergency and Critical Care Medicine, Paracelsus Medical University, 90419 Nuremberg, Germany. [4] Department of Anaesthesiology and Intensive Care Medicine, Sana Kliniken Stuttgart, 70174 Stuttgart, Germany. [5] Department of Anaesthesiology and Intensive Care Medicine, University of Cologne, 50937 Cologne, Germany. [6] Department of Anaesthesiology, Krankenhaus Barmherzige Brueder, 54292 Trier, Germany. [7] Department of Intensive Care and Intermediate Care, RWTH University Hospital Aachen, 52074 Aachen, Germany. [8] Department of Anaesthesiology, Surgical Intensive Care and Pain Medicine, St. Elisabeth Hospital, St.-Elisabeth-Str. 23, 94315 Straubing, Germany.

### Acknowledgements

The authors are very grateful to the participating centres and the responsible investigators. Beyond that we have to thank PD Dr. Daniel Chappell (Department of Anaesthesiology, University Hospital Munich, Germany), Dr. Miriam Imo, Dr. Markus Lorek, Dr. Aike Schweda, Dr. Mario Pahl and Dr. Christoph Messer (DBM Wissen schafft, Muehlhausen, Germany) for their excellent work and advice. The authors also thank Thomas Zwingers (estimate, Augsburg, Germany) for expert statistical review and advice of the revised manuscript.

**Participating centres** (ordered according to number of included patients): Universitätsklinikum Münster; Uniklinik Köln; Klinik für Anaesthesiologie, Campus Innenstadt, Klinikum der Universität München; Klinik für Notfall- und Internistische Intensivmedizin, Klinikum Nürnberg; Krankenhaus der Barmherzigen Brüder Trier; Uniklinik RWTH Aachen; St. Barbara-Klinik Hamm-Heessen; Universitätsklinikum Knappschaftskrankenhaus Bochum; Kreiskrankenhaus Mechernich; Klinikum Großburgwedel; Bethanien Krankenhaus Moers; HELIOS Klinikum Meiningen; Klinikum Barnim, Werner Forßmann; Krankenhaus Eberswalde; Südharz Klinikum Nordhausen; Klinik für Anaesthesiologie, Campus Grosshadern, Klinikum der Universität München; St. Elisabeth- Krankenhaus Köln; Ubbo-Emmius-Klinik Aurich; Krankenhaus Barmherzige Brüder München; Städtisches Klinikum Solingen; Universitätsklinikum Carl Gustav Carus Dresden; Krankenhaus Düren; Krankenhaus Hetzelstift Neustadt/ Weinstrasse; Harzklinikum Dorothea Christiane Erxleben Quedlinburg; Ev. Krankenhaus Bielefeld; Kliniken Landkreis Heidenheim; Lahn-Dill-Kliniken Wetzlar; Elisabeth-Krankenhaus Essen; RoMed Klinikum Rosenheim; Dietrich Bonhoeffer Klinikum Neubrandenburg; Zeisigwaldkliniken Bethanien Chemnitz; Krankenhaus Martha-Maria Nürnberg; Ortenau-Klinikum Lahr-Ettenheim; Klinikum Ingolstadt; Diakoniekrankenhaus Henriettenstiftung Hannover; Berufsgenossenschaftliche Unfallklinik Tübingen; HELIOS Klinikum Wuppertal; Krankenhaus St. Franziskus Mönchengladbach; St. Vincentius-Kliniken Karlsruhe; Oskar-Ziethen-Krankenhaus Berlin-Lichtenberg; Bürgerhospital Frankfurt; Klinik für Anaesthesiologie, Campus Herzklinik der Universität am Augustinum, Klinikum der Universität München; Klinikum Minden; Klinikum Sankt Georg Leipzig; Katharinenhospital, Klinikum Stuttgart; Carl-von-Basedow-Klinikum Saalekreis Merseburg; Hufeland Klinikum Bad Langensalza; St. Franziskus-Hospital Münster; Chirurgische Klinik, Campus Innenstadt, Klinikum der Universität München; Ev. Krankenhaus Bethesda; Mönchengladbach; Kliniken Miltenberg-Erlenbach; Klinikum München Pasing; Marienhaus Klinikum Neuwied; Marienhospital Gelsenkirchen; St. Franziskus-Hospital Flensburg; St. Franziskus-Hospital Köln; St. Josef Hospital Bad Driburg; St. Nikolaus-Stiftshospital Andernach; Universitätsklinikum des Saarlandes Homburg; Diakonie Krankenhaus Bad Kreuznach; Klinikum Herford; Klinikum Idar-Oberstein; Lukaskrankenhaus Neuss; Park-Krankenhaus Leipzig; Vinzentius-Krankenhaus Landau; Westpfalz-Klinikum Kusel.

### Competing interests

CE: Non-financial support for the submitted work from DBM Wissen schafft GmbH. A grant from Fresenius Kabi for logistics related to the submitted work. Unrelated to the submitted work are speaker's honorary, research support and travel reimbursement from Fresenius Kabi. No other relationships or activities that could appear to have influenced the submitted work. BZ: Non-financial support for the submitted work from DBM Wissen schafft GmbH. No other relationships or activities that could appear to have influenced the submitted work. HVA: Non-financial support for the submitted work from DBM Wissen schafft GmbH. No other relationships or activities that could appear to have influenced the submitted work. MC: Non-financial support for the submitted work from DBM Wissen schafft GmbH. No other relationships or activities that could appear to have influenced the submitted work. FS: Non-financial support for the submitted work from DBM Wissen schafft GmbH. No other relationships or activities that could appear to have influenced the submitted work. AS: Non-financial support for the submitted work from DBM Wissen schafft GmbH. No other relationships or activities that could appear to have influenced the submitted work. RD: Non-financial support for the submitted work from DBM Wissen schafft GmbH. No other relationships or activities that could appear to have influenced the submitted work. MJ: Non-financial support for the submitted work from DBM Wissen schafft GmbH. A grant from Fresenius Kabi for logistics related to the submitted work. Unrelated to the submitted work are unrestricted research grants from Serumwerk Bernburg, GRIFOLS Inc., CSL Behring and speaker's honorary and travel reimbursement from Fresenius Kabi, B. Braun, Serumwerk Bernburg, GRIFOLS Inc. and Baxter. Member of the GRIFOLS Inc. Albumin Advisory Board. No other relationships or activities that could appear to have influenced the submitted work.

### Funding

Fresenius Kabi supported data collection with an unrestricted grant. The sponsor did not influence the study design and the data collection, analysis, interpretation and writing of the manuscript and the decision to submit it for publication. The researchers are independent from the sponsor and all authors had full access to all of the data (including statistical reports and tables) in the study and can take responsibility for the integrity of the data and the accuracy of the data analysis.

## References

1. Rivers E, Nguyen B, Havstad S, Ressler J, Muzzin A, Knoblich B, et al. Early goal-directed therapy in the treatment of severe sepsis and septic shock. N Engl J Med. 2001;345(19):1368–77.

2. The ProCESS Investigators. A randomized trial of protocol-based care for early septic shock. N Engl J Med. 2014;370(18):1683–93. https://doi.org/10.1056/NEJMoa1401602.

3. Reinhart K, Perner A, Sprung CL, Jaeschke R, Schortgen F, Johan Groeneveld AB, et al. Consensus statement of the ESICM task force on colloid volume therapy in critically ill patients. Intensive Care Med. 2012;38(3):368–83. https://doi.org/10.1007/s00134-012-2472-9.

4. Zacharowski K, Aken H, Marx G, Jacob M, Schaffartzik W, Zenz M, et al. Comments on Reinhart et al.: Consensus statement of the ESICM task force on colloid volume therapy in critically ill patients. Intensive Care Med. 2012;38(9):1556–7. https://doi.org/10.1007/s00134-012-2639-4.

5. Brunkhorst FM, Engel C, Bloos F, Meier-Hellmann A, Ragaller M, Weiler N, et al. Intensive insulin therapy and pentastarch resuscitation in severe sepsis. N Engl J Med. 2008;358(2):125–39. https://doi.org/10.1056/NEJMoa070716.

6. Guidet B, Martinet O, Boulain T, Philippart F, Poussel JF, Maizel J, et al. Assessment of hemodynamic efficacy and safety of 6% hydroxyethyl-starch 130/0.4 vs. 0.9% NaCl fluid replacement in patients with severe sepsis: The CRYSTMAS study. Crit Care. 2012;16(R94):1–10.

7. Myburgh JA, Finfer S, Bellomo R, Billot L, Cass A, Gattas D, et al. Hydroxyethyl starch or saline for fluid resuscitation in intensive care. N Engl J Med. 2012;367(20):1901–11. https://doi.org/10.1056/NEJMoa1209759.

8. Perner A, Haase N, Guttormsen AB, Tenhunen J, Klemenzson G, Aneman A, et al. Hydroxyethyl starch 130/0.42 versus Ringer's acetate in severe sepsis. N Engl J Med. 2012;367(2):124–34. https://doi.org/10.1056/nejmoa1204242.

9. Shum HP, Lee FMH, Chan KC, Yan WW. Interaction between fluid balance and disease severity on patient outcome in the critically ill. J Crit Care. 2011;26(6):613–9. https://doi.org/10.1016/j.jcrc.2011.02.008.

10. Dellinger RP, Levy MM, Rhodes A, Annane D, Gerlach H, Opal SM, et al. Surviving sepsis campaign. Crit Care Med. 2013;41(2):580–637. https://doi.org/10.1097/ccm.0b013e31827e83af.

11. Chappell D, Jacob M. Twisting and ignoring facts on hydroxyethyl starch is not very helpful. Scand J Trauma Resusc Emerg Med. 2013;21(85):1–3. https://doi.org/10.1186/1757-7241-21-85.

12. Hartog CS, Natanson C, Sun J, Klein HG, Reinhart K. Concerns over use of hydroxyethyl starch solutions. BMJ. 2014;349:g5981. https://doi.org/10.1136/bmj.g5981.

13. Bellomo R, Ronco C, Kellum JA, Mehta RL, Palevsky P. Acute renal failure—definition, outcome measures, animal models, fluid therapy and information technology needs: the Second International Consensus Conference of the Acute Dialysis Quality Initiative (ADQI) Group. Crit Care. 2004;8(4):R204–12. https://doi.org/10.1186/cc2872.

14. Knaus WA, Draper EA, Wagner DP, Zimmerman JE. APACHE II: a severity of disease classification system. Crit Care Med. 1985;13(10):818–29.

15. Le Gall JR, Lemeshow S, Saulnier F. A new Simplified Acute Physiology Score (SAPS II) based on a European/North American multicenter study. JAMA. 1993;270(24):2957–63.

16. National Kidney Foundation. K/DOQI Clinical practice guidelines for chronic kidney disease: evaluation, classification and stratification. Am J Kidney Dis. 2002;39:S1–266.

17. Muckart DJ, Bhagwanjee S. American College of Chest Physicians/Society of Critical Care Medicine Consensus Conference definitions for sepsis and organ failure and guidelines for the use of innovative therapies in sepsis. Crit Care. 1992;20(6):864–74.

18. Brown SM, Lanspa MJ, Jones JP, Kuttler KG, Li Y, Carlson R, et al. Survival after shock requiring high-dose vasopressor therapy. Chest. 2013;143(3):664–71. https://doi.org/10.1378/chest.12-1106.

19. Asai T. Confidence in statistical analysis. Br J Anaesth. 2002;89(6):807–10.

20. Engel C, Brunkhorst FM, Bone H-G, Brunkhorst R, Gerlach H, Grond S, et al. Epidemiology of sepsis in Germany: results from a national prospective multicenter study. Intensive Care Med. 2007;33(4):606–18. https://doi.org/10.1007/s00134-006-0517-7.

21. Vincent J-L, Rello J, Marshall J, Silva E, Anzueto A, Martin CD, et al. International study of the prevalence and outcomes of infection in intensive care units. JAMA. 2009;302(21):2323–9. https://doi.org/10.1001/jama.2009.1754.

22. Vincent J-L, Sakr Y, Sprung CL, Ranieri VM, Reinhart K, Gerlach H, et al. Sepsis in European intensive care units: results of the SOAP study. Crit Care Med. 2006;34(2):344–53.

23. Retter A, Wyncoll D, Pearse R, Carson D, McKechnie S, Stanworth S, et al. Guidelines on the management of anaemia and red cell transfusion in adult critically ill patients. Br J Haematol. 2013;160(4):445–64. https://doi.org/10.1111/bjh.12143.

24. Sakr Y, Payen D, Reinhart K, Sipmann FS, Zavala E, Bewley J, et al. Effects of hydroxyethyl starch administration on renal function in critically ill patients. Br J Anaesth. 2007;98(2):216–24. https://doi.org/10.1093/bja/ael333.

25. Annane D, Siami S, Jaber S, Martin C, Elatrous S, Declère AD, et al. Effects of fluid resuscitation with colloids vs crystalloids on mortality in critically ill patients presenting with hypovolemic shock. The CRISTAL randomized trial. J Am Med Assoc. 2013;310:1809–17. https://doi.org/10.1001/jama.2013.280502.

26. Coriat P, Guidet B, de Hert S, Kochs E, Kozek S, van Aken H. Counter statement to open letter to the Executive Director of the European Medicines Agency concerning the licensing of hydroxyethyl starch solutions for fluid resuscitation. Br J Anaesth. 2014;113(1):194–5. https://doi.org/10.1093/bja/aeu217.

27. Schortgen F, Lacherade JC, Bruneel F, Cattaneo I, Hemery F, Lemaire F, Brochard L. Effects of hydroxyethylstarch and gelatin on renal function in severe sepsis: a multicentre randomised study. Lancet. 2001;357(9260):911–6. https://doi.org/10.1016/S0140-6736(00)04211-2.

28. Martin C, Jacob M, Vicaut E, Guidet B, Van Aken H, Kurz A. Effect of waxy maize-derived hydroxyethyl starch 130/0.4 on renal function in surgical patients. Anesthesiology. 2013;118(2):387–94. https://doi.org/10.1097/aln.0b013e31827e5569.

29. Qureshi SH, Rizvi SI, Patel NN, Murphy GJ. Meta-analysis of colloids versus crystalloids in critically ill, trauma and surgical patients. Br J Surg. 2016;103(1):14–26. https://doi.org/10.1002/bjs.9943.

30. Raiman M, Mitchell CG, Biccard BM, Rodseth RN. Comparison of hydroxyethyl starch colloids with crystalloids for surgical patients: a systematic review and meta-analysis. Eur J Anaesthesiol. 2016;33(1):42–8.

31. Cecconi M, Hofer C, Teboul J-L, Pettila V, Wilkman E, Molnar Z, et al. Fluid challenges in intensive care: the FENICE study: a global inception cohort study. Intensive Care Med. 2015;41(9):1529–37. https://doi.org/10.1007/s00134-015-3850-x.

32. Fewtrell MS, Kennedy K, Singhal A, Martin RM, Ness A, Hadders-Algra M, et al. How much loss to follow-up is acceptable in long-term randomised trials and prospective studies? Arch Dis Child. 2008;93(6):458–61.

# 16

# Blood platelets and sepsis pathophysiology: A new therapeutic prospect in critical ill patients?

Antoine Dewitte[1,2*], Sébastien Lepreux[1,3], Julien Villeneuve[4], Claire Rigothier[1,5], Christian Combe[1,5], Alexandre Ouattara[2,6] and Jean Ripoche[1]

### Abstract

Beyond haemostasis, platelets have emerged as versatile effectors of the immune response. The contribution of platelets in inflammation, tissue integrity and defence against infections has considerably widened the spectrum of their role in health and disease. Here, we propose a narrative review that first describes these new platelet attributes. We then examine their relevance to microcirculatory alterations in multi-organ dysfunction, a major sepsis complication. Rapid progresses that are made on the knowledge of novel platelet functions should improve the understanding of thrombocytopenia, a common condition and a predictor of adverse outcome in sepsis, and may provide potential avenues for management and therapy.

**Keywords:** Platelets, Sepsis, Inflammation, Intensive care

## Background

Sepsis is a syndrome based on a dysregulated immune response to infection also involving non-immunologic mechanisms, including neuroendocrine, cardiovascular and metabolic pathways [1–3]. Due to its prevalence and high mortality rate, sepsis is a major public health issue [4, 5]. The contribution of blood platelets to sepsis pathophysiology has been the subject of renewed attention. First, alterations of platelet count are commonly encountered in the intensive care unit (ICU). Using common platelet counts thresholds, thrombocytopenia accounts for 20–50% of patients for the whole part of intensive care settings [6–9]. Thrombocytopenia or the non-resolution of thrombocytopenia is associated with poor outcome [8, 10–15]. Second, platelets are well-known players in coagulation and likely to contribute to disseminated intravascular coagulation (DIC). Third, beyond the confines of haemostasis and thrombosis, platelets are now acknowledged as essential actors of the immune response, reacting to infection and disturbed tissue integrity and contributing to inflammation, pathogen killing and tissue repair [16–21]. These advances in platelet biology have opened perspectives on the knowledge of sepsis pathophysiology and on its management. The matter is a complex one as platelets are not only vectors of inflammation contributing to vascular and tissue injury in acute or chronic inflammation [18, 22, 23], but also play an important role in the resolution of inflammation, vascular protection and the repair of damaged tissues. The friend and foe dialogue between platelets and endothelium has been extensively studied and is thought to be relevant to sepsis complications. Here we examine this enlarged spectrum of platelet functions and their relevance to the pathophysiology of multi-organ dysfunction (MOD) and discuss some potential links between these advances and sepsis management.

## Sepsis as a dysregulated host response to infection

Recent definition of sepsis [24] emphasizes the non-homoeostatic host response to infection that drives life-threatening organ dysfunctions. Activation of innate immune responses in sepsis realizes a systemic inflammatory condition. The inflammatory phase is

*Correspondence: antoine.dewitte@chu-bordeaux.fr
[2] Department of Anaesthesia and Critical Care II, Magellan Medico-Surgical Center, CHU Bordeaux, 33000 Bordeaux, France
Full list of author information is available at the end of the article

characterized by the production of pro-inflammatory mediators and immune cell activation [25–29], and sepsis prognosis is linked to the magnitude and duration of this inflammatory response, high circulating cytokine levels being, for example, associated with poor outcome [30–32]. The triggering of innate immune responses by pathogens and pathogen-associated molecular patterns (PAMPs) has been identified as an early and primary mechanism [2, 31, 33–36]. Interestingly, mechanisms of non-septic systemic-associated inflammatory response syndrome (SIRS) as met in major surgery, severe trauma, extensive burns or pancreatitis may share common features with sepsis-associated SIRS, taking the form of a comparable early inflammatory storm that is triggered by alarmins released by damaged tissues [37]. However, the role played by this hyper-inflammatory phase in the progression of sepsis and its prognostic is to be understood in the context of an accompanying anti-inflammatory response and immunosuppression state, and much effort is made in elaborating a coherent vision of these opposite and complex events [38–43].

## Platelets: multifunctional tiny cytoplasmic fragments

Platelets are small (2–4 μm), anucleate, discoid-shaped cytoplasmic fragments released in the bloodstream during the fragmentation of polyploid megakaryocytes in bone marrow sinusoidal blood vessels [44]. In humans, a regulated steady platelet supply and clearance maintains numbers of 150,000–400,000 platelets per microlitre of blood. Platelet production is critically dependent on thrombopoietin (TPO) that acts for an important part on megakaryocyte progenitor proliferation/differentiation and on megakaryocyte maturation [45]. Platelets have a short lifespan, of up to 10 days. They are cleared out from the circulation by mechanisms involving lectin–carbohydrate recognition by splenic and liver macrophages and hepatocytes [46, 47].

Platelets harbour a large variety of mediators stored in a pool of morphologically distinct granules [48]. Granule cargo loading is carried out in megakaryocytes. Platelets also transport mediators, such as serotonin, that they uptake from plasma and can deliver at sites of activation. The cataloguing of platelet-derived mediators reflects the remarkable versatility of platelets in haemostasis, thrombosis and immune responses [49, 50].

The secretion of granule content following platelet activation by agonists is central to platelet functions. Platelet activation induces the expression of membrane proteins and the release of mediators via several mechanisms. Many of these mediators are preformed and stored in granules such as cytokines/chemokines and coagulation factors, others can be synthesized by translational

pathways, such as IL-1β, and others are released by yet incompletely defined mechanisms such as CD154. Activated platelets also release vesicles, which include platelet microparticles (PMPs) and exosomes [51]. Platelets represent a major source of circulating MPs [52].

In pathological conditions associated with platelet activation, multiple agonists are generated. In fact, apart from classical strong agonists such as thrombin or collagen, there is an expanding list of agonists that can contribute to platelet activation. These additional platelet agonists have allowed a re-appreciation of mechanisms and role of platelet activation in vascular inflammation and thrombotic events associated with a range of infectious and inflammatory conditions [53].

The archetypal function of platelets is haemostasis. Platelets encounter inhibitory signals that prevent their activation in the healthy vasculature, such as nitric oxide and prostacyclin, which are released by endothelial cells (ECs). Platelets circulate in close proximity to the vessel wall, and the disruption of EC lining overcomes inhibitory signals and drives platelet adherence, activation and aggregation, which temporarily plug the damaged vessel. In this process, platelets also activate and confine coagulation at site of damage, particularly via the exposure of an efficient catalytic phospholipidic surface [54].

Besides binding to damaged vessels and preventing bleeding, platelets support a large spectrum of more recently studied functions, as could be reflected by the diversity of platelet mediators [55–57]. Platelets are activated in conditions that disrupt tissue homoeostasis and exert, directly and indirectly, a complex control over the different stages of inflammation, contributing to pathogen clearance, wound repair and tissue regeneration (Figs. 1, 2). As such, platelets are now acknowledged as essential components of the innate immune response, monitoring and rapidly responding to noxious signals.

## Platelets as key players in the inflammatory reaction; critical links with coagulation

Activated platelets secrete a profusion of pro-inflammatory material, cytokines/chemokines, vasoactive amines, eicosanoids, and components of proteolytic cascades that directly or indirectly, through the activation of bystander target cells, fuel inflammation [23, 58, 59]. ECs and leucocytes are prime targets for platelets. Endothelium is a non-adhesive, non-thrombogenic surface in normal conditions; when stimulated by inflammatory mediators, ECs undergo profound changes, collectively designed as "EC activation", which include the expression of cell adhesion molecules and tissue factor, production of von Willebrand factor, cytokines/chemokines, proteases and vasoactive substances such as nitric oxide. Platelets adhere to activated ECs, following a multi-step process in which

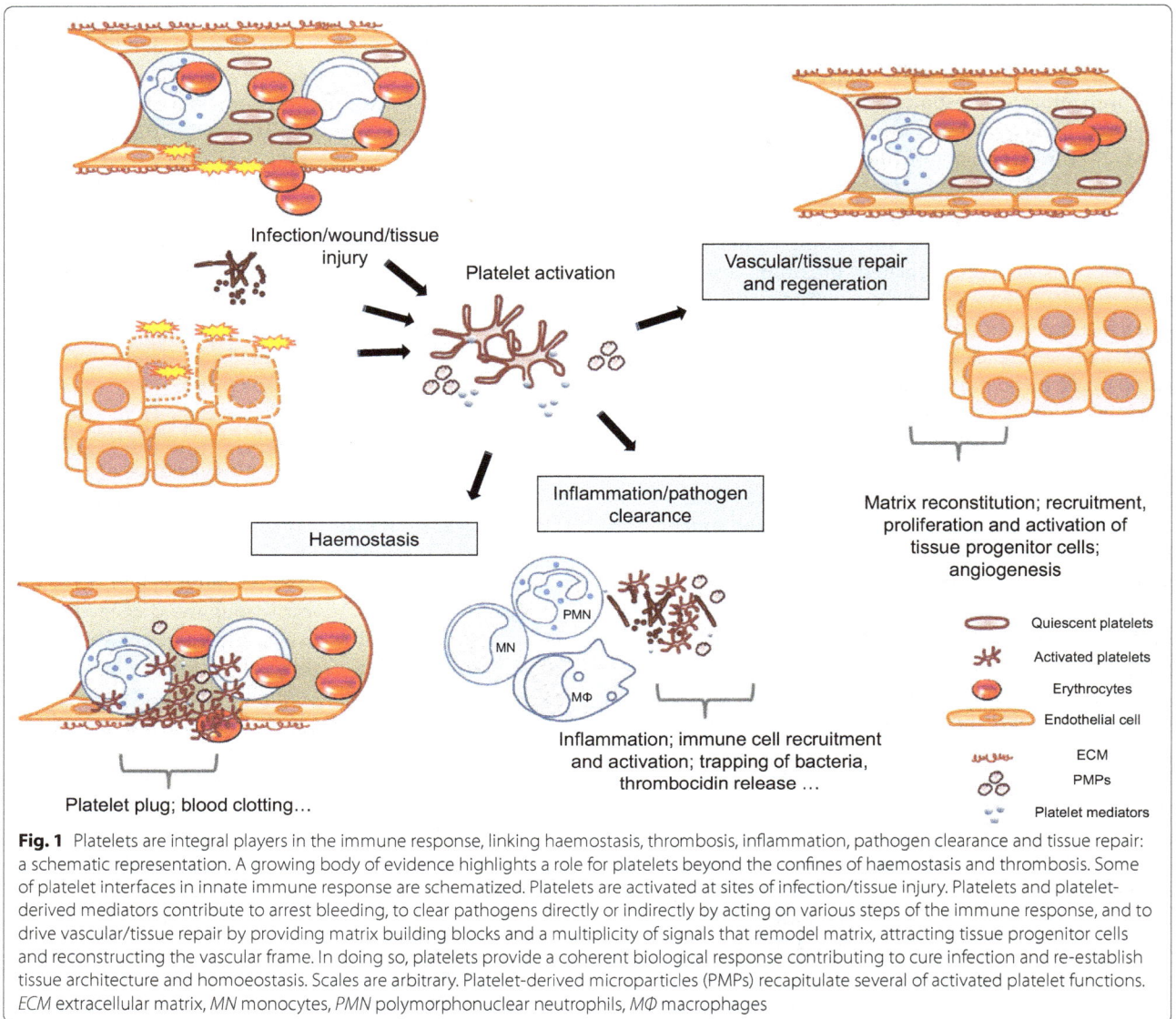

**Fig. 1** Platelets are integral players in the immune response, linking haemostasis, thrombosis, inflammation, pathogen clearance and tissue repair: a schematic representation. A growing body of evidence highlights a role for platelets beyond the confines of haemostasis and thrombosis. Some of platelet interfaces in innate immune response are schematized. Platelets are activated at sites of infection/tissue injury. Platelets and platelet-derived mediators contribute to arrest bleeding, to clear pathogens directly or indirectly by acting on various steps of the immune response, and to drive vascular/tissue repair by providing matrix building blocks and a multiplicity of signals that remodel matrix, attracting tissue progenitor cells and reconstructing the vascular frame. In doing so, platelets provide a coherent biological response contributing to cure infection and re-establish tissue architecture and homoeostasis. Scales are arbitrary. Platelet-derived microparticles (PMPs) recapitulate several of activated platelet functions. *ECM* extracellular matrix, *MN* monocytes, *PMN* polymorphonuclear neutrophils, *MΦ* macrophages

glycans play a critical role [60–62]. Inflammation can also alter the protective EC glycocalyx barrier, favouring platelet adhesion [63, 64]. During the adhesion process, platelets can be activated and in turn activate ECs. Platelet activation in inflammation can alter the vascular tone and lead to deleterious effects on vasculature integrity, by increasing vascular barrier permeability and contributing to the generation of cytopathic signals, for example by mediating reactive oxygen species generation by neutrophils [65]; these effects have to be paralleled with the opposed protective role of platelets (below) [66–69]. Leucocytes are a second critical target for platelets, the platelet/leucocyte dialogue being essential in inflammation; here, we focus on neutrophils and monocytes. Platelet/

leucocyte interactions are a critical step in leucocyte recruitment, activation and migration in inflammation [70]. Platelet/neutrophil or platelet/monocyte interactions can occur at the EC surface, in clot/thrombi and in circulating blood [18, 70, 71], and platelets direct neutrophil/monocyte migration to sites of tissue injury [72, 73]. Moreover, platelets activate neutrophils and monocytes upon interaction, via several mechanisms, including the triggering of TREM-1 on neutrophils, leading to various pro-inflammatory responses [65, 74–77]. The formation of platelet/leucocyte aggregates in blood depends on platelet activation and is an early phenomenon in sepsis progression. For example, platelet/neutrophils complexes are elevated at early phases, while being reduced in

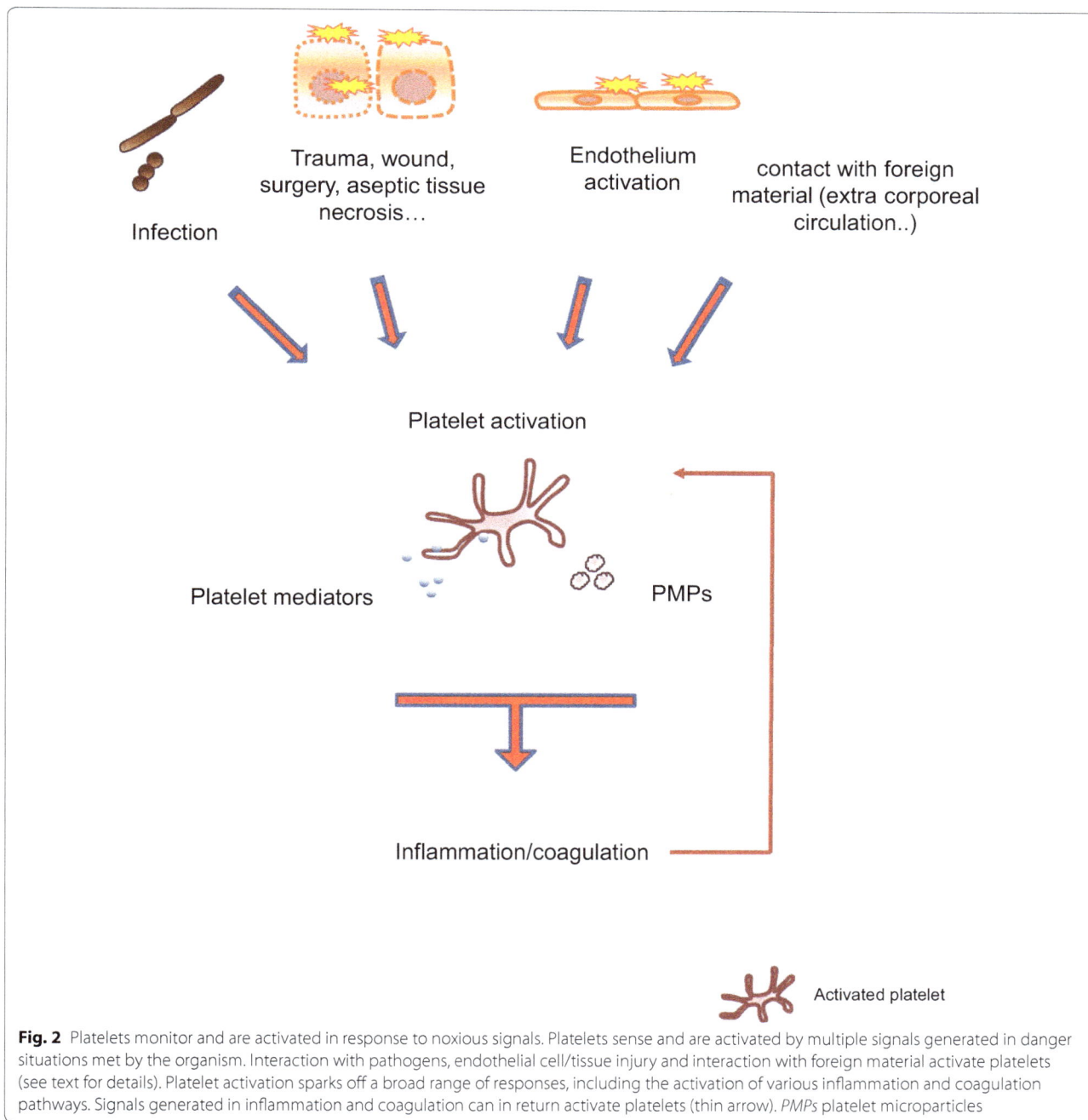

**Fig. 2** Platelets monitor and are activated in response to noxious signals. Platelets sense and are activated by multiple signals generated in danger situations met by the organism. Interaction with pathogens, endothelial cell/tissue injury and interaction with foreign material activate platelets (see text for details). Platelet activation sparks off a broad range of responses, including the activation of various inflammation and coagulation pathways. Signals generated in inflammation and coagulation can in return activate platelets (thin arrow). *PMPs* platelet microparticles

complicated sepsis possibly reflecting peripheral sequestration or sepsis-associated thrombocytopenia [78, 79], and endotoxin administration in humans leads to an increased circulating platelet/neutrophil aggregates that follows a brief decrease [80]. Amplification of inflammation results from the reciprocal activation between platelets and their target cells [66], and circulating monocyte/and neutrophil/platelet aggregates may contribute

to disseminate inflammatory signals [81]. Platelets also link several inflammatory cascades; for example, they propagate the activation of the complement system [82]. Commonly, cytokines have an induced expression that is regulated at the transcriptional/translational level. Most of platelet-derived inflammatory mediators are very rapidly released from activated platelets, making platelets instant providers of pro-inflammatory material. Cytokine bioactivity at organs remote from their source is debated as cytokine bioactivity may be hampered in plasma. Platelet transport may protect inflammatory mediators from otherwise degradation. Therefore, platelets play a central role in the inflammatory reaction. Importantly, they also contribute to the control and resolution of inflammation via several mechanisms, including the release of anti-inflammatory cytokines and inflammation pro-resolving mediators [83].

The activation of coagulation and inflammation cascades are consequences of platelet activation, and inflammation and coagulation pathways crosstalk [84]. For example, some platelet mediators have both inflammatory and pro-coagulant properties, such as polyphosphates [85]. Pro-inflammatory cytokines released by platelets can also activate the coagulation cascade at various steps [86]. Conversely, the activation of coagulation by platelets generates a number of inflammatory effectors, such as thrombin. Further, inflammatory mediators can impair anticoagulant and fibrinolysis pathway mechanisms, which may contribute to coagulation dysregulation in sepsis [87–89]. Platelet inflammatory mediators may thus contribute to sepsis coagulopathy [88–91]. DIC is a frequent and major complication of sepsis [41], and various mechanisms concur to involve platelets in DIC; only some can be mentioned. First, platelets support the generation of thrombin. Second, platelet links inflammation and coagulation. Third, platelets are major inducers of the release of pro-thrombotic scaffolds neutrophil extracellular traps (NETs) [92–96].

Notwithstanding, the involvement of PMPs in vascular inflammation and inflammatory disorders, including sepsis, has been emphasized [97–102]. PMPs retain many pro-inflammatory and pro-coagulant features of parent platelets and are thought to disseminate inflammatory and coagulation signals. Although they represent potential pathophysiological players in inflammatory disorders [52, 99, 100, 103, 104], their role in sepsis remains ill-understood.

### Platelets in vascular and tissue integrity

In normal wound healing, platelets establish regulatory crosstalks between soluble and cellular actors of tissue repair that concur to the various phases of inflammation and reestablishment of tissue homoeostasis [50, 83, 104, 105]. Platelets accumulate early, are activated at sites of tissue injury and intervene at each stage of tissue repair, the inflammatory, new tissue formation and remodelling stages. In fact, platelet-healing properties are already translated to the clinics [50, 55]. The best studied role of platelets in tissue homoeostasis is the preservation of resting and injured endothelium integrity, a critical point in MOD pathophysiology [71, 106–108]. The importance of

platelets is exemplified by the disruption of the endothelium barrier associated with thrombocytopenia [109]. How platelets contribute is incompletely understood. Mechanisms include gap filling, production of EC mitogenic factors and factors enhancing the vascular barrier [71, 107]. On injured endothelium, platelets adhere to the vascular wall at sites of damage and immediate proximity, a first step in a sequence of events that lead to the initiation and the propagation of haemostasis, thrombosis and bleeding arrest [110, 111]. Platelets provide material for endothelium repair, including EC growth-promoting, antiapoptotic mediators, and attractants for progenitor cells endowed with vascular healing properties [104]. They help restoring the disrupted vascular network, providing positive and negative regulators of angiogenesis and stimulating angiogenic mediator production by target cells. Platelets are also important contributors to extracellular matrix (ECM) repair as they are a rich source of ECM components, ECM remodelling proteins, and fibrocompetent cell activators. Platelets have however been found to both promote and prevent vascular permeability in inflammation. The differential regulation of vascular permeability by platelets has been studied for a large part in acute lung injury (ALI) models and will be presented in the corresponding section. Importantly, platelets are highly efficient at preventing bleeding in an inflammatory context [76, 107, 112]. The platelet count threshold needed for vasculoprotection in humans in normal or inflammatory conditions is an important question that remains to be answered [107]. More generally, platelets may play a broader role in organ regeneration. Platelets not only prevent blood loss but also provide key signals for matrix architecture reconstruction and for the recruitment, proliferation, survival and differentiation of cells endowed with new tissue formation, such as fibroblasts, smooth muscle cells and tissue-specific progenitors cells [113]. This is remarkably illustrated by the requirement of platelets in liver regeneration [114]. PMPs are also thought to contribute to vascular repair [115]. Hence, platelet activation is both necessary to tissue integrity and undesirable as it generates tissue-damaging signals. The complex network of signals that organize this fine-tuned equilibrium is only recently being biochemically dissected [55, 104]. Many questions remain on this balanced platelet friend or foe contribution, although they are of key importance to the pathophysiology of microvascular dysfunctions, such as in sepsis [68].

### Platelets contribute to the innate immune response against infection

The role of platelets in the defence against infection is increasingly stressed [83, 116]. Platelets are now acknowledged as *bona fide* pathogen sensors interacting directly or indirectly with a number of bacterial, viral, fungal and protozoan pathogens and their products, contributing to their clearance. Platelet interaction with bacteria depends on the nature and concentration of bacteria, interaction time, and involves multiple mechanisms. Toll like receptors-dependent and independent mechanisms, such as those involving Fcγ receptors, complement receptors or glycoproteins GPIIb-IIIa and GPIbα, contribute to platelet–bacteria interactions. Indirect interactions are also involved, such as via the binding of plasma proteins, including fibrinogen, von Willebrand factor, complement proteins or IgG, that bridge pathogens and platelets or via interaction with bacterial toxins. Interaction with pathogens can lead to platelet adhesion or to their activation, aggregation and release of platelet mediators [83, 117–120]. Mechanisms of pathogen clearance by platelets may be direct, through the release of various antimicrobial peptides and indirect via the release of platelet-derived mediators that coordinate chemotaxis and activation of immune cells [83, 116–118, 120, 121]. Infection is commonly associated with tissue injury. Injured and dying cells generate mediators such as alarmins that fuel inflammation [122]. Mediators generated by cell damage such as complement activation products and histones can activate platelets [123, 124]. Notwithstanding, platelets also contribute to the adaptive immune response to infection [17, 18, 22, 125].

The aforementioned role of platelets in the defence against pathogens suggests that they can interfere with the progression of infection. How can these observations be translated to sepsis pathophysiology [120, 124, 126]? Models suggest a protective role of platelets, as, for example, in streptococcal endocarditis, malaria or gram-negative pneumonia [127–129], and thrombocytopenia could be a risk factor for bacterial or fungal infection. Alternatively, platelets could contribute to spreading infection, via the transport of pathogens [130].

## Platelets in MOD pathophysiology
### Endothelium in MOD: a common pathophysiological denominator

The pathophysiology of sepsis and its complications remains uncertain as much caution has to be applied in extrapolating to clinical sepsis results obtained in rodent models which have their own inherent complexities [131–134]. Within these extrapolation limits, experimental models have, however, yielded significant knowledge. Numerous studies have emphasized the orchestrating role of endothelium in sepsis, and endothelium injury could be one of the *primum movens* pathophysiological events in sepsis complications [102, 135–148]. Markers of endothelium injury are elevated in sepsis patients, although variably associated with sepsis severity [29,

32, 149]. Inflammation, thrombosis, capillary perfusion alterations are among key features of MOD microvascular alterations [102, 136, 150, 151]. Platelet activation can be detected in sepsis patients and sepsis models, and studies reported association with sepsis severity [79, 124, 152, 153]. Many signals can activate ECs and platelets in sepsis, including pathogens and mediators generated by inflammation and coagulation. Activated platelets may thus contribute to MOD via their role in inflammation and coagulation (Fig. 3) [23, 56, 83, 124, 141, 144, 152, 154].

### Platelets in acute lung injury (ALI) in sepsis

There are arguments to involve platelets in ALI pathophysiology [155–158]. Dysregulated inflammation and coagulation are central pathophysiological events in ALI and lung vascular endothelium injury is a primary cause of the alteration of the alveolar-capillary barrier leading to pulmonary oedema [159] [160]. Platelets are sequestered early in lung microvascular beds in ALI models and may contribute to the initial insult of lung endothelium [155, 161–164]. EC activation/injury by inflammatory stimuli, PAMPs and alarmins can generate signals mediating platelet accumulation and activation. Entrapment and activation of platelets in pulmonary capillaries will consequently feed the deleterious cascade of pro-inflammatory and pro-coagulant events in the lung [71, 156, 158, 159, 165]. Platelets can also induce apoptosis in the lung in sepsis models [166]. Among these events, platelet/neutrophil interactions have received considerable attention. Neutrophils are of critical importance in MOD, neutrophil influx being a hallmark of ALI and their inappropriate activation leading to tissue damage signals [167]. Platelets play an important role in neutrophil recruitment and activation in the lung, and platelet-mediated neutrophil activation results in the release of cytokines, chemokines, reactive oxygen species and NET generation [71]. Indeed, experimental models highlight the deleterious role of platelet/neutrophil and also platelet/monocyte interactions in the alteration of the alveolar-capillary integrity [71, 108, 168]. Coagulation activation and alveolar fibrin deposition are common findings in ALI, and platelets are thought to be key contributors to the dysregulation of coagulation in ALI, through their role in coagulation and NET generation [169]. Therefore, several studies suggest a platelet involvement in ALI. In fact, platelet depletion, blocking of platelet/neutrophil interaction, NET dismantling or antiplatelet treatments are protective in experimental models [96, 162–164, 170]. Although in vitro experiments show pro-inflammatory and pro-coagulant effects of PMPs, there is little evidence for a specific deleterious role of PMPs in ALI, a study difficult to address due

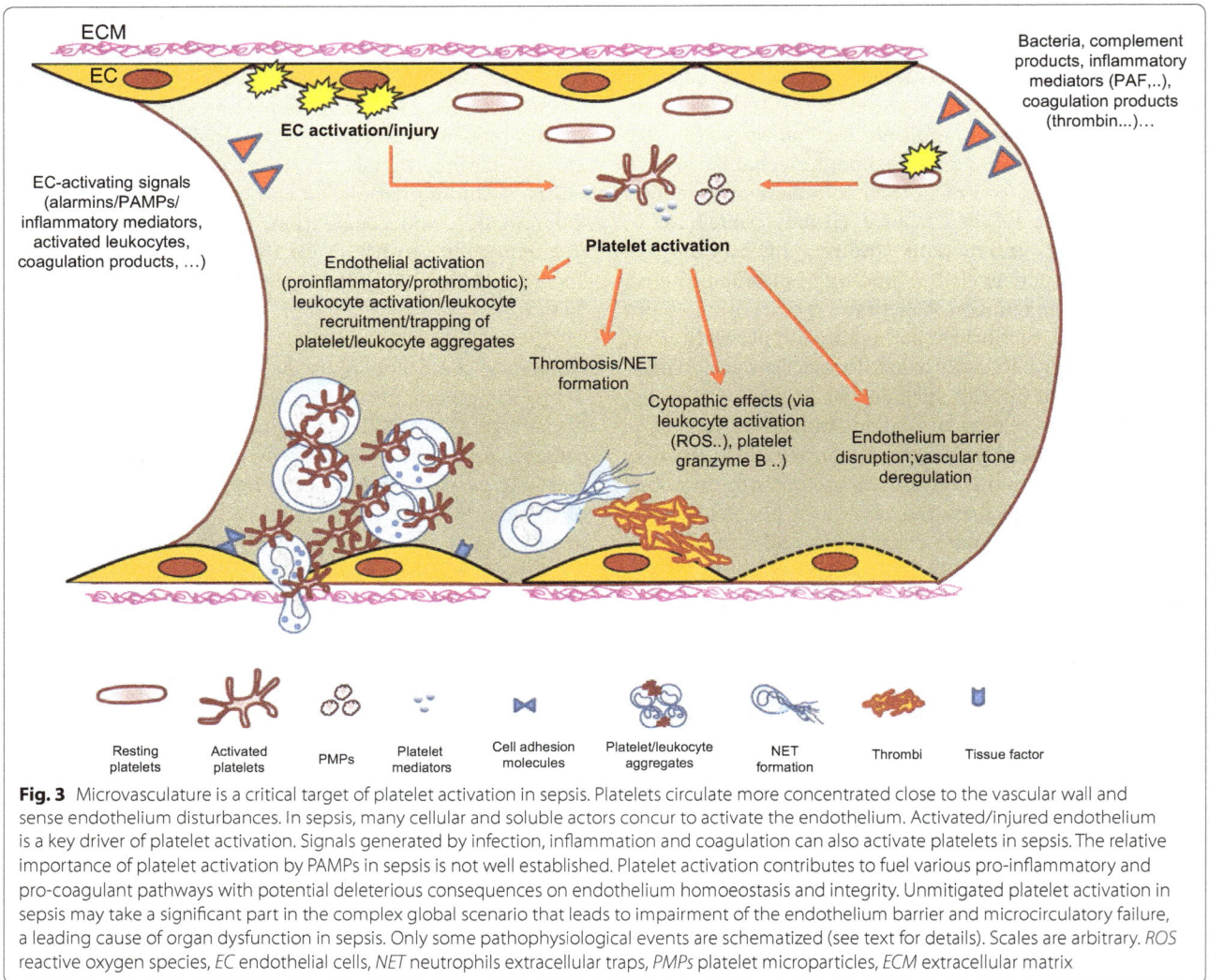

**Fig. 3** Microvasculature is a critical target of platelet activation in sepsis. Platelets circulate more concentrated close to the vascular wall and sense endothelium disturbances. In sepsis, many cellular and soluble actors concur to activate the endothelium. Activated/injured endothelium is a key driver of platelet activation. Signals generated by infection, inflammation and coagulation can also activate platelets in sepsis. The relative importance of platelet activation by PAMPs in sepsis is not well established. Platelet activation contributes to fuel various pro-inflammatory and pro-coagulant pathways with potential deleterious consequences on endothelium homoeostasis and integrity. Unmitigated platelet activation in sepsis may take a significant part in the complex global scenario that leads to impairment of the endothelium barrier and microcirculatory failure, a leading cause of organ dysfunction in sepsis. Only some pathophysiological events are schematized (see text for details). Scales are arbitrary. *ROS* reactive oxygen species, *EC* endothelial cells, *NET* neutrophils extracellular traps, *PMPs* platelet microparticles, *ECM* extracellular matrix

to microparticle identification uncertainties and to the simultaneous presence of microparticles from various origins with heterogeneous functions [158, 171].

Increased vascular permeability is the basis for oedema in inflammation. The concept that platelets protect the basal barrier of alveolar capillaries is supported by experimental evidences, and thrombocytopenia put the lung capillary integrity at risk, particularly in inflammatory conditions. Indeed, severe thrombocytopenia results in increased alveolar-capillary permeability [71, 107, 108]. However, as mentioned above, platelet activation in inflammation can also disrupt endothelium barrier integrity, and platelet depletion is protective in several ALI models [69, 71, 162, 172]. How this dual endothelial barrier-stabilizing versus barrier-destabilizing property of platelets is organized and contribute to ALI progression, as well as the specific role of PMPs, is not

understood. Such a differential effect of platelets in controlling endothelial barrier integrity is likely to be based on a complex balance between characteristics of inflammation in vascular beds, early or late phase, magnitude, role of other inflammatory players, i.e. leukocytes, and experimental models used. The changing relative importance during sepsis progression of platelet-activating signals, platelet count and proteome, interactions with leucocytes and ECs, underline the difficulty to dissect these mechanisms [69, 71, 76, 108, 173]. Moreover, platelets may play a positive role in the control and resolution of inflammation in lung injury, a mechanism that is only recently being understood [158]. The genetic background also plays a role in ALI-associated mortality and morbidity [174]. Platelet count is determined by genetic factors, and genetic studies point to an association between low platelet count and acute respiratory distress syndrome

(ARDS) risk. Genetic variants within the LRRC16A locus (6p22) are associated with a low platelet count. Interestingly, a low platelet count links a single nucleotide polymorphism within this locus to ARDS risk [175].

### Platelets and acute kidney injury (AKI) in sepsis

Acute kidney injury (AKI), a major sepsis complication, is accompanied by hemodynamic disturbances such as decreased glomerular filtration rate and microcirculation alterations [146, 176–180]. The extent of apoptosis and necrosis in tubular lesions is debated. Subtle, heterogeneous, potentially reversible, cytopathic and adaptive cellular events (metabolic changes, mitochondrial dysfunction, autophagy, cell cycle arrest, etc.) may characterize tubular lesions in sepsis AKI [181–184]. Beyond the classic paradigm of renal hypoperfusion, the role of immune response pathways and particularly inflammation in AKI progression is increasingly stressed [1, 178, 185–195]. Alarmins, PAMPs, inflammatory mediators and leukocytes can activate ECs in the renal microcirculation bed, leading to inflammation/thrombosis, metabolic alterations, oxidative stress, concurring to microvascular dysfunction. Due to the close dependence between TECs and tubular microvascularization, compromise blood flow and inflammation in the microvascular beds can lead to tubular epithelial cells (TECs) injury, driving inflammation, mitochondrial/metabolic alterations and various adaptive responses, including cell cycle arrest. Alarmins, PAMPs and inflammatory mediators may also impact TECs after being filtered, and TECs are active participants in kidney inflammation [192, 196–198].

In the highly vascularized kidney, platelet/endothelium interactions can be postulated to be of specific importance. In an AKI model in which selective kidney endothelial injury is realized, there are evidences for platelet contribution [199]. Platelets will be arrested and activated on the kidney endothelium activated by circulating deleterious signals. Inflammation-mediated alteration of EC glycocalyx can also favour platelet adhesion [141, 146, 200–203]. Platelets can also be activated by ischaemic blood flow disturbances in the septic kidney. Therefore, and although much remains to be understood, platelets may be pathophysiological players in sepsis AKI. On the other hand, as mentioned above, platelets contribute to the resolution of inflammation and vasculature integrity. Important questions remain with reference to the identification of soluble and cellular effectors that contribute to the resolution of inflammation and tubular regeneration in the kidney [204]. Microparticles, and PMPs more specifically, are elevated in sepsis and sepsis complicated by AKI [101, 102, 193]. However, their specific role remains to be addressed.

### Platelets and organ-to-organ crosstalk in sepsis

Despite the importance of the deleterious organ-to-organ communication in sepsis, underlying mechanisms are only beginning to be unravelled. Inflammatory signals are implicated in these communications [205]. Can platelets vectorize the exchange of pro-inflammatory and/or pro-coagulant signals that link injuries in distant organs? Interestingly, the activation of platelets at remote sites may mediate lung injury, as shown in mesenteric ischaemia/reperfusion models [206]. Platelets can mediate remote kidney damage induced by pneumonia [207]. Among platelet-derived mediators that could convey such a deleterious action, platelet factor 4 (CXCL4) and CD154 have been identified [208, 209]. When activated, platelets express CD154 and release a soluble form of CD154 [22, 210]; CD154 may bear a particular responsibility as, for example, the CD154/CD40 dyad plays a deleterious role in ALI, including pancreatitis-associated lung injury [211, 212], and as it could be brought to lung microcirculation via PMPs. Further, platelet CD154 mediates neutrophil recruitment in septic lung injury [213]. Although these results suggest a role for platelets, the extent and relative contribution of platelets, platelet-derived mediators, PMPs or circulating platelet/leucocyte aggregates in conveying deleterious signals at distance in patients with sepsis is unknown.

### Platelet count in sepsis and the dilemma of platelet transfusion

#### Platelet count and dynamics of platelet count as determinants of clinical outcome in sepsis patients

Thrombocytopenia is common in sepsis and more generally in critically ill patients and has long been recognized as an independent risk factor for mortality in ICU patients and a sensitive marker for disease severity; the severity of sepsis is a risk factor for thrombocytopenia [6, 8–15, 214–221]. For these reasons, the platelet count is included in the ICU severity of illness scoring system. Platelet count kinetics is often biphasic in ICU patients, characterized by a moderate initial decrease in the first days followed by a rise [11, 216, 222]. Early thrombocytopenia and new-onset thrombocytopenia during ICU hospitalization are associated with a poor prognostic; the magnitude and duration of thrombocytopenia and the absence of relative increase in the platelet count have been linked to the poor outcome [6, 9, 11, 216, 221–227]. In a large recent study, which included 931 sepsis patients, a low platelet count at admission in the ICU was associated with an increased mortality risk [29]. Notably, patients with low platelet counts were more severely ill at ICU admission. Understanding pathophysiological links between platelet count alterations and clinical outcomes is therefore an important issue for the intensive care physician.

## The multiple causes of thrombocytopenia in sepsis patients

The association between thrombocytopenia and clinical outcome does not establish causality, and identifying the causes of thrombocytopenia is essential to patient management. Management of the underlying condition is a primary focus, and an important issue is platelet transfusion. Platelet transfusion may be ineffectual and deleterious in patients with, for example, intravascular platelet activation and have their own risks [228–230]. In a recent report, sepsis was identified as associated with ineffectual platelet transfusion, as evaluated by inadequate platelet count increase [231].

Several mechanisms, acting alone or in combination, can be responsible for a low platelet count in sepsis, and all steps of platelet life may be concerned. Decreased platelet production in the bone marrow can result from pre-existing conditions or from the inhibitory effect of pathogen toxins, drugs or inflammatory mediators on haematopoiesis. Peripheral mechanisms are essential causes of thrombocytopenia [15, 214, 218, 227, 232, 233]. The reduction in platelet half-life and their consumption/destruction may be linked to the many events of platelet activation occurring in sepsis, intravascular coagulopathy and immune mechanisms. Drug-induced thrombocytopenia, hemophagocytosis, bleeding, hemodilution are also major explanatory factors. Laboratory artefact of pseudothrombocytopenia can be encountered, and assessing the reality of thrombocytopenia is an important point [230].

Systematic investigations with routinely available tests can help to delineate mechanisms of thrombocytopenia [218, 232, 234]. An early rise of reticulated platelets follows endotoxin administration in humans, and the percentage of immature platelet fraction that evaluates thrombopoietic rate could be a useful tool to witness early bone marrow reaction predicting sepsis development [80, 235]. Apart from altering platelet count, sepsis and sepsis medications can also result in platelet function defect, adding another pathophysiological interface [236, 237]. A detailed description of these mechanisms and diagnostic/management guidance has been excellently reviewed and is beyond the scope of the present work [154, 222, 230, 233, 238–242]. A difficulty in approaching thrombocytopenia and its management is related to the paradox of platelets being potentially both deleterious and beneficial during sepsis course. In a first point of view, platelet count reduction is related to sepsis via consumption mechanisms including pathogen and pathogen product-mediated activation, induction of apoptosis,

lysis and increased phagocytic clearance. Acute infections often lead to thrombocytopenia [58], and bloodstream infection is associated with lower platelet counts [221]. Coagulopathy, particularly DIC, platelet sequestration by leucocytes and by inflammatory vascular beds are also commonly stressed mechanisms of thrombocytopenia. Through these mechanisms, platelets can be perceived as bystanders whose destruction is related to the severity of infection and to the characteristics of the host response to the infectious challenge. In that case, the use of platelet transfusion may be perceived as being detrimental, via the fuelling of inflammation and coagulation. On the other hand, platelets are active players in pathogen clearance, leading to the possibility that a low platelet count and platelet function alteration may first favour infection. Further, platelets also protect vascular integrity; hence, maintaining an adequate threshold of platelet count seems a necessary target to prevent bleeding. In fact, platelet transfusions are mostly used to prevent or treat bleeding [228]. Conciliating such a paradox of platelets being both deleterious and beneficial is a challenging point for platelet-targeted therapeutic interventions in sepsis.

## Can platelets represent therapeutic targets and diagnostic tools in sepsis?

The clinical management of sepsis remains a difficult challenge, and pathophysiological advances have not yet been translated into effective therapeutic protocols [2]. Notably, strategies to counteract the runaway proinflammatory state in sepsis, such as inhibition of specific inflammatory mediators, have given disappointing results [243]. However, current knowledge on sepsis pathophysiology, highlighting multiple humoral and cellular factors in the inappropriate inflammatory response to infection, suggests that therapies targeting a single mediator will not demonstrate effectiveness [41]. Additional complexity is linked to individual disease susceptibilities and medical comorbidities that would necessitate individual approaches. Accumulating evidence therefore speaks for an integrated approach of sepsis treatment based on a better knowledge of its natural history.

The recently described involvement of platelets at the crossroads of several immune response pathways has led to the assumption that platelets or platelet-derived effectors represent therapeutic targets in sepsis. Platelet activation can drive multiple inflammatory and coagulation pathways, and targeting platelets offer the theoretical perspective of targeting simultaneously several deleterious pathways. Although the clinical relevance of animal models has many drawbacks, it is of interest that platelet depletion, inhibition of platelet functions and antiplatelet drugs show protection in experimental ALI or

AKI [124]. P2Y12 inhibitors reduce inflammatory and pro-thrombotic mechanisms after endotoxin administration in humans [244]. Several observational and retrospective clinical studies have shown that antiplatelet agents such as acetylsalicylic acid, platelet P2Y12 inhibitor clopidogrel or GPIIb/IIIa antagonists reduce mortality or complications in critically ill patients [245–255]. However, some studies are conflicting [249, 252, 256] (Table 1). There is therefore a strong need for large randomized controlled clinical trials to investigate the effects of antiplatelet therapy in sepsis. The complexity of such studies relates in part to the heterogeneity of sepsis patients in terms of nature of the causal germ, site and severity of infection, multiple comorbidities, gender, age and genetic background. There is also individual variability in the concentration of antiplatelet agents that efficiently inhibits platelet function. A defective response to clopidogrel or aspirin treatment may concern up to 30 or 40% individuals, respectively [257–259]. Also, antiplatelet treatments have differential effects on platelet functions. Platelets treated with aspirin can still be activated by strong agonists, such as thrombin or ADP. Hence, in a full-blown pro-inflammatory/pro-coagulant condition as met in sepsis, it remains to be determined whether platelet activation is efficiently inhibited by antiplatelet treatments. Platelets are an important blood reservoir of pro-inflammatory molecules and may contribute to the "cytokine storm" that characterizes sepsis. However, many cellular players, including leucocytes and EC, also produce such mediators, and the relative contribution of platelets is not understood. In a recent study, antiplatelet therapy did not significantly reduce plasma pro-inflammatory cytokines levels in sepsis patients [260]. Antiplatelet agents have also been shown to have indirect off-platelet effects, a mechanism which importance is not yet established [261]. Finally, the impairment of platelet function may have undesirable consequences, such as bleeding or the blunting of platelet protective functions.

As mentioned above, elucidating mechanisms of thrombocytopenia in sepsis are essential with reference to transfusion. Platelet transfusion is mostly used to prevent/treat bleeding [228, 229]. The risk of bleeding increases with the severity of thrombocytopenia [222]. The threshold of platelet count ensuring protection may be higher in sepsis patients, reflecting the severity of the disturbance of the vascular beds. Commonly advocated threshold of platelet count is in the range of $10–50 \times 10^9$/L, depending on clinical situations, additional bleeding risks, evidence for central thrombocytopenia. The risk of bleeding is, however, not straightforwardly linked to the depth of thrombocytopenia, in the context of a sustained production of platelets, and additional parameters in the critically ill patient may

interfere; indeed, the risk of bleeding is also increased for platelet counts between 50 and $100 \times 10^9$/L [8, 9, 222, 229]. In fact, there is a poor evidence-based clinical benefit of platelet transfusion in the non-bleeding ICU patient [154, 228–230, 242]. The lack of a clear understanding of thrombocytopenia causes makes the risk/benefit assessment difficult, as there is a theoretical risk to aggravate the underlying pathophysiology [229]. The main regulator of platelet production, TPO, is elevated in sepsis and related to the platelet count [262, 263], which may be linked to the reduction in platelet mass or stimulation of TPO production by inflammatory mediators. Experimental models show that TPO neutralization reduces the severity of organ damage [264]. However, in the clinics, the potential benefit of TPO administration in thrombocytopenic patients in sepsis has been recently suggested [265]. At this stage, results from randomized controlled trials remain necessary to evaluate TPO interest in sepsis.

If the interpretation of thrombocytopenia in sepsis patients is made difficult by the multiplicity of underlying mechanisms, the platelet count by itself may hold valuable information [242]. The platelet count may represent a surrogate marker of the severity of organ dysfunction. A low platelet count occurring even early in sepsis patients is indeed recognized as a sign of poor prognostic; however, a single platelet count at admission may have little pertinence [266], and the kinetics of platelet counts appears to have a deeper meaning. Two alterations of this kinetics have been shown to be of clinical interest in sepsis patients, suggesting that they must be given specific attention. Both the magnitude of the drop in platelet count rather that thrombocytopenia per se, and the non-resolution of thrombocytopenia are strong predictors of mortality in sepsis [9, 15, 267]. The onset and dynamics of thrombocytopenia have been stressed as potential diagnostic approaches in ICU patients [222].

## Conclusion

Platelets play key roles in various aspects of the immune response, suggesting that they take a significant part in sepsis pathophysiology. Therapeutic control of platelet functions would offer the perspective of targeting simultaneously several deleterious pathways in sepsis. The difficult extrapolation of experimental models to clinical sepsis and the conflicting results of clinical studies do not allow us today to introduce an antiplatelet agent in clinical practice. However, septic critically ill patients treated with long-term antiplatelet agent may benefit from the continuation of their treatment in the absence of bleeding risk, avoiding a rebound of platelet reactivity. The multiple facets of platelet involvement in sepsis therefore represent substantial challenges to the clinician and call for a deeper understanding of the relative importance of

**Table 1 Summary of cohort studies on antiplatelet agents and sepsis**

| Authors | Study year | Study type and setting | Patient number | Antiplatelet agent | Patients | Study conclusions | Potential limitations |
|---|---|---|---|---|---|---|---|
| Wang et al. [268] | 2016 | Meta analysis of cohort studies | 14,612 | ASA, clopidogrel, ticlopidine | ICU patients with ARDS predisposing conditions | Reduced mortality and lower incidence of ARDS | Non-sepsis patients included. Treatment bias of antiplatelet agents |
| Kor et al. [269] | 2012–2014 | Multicenter, double-blind, placebo-controlled, randomized clinical trial | 390 | ASA | Patients with elevated risk for developing ARDS in the emergency department | ASA did not reduce the risk of ARDS and 28-day or 1-year survival | Non-sepsis patients included. Low rate of ARDS development |
| Wiewel et al. [260] | 2011–2014 | Prospective observational study with propensity matching | 972 | Mostly ASA | Sepsis within 24 h after admission in 2 mixed medical/surgical ICU | Antiplatelet therapy was not associated with alterations in the presentation or outcome of sepsis or the host response | Treatment bias of ASA. Inadequate patient number and power |
| Osthoff et al. [270] | 2001–2013 | Retrospective cohort study with propensity matching | 689 | ASA | Patients with *S. aureus* and *E. coli* bloodstream infection admitted in a single medical/surgical ICU | Low-dose ASA at the time of bloodstream infection was strongly associated with a reduced short-term mortality in patients with *S. aureus* bloodstream infection | Treatment bias of ASA at the time of enrolment. Severity at presentation was not included in the analysis model. Inadequate patient number and power |
| Tsai et al. [255] | 2000–2010 | A nation-wide population-based cohort and nested case–control study | 683,421 | ASA, clopidogrel, ticlopidine | Sepsis | Antiplatelet agents were associated with a survival benefit in sepsis patients | Claims database |
| Chen et al. [253] | 2006–2012 | Secondary analysis of prospective cohort with propensity matching | 1149 | ASA | Patients admitted in a mixed ICU for at least 2 days | Decreased risk of ARDS | Non-sepsis patients included. Treatment bias of ASA |
| Boyle et al. [271] | 2010–2012 | Prospective observational study | 202 | ASA | ICU patients requiring invasive mechanical ventilation | Reduced risk of ICU mortality | Treatment bias of ASA. Non-sepsis patients included |
| Valerio-Rojas et al. [249] | 2007–2009 | Retrospective cohort with propensity matching | 651 | ASA, clopidogrel | ICU patients with sepsis | No decrease in hospital mortality but decreased incidence of ARDS | Inadequate patient number and power. Unmeasured bias and confounding |
| Otto et al. [251] | 2013 | Retrospective cohort | 886 | ASA, clopidogrel | Surgical ICU patients with sepsis and a minimum length of stay of 48 h and a history of atherosclerotic vascular diseases | ASA treatment reduced the ICU and hospital mortality. Combination of ASA with clopidogrel did not show any significant effect on mortality. Clopidogrel alone might have a similar benefit | Unmeasured bias and confounding |

**Table 1** continued

| Authors | Study year | Study type and setting | Patient number | Antiplatelet agent | Patients | Study conclusions | Potential limitations |
|---|---|---|---|---|---|---|---|
| Sossdorf et al. [250] | 2013 | Retrospective cohort | 979 | ASA | Septic patients admitted to a surgical ICU | Decreased mortality with ASA or NSAIDs was associated with decreased hospital mortality. No benefit when ASA and NSAIDs are given together | Unmeasured bias and confounding |
| Eisen et al. [248] | 2000–2009 | Retrospective cohort study with propensity matching | 7945 | ASA | ICU patients with SIRS/sepsis on ASA at the time of SIRS/sepsis | ASA was associated with survival | Treatment bias of ASA at the time of enrolment and confounders |
| O'Neal et al. [272] | 2006–2008 | Cross-sectional analysis of a prospective cohort | 575 | ASA and Statin | Patients admitted in a mixed ICU for at least 2 days | ASA was not associated with the diagnosis of ALI/ARDS, sepsis or hospital mortality | Treatment bias of ASA Unmeasured bias and confounding Non-sepsis patients included |
| Erlich et al. [246] | 2006 | Retrospective cohort | 161 | ASA, clopidogrel, ticlopidine | Adult patients admitted in a medical ICU with a major risk factor for ALI | Reduced incidence of ALI/ARDS | Treatment bias of ASA Non-sepsis patients included |
| Kor et al. [256] | 2009 | Second analysis of prospective multicenter observational study | 3855 | ASA | Consecutive, adult, non-surgical patients with at least one major risk factor for ALI | ASA was not associated with ICU or hospital mortality and ICU or hospital lengths | Treatment bias of ASA Non-sepsis patients included Unmeasured bias and confounding |
| Storey et al. [273] | 2006–2008 | Post hoc analysis PLATO study | 18,421 | Ticagrelor vs clopidogrel | Patients with acute coronary syndrome | Reduced mortality following pulmonary infection and sepsis in acute coronary syndrome with ticagrelor | Unmeasured bias and confounding |
| Winning et al. [245] | 2007–2009 | Retrospective cohort | 615 | ASA, clopidogrel | Consecutive patients admitted in a mixed ICU | Reduction in organ failure and mortality in critically ill patients with pre-existing medication | Non-sepsis patients included Treatment bias of ASA |
| Winning et al. [274] | 2002–2007 | Retrospective cohort | 224 | ASA, clopidogrel ticlopidine | Patients admitted for CAP not receiving statins and using antiplatelet drugs for more than 6 months | Reduction in need of intensive care treatment and length of hospital stay | Unmeasured bias and confounding |
| Gross et al. [275] | 2001–2005 | Retrospective cohort | 417,648 | Clopidogrel | All adult (≥ 18 years) Medicaid beneficiaries in Kentucky | Increased CAP incidence and no significant reduction in severity | Claims database |

*ASA* Acetylsalicylic acid, *ARDS* acute respiratory distress syndrome, *ALI* acute lung injury, *CAP* community-acquired pneumonia, *NSAID* non-steroidal anti-inflammatory drug

platelet contribution to determine their ultimate clinical significance.

## Abbreviations

ALI: acute lung injury; ARDS: acute respiratory distress syndrome; PAMPs: pathogen-associated molecular patterns; DIC: disseminated intravascular coagulation; EC: endothelial cell; ICU: intensive care unit; MOD: multi-organ dysfunction; PMPs: platelet microparticles; SIRS: systemic inflammatory response syndrome; TEC: tubular epithelial cell; AKI: acute kidney injury; ECM: extracellular matrix; NET: neutrophil extracellular traps; TPO: thrombopoietin; TREM-1: triggering receptor expressed on myeloid cells 1.

## Authors' contributions

AD and JR conceived, designed and coordinated this review. SL, JV, CR, CC and AO helped to critically revise the manuscript. All authors read and approved the final manuscript.

## Author details

[1] INSERM U1026, BioTis, Univ. Bordeaux, 33000 Bordeaux, France. [2] Department of Anaesthesia and Critical Care II, Magellan Medico-Surgical Center, CHU Bordeaux, 33000 Bordeaux, France. [3] Department of Pathology, CHU Bordeaux, 33000 Bordeaux, France. [4] Cell and Developmental Biology Department, Centre for Genomic Regulation, The Barcelona Institute for Science and Technology, 08003 Barcelona, Spain. [5] Department of Nephrology, Transplantation and Haemodialysis, CHU Bordeaux, 33000 Bordeaux, France. [6] INSERM U1034, Biology of Cardiovascular Diseases, Univ. Bordeaux, 33600 Pessac, France.

## Competing interests

The authors declare that they have no competing interests.

## Funding

JV acknowledges support from a Marie Curie international outgoing fellowship within the 7th European Community Framework Programme.

## References

1. Singer M, De Santis V, Vitale D, Jeffcoate W. Multiorgan failure is an adaptive, endocrine-mediated, metabolic response to overwhelming systemic inflammation. Lancet. 2004;364(9433):545–8.
2. Angus DC, van der Poll T. Severe sepsis and septic shock. N Engl J Med. 2013;369(21):2063.
3. Deutschman CS, Tracey KJ. Sepsis: current dogma and new perspectives. Immunity. 2014;40(4):463–75.
4. Gaieski DF, Edwards JM, Kallan MJ, Carr BG. Benchmarking the incidence and mortality of severe sepsis in the United States. Crit Care Med. 2013;41(5):1167–74.
5. Fleischmann C, Scherag A, Adhikari NK, Hartog CS, Tsaganos T, Schlattmann P, et al. Assessment of Global Incidence and Mortality of Hospital-treated Sepsis. Current Estimates and Limitations. Am J Respir Crit Care Med. 2016;193(3):259–72.
6. Baughman RP, Lower EE, Flessa HC, Tollerud DJ. Thrombocytopenia in the intensive care unit. Chest. 1993;104(4):1243–7.
7. Drews RE, Weinberger SE. Thrombocytopenic disorders in critically ill patients. Am J Respir Crit Care Med. 2000;162(2 Pt 1):347–51.
8. Vanderschueren S, De Weerdt A, Malbrain M, Vankersschaever D, Frans E, Wilmer A, et al. Thrombocytopenia and prognosis in intensive care. Crit Care Med. 2000;28(6):1871–6.
9. Strauss R, Wehler M, Mehler K, Kreutzer D, Koebnick C, Hahn EG. Thrombocytopenia in patients in the medical intensive care unit: bleeding prevalence, transfusion requirements, and outcome. Crit Care Med. 2002;30(8):1765–71.
10. Smith-Erichsen N. Serial determinations of platelets, leucocytes and coagulation parameters in surgical septicemia. Scand J Clin Lab Invest Suppl. 1985;178:7–14.
11. Akca S, Haji-Michael P, de Mendonca A, Suter P, Levi M, Vincent JL. Time course of platelet counts in critically ill patients. Crit Care Med. 2002;30(4):753–6.
12. Crowther MA, Cook DJ, Meade MO, Griffith LE, Guyatt GH, Arnold DM, et al. Thrombocytopenia in medical-surgical critically ill patients: prevalence, incidence, and risk factors. J Crit Care. 2005;20(4):348–53.
13. Moreau D, Timsit JF, Vesin A, Garrouste-Orgeas M, de Lassence A, Zahar JR, et al. Platelet count decline: an early prognostic marker in critically ill patients with prolonged ICU stays. Chest. 2007;131(6):1735–41.
14. Hui P, Cook DJ, Lim W, Fraser GA, Arnold DM. The frequency and clinical significance of thrombocytopenia complicating critical illness: a systematic review. Chest. 2011;139(2):271–8.
15. Venkata C, Kashyap R, Farmer JC, Afessa B. Thrombocytopenia in adult patients with sepsis: incidence, risk factors, and its association with clinical outcome. J Intensive Care. 2013;1(1):9.
16. Semple JW, Freedman J. Platelets and innate immunity. Cell Mol Life Sci. 2010;67(4):499–511.
17. Semple JW, Italiano JE Jr, Freedman J. Platelets and the immune continuum. Nat Rev Immunol. 2011;11(4):264–74.
18. Vieira-de-Abreu A, Campbell RA, Weyrich AS, Zimmerman GA. Platelets: versatile effector cells in hemostasis, inflammation, and the immune continuum. Semin Immunopathol. 2012;34(1):5–30.
19. Herter JM, Rossaint J, Zarbock A. Platelets in inflammation and immunity. J Thromb Haemost. 2014;12(11):1764–75.
20. Morrell CN, Aggrey AA, Chapman LM, Modjeski KL. Emerging roles for platelets as immune and inflammatory cells. Blood. 2014;123(18):2759–67.
21. Xu XR, Zhang D, Oswald BE, Carrim N, Wang X, Hou Y, et al. Platelets are versatile cells: new discoveries in hemostasis, thrombosis, immune responses, tumor metastasis and beyond. Crit Rev Clin Lab Sci. 2016;53(6):409–30.
22. Dewitte A, Tanga A, Villeneuve J, Lepreux S, Ouattara A, Desmouliere A, et al. New frontiers for platelet CD154. Exp Hematol Oncol. 2015;4:6.
23. Thomas MR, Storey RF. The role of platelets in inflammation. Thromb Haemost. 2015;114(3):449–58.
24. Singer M, Deutschman CS, Seymour CW, Shankar-Hari M, Annane D, Bauer M, et al. The third international consensus definitions for sepsis and septic shock (sepsis-3). JAMA. 2016;315(8):801–10.
25. Riedemann NC, Guo RF, Ward PA. The enigma of sepsis. J Clin Investig. 2003;112(4):460–7.
26. Pierrakos C, Vincent JL. Sepsis biomarkers: a review. Crit Care. 2010;14(1):R15.
27. Aziz M, Jacob A, Yang WL, Matsuda A, Wang P. Current trends in inflammatory and immunomodulatory mediators in sepsis. J Leukoc Biol. 2013;93(3):329–42.
28. Parlato M, Cavaillon JM. Host response biomarkers in the diagnosis of sepsis: a general overview. Methods Mol Biol. 2015;1237:149–211.
29. Claushuis TA, van Vught LA, Scicluna BP, Wiewel MA, Klein Klouwenberg PM, Hoogendijk AJ, et al. Thrombocytopenia is associated with a dysregulated host response in critically ill sepsis patients. Blood. 2016;127(24):3062–72.
30. Hatherill M, Tibby SM, Turner C, Ratnavel N, Murdoch IA. Procalcitonin and cytokine levels: relationship to organ failure and mortality in pediatric septic shock. Crit Care Med. 2000;28(7):2591–4.
31. Marshall JC. Inflammation, coagulopathy, and the pathogenesis of multiple organ dysfunction syndrome. Crit Care Med. 2001;29(7 Suppl):S99–106.

32. Mikacenic C, Hahn WO, Price BL, Harju-Baker S, Katz R, Kain KC, et al. Biomarkers of endothelial activation are associated with poor outcome in critical illness. PLoS ONE. 2015;10(10):e0141251.

33. Rittirsch D, Flierl MA, Ward PA. Harmful molecular mechanisms in sepsis. Nat Rev Immunol. 2008;8(10):776–87.

34. Stearns-Kurosawa DJ, Osuchowski MF, Valentine C, Kurosawa S, Remick DG. The pathogenesis of sepsis. Annu Rev Pathol. 2011;6:19–48.

35. Wiersinga WJ, Leopold SJ, Cranendonk DR, van der Poll T. Host innate immune responses to sepsis. Virulence. 2014;5(1):36–44.

36. Raymond SL, Holden DC, Mira JC, Stortz JA, Loftus TJ, Mohr AM, et al. Microbial recognition and danger signals in sepsis and trauma. Biochim Biophys Acta. 2017;1863(10 Pt B):2564–73.

37. Xiao W, Mindrinos MN, Seok J, Cuschieri J, Cuenca AG, Gao H, et al. A genomic storm in critically injured humans. J Exp Med. 2011;208(13):2581–90.

38. Munford RS, Pugin J. Normal responses to injury prevent systemic inflammation and can be immunosuppressive. Am J Respir Crit Care Med. 2001;163(2):316–21.

39. Hotchkiss RS, Karl IE. The pathophysiology and treatment of sepsis. N Engl J Med. 2003;348(2):138–50.

40. Ward NS, Casserly B, Ayala A. The compensatory anti-inflammatory response syndrome (CARS) in critically ill patients. Clin Chest Med. 2008;29(4):617–25.

41. Iskander KN, Osuchowski MF, Stearns-Kurosawa DJ, Kurosawa S, Stepien D, Valentine C, et al. Sepsis: multiple abnormalities, heterogeneous responses, and evolving understanding. Physiol Rev. 2013;93(3):1247–88.

42. Hotchkiss RS, Monneret G, Payen D. Sepsis-induced immunosuppression: from cellular dysfunctions to immunotherapy. Nat Rev Immunol. 2013;13(12):862–74.

43. Delano MJ, Ward PA. The immune system's role in sepsis progression, resolution, and long-term outcome. Immunol Rev. 2016;274(1):330–53.

44. Machlus KR, Italiano JE Jr. The incredible journey: from megakaryocyte development to platelet formation. J Cell Biol. 2013;201(6):785–96.

45. Hitchcock IS, Kaushansky K. Thrombopoietin from beginning to end. Br J Haematol. 2014;165(2):259–68.

46. Josefsson EC, Dowling MR, Lebois M, Kile BT. The regulation of platelet life span. In: Michelson AD, editor. Platelets. Cambridge: Academic Press; 2013. p. 51–66.

47. Grozovsky R, Giannini S, Falet H, Hoffmeister KM. Regulating billions of blood platelets: glycans and beyond. Blood. 2015;126(16):1877–84.

48. Rendu F, Brohard-Bohn B. The platelet release reaction: granules' constituents, secretion and functions. Platelets. 2001;12(5):261–73.

49. Coppinger JA, Cagney G, Toomey S, Kislinger T, Belton O, McRedmond JP, et al. Characterization of the proteins released from activated platelets leads to localization of novel platelet proteins in human atherosclerotic lesions. Blood. 2004;103(6):2096–104.

50. Nurden AT, Nurden P, Sanchez M, Andia I, Anitua E. Platelets and wound healing. Front Biosci. 2008;13:3532–48.

51. Nieuwland R, Sturk A. Platelet-derived microparticles. In: Michelson AD, editor. Platelets. Cambridge: Academic Press; 2013. p. 403–13.

52. Melki I, Tessandier N, Zufferey A, Boilard E. Platelet microvesicles in health and disease. Platelets. 2017;28(3):214–21.

53. Morrell CN, Maggirwar SB. Recently recognized platelet agonists. Curr Opin Hematol. 2011;18(5):309–14.

54. Monroe DM, Hoffman M, Roberts HR. Platelets and thrombin generation. Arterioscler Thromb Vasc Biol. 2002;22(9):1381–9.

55. Nurden AT. Platelets, inflammation and tissue regeneration. Thromb Haemost. 2011;105(Suppl 1):S13–33.

56. Garraud O, Hamzeh-Cognasse H, Pozzetto B, Cavaillon JM, Cognasse F. Bench-to-bedside review: platelets and active immune functions-new clues for immunopathology? Crit Care. 2013;17(4):236.

57. Nurden AT. The biology of the platelet with special reference to inflammation, wound healing and immunity. Front Biosci (Landmark Ed). 2018;01(23):726–51.

58. Kapur R, Zufferey A, Boilard E, Semple JW. Nouvelle cuisine: platelets served with inflammation. J Immunol. 2015;194(12):5579–87.

59. Manne BK, Xiang SC, Rondina MT. Platelet secretion in inflammatory and infectious diseases. Platelets. 2017;28(2):155–64.

60. Chen J, Lopez JA. Interactions of platelets with subendothelium and endothelium. Microcirculation. 2005;12(3):235–46.

61. Siegel-Axel DI, Gawaz M. Platelets and endothelial cells. Semin Thromb Hemost. 2007;33(2):128–35.

62. Etulain J, Schattner M. Glycobiology of platelet-endothelial cell interactions. Glycobiology. 2014;24(12):1252–9.

63. Kolarova H, Ambruzova B, Svihalkova Sindlerova L, Klinke A, Kubala L. Modulation of endothelial glycocalyx structure under inflammatory conditions. Mediat Inflamm. 2014;2014:694312.

64. Schmidt EP, Kuebler WM, Lee WL, Downey GP. Adhesion molecules: master controllers of the circulatory system. Compr Physiol. 2016;6(2):945–73.

65. Page C, Pitchford S. Neutrophil and platelet complexes and their relevance to neutrophil recruitment and activation. Int Immunopharmacol. 2013;17(4):1176–84.

66. May AE, Seizer P, Gawaz M. Platelets: inflammatory firebugs of vascular walls. Arterioscler Thromb Vasc Biol. 2008;28(3):s5–10.

67. Lowenberg EC, Meijers JC, Levi M. Platelet-vessel wall interaction in health and disease. Neth J Med. 2010;68(6):242–51.

68. Stokes KY, Granger DN. Platelets: a critical link between inflammation and microvascular dysfunction. J Physiol. 2012;590(Pt 5):1023–34.

69. Rondina MT, Weyrich AS, Zimmerman GA. Platelets as cellular effectors of inflammation in vascular diseases. Circ Res. 2013;112(11):1506–19.

70. Ed Rainger G, Chimen M, Harrison MJ, Yates CM, Harrison P, Watson SP, et al. The role of platelets in the recruitment of leukocytes during vascular disease. Platelets. 2015;26(6):507–20.

71. Middleton EA, Weyrich AS, Zimmerman GA. Platelets in pulmonary immune responses and inflammatory lung diseases. Physiol Rev. 2016;96(4):1211–59.

72. Sreeramkumar V, Adrover JM, Ballesteros I, Cuartero MI, Rossaint J, Bilbao I, et al. Neutrophils scan for activated platelets to initiate inflammation. Science. 2014;346(6214):1234–8.

73. Zuchtriegel G, Uhl B, Puhr-Westerheide D, Pornbacher M, Lauber K, Krombach F, et al. Platelets guide leukocytes to their sites of extravasation. PLoS Biol. 2016;14(5):e1002459.

74. Peters MJ, Dixon G, Kotowicz KT, Hatch DJ, Heyderman RS, Klein NJ. Circulating platelet-neutrophil complexes represent a subpopulation of activated neutrophils primed for adhesion, phagocytosis and intracellular killing. Br J Haematol. 1999;106(2):391–9.

75. Haselmayer P, Grosse-Hovest L, von Landenberg P, Schild H, Radsak MP. TREM-1 ligand expression on platelets enhances neutrophil activation. Blood. 2007;110(3):1029–35.

76. Gros A, Ollivier V, Ho-Tin-Noe B. Platelets in inflammation: regulation of leukocyte activities and vascular repair. Front Immunol. 2014;5:678.

77. Kral JB, Schrottmaier WC, Salzmann M, Assinger A. Platelet interaction with innate immune cells. Transfus Med Hemother. 2016;43(2):78–88.

78. Gawaz M, Fateh-Moghadam S, Pilz G, Gurland HJ, Werdan K. Platelet activation and interaction with leucocytes in patients with sepsis or multiple organ failure. Eur J Clin Investig. 1995;25(11):843–51.

79. Russwurm S, Vickers J, Meier-Hellmann A, Spangenberg P, Bredle D, Reinhart K, et al. Platelet and leukocyte activation correlate with the severity of septic organ dysfunction. Shock. 2002;17(4):263–8.

80. Stohlawetz P, Folman CC, von dem Borne AE, Pernerstorfer T, Eichler HG, Panzer S, et al. Effects of endotoxemia on thrombopoiesis in men. Thromb Haemost. 1999;81(4):613–7.

81. Michelson AD, Barnard MR, Krueger LA, Valeri CR, Furman MI. Circulating monocyte-platelet aggregates are a more sensitive marker of in v vo platelet activation than platelet surface P-selectin: studies in baboons, human coronary intervention, and human acute myocardial infarction. Circulation. 2001;104(13):1533–7.

82. Ioannou A, Kannan L, Tsokos GC. Platelets, complement and tissue inflammation. Autoimmunity. 2013;46(1):1–5.

83. Stocker TJ, Ishikawa-Ankerhold H, Massberg S, Schulz C. Small but mighty: platelets as central effectors of host defense. Thromb Haemost. 2017;117(4):651–61.

84. Engelmann B, Massberg S. Thrombosis as an intravascular effector of innate immunity. Nat Rev Immunol. 2013;13(1):34–45.

85. Muller F, Mutch NJ, Schenk WA, Smith SA, Esterl L, Spronk HM, et al. Platelet polyphosphates are proinflammatory and procoagulant mediators in vivo. Cell. 2009;139(6):1143–56.

86. Esmon CT. The interactions between inflammation and coagulation. Br J Haematol. 2005;131(4):417–30.

87. Esmon CT. Coagulation inhibitors in inflammation. Biochem Soc Trans. 2005;33(Pt 2):401–5.

88. Semeraro N, Ammollo CT, Semeraro F, Colucci M. Sepsis-associated disseminated intravascular coagulation and thromboembolic disease. Mediterr J Hematol Infect Dis. 2010;2(3):e2010024.

89. Levi M, van der Poll T. Coagulation and sepsis. Thromb Res. 2017;149:38–44.

90. Simmons J, Pittet JF. The coagulopathy of acute sepsis. Curr Opin Anaesthesiol. 2015;28(2):227–36.

91. Davis RP, Miller-Dorey S, Jenne CN. Platelets and coagulation in infection. Clin Transl Immunol. 2016;5(7):e89.

92. Ma AC, Kubes P. Platelets, neutrophils, and neutrophil extracellular traps (NETs) in sepsis. J Thromb Haemost. 2008;6(3):415–20.

93. Ghasemzadeh M, Hosseini E. Platelet-leukocyte crosstalk: linking proinflammatory responses to procoagulant state. Thromb Res. 2013;131(3):191–7.

94. Carestia A, Kaufman T, Schattner M. Platelets: new bricks in the building of neutrophil extracellular traps. Front Immunol. 2016;7:271.

95. Swystun LL, Liaw PC. The role of leukocytes in thrombosis. Blood. 2016;128(6):753–62.

96. McDonald B, Davis RP, Kim SJ, Tse M, Esmon CT, Kolaczkowska E, et al. Platelets and neutrophil extracellular traps collaborate to promote intravascular coagulation during sepsis in mice. Blood. 2017;129(10):1357–67.

97. Nieuwland R, Berckmans RJ, McGregor S, Boing AN, Romijn FP, Westendorp RG, et al. Cellular origin and procoagulant properties of microparticles in meningococcal sepsis. Blood. 2000;95(3):930–5.

98. George FD. Microparticles in vascular diseases. Thromb Res. 2008;122(Suppl 1):S55–9.

99. Italiano JE Jr, Mairuhu AT, Flaumenhaft R. Clinical relevance of microparticles from platelets and megakaryocytes. Curr Opin Hematol. 2010;17(6):578–84.

100. Reid VL, Webster NR. Role of microparticles in sepsis. Br J Anaesth. 2012;109(4):503–13.

101. Tokes-Fuzesi M, Woth G, Ernyey B, Vermes I, Muhl D, Bogar L, et al. Microparticles and acute renal dysfunction in septic patients. J Crit Care. 2013;28(2):141–7.

102. Souza AC, Yuen PS, Star RA. Microparticles: markers and mediators of sepsis-induced microvascular dysfunction, immunosuppression, and AKI. Kidney Int. 2015;87(6):1100–8.

103. Ripoche J. Blood platelets and inflammation: their relationship with liver and digestive diseases. Clin Res Hepatol Gastroenterol. 2011;35(5):353–7.

104. Gawaz M, Vogel S. Platelets in tissue repair: control of apoptosis and interactions with regenerative cells. Blood. 2013;122(15):2550–4.

105. Golebiewska EM, Poole AW. Platelet secretion: from haemostasis to wound healing and beyond. Blood Rev. 2015;29(3):153–62.

106. Nachman RL, Rafii S. Platelets, petechiae, and preservation of the vascular wall. N Engl J Med. 2008;359(12):1261–70.

107. Ho-Tin-Noe B, Demers M, Wagner DD. How platelets safeguard vascular integrity. J Thromb Haemost. 2011;9(Suppl 1):56–65.

108. Weyrich AS, Zimmerman GA. Platelets in lung biology. Annu Rev Physiol. 2013;75:569–91.

109. Kitchens CS, Weiss L. Ultrastructural changes of endothelium associated with thrombocytopenia. Blood. 1975;46(4):567–78.

110. Broos K, Feys HB, De Meyer SF, Vanhoorelbeke K, Deckmyn H. Platelets at work in primary hemostasis. Blood Rev. 2011;25(4):155–67.

111. Versteeg HH, Heemskerk JW, Levi M, Reitsma PH. New fundamentals in hemostasis. Physiol Rev. 2013;93(1):327–58.

112. Goerge T, Ho-Tin-Noe B, Carbo C, Benarafa C, Remold-O'Donnell E, Zhao BQ, et al. Inflammation induces hemorrhage in thrombocytopenia. Blood. 2008;111(10):4958–64.

113. Mazzucco L, Borzini P, Gope R. Platelet-derived factors involved in tissue repair-from signal to function. Transfus Med Rev. 2010;24(3):218–34.

114. Rafii S, Cao Z, Lis R, Siempos II, Chavez D, Shido K, et al. Platelet-derived SDF-1 primes the pulmonary capillary vascular niche to drive lung alveolar regeneration. Nat Cell Biol. 2015;17(2):123–36.

115. Morel O, Toti F, Morel N, Freyssinet JM. Microparticles in endothelial cell and vascular homeostasis: are they really noxious? Haematologica. 2009;94(3):313–7.

116. Yeaman MR. Platelets: at the nexus of antimicrobial defence. Nat Rev Microbiol. 2014;12(6):426–37.

117. Cox D, Kerrigan SW, Watson SP. Platelets and the innate immune system: mechanisms of bacterial-induced platelet activation. J Thromb Haemost. 2011;9(6):1097–107.

118. Kerrigan SW. The expanding field of platelet-bacterial interconnections. Platelets. 2015;26(4):293–301.

119. de Stoppelaar SF, Claushuis TA, Schaap MC, Hou B, van der Poll T, Nieuwland R, et al. Toll-like receptor signalling is not involved in platelet response to streptococcus pneumoniae in vitro or in vivo. PLoS ONE. 2016;11(6):e0156977.

120. Hamzeh-Cognasse H, Damien P, Chabert A, Pozzetto B, Cognasse F, Garraud O. Platelets and infections—complex interactions with bacteria. Front Immunol. 2015;6:82.

121. Fitzgerald JR, Foster TJ, Cox D. The interaction of bacterial pathogens with platelets. Nat Rev Microbiol. 2006;4(6):445–57.

122. Chan JK, Roth J, Oppenheim JJ, Tracey KJ, Vogl T, Feldmann M, et al. Alarmins: awaiting a clinical response. J Clin Investig. 2012;122(8):2711–9.

123. Semeraro F, Ammollo CT, Morrissey JH, Dale GL, Friese P, Esmon NL, et al. Extracellular histones promote thrombin generation through platelet-dependent mechanisms: involvement of platelet TLR2 and TLR4. Blood. 2011;118(7):1952–61.

124. de Stoppelaar SF, van 't Veer C, van der Poll T. The role of platelets in sepsis. Thromb Haemost. 2014;112(4):666–77.

125. Elzey BD, Sprague DL, Ratliff TL. The emerging role of platelets in adaptive immunity. Cell Immunol. 2005;238(1):1–9.

126. Middleton E, Rondina MT. Platelets in infectious disease. Hematol Am Soc Hematol Educ Program. 2016;2016(1):256–61.

127. Dankert J, van der Werff J, Zaat SA, Joldersma W, Klein D, Hess J. Involvement of bactericidal factors from thrombin-stimulated platelets in clearance of adherent viridans streptococci in experimental infective endocarditis. Infect Immun. 1995;63(2):663–71.

128. McMorran BJ, Marshall VM, de Graaf C, Drysdale KE, Shabbar M, Smyth GK, et al. Platelets kill intraerythrocytic malarial parasites and mediate survival to infection. Science. 2009;323(5915):797–800.

129. de Stoppelaar SF, van 't Veer C, Claushuis TA, Albersen BJ, Roelofs JJ, van der Poll T. Thrombocytopenia impairs host defense in gram-negative pneumonia-derived sepsis in mice. Blood. 2014;124(25):3781–90.

130. Kahn F, Hurley S, Shannon O. Platelets promote bacterial dissemination in a mouse model of streptococcal sepsis. Microbes Infect. 2013;15(10–11):669–76.

131. Rittirsch D, Hoesel LM, Ward PA. The disconnect between animal models of sepsis and human sepsis. J Leukoc Biol. 2007;81(1):137–43.

132. Doi K, Leelahavanichkul A, Yuen PS, Star RA. Animal models of sepsis and sepsis-induced kidney injury. J Clin Investig. 2009;119(10):2868–78.

133. Ward PA. New approaches to the study of sepsis. EMBO Mol Med. 2012;4(12):1234–43.

134. Fink MP. Animal models of sepsis. Virulence. 2014;5(1):143–53.

135. Vincent JL. Microvascular endothelial dysfunction: a renewed appreciation of sepsis pathophysiology. Crit Care. 2001;5(2):S1–5.

136. Aird WC. The role of the endothelium in severe sepsis and multiple organ dysfunction syndrome. Blood. 2003;101(10):3765–77.

137. Bateman RM, Sharpe MD, Ellis CG. Bench-to-bedside review: microvascular dysfunction in sepsis–hemodynamics, oxygen transport, and nitric oxide. Crit Care. 2003;7(5):359–73.

138. Peters K, Unger RE, Brunner J, Kirkpatrick CJ. Molecular basis of endothelial dysfunction in sepsis. Cardiovasc Res. 2003;60(1):49–57.

139. Warkentin TE, Aird WC, Rand JH. Platelet-endothelial interactions: sepsis, HIT, and antiphospholipid syndrome. Hematol Am Soc Hematol Educ Program. 2003;2003:497–519.

140. Matsuda N, Hattori Y. Vascular biology in sepsis: pathophysiological and therapeutic significance of vascular dysfunction. J Smooth Muscle Res. 2007;43(4):117–37.

141. Schouten M, Wiersinga WJ, Levi M, van der Poll T. Inflammation, endothelium, and coagulation in sepsis. J Leukoc Biol. 2008;83(3):536–45.

142. Gando S. Microvascular thrombosis and multiple organ dysfunction syndrome. Crit Care Med. 2010;38(2 Suppl):S35–42.

143. Goldenberg NM, Steinberg BE, Slutsky AS, Lee WL. Broken barriers: a new take on sepsis pathogenesis. Sci Transl Med. 2011;3(88):88ps25.

144. Tyml K. Critical role for oxidative stress, platelets, and coagulation in capillary blood flow impairment in sepsis. Microcirculation. 2011;18(2):152–62.

145. Boisrame-Helms J, Kremer H, Schini-Kerth V, Meziani F. Endothelial dysfunction in sepsis. Curr Vasc Pharmacol. 2013;11(2):150–60.

146. De Backer D, Orbegozo Cortes D, Donadello K, Vincent JL. Pathophysiology of microcirculatory dysfunction and the pathogenesis of septic shock. Virulence. 2014;5(1):73–9.

147. Opal SM, van der Poll T. Endothelial barrier dysfunction in septic shock. J Int Med. 2015;277(3):277–93.

148. Ince C, Mayeux PR, Nguyen T, Gomez H, Kellum JA, Ospina-Tascon GA, et al. The endothelium in sepsis. Shock. 2016;45(3):259–70.

149. Xing K, Murthy S, Liles WC, Singh JM. Clinical utility of biomarkers of endothelial activation in sepsis–a systematic review. Crit Care. 2012;16(1):R7.

150. Ait-Oufella H, Maury E, Lehoux S, Guidet B, Offenstadt G. The endothelium: physiological functions and role in microcirculatory failure during severe sepsis. Intensive Care Med. 2010;36(8):1286–98.

151. Vincent JL, De Backer D. Circulatory shock. N Engl J Med. 2013;369(18):1726–34.

152. Gawaz M, Dickfeld T, Bogner C, Fateh-Moghadam S, Neumann FJ. Platelet function in septic multiple organ dysfunction syndrome. Intensive Care Med. 1997;23(4):379–85.

153. Hurley SM, Lutay N, Holmqvist B, Shannon O. The dynamics of platelet activation during the progression of streptococcal sepsis. PLoS ONE. 2016;11(9):e0163531.

154. Levi M. Platelets in critical illness. Semin Thromb Hemost. 2016;42(3):252–7.

155. Heffner JE, Sahn SA, Repine JE. The role of platelets in the adult respiratory distress syndrome. Culprits or bystanders? Am Rev Respir Dis. 1987;135(2):482–92.

156. Bozza FA, Shah AM, Weyrich AS, Zimmerman GA. Amicus or adversary: platelets in lung biology, acute injury, and inflammation. Am J Respir Cell Mol Biol. 2009;40(2):123–34.

157. Reilly JP, Christie JD. Linking genetics to ARDS pathogenesis: the role of the platelet. Chest. 2015;147(3):585–6.

158. Yadav H, Kor DJ. Platelets in the pathogenesis of acute respiratory distress syndrome. Am J Physiol Lung Cell Mol Physiol. 2015;28:ajplung 00266.

159. Ware LB, Matthay MA. The acute respiratory distress syndrome. N Engl J Med. 2000;342(18):1334–49.

160. Bhattacharya J, Matthay MA. Regulation and repair of the alveolar-capillary barrier in acute lung injury. Annu Rev Physiol. 2013;75:593–615.

161. Kiefmann R, Heckel K, Schenkat S, Dorger M, Wesierska-Gadek J, Goetz AE. Platelet-endothelial cell interaction in pulmonary micro-circulation: the role of PARS. Thromb Haemost. 2004;91(4):761–70.

162. Zarbock A, Singbartl K, Ley K. Complete reversal of acid-induced acute lung injury by blocking of platelet-neutrophil aggregation. J Clin Investig. 2006;116(12):3211–9.

163. Looney MR, Nguyen JX, Hu Y, Van Ziffle JA, Lowell CA, Matthay MA. Platelet depletion and aspirin treatment protect mice in a two-event model of transfusion-related acute lung injury. J Clin Investig. 2009;119(11):3450–61.

164. Ortiz-Munoz G, Mallavia B, Bins A, Headley M, Krummel MF, Looney MR. Aspirin-triggered 15-epi-lipoxin A4 regulates neutrophil-platelet aggregation and attenuates acute lung injury in mice. Blood. 2014;124(17):2625–34.

165. Katz JN, Kolappa KP, Becker RC. Beyond thrombosis: the versatile platelet in critical illness. Chest. 2011;139(3):658–68.

166. Sharron M, Hoptay CE, Wiles AA, Garvin LM, Geha M, Benton AS, et al. Platelets induce apoptosis during sepsis in a contact-dependent manner that is inhibited by GPIIb/IIIa blockade. PLoS ONE. 2012;7(7):e41549.

167. Brown KA, Brain SD, Pearson JD, Edgeworth JD, Lewis SM, Treacher DF. Neutrophils in development of multiple organ failure in sepsis. Lancet. 2006;368(9530):157–69.

168. Zarbock A, Ley K. The role of platelets in acute lung injury (ALI). Front Biosci (Landmark Ed). 2009;01(14):150–8.

169. Idell S. Coagulation, fibrinolysis, and fibrin deposition in acute lung injury. Crit Care Med. 2003;31(4 Suppl):S213–20.

170. Caudrillier A, Kessenbrock K, Gilliss BM, Nguyen JX, Marques MB, Monestier M, et al. Platelets induce neutrophil extracellular traps in transfusion-related acute lung injury. J Clin Investig. 2012;122(7):2661–71.

171. McVey M, Tabuchi A, Kuebler WM. Microparticles and acute lung injury. Am J Physiol Lung Cell Mol Physiol. 2012;303(5):L364–81.

172. Asaduzzaman M, Lavasani S, Rahman M, Zhang S, Braun OO, Jeppsson B, et al. Platelets support pulmonary recruitment of neutrophils in abdominal sepsis. Crit Care Med. 2009;37(4):1389–96.

173. Cloutier N, Pare A, Farndale RW, Schumacher HR, Nigrovic PA, Lacroix S, et al. Platelets can enhance vascular permeability. Blood. 2012;120(6):1334–43.

174. Reddy AJ, Kleeberger SR. Genetic polymorphisms associated with acute lung injury. Pharmacogenomics. 2009;10(9):1527–39.

175. Wei Y, Wang Z, Su L, Chen F, Tejera P, Bajwa EK, et al. Platelet count mediates the contribution of a genetic variant in LRRC16A to ARDS risk. Chest. 2015;147(3):607–17.

176. De Backer D, Creteur J, Preiser JC, Dubois MJ, Vincent JL. Microvascular blood flow is altered in patients with sepsis. Am J Respir Crit Care Med. 2002;166(1):98–104.

177. Schrier RW, Wang W. Acute renal failure and sepsis. N Engl J Med. 2004;351(2):159–69.

178. Langenberg C, Wan L, Egi M, May CN, Bellomo R. Renal blood flow in experimental septic acute renal failure. Kidney Int. 2006;69(11):1996–2002.

179. Shum HP, Yan WW, Chan TM. Recent knowledge on the pathophysiology of septic acute kidney injury: a narrative review. J Crit Care. 2016;31(1):82–9.

180. Post EH, Kellum JA, Bellomo R, Vincent JL. Renal perfusion in sepsis: from macro- to microcirculation. Kidney Int. 2017;91(1):45–60.

181. Wan L, Bagshaw SM, Langenberg C, Saotome T, May C, Bellomo R. Pathophysiology of septic acute kidney injury: what do we really know? Crit Care Med. 2008;36(4 Suppl):S198–203.

182. Lerolle N, Nochy D, Guerot E, Bruneval P, Fagon JY, Diehl JL, et al. Histopathology of septic shock induced acute kidney injury: apoptosis and leukocytic infiltration. Intensive Care Med. 2010;36(3):471–8.

183. Jacobs R, Honore PM, Joannes-Boyau O, Boer W, De Regt J, De Waele E, et al. Septic acute kidney injury: the culprit is inflammatory apoptosis rather than ischemic necrosis. Blood Purif. 2011;32(4):262–5.

184. Takasu O, Gaut JP, Watanabe E, To K, Fagley RE, Sato B, et al. Mechanisms of cardiac and renal dysfunction in patients dying of sepsis. Am J Respir Crit Care Med. 2013;187(5):509–17.

185. Langenberg C, Bellomo R, May C, Wan L, Egi M, Morgera S. Renal blood flow in sepsis. Crit Care. 2005;9(4):R363–74.

186. Prowle JR, Ishikawa K, May CN, Bellomo R. Renal blood flow during acute renal failure in man. Blood Purif. 2009;28(3):216–25.

187. Chvojka J, Sykora R, Karvunidis T, Radej J, Krouzecky A, Novak I, et al. New developments in septic acute kidney injury. Physiol Res. 2010;59(6):859–69.

188. Murugan R, Karajala-Subramanyam V, Lee M, Yende S, Kong L, Carter M, et al. Acute kidney injury in non-severe pneumonia is associated with an increased immune response and lower survival. Kidney Int. 2010;77(6):527–35.

189. Kellum JA. Impaired renal blood flow and the 'spicy food' hypothesis of acute kidney injury. Crit Care Med. 2011;39(4):901–3.

190. Zarjou A, Agarwal A. Sepsis and acute kidney injury. J Am Soc Nephrol. 2011;22(6):999–1006.

191. Basile DP, Anderson MD, Sutton TA. Pathophysiology of acute kidney injury. Compr Physiol. 2012;2(2):1303–53.

192. Gomez H, Ince C, De Backer D, Pickkers P, Payen D, Hotchkiss J, et al. A unified theory of sepsis-induced acute kidney injury: inflammation, microcirculatory dysfunction, bioenergetics, and the tubular cell adaptation to injury. Shock. 2014;41(1):3–11.

193. Umbro I, Gentile G, Tinti F, Muiesan P, Mitterhofer AP. Recent advances in pathophysiology and biomarkers of sepsis-induced acute kidney injury. J Infect. 2015;72:131–42.

194. Gomez H, Kellum JA. Sepsis-induced acute kidney injury. Curr Opin Crit Care. 2016;22(6):546–53.

195. Bellomo R, Kellum JA, Ronco C, Wald R, Martensson J, Maiden M, et al. Acute kidney injury in sepsis. Intensive Care Med. 2017;43(6):816–28.

196. Bonventre JV, Yang L. Cellular pathophysiology of ischemic acute kidney injury. J Clin Investig. 2011;121(11):4210–21.

197. Zarbock A, Gomez H, Kellum JA. Sepsis-induced acute kidney injury revisited: pathophysiology, prevention and future therapies. Curr Opin Crit Care. 2014;20(6):588–95.

198. Glodowski SD, Wagener G. New insights into the mechanisms of acute kidney injury in the intensive care unit. J Clin Anesth. 2015;27(2):175–80.

199. Schwarzenberger C, Sradnick J, Lerea KM, Goligorsky MS, Nieswandt B, Hugo CP, et al. Platelets are relevant mediators of renal injury induced by primary endothelial lesions. Am J Physiol Renal Physiol. 2015;308(11):F1238–46.

200. Wiesinger A, Peters W, Chappell D, Kentrup D, Reuter S, Pavenstadt H, et al. Nanomechanics of the endothelial glycocalyx in experimental sepsis. PLoS ONE. 2013;8(11):e80905.

201. Becker BF, Jacob M, Leipert S, Salmon AH, Chappell D. Degradation of the endothelial glycocalyx in clinical settings: searching for the shed-dases. Br J Clin Pharmacol. 2015;80(3):389–402.

202. Chelazzi C, Villa G, Mancinelli P, De Gaudio AR, Adembri C. Glycocalyx and sepsis-induced alterations in vascular permeability. Crit Care. 2015;28(19):26.

203. Martin L, Koczera P, Zechendorf E, Schuerholz T. The endothelial glyco-calyx: new diagnostic and therapeutic approaches in sepsis. Biomed Res Int. 2016;2016:3758278.

204. Zuk A, Bonventre JV. Acute kidney injury. Annu Rev Med. 2016;14(67):293–307.

205. Doi K, Rabb H. Impact of acute kidney injury on distant organ func-tion: recent findings and potential therapeutic targets. Kidney Int. 2016;89(3):555–64.

206. Lapchak PH, Kannan L, Ioannou A, Rani P, Karian P, Dalle Lucca JJ, et al. Platelets orchestrate remote tissue damage after mesen-teric ischemia-reperfusion. Am J Physiol Gastrointest Liver Physiol. 2012;302(8):G888–97.

207. Singbartl K, Bishop JV, Wen X, Murugan R, Chandra S, Filippi MD, et al. Differential effects of kidney-lung cross-talk during acute kidney injury and bacterial pneumonia. Kidney Int. 2011;80(6):633–44.

208. Lapchak PH, Ioannou A, Kannan L, Rani P, Dalle Lucca JJ, Tsokos GC. Platelet-associated CD40/CD154 mediates remote tissue damage after mesenteric ischemia/reperfusion injury. PLoS ONE. 2012;7(2):e32260.

209. Lapchak PH, Ioannou A, Rani P, Lieberman LA, Yoshiya K, Kannan L, et al. The role of platelet factor 4 in local and remote tissue damage in a mouse model of mesenteric ischemia/reperfusion injury. PLoS ONE. 2012;7(7):e39934.

210. Henn V, Slupsky JR, Grafe M, Anagnostopoulos I, Forster R, Muller-Berghaus G, et al. CD40 ligand on activated platelets triggers an inflam-matory reaction of endothelial cells. Nature. 1998;391(6667):591–4.

211. Frossard JL, Kwak B, Chanson M, Morel P, Hadengue A, Mach F. Cd40 ligand-deficient mice are protected against cerulein-induced acute pancreatitis and pancreatitis-associated lung injury. Gastroenterology. 2001;121(1):184–94.

212. Hashimoto N, Kawabe T, Imaizumi K, Hara T, Okamoto M, Kojima K, et al. CD40 plays a crucial role in lipopolysaccharide-induced acute lung injury. Am J Respir Cell Mol Biol. 2004;30(6):808–15.

213. Rahman M, Zhang S, Chew M, Ersson A, Jeppsson B, Thorlacius H. Plate-let-derived CD40L (CD154) mediates neutrophil upregulation of Mac-1 and recruitment in septic lung injury. Ann Surg. 2009;250(5):783–90.

214. Stephan F, Hollande J, Richard O, Cheffi A, Maier-Redelsperger M, Flahault A. Thrombocytopenia in a surgical ICU. Chest. 1999;115(5):1363–70.

215. Mavrommatis AC, Theodoridis T, Orfanidou A, Roussos C, Christopou-lou-Kokkinou V, Zakynthinos S. Coagulation system and platelets are fully activated in uncomplicated sepsis. Crit Care Med. 2000;28(2):451–7.

216. Nijsten MW, ten Duis HJ, Zijlstra JG, Porte RJ, Zwaveling JH, Paling JC, et al. Blunted rise in platelet count in critically ill patients is associated with worse outcome. Crit Care Med. 2000;28(12):3843–6.

217. Sharma B, Sharma M, Majumder M, Steier W, Sangal A, Kalawar M. Thrombocytopenia in septic shock patients–a prospective obser-vational study of incidence, risk factors and correlation with clinical outcome. Anaesth Intensive Care. 2007;35(6):874–80.

218. Thiolliere F, Serre-Sapin AF, Reignier J, Benedit M, Constantin JM, Lebert C, et al. Epidemiology and outcome of thrombocytopenic patients in the intensive care unit: results of a prospective multicenter study. Intensive Care Med. 2013;39(8):1460–8.

219. Williamson DR, Lesur O, Tetrault JP, Nault V, Pilon D. Thrombocytope-nia in the critically ill: prevalence, incidence, risk factors, and clinical outcomes. Can J Anaesth. 2013;60(7):641–51.

220. Aydemir H, Piskin N, Akduman D, Kokturk F, Aktas E. Platelet and mean platelet volume kinetics in adult patients with sepsis. Platelets. 2015;26(4):331–5.

221. Thiery-Antier N, Binquet C, Vinault S, Meziani F, Boisrame-Helms J, Que-not JP. Is thrombocytopenia an early prognostic marker in septic shock? Crit Care Med. 2016;44(4):764–72.

222. Greinacher A, Selleng K. Thrombocytopenia in the intensive care unit patient. Hematol Am Soc Hematol Educ Program. 2010;2010:135–43.

223. Brun-Buisson C, Doyon F, Carlet J, Dellamonica P, Gouin F, Lepoutre A, et al. Incidence, risk factors, and outcome of severe sepsis and septic shock in adults. A multicenter prospective study in intensive care units. French ICU Group for Severe Sepsis. JAMA. 1995;274(12):968–74.

224. Martin CM, Priestap F, Fisher H, Fowler RA, Heyland DK, Keenan SP, et al. A prospective, observational registry of patients with severe sepsis: the Canadian Sepsis Treatment and Response Registry. Crit Care Med. 2009;37(1):81–8.

225. Selleng S, Malowsky B, Strobel U, Wessel A, Ittermann T, Wollert HG, et al. Early-onset and persisting thrombocytopenia in post-cardiac sur-gery patients is rarely due to heparin-induced thrombocytopenia, even when antibody tests are positive. J Thromb Haemost. 2010;8(1):30–6.

226. Vandijck DM, Blot SI, De Waele JJ, Hoste EA, Vandewoude KH, Decruyen-aere JM. Thrombocytopenia and outcome in critically ill patients with bloodstream infection. Heart Lung. 2010;39(1):21–6.

227. Lim SY, Jeon EJ, Kim HJ, Jeon K, Um SW, Koh WJ, et al. The incidence, causes, and prognostic significance of new-onset thrombocytopenia in intensive care units: a prospective cohort study in a Korean hospital. J Korean Med Sci. 2012;27(11):1418–23.

228. Lieberman L, Bercovitz RS, Sholapur NS, Heddle NM, Stanworth SJ, Arnold DM. Platelet transfusions for critically ill patients with thrombo-cytopenia. Blood. 2014;123(8):1146–51 **(quiz 280)**.

229. Pene F, Benoit DD. Thrombocytopenia in the critically ill: considering pathophysiology rather than looking for a magic threshold. Intensive Care Med. 2013;39(9):1656–9.

230. Greinacher A, Selleng S. How I evaluate and treat thrombocytopenia in the intensive care unit patient. Blood. 2016;128(26):3032–42.

231. Ning S, Barty R, Liu Y, Heddle NM, Rochwerg B, Arnold DM. Platelet transfusion practices in the icu: data from a large transfusion registry. Chest. 2016;150(3):516–23.

232. Antier N, Quenot JP, Doise JM, Noel R, Demaistre E, Devilliers H. Mecha-nisms and etiologies of thrombocytopenia in the intensive care unit: impact of extensive investigations. Ann Intensive Care. 2014;4:24.

233. Larkin CM, Santos-Martinez MJ, Ryan T, Radomski MW. Sepsis-associated thrombocytopenia. Thromb Res. 2016;141:11–6.

234. Pigozzi L, Aron JP, Ball J, Cecconi M. Understanding platelet dysfunction in sepsis. Intensive Care Med. 2016;42(4):583–6.

235. De Blasi RA, Cardelli P, Costante A, Sandri M, Mercieri M, Arcioni R. Immature platelet fraction in predicting sepsis in critically ill patients. Intensive Care Med. 2013;39(4):636–43.

236. Levi M. Platelets at a crossroad of pathogenic pathways in sepsis. J Thromb Haemost. 2004;2(12):2094–5.

237. Yaguchi A, Lobo FL, Vincent JL, Pradier O. Platelet function in sepsis. J Thromb Haemost. 2004;2(12):2096–102.

238. Goyette RE, Key NS, Ely EW. Hematologic changes in sepsis and their therapeutic implications. Semin Respir Crit Care Med. 2004;25(6):645–59.

239. Arnold DM, Lim W. A rational approach to the diagnosis and manage-ment of thrombocytopenia in the hospitalized patient. Semin Hematol. 2011;48(4):251–8.

240. Thiele T, Selleng K, Selleng S, Greinacher A, Bakchoul T. Thrombocyto-penia in the intensive care unit-diagnostic approach and management. Semin Hematol. 2013;50(3):239–50.

241. Smock KJ, Perkins SL. Thrombocytopenia: an update. Int J Lab Hematol. 2014;36(3):269–78.

242. Thachil J, Warkentin TE. How do we approach thrombocytopenia in critically ill patients? Br J Haematol. 2017;177(1):27–38.

243. Remick DG. Cytokine therapeutics for the treatment of sepsis: why has nothing worked? Curr Pharm Des. 2003;9(1):75–82.

244. Thomas MR, Outteridge SN, Ajjan RA, Phoenix F, Sangha GK, Faulkner RE, et al. Platelet P2Y12 inhibitors reduce systemic inflammation and its prothrombotic effects in an experimental human model. Arterioscler Thromb Vasc Biol. 2015;35(12):2562–70.

245. Winning J, Neumann J, Kohl M, Claus RA, Reinhart K, Bauer M, et al. Antiplatelet drugs and outcome in mixed admissions to an intensive care unit. Crit Care Med. 2010;38(1):32–7.

246. Erlich JM, Talmor DS, Cartin-Ceba R, Gajic O, Kor DJ. Prehospitalization antiplatelet therapy is associated with a reduced incidence of acute lung injury: a population-based cohort study. Chest. 2011;139(2):289–95.

247. Losche W, Boettel J, Kabisch B, Winning J, Claus RA, Bauer M. Do aspirin and other antiplatelet drugs reduce the mortality in critically ill patients? Thrombosis. 2012;2012:720254.

248. Eisen DP, Reid D, McBryde ES. Acetyl salicylic acid usage and mortality in critically ill patients with the systemic inflammatory response syndrome and sepsis. Crit Care Med. 2012;40(6):1761–7.

249. Valerio-Rojas JC, Jaffer IJ, Kor DJ, Gajic O, Cartin-Ceba R. Outcomes of severe sepsis and septic shock patients on chronic antiplatelet treatment: a historical cohort study. Crit Care Res Pract. 2013;2013:782573.

250. Sossdorf M, Otto GP, Boettel J, Winning J, Losche W. Benefit of low-dose aspirin and non-steroidal anti-inflammatory drugs in septic patients. Crit Care. 2013;17(1):402.

251. Otto GP, Sossdorf M, Boettel J, Kabisch B, Breuel H, Winning J, et al. Effects of low-dose acetylsalicylic acid and atherosclerotic vascular diseases on the outcome in patients with severe sepsis or septic shock. Platelets. 2013;24(6):480–5.

252. Akinosoglou K, Alexopoulos D. Use of antiplatelet agents in sepsis: a glimpse into the future. Thromb Res. 2014;133(2):131–8.

253. Chen W, Janz DR, Bastarache JA, May AK, O'Neal HR Jr, Bernard GR, et al. Prehospital aspirin use is associated with reduced risk of acute respiratory distress syndrome in critically ill patients: a propensity-adjusted analysis. Crit Care Med. 2015;43(4):801–7.

254. Toner P, McAuley DF, Shyamsundar M. Aspirin as a potential treatment in sepsis or acute respiratory distress syndrome. Crit Care. 2015;19:374.

255. Tsai MJ, Ou SM, Shih CJ, Chao PW, Wang LF, Shih YN, et al. Association of prior antiplatelet agents with mortality in sepsis patients: a nationwide population-based cohort study. Intensive Care Med. 2015;41(5):806–13.

256. Kor DJ, Erlich J, Gong MN, Malinchoc M, Carter RE, Gajic O, et al. Association of prehospitalization aspirin therapy and acute lung injury: results of a multicenter international observational study of at-risk patients. Crit Care Med. 2011;39(11):2393–400.

257. Gum PA, Kottke-Marchant K, Poggio ED, Gurm H, Welsh PA, Brooks L, et al. Profile and prevalence of aspirin resistance in patients with cardiovascular disease. Am J Cardiol. 2001;88(3):230–5.

258. Nguyen TA, Diodati JG, Pharand C. Resistance to clopidogrel: a review of the evidence. J Am Coll Cardiol. 2005;45(8):1157–64.

259. Macchi L, Sorel N, Christiaens L. Aspirin resistance: definitions, mechanisms, prevalence, and clinical significance. Curr Pharm Des. 2006;12(2):251–8.

260. Wiewel MA, de Stoppelaar SF, van Vught LA, Frencken JF, Hoogendijk AJ, Klein Klouwenberg PM, et al. Chronic antiplatelet therapy is not associated with alterations in the presentation, outcome, or host response biomarkers during sepsis: a propensity-matched analysis. Intensive Care Med. 2016;42(3):352–60.

261. Muhlestein JB. Effect of antiplatelet therapy on inflammatory markers in atherothrombotic patients. Thromb Haemost. 2010;103(1):71–82.

262. Zakynthinos SG, Papanikolaou S, Theodoridis T, Zakynthinos EG, Christopoulou-Kokkinou V, Katsaris G, et al. Sepsis severity is the major determinant of circulating thrombopoietin levels in septic patients. Crit Care Med. 2004;32(4):1004–10.

263. Lupia E, Goffi A, Bosco O, Montrucchio G. Thrombopoietin as biomarker and mediator of cardiovascular damage in critical diseases. Mediat Inflamm. 2012;2012:390892.

264. Cuccurullo A, Greco E, Lupia E, De Giuli P, Bosco O, Martin-Conte E, et al. Blockade of thrombopoietin reduces organ damage in experimental endotoxemia and polymicrobial sepsis. PLoS ONE. 2016;11(3):e0151088.

265. Wu Q, Ren J, Wu X, Wang G, Gu G, Liu S, et al. Recombinant human thrombopoietin improves platelet counts and reduces platelet transfusion possibility among patients with severe sepsis and thrombocytopenia: a prospective study. J Crit Care. 2014;29(3):362–6.

266. Van Deuren M, Neeleman C, Van 't Hek LG, Van der Meer JW. A normal platelet count at admission in acute meningococcal disease does not exclude a fulminant course. Intensive Care Med. 1998;24(2):157–61.

267. Agrawal S, Sachdev A, Gupta D, Chugh K. Platelet counts and outcome in the pediatric intensive care unit. Indian J Crit Care Med. 2008;12(3):102–8.

268. Wang L, Li H, Gu X, Wang Z, Liu S, Chen L. Effect of antiplatelet therapy on acute respiratory distress syndrome and mortality in critically ill patients: a meta-analysis. PLoS ONE. 2016;11(5):e0154754.

269. Kor DJ, Carter RE, Park PK, Festic E, Banner-Goodspeed VM, Hinds R, et al. Effect of aspirin on development of ARDS in at-risk patients presenting to the emergency department: the LIPS-A randomized clinical trial. JAMA. 2016;315(22):2406–14.

270. Osthoff M, Sidler JA, Lakatos B, Frei R, Dangel M, Weisser M, et al. Low-dose acetylsalicylic acid treatment and impact on short-term mortality in *Staphylococcus aureus* bloodstream infection: a propensity score-matched cohort study. Crit Care Med. 2016;44(4):773–81.

271. Boyle AJ, Di Gangi S, Hamid UI, Mottram LJ, McNamee L, White G, et al. Aspirin therapy in patients with acute respiratory distress syndrome (ARDS) is associated with reduced intensive care unit mortality: a prospective analysis. Crit Care. 2015;19:109.

272. O'Neal HR Jr, Koyama T, Koehler EA, Siew E, Curtis BR, Fremont RD, et al. Prehospital statin and aspirin use and the prevalence of severe sepsis and acute lung injury/acute respiratory distress syndrome. Crit Care Med. 2011;39(6):1343–50.

273. Storey RF, James SK, Siegbahn A, Varenhorst C, Held C, Ycas J, et al. Lower mortality following pulmonary adverse events and sepsis with ticagrelor compared to clopidogrel in the PLATO study. Platelets. 2014;25(7):517–25.

274. Winning J, Reichel J, Eisenhut Y, Hamacher J, Kohl M, Deigner HP, et al. Anti-platelet drugs and outcome in severe infection: clinical impact and underlying mechanisms. Platelets. 2009;20(1):50–7.

275. Gross AK, Dunn SP, Feola DJ, Martin CA, Charnigo R, Li Z, et al. Clopidogrel treatment and the incidence and severity of community acquired pneumonia in a cohort study and meta-analysis of antiplatelet therapy in pneumonia and critical illness. J Thromb Thrombolysis. 2013;35(2):147–54.

# 17

# Early goal-directed therapy using a physiological holistic view: the ANDROMEDA-SHOCK—a randomized controlled trial

Glenn Hernández[1*], Alexandre Biasi Cavalcanti[2], Gustavo Ospina-Tascón[3], Fernando Godinho Zampieri[2], Arnaldo Dubin[4], F. Javier Hurtado[5], Gilberto Friedman[6], Ricardo Castro[1], Leyla Alegría[1], Maurizio Cecconi[7], Jean-Louis Teboul[8] and Jan Bakker[1,9,10,11]The ANDROMEDA-SHOCK Study Investigators

## Abstract

**Background:** Septic shock is a highly lethal condition. Early recognition of tissue hypoperfusion and its reversion are key factors for limiting progression to multiple organ dysfunction and death. Lactate-targeted resuscitation is the gold-standard under current guidelines, although it has several pitfalls including that non-hypoxic sources of lactate might predominate in an unknown proportion of patients. Peripheral perfusion-targeted resuscitation might provide a real-time response to increases in flow that could lead to a more timely decision to stop resuscitation, thus avoiding fluid overload and the risks of over-resuscitation. This article reports the rationale, study design and analysis plan of the ANDROMEDA-SHOCK Study.

**Methods:** ANDROMEDA-SHOCK is a randomized controlled trial which aims to determine if a peripheral perfusion-targeted resuscitation is associated with lower 28-day mortality compared to a lactate-targeted resuscitation in patients with septic shock with less than 4 h of diagnosis. Both groups will be treated with the same sequential approach during the 8-hour study period pursuing normalization of capillary refill time versus normalization or a decrease of more than 20% of lactate every 2 h. The common protocol starts with fluid responsiveness assessment and fluid loading in responders, followed by a vasopressor and an inodilator test if necessary. The primary outcome is 28-day mortality, and the secondary outcomes are: free days of mechanical ventilation, renal replacement therapy and vasopressor support during the first 28 days after randomization; multiple organ dysfunction during the first 72 h after randomization; intensive care unit and hospital lengths of stay; and all-cause mortality at 90-day. A sample size of 422 patients was calculated to detect a 15% absolute reduction in mortality in the peripheral perfusion group with 90% power and two-tailed type I error of 5%. All analysis will follow the intention-to-treat principle.

**Conclusions:** If peripheral perfusion-targeted resuscitation improves 28-day mortality, this could lead to simplified algorithms, assessing almost in real-time the reperfusion process, and pursuing more physiologically sound objectives. At the end, it might prevent the risk of over-resuscitation and lead to a better utilization of intensive care unit resources.

**Keywords:** Septic shock, Resuscitation, Peripheral perfusion, Lactate, Fluid responsiveness

*Correspondence: glennguru@gmail.com
[1] Departamento de Medicina Intensiva, Facultad de Medicina, Pontificia Universidad Católica de Chile, Diagonal Paraguay 362, Santiago, Chile
Full list of author information is available at the end of the article

## Background

Septic shock is a potentially lethal condition associated with a mortality risk of up to 30–60% [1, 2]. Early recognition of tissue hypoperfusion and its reversion are key factors for limiting progression to multiple organ dysfunction and death [1–6].

Hyperlactatemia has been traditionally considered as a hallmark of ongoing tissue hypoxia and anaerobic metabolism [7, 8]. A recent study targeting a decrease in lactate levels as a resuscitation goal in critically ill patients showed a significant improvement in organ failure and outcomes associated with this endpoint [9]. Therefore, normalization of lactate levels has been recommended as a resuscitation target by current guidelines [10]. However, other non-hypoperfusion-related causes of hyperlactatemia might predominate in an unknown number of patients [11, 12]. In that setting, sustained efforts to increase cardiac output (CO) with fluids or vasoactive drugs could lead to detrimental effects of over-resuscitation [13, 14]. In addition, lactate exhibits a biphasic recovery rate even after a successful resuscitation [15], introducing an important confounder for practitioners.

Monitoring peripheral perfusion is particularly attractive because of its easy clinical accessibility and more importantly, because it could reflect the adequacy of intraabdominal visceral organ perfusion [16, 17]. The skin territory lacks auto-regulatory flow control, and therefore, sympathetic activation impairs skin perfusion during circulatory dysfunction [17], a phenomenon that could be evaluated by peripheral perfusion assessment. A robust body of evidence confirms that abnormal peripheral perfusion after initial resuscitation is associated with increased morbidity and mortality [18–23], whereby it could be used as a potential resuscitation goal [24]. In fact, the presence of a cold clammy skin, mottling or prolonged capillary refill time (CRT) has been suggested as indicators to initiate fluid resuscitation in patients with septic shock [17]. Interestingly, CRT was the first parameter to be normalized in patients surviving from septic shock and predicted lactate normalization at 24 h [18]. A recent pilot study suggests that targeting peripheral perfusion during septic shock resuscitation is safe and associated with less fluid administration and organ dysfunctions [25]. Therefore, the excellent prognosis associated with CRT recovery, its rapid-response time to fluid loading, its relative simplicity, its availability in resource-limited settings and its capacity to change in parallel with perfusion of physiologically relevant territories such as the hepatosplanchnic region [16] constitute strong reasons to evaluate the usefulness of CRT to guide resuscitation in septic shock patients.

Consequently, we decided to conduct a randomized controlled trial (RCT) comparing peripheral perfusion-targeted resuscitation (PPTR) versus lactate-targeted resuscitation (LTR) in patients with septic shock, hypothesizing that resuscitation aimed at peripheral perfusion will be associated with lower mortality rates. We also hypothesize that patients assigned to PPTR will require less volume of fluids with subsequent lower positive fluid balances. Accordingly, PPTR should be associated with less organ dysfunctions, especially at respiratory, renal and gastrointestinal levels.

## Methods

### Primary objective

To determine if PPTR is associated with lower mortality rates at 28 day than a LTR in patients with septic shock.

### Secondary objectives

To determine if a PPTR is associated with less severe multiple organ dysfunction; more mechanical ventilation (MV) free days; and less vasopressor load and renal replacement therapies (RRT) than a LTR strategy in patients with septic shock.

### Outcomes

Primary outcome will be all-cause mortality at 28-day.
  Secondary outcomes:

* Free days of MV, RRT and vasopressor support during the first 28 days after randomization;
* Multiple organ dysfunction during the first 72 h after randomization [26];
* Intensive care unit (ICU) and hospital lengths of stay;
* All-cause mortality at 90-day.

Tertiary outcomes:

* Amount of resuscitation fluids at 8 and 24-hours;
* Total fluid balance at 8, 24, 48 and 72-h;
* Occurrence of intraabdominal hypertension (IAH) during the first 72 h after randomization (%);
* Use of RRT (%)
* In-hospital mortality

### Study design

ANDROMEDA-SHOCK is a prospective, multicenter, parallel-group, randomized trial aimed to compare an 8-h protocol of PPTR vs. LTR in patients with septic shock [27].

### Patients

Consecutive adult patients ($\geq 18$ years) with septic shock will be considered eligible. Septic shock is defined as suspected or confirmed infection, plus hyperlactatemia ($\geq 2.0$ mmol per liter) and vasopressor requirements due to refractory hypotension [27]. This latter is character-ized as a systolic blood pressure (SBP) < 90 mmHg or a mean arterial pressure (MAP) < 65 mmHg after an intra-venous fluid load of at least 20 ml/kg, administered over the course of 60 min.

Patients will be excluded in case of:

- pregnancy;
- anticipated surgery or dialysis procedure during the first 8 h after septic shock diagnosis;
- Do-Not-Attempt-Resuscitation status;
- active bleeding;
- acute hematological malignancy;
- concomitant severe acute respiratory distress syn-drome (ARDS);
- more than 4 h after the onset of septic shock criteria.

An active daily screening for potentially eligible patients will be performed at all the participating ICUs.

### Randomization

Eligible patients will be randomly allocated to PPTR or LTR groups. PPTR will be aimed to normalize CRT, while LTR will target lactate normalization or a decreasing rate > 20% per 2 h of lactate levels during the 8 h of the study period (Fig. 1).

A randomization sequence with an allocation of 1:1 will be generated by a computer program. Study-group assignment will be performed by means of randomized permuted blocks of eight. Allocation concealment will be maintained by means of central randomization.

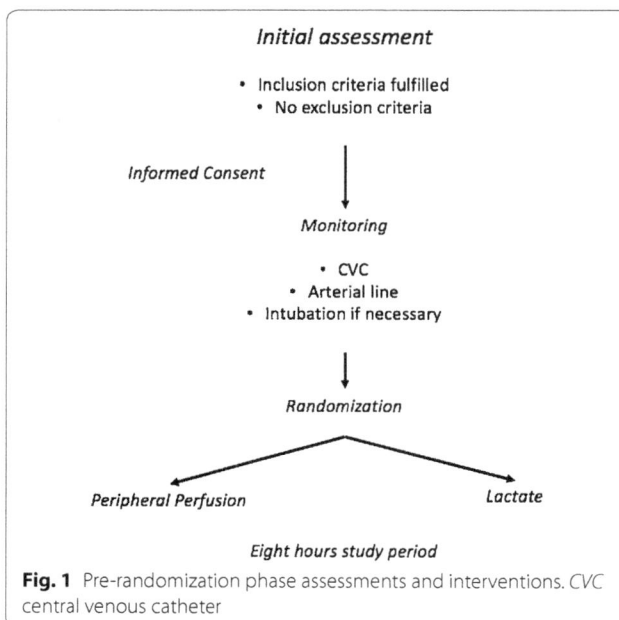

**Fig. 1** Pre-randomization phase assessments and interventions. *CVC* central venous catheter

Investigators at the sites will call a representative of the Study Coordinating Center (SCC) available 24 h/7 days through a dedicated phone number. The group to which the patient is allocated will only be disclosed after the information is recorded by the SCC. Such a measure prevents the investigator and the medical team from predicting to which treatment group the patient will be allocated.

### Interventions
#### General management protocol

Both study groups will be treated with a common gen-eral management protocol. Sepsis source identification and control, and antimicrobial therapy will be given at the discretion of the treating physician. A central venous catheter (CVC) and an arterial line will be inserted in all cases, while the use of CO monitoring (pulmonary artery catheter or transpulmonary thermodilution techniques) is recommended for patients with a past medical history of heart failure or concomitant ARDS but leaving deci-sion at discretion of the attending physician. Echocardi-ography will be performed routinely as soon as possible after admission to evaluate basal cardiac function, and to add in assessing fluid responsiveness (FR) [28]. Other dynamic predictors of response to fluids such as pulse pressure variation (PPV), stroke volume variation (SVV) or end-expiratory occlusion test (EEOT) will be used whenever applicable (see below) [28, 29]. MV will be pro-vided (when needed) under light sedation (midazolam, propofol or dexmedetomidine) and analgesia (fenta-nyl, alfentanil, morphine); tidal volume (Vt) will be lim-ited to 6–8 mL/kg and positive-end-expiratory-pressure (PEEP) will be set according to individual requirements [10]. Glycemic control will be adjusted to maintain glu-cose levels < 150 mg/dL. Norepinephrine (NE) will be the vasopressor of choice, and its dose will be adjusted to maintain a MAP ≥ 65 mmHg in all patients. Hemoglobin concentrations will be maintained at 8 g/dL or higher to optimize arterial $O_2$ content. The use of other therapies such as epinephrine, vasopressin analogues, steroids or different blood purification techniques like high-volume hemofiltration (HVHF) will be provided according to the usual practice at the involved centers in patients evolv-ing with refractory septic shock. Finally, stress ulcer and venous thrombosis prophylaxis will be managed accord-ing to international recommendations [10].

#### Study protocol

A sequential approach to resuscitation will be followed in both groups as shown in Fig. 2. After fulfilling inclu-sion criteria and discarding all exclusion conditions, an informed consent will be obtained. Basal measurements including hemodynamics and blood sampling will be

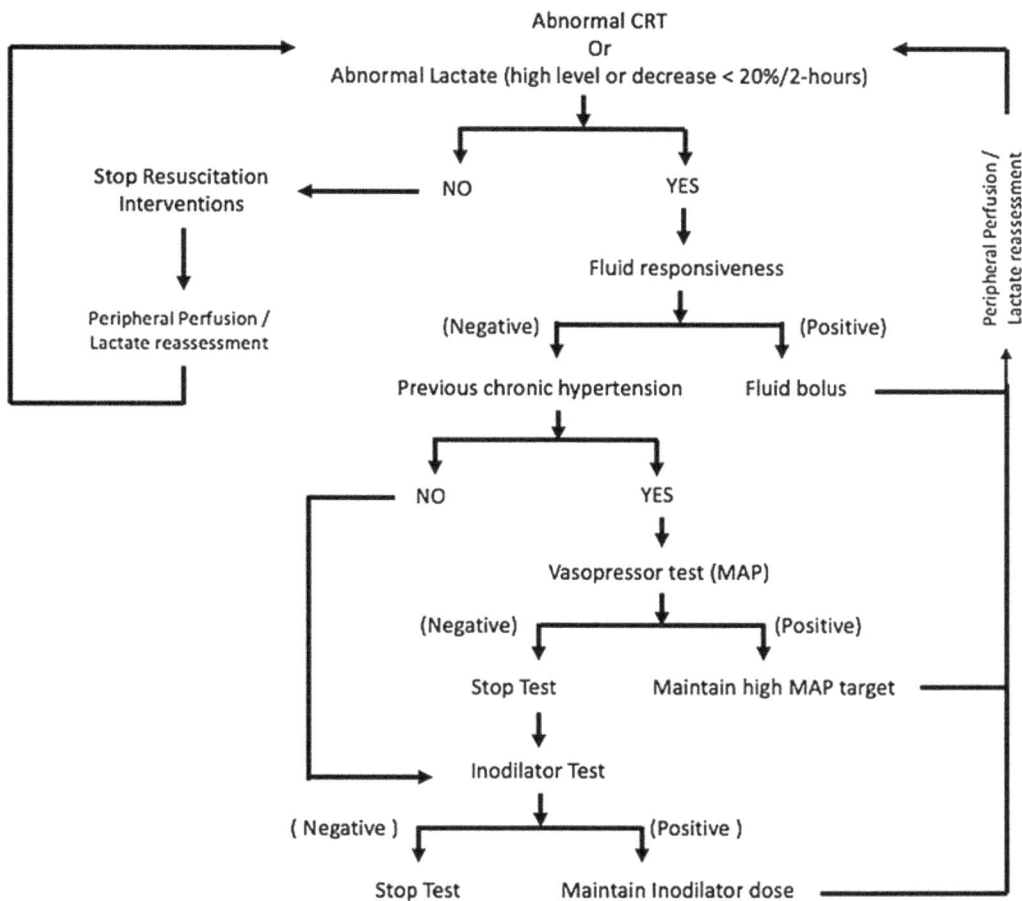

**Fig. 2** Resuscitation protocol for both groups. The figure describes the sequential approach to resuscitation. The process starts with fluid loading according to the status of fluid responsiveness. If the goal is not obtained, the second step is a vasopressor test, and then an inodilator test. *CRT,* capillary refill time

performed at Time 0 (T0) representing the starting point just after randomization. The intervention period will be extended for 8 h. All other treatments, during the intervention period and after, will be at the discretion of the treating clinicians according to their local usual clinical practices.

## Tests and procedures during the study period
### Capillary refill time assessment
CRT will be measured by applying firm pressure to the ventral surface of the right index finger distal phalanx with a glass microscope slide. The pressure will be increased until the skin is blank and then maintained for 10 s. The time for return of the normal skin color will be registered with a chronometer. A CRT > 3 s will be considered as abnormal [30].

### Lactate measurements
A lactate value ≥ 2.0 mmol per liter will be considered as abnormal. Arterial lactate levels will be measured at each center, either at point of care or central laboratories (point of care: GEM 4000, Instrumentation Lab, IL, USA; central laboratories: Cobas b221, Roche Diagnostics International; Basel, CH).

### Fluid responsiveness (Fig. 3)
FR will be assessed using a structured approach outlined in Fig. 2. Dynamic predictors of FR will be evaluated depending on the individual status, i.e., considering if under MV or spontaneous breathing, Vt, respiratory rate (RR), respiratory system compliance and the presence of arrhythmias. The protocol for patients under MV is shown in Fig. 3 [28, 29].

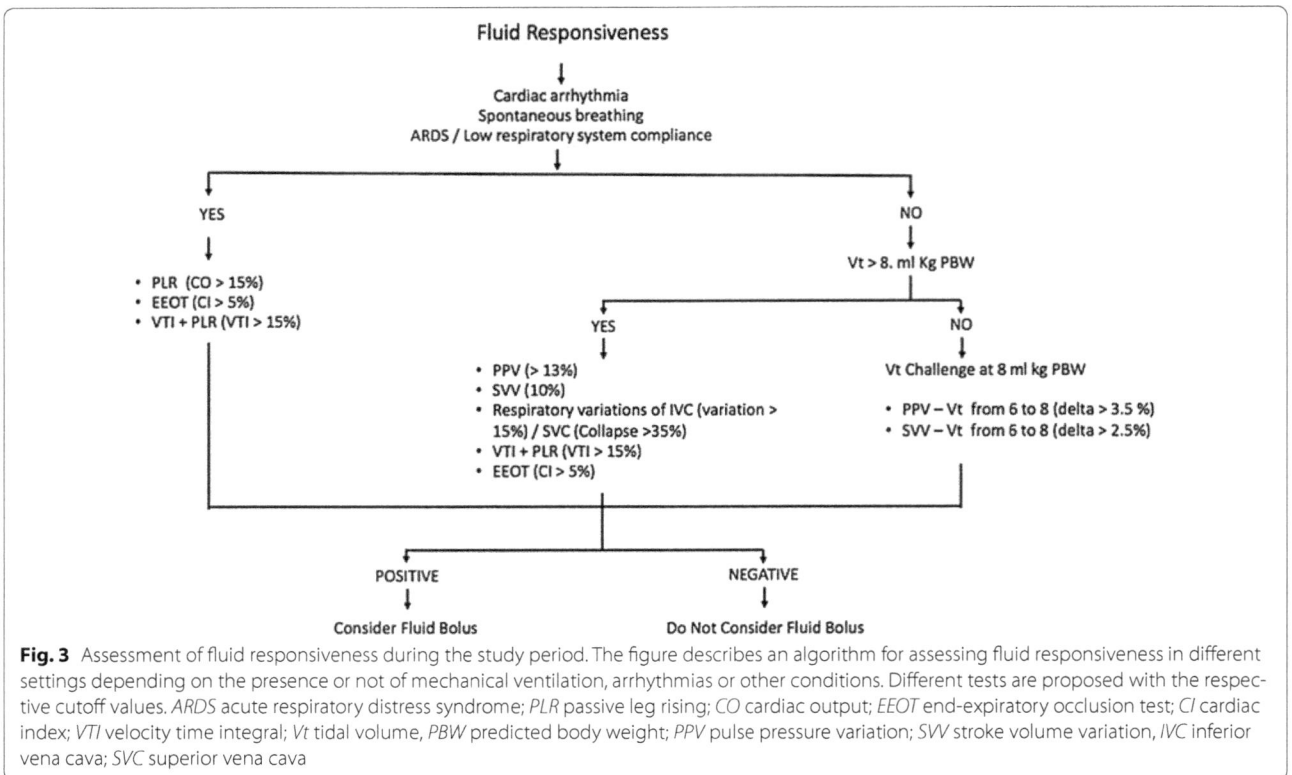

**Fig. 3** Assessment of fluid responsiveness during the study period. The figure describes an algorithm for assessing fluid responsiveness in different settings depending on the presence or not of mechanical ventilation, arrhythmias or other conditions. Different tests are proposed with the respective cutoff values. *ARDS* acute respiratory distress syndrome; *PLR* passive leg rising; *CO* cardiac output; *EEOT* end-expiratory occlusion test; *CI* cardiac index; *VTI* velocity time integral; *Vt* tidal volume, *PBW* predicted body weight; *PPV* pulse pressure variation; *SVV* stroke volume variation, *IVC* inferior vena cava; *SVC* superior vena cava

### Fluid challenges

In FR$^+$ patients, the first resuscitation step will be to administer a fluid bolus (FB) of 500 ml of crystalloids every 30 min until normalizing CRT in the PPTR group. In the LTR group, FB will be stopped if at 2 h lactate is normalized or has decreased > 20%, or previously if after any of the fluid boluses, central venous pressure (CVP) has increased $\geq$ 5 mmHg or the patients have become fluid unresponsive (FR$^-$).

### Safety measures during fluid challenges

CVP and FR will be reevaluated after any fluid challenge. If CVP increases < 5 mmHg and FR is still +, another FB will be administered and so on while the perfusion (CRT or lactate) goal are not attained. If CVP increases $\geq$ 5 mmHg or FR is or become negative, fluids will be stopped and the patient will be moved to the next step.

### Vasopressor test

An open-label vasopressor test will be performed increasing MAP up to 80–85 mmHg by using progressive incremental doses of NE in patients with previous history of chronic hypertension and persistently abnormal CRT or unfulfilled lactate goals accompanied by a fluid unresponsive state. Parameters will be reassessed 1 h after in

the PPTR and 2 h after in the LTR. If after the vasopressor test, CRT improves, and lactate goals are achieved in PPTR and LTR, respectively, NE will be titrated to maintain this new MAP goal throughout the study period. If goals are not achieved despite increasing MAP, or NE dose surpasses 0.8 mcg/kg/min or adverse effects are observed (heart rate (HR) > 140 ppm, arrhythmias or evident cardiac ischemia), NE dose will be reduced to the level before the vasopressor test, and the protocol will move to the next step.

### Inodilator test

An open-label test of dobutamine at fixed 5 mcg/kg/min or milrinone at fixed 0.25 mcg/kg/min doses (at discretion of the attending physician) will be started in patients with persistent abnormal CRT or non-achieved lactate goals, and negative FR status. CRT and lactate goals will be rechecked such as in the vasopressor test. If such resuscitation goals are not reached, drugs will be discontinued and no further action will be taken during the study period, except for rechecking FR every hour and restart fluid challenges if the patient gets again FR +. Dobutamine or milrinone doses will be maintained throughout the study period in those favorably responding to the open-label inodilators test. As a safety measure, inodilators will be stopped if HR increases > 15%, or arrhythmias, ischemia or hypotension develop.

## Management of peripheral perfusion-targeted resuscitation

As a safety measure, if signs of inadequate macrohemodynamics persist such as HR > 120 BPM or unstable MAP with increases in vasopressors during the last hour, resuscitation will be continued even if CRT is normal.

After CRT normalization at any step, it will be reassessed hourly during the study period. If at any point it turns abnormal again, the resuscitation sequence will be restarted (Fig. 2)

## Management of lactate-targeted resuscitation

Lactate will be assessed every 2 h during the 8-h study period. If after achieving lactate goals, it becomes again abnormal or the decrease rate slow down under 20%/2 h at any of the following controls, the resuscitation sequence will be restarted (Fig. 2).

### Safety measures

The protocol can be stopped at any moment for safety considerations during the 8-h study period if the attending intensivist considers that the patient has developed unexpected and severe complications or evolves into refractory shock, conditions that under his judgment require liberalization of management. This action has to be reported on the case report form (CRF), and the patient will be followed up with major outcomes, and included in the intention-to-treat (ITT) analysis. Specific safety measures for fluid administration, vasopressor test and inodilator use are specified above.

### Suspected unexpected serious adverse reactions (SUSAR)

Any adverse event that occurs in a clinical trial subject, which is assessed by the study investigator as being unexpected, serious and as having a reasonable possibility of a causal relationship with the study procedure will be reported. Reports of these reactions are subject to expedited submission to health authorities. SUSAR's will be analyzed by both the SCC and the data safety monitoring committee (DSMC).

### Blinding

Since the intervention will be administered to critically ill patients (mostly sedated), blinding of these patients is not necessary. Because this is a non-pharmacological intervention, blinding of the medical team is not feasible.

### Data collection and management

Study follow-up and the variables that will be collected are described below.

### Baseline

Demographics, comorbidities, acute physiology and chronic health evaluation (APACHE) II [31], sepsis source and treatment

pre-ICU resuscitation and fluid balance

Sequential Organ Failure Assessment (SOFA) [26] + and Acute Kidney Injury Network (AKI) criteria [32]

*Hemodynamics*: HR, SBP, diastolic blood pressure (DBP), MAP, CVP, FR status, intraabdominal pressure (IAP), NE levels, diuresis.

*Perfusion*: lactate, central venous $O_2$ saturation ($ScvO_2$), central venous arterial $pCO_2$ gradient ($P(cv-a)CO_2$), Hb, central venous and arterial blood gases, CRT, mottling score.

### Evolution

SOFA and AKI criteria at 8, 24, 48 and 72 h
Hemodynamics hourly up to 8 h
Fluid administration and balance at 8, 24, 48 and 72 h
Complete perfusion assessment when the targeted parameter is normalized and then at 8, 24, 48 and 72 h
Register of vasoactive drugs and dobutamine/milrinone use
Register of MV and RRT
Source control re-analysis at 4 h
Rescue therapies: HVHF, vasopressin, epinephrine, steroids, others.
Echocardiography at least once during the study period
Follow-up till 28 days for use of MV, RRT and vasopressors
All-cause mortality at hospital discharge, 28 and 90 days
Cause of death.

### Quality control

Several procedures will assure data quality, including (1) all investigators will attend a training session before the start of the study to standardize procedures, including data collection (2) the investigators may contact the SCC to solve issues or problems that may arise; (3) CRFs provided by the centers will be subjected to various checks by members of the SCC for missing data, plausible, possible or non-permitted value ranges, and logic checks on a weekly basis. (4) centers will be notified of the inconsistencies or missing data as queries and asked to correct them; (5) the SCC will review detailed reports on screening, enrollment, follow-up, inconsistencies and completeness of data. Immediate actions will follow to solve problems that arise; (6) only after the CRFs are cleared by the SCC, data will be entered in the final electronic database by the data digitizer.

## Sample size

Mortality in patients with increased lactate levels in circulatory dysfunction has been shown to exceed 40% [9]. In addition, several studies have shown that abnormal peripheral perfusion is associated with a mortality exceeding 40% as well, whereas a normal CRT in the early phase of septic shock has been associated with a less than 10% mortality [19, 30].

A total sample size of 420 patients (210 per group), analyzing the data using the ITT principle, is expected to provide approximately 90% power to detect a reduction in 28-day mortality from 45 to 30%, considering logistic regression, with a two-sided alpha level of 5%. We consider a decrease of 15% in mortality to have direct clinical implementation effect. Similar effects on mortality have been shown in early resuscitation studies. In addition, limiting fluid administration in patients with septic shock and normal peripheral perfusion has been shown to decrease organ failure, which is the leading cause of death in these patients [25].

However, if a smaller decrease in mortality (such as 10%) is observed at interim analyses, our initial calculated sample size would have only a 57% power to detect benefit. Therefore, we will use an adaptive approach [33] that will allow for a sample-size re-estimation at a pre-planned interim analysis after 75% of the sample has been recruited. The sample-size re-estimation will be conducted by the DSMC only if the size effect observed in the interim analysis is between 10 and 15% absolute reduction in mortality [32].

## Statistical analysis plan

We will report a detailed statistical analysis plan in a separate document.

Briefly, all analysis will follow the intention-to-treat principle.

## Primary outcome

We will assess the effect of PPTR compared to LTR on the primary outcome using time-to-event analysis. Results of our main analysis will be calculated with Cox proportional hazards models, with adjustment for five pre-specified baseline covariates. APACHE II score, SOFA score, lactate level, CRT and source of infection, as fixed (individual-level) effects. Results will be reported as hazard ratios with 95% confidence intervals (CI) and $p$ values. We will also present Kaplan–Meier curves.

## Secondary outcomes

We identified several secondary outcomes. First, binary outcomes will be compared through Chi-squared tests, and we will present the results risk ratios (RR), with 95% CI and $p$ values.

Continuous outcomes with normal distribution will be analyzed with $t$ test and reported as mean difference 95% CI and $p$ value. Continuous outcomes with asymmetrical distribution will be analyzed using bootstrapping techniques and reported as absolute difference between medians, 95% CI and $p$ values.

## Subgroup analyses

We will analyze the effects of resuscitation strategies on the primary outcome in the following subgroups:

(a) Patients with lactate > 4.0 mmol/L as set by SSC [10]
(b) Patients without a confirmed source of infection (as this could increase the translation of the study to other critically ill).
(c) Patients with low APACHE II/SOFA scores
(d) Patients with a more than 10% difference in lactate levels between the very first one measured and the baseline when starting the study.

## Ethical aspects

Each investigator center will submit the study protocol to its Institutional Review Board (IRB). The study will start only after being approved by the IRB. Written informed consent will be obtained from a legal representative of all participants. This study is in compliance with local and international declarations.

## Trial organization and management
### Study Coordinating Center

A team based on the Departmento de Medicina Intensiva, Facultad de Medicina of Pontificia Universidad Católica, Chile, will manage the trial on a day-to-day basis. The SCC is comprised by the chief and co-chair investigators, four project managers, a statistician and a data digitizer. The statistician is based on the Research Institute HCor, São Paulo, Brazil.

The responsibilities of the SCC include:

1. *Planning and conducting the study* designing the protocol; designing the CRF; designing the operation guide; managing and controlling data quality; designing, testing and maintaining the electronic database; data quality control; assisting the steering committee;
2. *Managing the research centers* selecting and training the research centers; helping the centers prepare a regulatory report to be submitted to the IRBs and assisting the centers with the submission; monitoring recruitment rates and the actions to increase recruitment; monitoring follow-up and implementing actions to prevent follow-up losses; auditing; sending study materials to the research centers; producing

a monthly study newsletter; developing supporting material for the study;

3. *Statistical analysis and research reporting* complete statistical analysis; helping to write the final manuscript.

### Trial Steering Committee

The Trial Steering Committee (TSC) is responsible for the overall study supervision, assisting in developing the study protocol and preparing the final manuscript. All other study committees report to the TSC. The TSC members are investigators trained in designing and conducting randomized clinical trials in critically ill patients.

### Study centers

The study centers for ANDROMEDA-SHOCK were selected through a rigorous process. This started with a survey of professional and technical resources as well as processes of care. Centers were contacted trying to make this process representative across public, private and university hospitals, different countries and cultures, and hospital size.

At the end, 34 centers were selected and all applied for IRB approval, leaving finally 26 active centers to start on March 1, 2017, in 5 countries. Brazil is still pending

Details of the centers which accepted to participating in the trial at the time of this manuscript submission are given in the Appendix.

### Publication policy

The ANDROMEDA-SHOCK study success depends on all its collaborators. Therefore, the primary results of the trial will be published under the name of ANDROMEDA-SHOCK Investigators. The contributions of all collaborators, their names and respective institutions, will be acknowledged in the manuscript. To safeguard the scientific integrity of the study, data from this study will be submitted to publication only after the final approval from the TSC.

### Data Safety Monitoring Committee

The DSMC is set up with independent epidemiologists and intensivists. The DSMC is in charge of providing recommendations for the SCC of continuing the study as planned or discontinuing the recruitment based on evidence that the intervention causes increased mortality in the experimental group (PPTR) as compared to the control group (LTR). Interim analyses will be conducted after recruitment of the first 100 patients and at 75% of the sample.

In addition, the DSMC will discuss and potentially recommend a re-estimation of the sample size according to the interim analysis after recruitment of 75% of the

patients. A sample-size re-estimation design is a flexible, adaptive design with the primary purpose of allowing sample size of a study to be reassessed in the mid-course of the study to ensure adequate power.

### Discussion

ANDROMEDA-SHOCK is a relevant study in septic shock for several reasons: (1) it determines the value of a simple, bedside, universally available parameter to be used as a resuscitation goal in early septic shock; (2) it proposes an early goal-directed resuscitation strategy based on a holistic physiological view of the reperfusion process; (3) it challenges the gold-standard parameter of lactate since this latter is not universally available and has many interpretation difficulties.

If our hypothesis proves to be correct, resuscitation algorithms might be simplified, assessing almost in real-time the reperfusion process, and in pursuing more physiologically sound objectives through a peripheral perfusion-based strategy, it could prevent the risk of over-resuscitation and lead to a better utilization of ICU resources.

### Study status

ANDROMEDA-SHOCK study started recruiting on March 1 in 26 centers from five countries. At the submission of this manuscript, already 388 patients have been recruited.

### Abbreviations

CO: cardiac output; CRT: capillary refill time; RCT: randomized controlled trial; PPTR: peripheral perfusion-targeted resuscitation; LTR: lactate-targeted resuscitation; MV: mechanical ventilation; RRT: renal replacement therapy; ICU: intensive care unit; IAH: intraabdominal hypertension; SBP: systolic blood pressure; MAP: mean arterial pressure; SCC: Study Coordinating Center; CVC: central venous catheter; FR: fluid responsiveness; PPV: pulse pressure variation; SVV: stroke volume variation; EEOT: end-expiratory occlusion test; Vt: tidal volume; PEEP: positive-end-expiratory-pressure; NE: norepinephrine; HVHF: high-volume hemofiltration; RR: respiratory rate; VTI: aortic velocity time integral; PLR: passive leg raising; HR: heart rate; CRF: case report form; ITT: intention-to-treat; DSMC: data safety monitoring committee; APACHE: acute physiology and chronic health evaluation; AKI: acute kidney injury network; DBP: diastolic blood pressure; SUSAR: suspected unexpected serious adverse reactions; IAP: intraabdominal pressure; $ScvO_2$: central venous oxygen saturation; P(cv-a) $CO_2$: central venous-arterial $PCO_2$ gradient; IRB: Institutional Review Board; TSC: Trial Steering Committee.

### Authors' contributions

JB and GH are guarantors of the entire manuscript; JB, JLT, GH, GOT, AD, GF, MC, JH, AC, RC, LA designed the study; All the authors will help in the data interpretation and the final manuscript draft. All authors read and approved this final manuscript.

### Author details

[1] Departamento de Medicina Intensiva, Facultad de Medicina, Pontificia Universidad Católica de Chile, Diagonal Paraguay 362, Santiago, Chile. [2] Research Institute HCor, Hospital do Coração, R. Des. Eliseu Guilherme, 147 - Paraíso, São Paulo, Brazil. [3] Department of Intensive Care Medicine, Fundación Valle del Lili, Universidad ICESI, Carrera 98 # 18-49, Cali, Colombia. [4] Servicio de Terapia Intensiva, Sanatorio Otamendi y Miroli, Azcuénaga 894, Ciudad Autónoma de

Buenos Aires, Argentina. [5] Centro de Tratamiento Intensivo, Hospital Español, Escuela de Medicina, Universidad de la República, Avda. Gral. Garibaldi, 1729 esq. Rocha, Montevideo, Uruguay. [6] Departamento de Medicina Interna, Faculdade de Medicina, Universidade Federal do Rio Grande do Sul, R. Ramiro Barcelos 2350 – Santa Cecilia, Porto Alegre, Brazil. [7] St George's University Hospitals NHS Foundation Trust, Rd, London SW17 0QT, UK. [8] Service de Réanimation médicale, Hôpitaux universitaires Paris-Sud, Assistance Publique-Hôpitaux de Paris, Paris, France. [9] Division of Pulmonary, Allergy and Critical Care Medicine, Columbia University Medical Center, 630 W 168th St, New York, USA. [10] Department Intensive Care Adults, Erasmus MC University Medical Center, Rotterdam, CA, The Netherlands. [11] Division of Pulmonary, and Critical Care Medicine, New York University-Langone, New York, USA.

## Acknowledgements
We acknowledge the support from the Departamento de Medicina Intensiva, Facultad de Medicina, Pontificia Universidad Católica de Chile.


## Competing interests
The authors declare that they have no competing interests.


## Funding
The study is financed in part by an internal grant from the Departamento de Medicina Intensiva, Facultad de Medicina, Pontificia Universidad Católica de Chile.

## ANDROMEDA–SHOCK Investigators consists of: Writing and Steering Committee
Glenn Hernandez (chair), Gustavo Ospina-Tascón, Alexandre Cavalcanti, Arnaldo Dubin, Javier Hurtado, Gilberto Friedman, Ricardo Castro, Leyla Alegría, Jean-Louis Teboul, Maurizio Cecconi, Fernando Zampieri, Lucas Petri Damiani, Jan Bakker (co-chair). **Study Coordinating Center:** Glenn Hernandez, Leyla Alegría, Giorgio Ferri, Nicolás Rodriguez, Patricia Holger, Natalia Soto, Mario Pozo, Lucas Petri Damiani, Jan Bakker. **Data Safety Monitoring Committee:** Deborah Cook, Jean-Louis Vincent, Andrew, Rhodes, Bryan Kavanagh, Phil Dellinger, Wim Rietdijk. **Study Centers:** Chile: Pontificia Universidad Católica de Chile, Santiago: David Carpio, Nicolás Pavéz, Elizabeth Henriquez, Sebastian Bravo, Emilio Daniel Valenzuela; Hospital Barros-Luco Trudeau, Santiago: Maria Alicia Cid, Ronald Pairumani, Macarena Larroulet, Edward Petruska, Claudio Sarabia; Hospital San Juan de Dios, Santiago: David Gallardo, Juan Eduardo Sanchez, Hugo González, José Miguel Arancibia, Alex Muñoz, Germán Ramirez, Florencia Aravena; Hospital Dr. Sótero del Río, Santiago: Andrés Aquevedo, Fabián Zambrano; Hospital Del Salvador, Santiago: Milan Bozinovic, Felipe Valle, Manuel Ramirez, Victor Rossel, Pilar Muñoz, Carolina Ceballos; Hospital Herminda Martinez, Chillán: Christian Esveile, Cristian Carmona, Eva Candia, Daniela Mendoza; Hospital San Juan de Dios, Curicó: Aída Sanchez; Hospital Guillermo Grant Benavente, Concepción: Paula Fernández, Daniela Ponce, Jaime Lastra, Bárbara Nahuelpán, Fabrizio Fasce; Hospital Clínico Universidad de Chile, Santiago: Cecilia Luengo, Nicolas Medel, Cesar Cortés. **Argentina:** Clínica La Pequeña Familia, Junín: Luz Campassi; Sanatorio Otamendi y Miroli, Buenos Aires: Arnaldo Dubin, Paolo Rubatto, Brenda Nahime Horna, Mariano Furche; Hospital Provincial del Centenario, Rosario: Juan Carlos Pendino, Lisandro Bettini; Sanatorio Parque, Rosario: Carlos Lovesio, María Cecilia González, Jésica Rodriguez; Hospital Interzonal San Martín, La Plata: Elisa Estenssoro, Héctor Canales, Francisco Caminos; Sanatorio Allende Nueva Córdoba: Cayetano Galletti, Estefanía Minoldo, María José Aramburu, Daniela Olmos; **Uruguay:** Hospital Español Juan J Crottogini, Montevideo: Javier Hurtado, Nicolás Nin, Jordán Tenzi, Carlos Quiroga, Pablo Lacuesta, Agustín Gaudín, Richard Pais, Ana Silvestre, Germán Olivera; Hospital de Clínicas, Montevideo: Gloria Rieppi, Dolores Berrutti. **Ecuador:** Hospital Universitario del Rio, Cuenca: Marcelo Ochoa, Paul Cobos, Fernando Vintimilla; Hospital Eugenio Espejo, Quito: Vanessa Ramirez, Milton Tobar, Manuel Jibaja, Fernanda García, Fabricio Picoita, Nelson Remache; Hospital San Francisco de Quito, Quito: Vladimir Granda, Fernando Paredes, Eduardo Barzallo, Paul Garcés; Hospital Carlos Andrade Marín, Quito: Fausto Guerrero, Santiago Salazar, German Torres, Cristian Tana, José Calahorrano, Freddy Solis; Hospital IESS Ibarra, Ibarra: Pedro Torres, Luís Herrera, Antonio Ornes, Verónica Peréz, Glenda Delgado, Alexei Carbonell, Eliana Espinosa, José Moreira; Hospital General Docente Calderón, Quito: Diego Barahona, Blanca Salcedo, Ivonne Villacres, Jhonny Suing, Marco Lopez, Luis Gomez, Guillermo Toctaquiza, Mario Cadena Zapata, Milton Alonso Orazabal, Ruben Pardo Espejo, Jorge Jimenez, Alexander Calderón. Hospital Enrique Garcés, Quito: Gustavo Paredes, José Luis Barberán, Tatiana Moya. **Colombia:** Hospital San Vicente de Paul, Medellín: Horacio Atehortua, Rodolfo Sabogal; Hospital de Santa Clara, Bogotá: Guillermo Ortiz, Antonio Lara; Hospital Universitario de Ñarino E.S.E, Pasto: Fabio Sanchez, Alvaro Hernán Portilla, Humberto Dávila, Jorge Antonio Mora; Fundación Valle del Lili, Cali: Gustavo-Ospina Tascón, Luis Eduardo Calderón, Ingrid Alvarez, Elena Escobar, Alejandro Bejarano, *Luis Alfonso Bustamante.*

## References
1. Vincent JL, De Backer D. Circulatory shock. N Engl J Med. 2013;369:1726–34.
2. Cecconi M, De Backer D, Antonelli M, Beale R, Bakker J, Hofer C, et al. Consensus on circulatory shock and hemodynamic monitoring. Task force of the European Society of Intensive Care Medicine. Intensiv Care Med. 2014;40:1795–815.
3. Shoemaker WC, Appel PL, Kram HB. Tissue oxygen debt as a determinant of lethal and nonlethal postoperative organ failure. Crit Care Med. 1988;16:1117–20.
4. Vallet B. Vascular reactivity and tissue oxygenation. Intensiv Care Med. 1998;24:3–11.
5. Bellomo R, Reade MC, Warrillow SJ. The pursuit of a high central venous oxygen saturation in sepsis: growing concerns. Crit Care. 2008;12:130.
6. PRISM Investigators, Rowan KM, Angus DC, Bailey M, Barnato AE, Bellomo R, et al. Early, goal-directed therapy for septic shock—a patient-level meta-analysis. N Engl J Med. 2017;376:2223–34.
7. Bakker J, Gris P, Coffernils M, Kahn R, Vincent J. Serial blood lactate levels can predict the development of multiple organ failure following septic shock. Am J Surg. 1996;171:221–6.
8. Friedman G, De Backer D, Shahla M, Vincent JL. Oxygen supply dependency can characterize septic shock. Intensiv Care Med. 1998;24:118–23.
9. Jansen TC, van Bommel J, Schoonderbeek FJ, Sleeswijk Visser SJ, van der Klooster JM, Lima AP, et al. Early lactate-guided therapy in intensive care unit patients: a multicenter, open-label, randomized controlled trial. Am J Respir Crit Care Med. 2010;182:752–61.
10. Rhodes A, Evans LE, Alhazzani W, Levy MM, Antonelli M, Ferrer R, et al. Surviving sepsis campaign: international guidelines for management of sepsis and septic shock: 2016. Intensiv Care Med. 2017;43:304–77.
11. Garcia-Alvarez M, Marik P, Bellomo R. Sepsis-associated hyperlactatemia. Crit Care. 2014;18:503.
12. Hernandez G, Bruhn A, Castro R, Regueira T. The holistic view on perfusion monitoring in septic shock. Curr Opinion Crit Care. 2012;18:280–6.
13. Marik PE, Linde-Zwirble WT, Bittner EA, Sahatjian J, Hansell D. Fluid administration in severe sepsis and septic shock, patterns and outcomes: an analysis of a large national database. Intensiv Care Med. 2017;43:625–32.
14. Hjortrup PB, Haase N, Bundgaard H, Thomsen SL, Winding R, Pettilä V, et al. Restricting volumes of resuscitation fluid in adults with septic shock after initial management: the CLASSIC randomised, parallel-group, multicentre feasibility trial. Intensiv Care Med. 2016;42:1695–705.
15. Hernandez G, Luengo C, Bruhn A, Kattan E, Friedman G, Ospina-Tascon GA, et al. When to stop septic shock resuscitation: clues from a dynamic perfusion monitoring. Ann Intensive Care. 2014;4:30.
16. Brunauer A, Koköfer A, Bataar O, Gradwohl-Matis I, Dankl D, Bakker J, et al. Changes in peripheral perfusion relate to visceral organ perfusion in early septic shock: a pilot study. J Crit Care. 2016;35:105–9.
17. Lima A, Bakker J. Clinical assessment of peripheral circulation. Curr Opin Crit Care. 2015;21:226–31.
18. Hernandez G, Pedreros C, Veas E, Bruhn A, Romero C, Rovegno M, et al. Evolution of peripheral vs metabolic perfusion parameters during septic shock resuscitation. J Crit Care. 2012;27:283–8.
19. Ait-Oufella H, Lemoinne S, Boelle PY, Galbois A, Baudel JL, Lemant J, et al. Mottling score predicts survival in septic shock. Intensive Care Med. 2011;37:801–7.
20. Lima A, Jansen TC, Van Bommel J, Ince C, Bakker J. The prognostic value of

the subjective assessment of peripheral perfusion in critically ill patients. Crit Care Med. 2009;37:934–8.

21. Coudroy R, Jamet A, Frat JP, Veinstein A, Chatellier D, Goudet V, et al. Incidence and impact of skin mottling over the knee and its duration on outcome in critically ill patients. Intensive Care Med. 2015;41:452–9.

22. Ait-Oufella H, Bige N, Boelle PY, Pichereau C, Alves M, Bertinchamp R, et al. Capillary refill time exploration during septic shock. Intensive Care Med. 2014;40:958–64.

23. van Genderen ME, Paauwe J, de Jonge J, van der Valk RJ, Lima A, Bakker J, et al. Clinical assessment of peripheral perfusion to predict postoperative complications after major abdominal surgery early: a prospective observational study in adults. Crit Care. 2014;18:R114.

24. Dünser MW, Takala J, Brunauer A, Bakker J. Re-thinking resuscitation: leaving blood pressure cosmetics behind and moving forward to permissive hypotension and a tissue perfusion-based approach. Crit Care. 2013;17:326.

25. van Genderen ME, Engels N, van der Valk RJP, Lima A, Klijn E, Bakker J, et al. Early peripheral perfusion-guided fluid therapy in patients with septic shock. Am J Respir Crit Care Med. 2015;191:477–80.

26. Vincent JL, Moreno R, Takala J, Willatts S, De Mendonca A, Bruining H, et al. The SOFA (Sepsis-related Organ Failure Assessment) score to describe organ dysfunction/failure. On behalf of the work-ing group on sepsis-related problems of the European Society of Intensive Care Medicine. Intensive Care Med. 1996;22:707–10.

27. Singer M, Deutschman CS, Seymour CW, Shankar-Hari M, Annane D, Bauer M, et al. The third international consensus definitions for sepsis and septic shock (Sepsis-3). JAMA. 2016;315:801–10.

28. Miller A, Mandeville J. Predicting and measuring fluid responsiveness with echocardiography. Echo Res Pract. 2016;3:G1–12.

29. Monnet X, Teboul JL. Assessment of volume responsiveness during mechanical ventilation: recent advances. Crit Care. 2013;17:217.

30. Lara B, Enberg L, Ortega M, Leon P, Kripper C, Aguilera P, et al. Capillary refill time during fluid resuscitation in patients with sepsis-related hyper-lactatemia at the emergency department is related to mortality. PLoS ONE. 2017;12:e0188548.

31. Knaus WA, Draper EA, Wagner DP, Zimmerman JE. APACHE II: a severity of disease classification system. Crit Care Med. 1985;13:818–29.

32. Kellum JA, Lameire N. KDIGO AKI Guideline Work Group. Diagnosis, evaluation, and management of acute kidney injury: a KDIGO summary (Part 1). Crit Care. 2013;17:204.

33. Bhatt DL, Mehta C. Adaptive designs for clinical trials. N Engl J Med. 2016;375:65–74.

# 18

# Fluoroscopy-guided simultaneous distal perfusion as a preventive strategy of limb ischemia in patients undergoing extracorporeal membrane oxygenation

Woo Jin Jang[1], Yang Hyun Cho[2], Taek Kyu Park[3], Young Bin Song[3], Jin-Oh Choi[3], Joo-Yong Hahn[3], Seung-Hyuk Choi[3], Hyeon-Cheol Gwon[3], Eun-Seok Jeon[3], Woo Jung Chun[1], Ju Hyeon Oh[1] and Jeong Hoon Yang[3]*

## Abstract

**Background:** Limited data are available regarding prevention of limb ischemia in femorally cannulated patients on venoarterial extracorporeal membrane oxygenation (VA-ECMO). We investigated the association between strategy of distal perfusion catheter (DPC) insertion and vascular complications like limb ischemia in patients undergoing VA-ECMO.

**Methods:** We evaluated 230 patients from two tertiary hospitals who received VA-ECMO via femoral cannulation between August 2014 and July 2017. The patients were divided into two groups according to DPC insertion strategy: patients who underwent DPC insertion at the time of primary cannulation (DPC group, $n = 96$) and patients who were provisionally treated with DPC (No-DPC group, $n = 134$). The primary outcome was limb ischemia.

**Results:** Of the 96 patients in the DPC group, 61 (63.5%) underwent insertion under fluoroscopic guidance. The DPC group had a significantly lower incidence of limb ischemia (2.1% vs. 8.2%, $p = 0.047$) and a lower tendency of in-hospital mortality (38.5% vs. 50.7%, $p = 0.067$) than the No-DPC group. In the multivariable analysis, fluoroscopy-guided simultaneous insertion of the DPC (odds ratio 0.11; 95% confidence interval 0.01–0.98; $p = 0.048$) was a significant predictor of reduction of limb ischemia.

**Conclusions:** Simultaneous insertion of a DPC, particularly under fluoroscopy guidance, can be considered as a preventive strategy for limb ischemia in femorally cannulated patients on VA-ECMO.

**Keywords:** Distal perfusion catheter, Limb ischemia, Extracorporeal membrane oxygenation

# Background

Venoarterial extracorporeal membrane oxygenation (VA-ECMO) has been widely used as a salvage therapy in critically ill patients with refractory cardiogenic shock

*Correspondence: jhysmc@gmail.com
[3] Division of Cardiology, Department of Critical Care Medicine and Medicine, Heart Vascular Stroke Institute, Samsung Medical Center, Sungkyunkwan University School of Medicine, 81, Irwon-dong, Gangnam-gu, Seoul 135-710, Republic of Korea
Full list of author information is available at the end of the article

[1]. The femoral vessel approach for VA-ECMO insertion is regarded as the default route because the equipment can be placed rapidly and easily [2]. In patients undergoing VA-ECMO using transfemoral cannulation, limb ischemia is a lethal complication that can be influenced by vessel size, increased vascular tone due to hemodynamic instability, size of the indwelling arterial cannula, and use of vasopressors [3–6]. To prevent limb ischemia after cannulation, the guidance of an antegrade distal perfusion catheter (DPC) into the proximal superficial femoral artery (SFA) has been assisted by various techniques such as ultrasound and fluoroscopy

[2, 7]. However, the optimal timing of and strategy for DPC insertion have not been fully elucidated for patients undergoing VA-ECMO via femoral cannulation. Therefore, we investigated whether simultaneous insertion of a DPC, particularly fluoroscopy-guided DPC insertion, at the time of primary ECMO cannulation can reduce critical limb ischemia compared with a provisional approach.

## Methods

### Study population

We investigated 257 consecutive patients who underwent VA-ECMO from a retrospective multicenter registry at Samsung Medical Center, Seoul, South Korea, and Samsung Changwon Hospital, Gyeongnam, South Korea, from August 2014 through July 2017. Of these, we included only patients who were placed on peripheral VA-ECMO via femoral cannulation and excluded patients who were under 18 years of age or who underwent ECMO using central aortic or axilla-arterial cannulation. Ultimately, 230 patients were enrolled in this study and were divided into two groups according to timing of DPC insertion: patients who underwent DPC insertion at the time of the primary cannulation (DPC group) and patients who did not undergo DPC insertion at the primary femoral cannulation including provisional DPC insertion after the onset of distal limb ischemia (No-DPC group) (Fig. 1). The local institutional review board of each participating hospital approved this study and waived the requirement for informed consent.

### Extracorporeal membrane oxygenation implantation and management

The decision to implant ECMO was made by an experienced team, and the ECMO was placed by either cardiovascular surgeons or interventional cardiologists. The Capiox Emergency Bypass System (Capiox EBS™; Terumo, Inc., Tokyo, Japan) and Permanent Life Support (PLS) System (MAQUET, Rastatt, Germany) were used. Heparin was intravenously administered as a bolus of 5000 units, followed by continuous intravenous infusion to maintain an activated clotting time between 150 and 180 s. After initiation of ECMO, the pump blood flow rate was initially set above 2.2 L/min/body surface area ($m^2$) and subsequently adjusted to maintain a mean arterial pressure above 65 mmHg. Blood pressure was continuously monitored through an arterial catheter, and arterial blood gas analysis was performed in the artery of the right arm to estimate cerebral oxygenation. Additional fluids, blood transfusion, and/or catecholamines (i.e., norepinephrine, epinephrine, or dobutamine) were supplied to maintain intravascular volume and/or to achieve a mean arterial pressure above 65 mmHg if necessary [8].

### Cannulation of extracorporeal membrane oxygenation and distal perfusion catheter

Percutaneous cannulation of the femoral artery and vein was mainly performed by the attending staff interventional cardiologist or cardiovascular surgeon using the Seldinger technique. The femoral vessels (either unilateral, one-side arterial, or one-side venous) were accessed

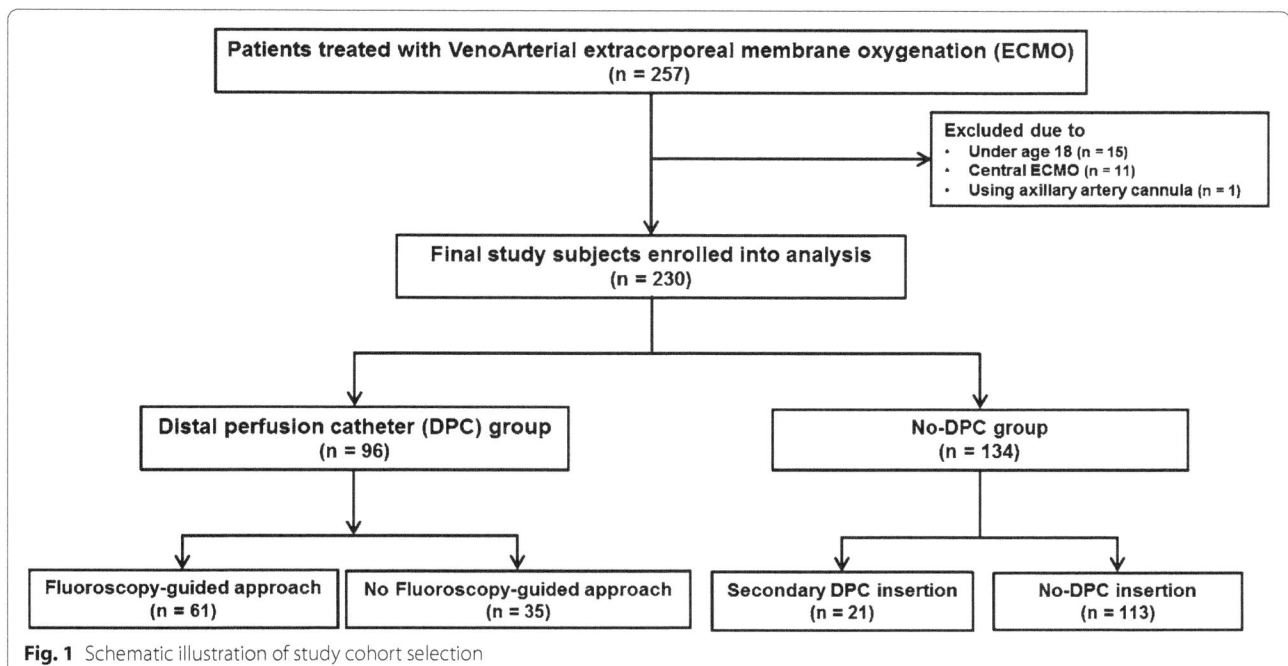

**Fig. 1** Schematic illustration of study cohort selection

retrograde using an angiogram needle. The venous cannula was either 55 or 68 cm in length and from 21 to 28 Fr.; the arterial cannula was 24 cm and from 14 to 21 Fr. The final selection of cannula was based on manufacturer pressure–flow curves for each cannula size and patient size. Femoral cut-down procedures were performed when it was difficult to puncture the femoral artery percutaneously, for example, in patients with peripheral artery disease or severe obesity. At bedside, the DPC placement site was accessed antegrade using a micropuncture needle followed by a 0.018-inch nitinol wire (Cook Medical Inc, Bloomington, IN, USA) at the proximal SFA ipsilateral to the arterial cannula. A 6- or 7-Fr. sheath was then advanced into the mid-SFA. In the catheterization laboratory, we first inserted another sheath at the common femoral artery (CFA) contralateral to the arterial ECMO cannula and advanced a hydrophilic wire from the CFA sheath (through the aortic bifurcation and the ipsilateral common iliac artery, then between the arterial ECMO cannula and the vessel wall of the ipsilateral common iliac artery) to the distal portion of the ipsilateral SFA. The DPC was then safely inserted into the distal portion of the arterial cannula (ipsilateral to the SFA) using a micropuncture needle as the reference point of the previously placed hydrophilic wire. The catheter was attached to the side port of the arterial cannula using 6-inch extension tubing with an intervening three-way stopcock (Fig. 2).

### Data collection, definitions, and study outcomes

Baseline characteristics, procedural characteristics, laboratory data, and clinical outcome data were obtained by reviewing medical records or by telephone contact, if necessary. Laboratory findings, including creatinine and lactate, were collected just before VA-ECMO insertion. The primary outcome was limb ischemia, which was defined as cases requiring surgical management or involving neurologic sequelae. In-hospital mortality, successful weaning rate of ECMO, thrombotic events, major bleeding, and catheter-related complications (defined as a composite of limb ischemia, major bleeding, and thrombotic events) were assessed in addition to the primary outcome. Major bleeding was defined as cases involving hemodynamic instability or those that occurred in a critical area or organ such as intracranial, retroperitoneal, pericardial, or intramuscular with compartment syndrome.

### Statistical analysis

Continuous variables were compared using Student's $t$ test or the Wilcoxon rank-sum test. The results were presented as mean ± standard deviation or median with interquartile range. Categorical data were tested using Fisher's exact test or the Chi-square test. Multivariable logistic regression analysis was performed via a stepwise backward selection process to determine the independent predictors of limb ischemia. Clinical variables (i.e., fluoroscopy-guided simultaneous DPC, age $\geq$ 65 years, gender, duration of ECMO > 5 days, and large arterial cannula) were included in the regression models. All variables associated with limb ischemia were analyzed using univariate analysis. Factors with $p < 0.2$ and those that were clinically relevant were included in the multivariable analysis. All tests were two-tailed, and $p$ value < 0.05 was considered statistically significant. Statistical analyses were performed using SPSS software, version 23 (IBM, Armonk, New York, USA).

## Results

### Baseline, procedural, and laboratory characteristics

The baseline and procedural characteristics of the study population are shown in Table 1. There were no significant differences between the DPC group and the No-DPC group except body mass index (BMI) in baseline characteristics. Of the 134 patients in the No-DPC group, 21 (15.7%) underwent secondary DPC insertion. ECMO was mainly inserted in either catheterization laboratory room, intensive care unit, or emergency room. Extracorporeal cardiopulmonary resuscitation (ECPR) was more frequently performed in the No-DPC group than in the DPC group ($p = 0.003$). The size of femoral arterial cannula was similar between the DPC group and the No-DPC group ($p = 0.080$), but venous cannular size was larger in the DPC group than in the No-DPC group ($p = 0.019$). Anticoagulation therapy ($p = 0.004$) and left ventricular venting during ECMO support ($p = 0.029$) were more frequently performed in the DPC group than in the No-DPC group, and large arterial cannula ($p = 0.066$) tended to be used less frequently in the DPC group compared to the No-DPC group. The median duration of ECMO support was 3 days [interquartile range (IQR) 1–7 days]. The median total length of stay in the intensive care unit was 6 days (IQR 1–16 days), and the median total length of stay in the hospital was 20 days (IQR 6–45 days).

### Limb ischemia and other catheter-related complications in VA-ECMO patients

Thirty-four cases of ischemic complication (13 limb ischemia, 18 thrombotic events, and 3 ischemic strokes) occurred. Of the 13 patients with distal limb ischemia, 3 were recovered through medical treatment, while 3

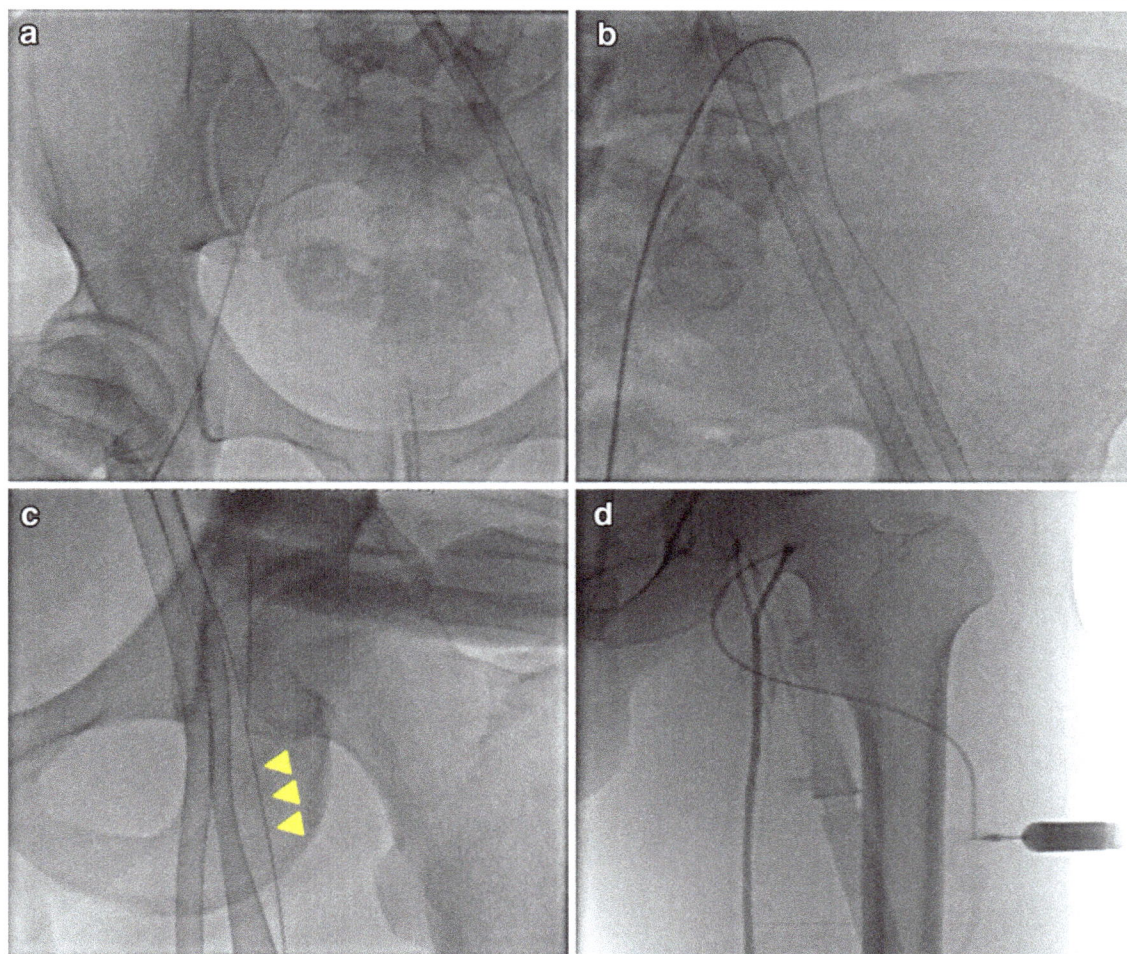

**Fig. 2** Percutaneous insertion of a distal perfusion catheter. **a** Under fluoroscopy guidance, a sheath at the contralateral common femoral artery (CFA) was inserted using a micropuncture needle followed by a 0.018-inch nitinol wire. **b** A hydrophilic wire was advanced from the sheath of the contralateral CFA (through the aortic bifurcation and the ipsilateral common iliac artery, between the arterial ECMO cannula and the vessel wall of the ipsilateral common iliac artery) to the distal portion of the ipsilateral superficial femoral artery (SFA). **c** The proximal SFA ipsilateral to the arterial cannula was punctured using a micropuncture needle followed by a 0.018-inch nitinol wire as the reference point of the previously placed wire (yellow arrow heads). A distal perfusion catheter (6- or 7-Fr. sheath) was inserted antegrade and advanced safely into the mid-SFA. **d** The distal perfusion catheter was attached to the side port of the arterial cannula using 6-inch extension tubing with an intervening three-way stopcock

underwent fasciotomy, 3 received surgical thrombectomy, and 4 underwent surgical amputation of the distal lower limb implanted with ECMO. Limb ischemia was less frequent in the DPC group than in the No-DPC group (2.1% vs. 8.2%; $p = 0.047$). The incidences of major bleeding (8.3% vs. 4.5%; $p = 0.228$), thrombotic events (5.2% vs. 9.7%; $p = 0.211$), and catheter-related complications (24.0% vs. 19.4%; $p = 0.405$) were not different between the two groups. The rate of successful ECMO weaning was greater in the DPC group than in the No-DPC group (79.2% vs. 61.9%; $p = 0.005$), and the DPC group had a lower tendency of in-hospital mortality than the No-DPC group (38.5% vs. 50.7%; $p = 0.067$) (Table 2).

### Fluoroscopy-guided distal perfusion and predictors on lower limb ischemia

Of the 96 patients in the DPC group, 61 (63.5%) underwent DPC insertion under fluoroscopic guidance (Table 1). Fluoroscopy-guided DPC group had a numerically low incidence of catheter-related complication including limb ischemia, cannular site bleeding, and thrombotic event compared to no fluoroscopy-guided DPC group (Table 2). Furthermore, the incidence of limb ischemia tended to be lower in the fluoroscopy-guided DPC group than in the No-DPC group ($p = 0.057$). We performed multivariable logistic regression analysis to identify predictors of limb ischemia in patients

**Table 1  Baseline and procedural characteristics**

| | DPC group (n = 96) | | | No-DPC group (n = 134) | p value DPC versus No-DPC |
|---|---|---|---|---|---|
| | Fluoroscopy-guided (n = 61) | No fluoroscopy-guided (n = 35) | p value | | |
| Age (years) | 55.2 ± 16.7 | 55.7 ± 16.2 | 0.143 | 58.5 ± 13.7 | 0.106 |
| Gender (male) | 39 (63.9) | 20 (57.1) | 0.735 | 89 (66.4) | 0.439 |
| Body mass index (kg/m$^2$) | 23.0 ± 3.1 | 25.0 ± 3.9 | <0.001 | 25.6 ± 3.9 | <0.001 |
| Diabetes mellitus | 16 (26.2) | 10 (28.6) | 0.260 | 46 (34.3) | 0.243 |
| Hypertension | 22 (36.1) | 10 (28.6) | 0.790 | 51 (38.1) | 0.462 |
| Dyslipidemia | 11 (18.0) | 2 (5.7) | 0.016 | 9 (6.7) | 0.083 |
| Current smoker | 13 (21.3) | 12 (34.3) | 0.959 | 29 (21.6) | 0.438 |
| Chronic kidney disease | 4 (6.6) | 2 (5.7) | 0.688 | 11 (8.2) | 0.576 |
| Peripheral vascular disease | 2 (3.3) | 0 (0) | 0.670 | 3 (2.2) | 0.936 |
| Previous MI | 10 (16.4) | 7 (20.0) | 0.396 | 29 (21.6) | 0.462 |
| Previous PCI | 9 (14.8) | 7 (20.0) | 0.217 | 30 (22.4) | 0.285 |
| Previous CABG | 1 (1.6) | 1 (2.9) | 0.136 | 9 (6.7) | 0.104 |
| Previous CVA | 5 (8.5) | 2 (5.7) | 0.858 | 10 (7.5) | 0.961 |
| Clinical presentation | | | 0.002 | | 0.061 |
| Ischemic cardiomyopathy | 32 (52.5) | 10 (28.6) | | 58 (43.3) | |
| Non-ischemic cardiomyopathy | 13 (21.3) | 5 (14.3) | | 21 (15.7) | |
| Septic shock | 0 (0) | 6 (17.1) | | 4 (3.0) | |
| Refractory arrhythmia | 8 (13.1) | 1 (2.9) | | 4 (3.0) | |
| Other causes | 8 (13.1) | 13 (37.1) | | 47 (35.1) | |
| Purpose of ECMO implantation | | | 0.035 | | 0.121 |
| Bridge to recovery | 49 (80.3) | 32 (91.4) | | 122 (91.0) | |
| Bridge to transplantation | 12 (19.7) | 3 (8.6) | | 12 (9.0) | |
| ECPR | 24 (39.3) | 17 (48.6) | 0.002 | 84 (62.7) | 0.003 |
| Initial ECMO pump flow (L/min) | 3.0 ± 0.8 | 3.3 ± 0.5 | 0.722 | 3.1 ± 1.1 | 0.729 |
| Operating site of ECMO | | | <0.001 | | <0.001 |
| Intensive care unit | 0 (0) | 21 (60.0) | | 31 (23.1) | |
| Catheterization laboratory room | 56 (91.8) | 0 (0) | | 33 (24.6) | |
| Emergency room | 4 (6.6) | 7 (20.0) | | 27 (20.1) | |
| Operating room | 0 (0) | 4 (11.4) | | 17 (12.7) | |
| Others | 1 (1.6) | 3 (8.6) | | 26 (19.4) | |
| Arterial catheter size (Fr.) | 15.3 ± 0.7 | 15.4 ± 0.9 | 0.061 | 15.3 ± 0.8 | 0.080 |
| Venous catheter sized (Fr.) | 22.4 ± 1.5 | 21.9 ± 0.7 | 0.010 | 21.5 ± 2.4 | 0.019 |
| Large arterial cannula[a] | 10 (16.4) | 9 (25.7) | 0.055 | 41 (30.6) | 0.066 |
| During ECMO support | | | | | |
| Anticoagulation therapy | 52 (85.2) | 25 (71.4) | 0.001 | 84 (62.7) | 0.004 |
| Left ventricular venting | 16 (26.2) | 3 (8.6) | 0.003 | 13 (9.7) | 0.029 |
| Distal perfusion | 61 (100.0) | 35 (100.0) | <0.001 | 21 (15.7) | <0.001 |
| Continuous renal replacement therapy | 18 (29.5) | 16 (45.7) | 0.177 | 53 (39.6) | 0.524 |
| Intra-aortic balloon pump | 2 (3.3) | 1 (2.9) | 0.696 | 6 (4.5) | 0.602 |
| Mechanical ventilation | 47 (77.0) | 27 (77.1) | 0.318 | 94 (70.1) | 0.243 |
| Laboratory findings | | | | | |
| Creatinine (mg/dL) (just before ECMO insertion) | 1.4 (1.0–1.54) | 1.2 (0.8–1.4) | 0.391 | 1.3 (0.9–1.9) | 0.779 |
| Lactate (mmol/L) (just before ECMO insertion) | 4.9 (2.8–9.2) | 5.7 (2.0–10.4) | 0.051 | 5.3 (2.1–10.1) | 0.683 |
| Lactate (mmol/L) (24 h after ECMO insertion) | 1.9 (1.4–3.1) | 2.2 (1.1–4.9) | 0.300 | 2.1 (0.0–3.9) | 0.700 |
| Duration of ECMO support (day) | 3.4 (2.1–7.5) | 4.0 (2.0–6.3) | 0.013 | 2.0 (1.0–5.0) | 0.052 |
| Length of ICU stay (day) | 10.0 (3.5–19.0) | 6.0 (1.0–15.5) | 0.518 | 5.0 (1.0–10.0) | 0.012 |
| Length of hospital stay (day) | 27.0 (14.0–73.0) | 24.0 (7.5–49.8) | 0.271 | 14.0 (5.0–34.0) | 0.030 |

Values are mean ± standard deviation, median (interquartile range), or n (%)

*CABG* coronary artery bypass grafting, *CVA* cerebrovascular accident, *DPC* distal perfusion catheter, *ECPR* extracorporeal cardiopulmonary resuscitation, *ICU* intensive care unit, *MI* myocardial infarction, *PCI* percutaneous coronary intervention, *ECMO* extracorporeal membrane oxygenation

[a] We considered patient used 16–21-Fr. catheter as patient used large arterial catheter

**Table 2 Clinical outcomes and complications**

| | DPC group (n = 96) | | | No-DPC group (n = 134) | p value DPC versus No-DPC |
|---|---|---|---|---|---|
| | Fluoroscopy-guided (n = 61) | No fluoroscopy-guided (n = 35) | p value | | |
| Limb ischemia | 1 (1.6) | 1 (2.9) | 0.688 | 11 (8.2) | 0.047 |
| Major bleeding | 5 (8.2) | 3 (8.6) | 0.949 | 6 (4.5) | 0.228 |
| Thrombotic event | 2 (3.3) | 3 (8.6) | 0.261 | 13 (9.7) | 0.211 |
| Catheter-related complication[a] | 12 (19.7) | 11 (31.4) | 0.194 | 26 (19.4) | 0.405 |
| Successful weaning from ECMO | 49 (80.3) | 27 (77.1) | 0.711 | 83 (61.9) | 0.005 |
| In-hospital mortality | 22 (36.1) | 15 (42.9) | 0.510 | 68 (50.7) | 0.067 |

Values are n (%)

DPC distal perfusion catheter, ECMO extracorporeal membrane oxygenation

[a] Catheter-related complication was defined as a composite of limb ischemia, cannular site bleeding, and thrombotic event

undergoing VA-ECMO. Simultaneous DPC insertion (OR 0.13, 95% CI 0.03–0.68, $p = 0.016$) and ICU stay ≥ 11 days (OR 4.34, 95% CI 1.26–14.97, $p = 0.020$) on model I, and fluoroscopy-guided simultaneous DPC insertion (OR 0.11, 95% CI 0.01–0.98, $p = 0.048$) and ICU stay ≥ 11 days (OR 3.71, 95% CI 1.12–12.32, $p = 0.032$) on model II were significant prognostic factors for lower limb ischemia (Table 3).

## Discussion

We investigated the association between the method and timing of distal perfusion and vascular complications, including limb ischemia, major bleeding, and thrombotic events, in patients undergoing VA-ECMO. Our main finding is that simultaneous DPC insertion at the time of primary ECMO cannulation reduced the incidence of lower limb ischemia. In the multivariable analysis, fluoroscopy-guided simultaneous insertion of DPC, duration of ECMO implantation > 5 days, and use of a large arterial cannula (over 16 Fr.) were significant predictors of limb ischemia. In general, our findings correspond well with earlier studies that established an association between distal perfusion and adverse clinical outcomes [2, 9]. The present study showed for the first time that fluoroscopy-guided DPC insertion via a contralateral approach might be a safe and effective strategy to prevent limb ischemia in femorally cannulated patients on VA-ECMO.

VA-ECMO implantation for patients with refractory cardiopulmonary failure is quick and convenient when using a percutaneous femoral approach, but limb ischemia and other catheter-related complications frequently develop due to partial luminal obstruction or injury to the common femoral artery or vein. Muehrcke et al. [10] reported an ischemia rate of 70% in an ECMO population of 24 patients without DPC placement at the time of cannulation. Their cannulation protocol

**Table 3 Predictors of lower limb ischemia**

| | Odds ratio | 95% CI | p value |
|---|---|---|---|
| Model I | | | |
| Simultaneous DPC insertion | 0.13 | 0.03–0.68 | 0.016 |
| Age ≥ 65 years | 0.27 | 0.06–1.35 | 0.111 |
| Male | 1.37 | 0.40–4.76 | 0.618 |
| BMI ≥ 25 kg/m² | 0.46 | 0.13–1.66 | 0.235 |
| Diabetes mellitus | 0.91 | 0.25–3.35 | 0.891 |
| Clinical presentation | 0.77 | 0.52–1.14 | 0.189 |
| ICU stay ≥ 11 days | 4.34 | 1.26–14.97 | 0.020 |
| Model II | | | |
| Fluoroscopy-guided DPC insertion | 0.11 | 0.01–0.98 | 0.048 |
| Age ≥ 65 years | 0.28 | 0.06–1.36 | 0.114 |
| Male | 1.46 | 0.42–5.10 | 0.554 |
| BMI ≥ 25 kg/m² | 0.48 | 0.14–1.70 | 0.255 |
| Diabetes mellitus | 0.93 | 0.25–3.45 | 0.910 |
| Clinical presentation | 0.73 | 0.49–1.10 | 0.131 |
| ICU stay ≥ 11 days | 3.71 | 1.12–12.32 | 0.032 |

Model I: adjusted with simultaneous DPC insertion, age ≥ 65 years, male, BMI ≥ 25 kg/m², diabetes mellitus, clinical presentation, and ICU stay ≥ 11 days

Model II: adjusted with fluoroscopy-guided simultaneous DPC insertion, age ≥ 65 years, male, BMI ≥ 25 kg/m², diabetes mellitus, clinical presentation, and ICU stay ≥ 11 days

BMI body mass index, CI confidence interval, DPC distal perfusion catheter, ICU intensive care unit

was modified to include simultaneous DPC placement, with noted improvement in limb salvage. Foley et al. [5] reported an ischemia rate of 21% in 58 patients without DPCs, although they found no difference in limb ischemia or mortality between prophylactic and expectant placement of a DPC. These findings strongly suggest that limb ischemia can be avoided in a large number of patients undergoing ECMO if the physician can safely insert a DPC. Additionally, Lamb et al. [2] reported that placement of a DPC at the time of cannulation and intensive monitoring of limb perfusion may decrease the incidence of ischemic complication. Ranney et al. [9] investigated the indication and timing of DPC placement and reported that DPC placement at the time of primary cannulation may lower the incidence of limb ischemia. However, both studies had a limited number of patients and focused only on the occurrence of complicated limb ischemia in ECMO patients; therefore, no definite conclusion can be drawn from these studies. The strength of our study is in the comparison of overall clinical outcomes and ECMO-related vascular complications, as well as limb ischemia, between two timings of DPC insertion using a large, dedicated ECMO registry.

In the real-world practice, additional procedures, like DPC insertion, could be harmful in critically ill patients who are vulnerable to bleeding or who had received anticoagulation therapy while on ECMO. Therefore, finding a method to insert the DPC that avoids bleeding complications caused by multiple needle thrusts would make it possible to avoid fatal complications in the lower limb. In the present study, DPCs were preferentially inserted in all VA-ECMO patients unless limited by technical considerations, typically an inability to cannulate the SFA, and no procedural-related limb complication occurred in patients treated with fluoroscopy-guided DPC insertion. Our findings suggest that simultaneous DPC insertion at the time of primary ECMO cannulation should be considered to prevent limb ischemia, and image-guided insertion methods, such as fluoroscopy, are more effective and safe.

### Study limitations
This study has several limitations. First, its design was non-randomized, retrospective, and observational, which may have affected the results due to confounding factors. Second, the selection of treatment strategy for the cannulated limb was at the discretion of the operator and could have influenced the results by introducing bias. Third, the impact of limb ischemia on long-term outcomes and the influence of eventual distal perfusion in the No-DPC group were not assessed in this study. Fourth, patients undergoing simultaneous DPC insertion may be comparatively more stable to those who do not undergo the procedure. The DPC and No-DPC groups were different in baseline BMI, rate of ECPR, and operating site of ECMO in the present study. This might have influenced study outcomes and produced a higher rate of ECMO weaning in patients undergoing simultaneous DPC insertion. Finally, we did not compare our fluoroscopy-guided contralateral DPC strategy with previous methods such as ultrasound-guided DPC insertion or ipsilateral DPC insertion. Therefore, this method cannot be chosen with certainty as the best method of DPC insertion.

### Conclusion
Simultaneous insertion of DPC at the time of primary ECMO cannulation using a femoral approach could prevent advanced limb ischemia. In particular, fluoroscopy-guided DPC insertion via a contralateral approach can be considered as a new strategy for prevention of disastrous vascular complications.

### Abbreviations
DPC: distal perfusion catheter; SFA: superficial femoral artery; VA-ECMO: venoarterial extracorporeal membrane oxygenation.

### Authors' contributions
WJJ and JHY had full access to all of the data and take responsibility for the integrity of the data and the accuracy of the data analysis. WJJ, YHC, and JHY contributed to the study concept and design. All authors contributed to the acquisition, analysis, or interpretation of data. WJJ and JHY drafted the manuscript. WJJ, YHC, and JHY contributed to critical revision of the manuscript for important intellectual content. WJJ and JHY performed statistical analysis. SHC and JHY were responsible for study supervision. All authors gave final approval of the version to be published and agreed to be accountable for all aspects of the work, thereby ensuring that questions related to the accuracy or integrity of any part of the work are appropriately investigated and resolved. All authors read and approved the final manuscript.

### Author details
[1] Division of Cardiology, Department of Internal Medicine, Samsung Changwon Hospital, Sungkyunkwan University School of Medicine, Changwon, Republic of Korea. [2] Department of Thoracic and Cardiovascular Surgery, Samsung Medical Center, Sungkyunkwan University School of Medicine, Seoul, Republic of Korea. [3] Division of Cardiology, Department of Critical Care Medicine and Medicine, Heart Vascular Stroke Institute, Samsung Medical Center, Sungkyunkwan University School of Medicine, 81, Irwon-dong, Gangnam-gu, Seoul 135-710, Republic of Korea.

### Acknowledgements
None.

### Competing interests
The authors declare that they have no competing interests.

### Funding
None.

### References
1. Kar B, Gregoric ID, Basra SS, Idelchik GM, Loyalka P. The percutaneous ventricular assist device in severe refractory cardiogenic shock. J Am Coll Cardiol. 2011;57:688–96.
2. Lamb KM, DiMuzio PJ, Johnson A, Batista P, Moudgill N, McCullough M, et al. Arterial protocol including prophylactic distal perfusion catheter decreases limb ischemia complications in patients undergoing extracorporeal membrane oxygenation. J Vasc Surg. 2017;65:1074–9.
3. Bisdas T, Beutel G, Warnecke G, Hoeper MM, Kuehn C, Haverich A, et al. Vascular complications in patients undergoing femoral cannulation for extracorporeal membrane oxygenation support. Ann Thorac Surg. 2011;92:626–31.
4. Huang SC, Yu HY, Ko WJ, Chen YS. Pressure criterion for placement of distal perfusion catheter to prevent limb ischemia during adult extracorporeal life support. J Thorac Cardiovasc Surg. 2004;128:776–7.

5.  Foley PJ, Morris RJ, Woo EY, Acker MA, Wang GJ, Fairman RM, et al. Limb ischemia during femoral cannulation for cardiopulmonary support. J Vasc Surg. 2010;52:850–3.

6.  Aziz F, Brehm CE, El-Banyosy A, Han DC, Atnip RG, Reed AB. Arterial complications in patients undergoing extracorporeal membrane oxygenation via femoral cannulation. Ann Vasc Surg. 2014;28:178–83.

7.  Zimpfer D, Heinisch B, Czerny M, Hoelzenbein T, Taghavi S, Wolner E, et al. Late vascular complications after extracorporeal membrane oxygenation support. Ann Thorac Surg. 2006;81:892–5.

8.  Park TK, Yang JH, Jeon K, Choi SH, Choi JH, Gwon HC, et al. Extracorporeal membrane oxygenation for refractory septic shock in adults. Eur J Cardiothorac Surg. 2015;47:e68–74.

9.  Ranney DN, Benrashid E, Meza JM, Keenan JE, Bonadonna D, Mureebe L, et al. Vascular complications and use of a distal perfusion cannula in femorally cannulated patients on extracorporeal membrane oxygenation. ASAIO J. 2018;64:328–33.

10. Muehrcke DD, McCarthy PM, Stewart RW, Seshagiri S, Ogella DA, Foster RC, et al. Complications of extracorporeal life support systems using heparin-bound surfaces. The risk of intracardiac clot formation. J Thorac Cardiovasc Surg. 1995;110:843–51.

# 19

# Iron metabolism in critically ill patients developing anemia of inflammation: a case control study

Margit Boshuizen[1,2]* ⓘ, Jan M. Binnekade[1], Benjamin Nota[3], Kirsten van de Groep[4,5], Olaf L. Cremer[4], Pieter R. Tuinman[6], Janneke Horn[1], Marcus J. Schultz[1], Robin van Bruggen[2†] and Nicole P. Juffermans[1†]Molecular Diagnosis and Risk Stratification of Sepsis (MARS) Consortium

## Abstract

**Background:** Anemia occurring as a result of inflammatory processes (anemia of inflammation, AI) has a high prevalence in critically ill patients. Knowledge on changes in iron metabolism during the course of AI is limited, hampering the development of strategies to counteract AI. This case control study aimed to investigate iron metabolism during the development of AI in critically ill patients.

**Methods:** Iron metabolism in 30 patients who developed AI during ICU stay was compared with 30 septic patients with a high Hb and 30 non-septic patients with a high Hb. Patients were matched on age and sex. Longitudinally collected plasma samples were analyzed for levels of parameters of iron metabolism. A linear mixed model was used to assess the predictive values of the parameters.

**Results:** In patients with AI, levels of iron, transferrin and transferrin saturation showed an early decrease compared to controls with a high Hb, already prior to the development of anemia. Ferritin, hepcidin and IL-6 levels were increased in AI compared to controls. During AI development, erythroferrone decreased. Differences in iron metabolism between groups were not influenced by APACHE IV score.

**Conclusions:** The results show that in critically ill patients with AI, iron metabolism is already altered prior to the development of anemia. Levels of iron regulators in AI differ from septic controls with a high Hb, irrespective of disease severity. AI is characterized by high levels of hepcidin, ferritin and IL-6 and low levels of iron, transferrin and erythroferrone.

**Keywords:** Critical care, Anemia, Iron, Inflammation, Sepsis, Hepcidin

## Background

Anemia is a hallmark of critical illness, occurring in up to 95% of critically ill patients [1, 2]. The cause of anemia in these patients is often multifactorial including blood loss, low nutrient intake and iatrogenic factors, such as hemodilution and frequent blood sampling. Another major cause of anemia in critically ill patients is anemia of inflammation (AI) [3]. Although distinguishing AI from anemia due to iron deficiency is a diagnostic challenge, the contribution of inflammation to the development of anemia is thought to play a role in up to 75% of critically ill patients [4, 5]. AI is characterized by a decreased production of red blood cells, a shortened red blood cell life span and alterations in iron metabolism, which will impact erythropoiesis [4, 6].

Levels of transferrin, the iron transporter in the circulation, are low in AI, as well as levels of iron [7]. The main regulator of iron levels in the circulation is hepcidin. Hepcidin inhibits iron uptake and transport by

*Correspondence: m.boshuizen@amc.uva.nl
†Robin van Bruggen and Nicole P. Juffermans contributed equally to this work
[1] Department of Intensive Care Medicine, Academic Medical Center, University of Amsterdam, Meibergdreef 9, 1105 AZ Amsterdam, The Netherlands
Full list of author information is available at the end of the article

internalization of the iron export channel ferroportin on enterocytes, hepatocytes and macrophages, resulting in low levels of iron available for erythropoiesis [8, 9]. Hepcidin production in the liver increases in response to cytokines, such as interleukin 6 (IL-6), whereas both low plasma iron levels and anemia suppress hepcidin. Hepcidin is also regulated by erythroferrone (ERFE), a hormone produced by erythroblasts in response to erythropoietin, which suppresses hepcidin production [10, 11]. During inflammation, cytokines such as IFN-γ inhibit erythropoiesis, resulting in a reduction of the number of erythroblasts [12] and as a result a low ERFE level. Taken together, in AI, due to the high levels of hepcidin, there is not an absolute iron deficiency but rather a decreased iron availability. Consequently, both oral and intravenous supplementation of iron to support erythropoiesis in critically ill patients with anemia has not been unequivocally successful [13–15]. As other means to treat anemia in critically ill, such as supplementation of recombinant erythropoietin, have shown benefit [16], but also harm [6, 17], correction of anemia is usually done by blood transfusions. However, as transfusion is associated with lung injury, infections and increased mortality [2], other strategies to increase iron availability for erythropoiesis are warranted. These may include reducing hepcidin activity, which has been suggested to be beneficial in experimental models [18, 19].

Currently, knowledge on changes in iron metabolism during the course of critical illness is limited, which hampers the development of new strategies to correct AI. In this case control study, we investigated several parameters of iron metabolism in critically ill septic patients who developed anemia during their stay on the ICU. These patients are classified as AI and compared to critically ill control patients with sepsis and without sepsis who have a high hemoglobin level (Hb).

## Methods

### Study design

This is a sub-study of the Molecular Diagnosis and Risk Stratification of Sepsis (MARS) project, which was a prospective observational cohort study on molecular diagnostics of sepsis, conducted in the ICU of 2 tertiary hospitals (ClinicalTrials.gov NCT01905033). All patients admitted to the ICUs between January 2011 and July 2013 older than 18 years and with an expected stay longer than 24 h were included. Trained ICU research physicians prospectively collected demographic data, including Acute Physiology and Chronic Health Evaluation, (APACHE IV score), admission type, daily disease severity scores (Sequential Organ Failure Assessment, SOFA) and outcome. For this study, an opt-out consent method was approved by the Medical Ethical Committees of both

centers (IRB No. 10-056C). Participants were informed about the study by a brochure provided at ICU admission attached with an opt-out card that could be completed by the patient or legal representative in case of unwillingness to participate.

### Patient selection

For the current study, three groups of critically ill patients were identified. Patients were classified as developing AI when anemia (Hb < 6 mmol/L) occurred during their ICU stay while complying to the diagnosis of sepsis (termed: AI group). Sepsis was used as criterion for inflammation to be able to identify patients with severe inflammation from the database. Patients with AI were compared to sepsis patients who had a high Hb (Hb level ≥ 7 mmol/L) (termed: septic controls, high Hb) and to patients without sepsis who had a high Hb (termed: non-septic controls, high Hb, $n = 30$ per group) (Additional file 1: Table S1). Hb levels of AI patients and controls were chosen in order to create a clear distinction between patient groups. Anemia was defined as Hb < 6 mmol/L, because these patients near the transfusion trigger and are therefore the clinically relevant anemic patients. The control patients were used to determine the influence of the presence of sepsis on iron metabolism as well as the "background" influence of being critically ill. Sample size of 30 patients per group was chosen based on a previous study that shows statistically significant results with similar patient numbers [20].

For all groups, the following patients were excluded: patients who received red blood cell transfusions prior to or during the inclusion period, patients with conditions which may induce or alter chronic anemia (chronic renal failure, hematological disease, chemotherapy, acquired immunodeficiency syndrome), patients receiving iron or erythropoietin therapy and postoperative patients (in order to avoid patients who became anemic due to blood loss due to invasive procedures). Daily patient files were screened on blood loss, due to surgery or other invasive procedures or gastrointestinal bleeding. Patients with reported blood loss due to invasive procedures or gastrointestinal bleeding directly prior to ICU admission or during the sampling period on the ICU were excluded.

Patients with AI were matched to controls for age and sex using the Optimal Matching method from the MatchIt package of R statistics [21]. Longitudinal blood samples were taken from the biobank of collected samples. Infection was scored and classified using a four point scale (none, possible probable or definite) according to the Center for Disease Control and Prevention [22] and International Sepsis Forum Consensus Conference definitions [23, 24]. Sepsis was defined as a definite or probable infection accompanied by at least one additional parameter as described in the 2001 International Sepsis Definitions Conference [25] (Additional file 2: Table S2). All included sepsis patients had a SOFA ≥ 2 at ICU admission, approximating the new sepsis-3 criteria [26]. To determine whether patients were suffering from iron deficiency, the algorithm of Weiss was used [3].

### Sample selection and analysis

The first blood sampling moment in all groups was on ICU admission. The second sampling moment for AI patients was on the day they developed anemia, the third sampling moment was 2 days later. Control patients were sampled on the first and third day of complying to their classification (Additional file 1: Table S1).

Samples were centrifuged at 1500 g for 15 min at room temperature and plasma was stored at − 80 °C. Measurements were done in heparin anti-coagulated plasma. Serum iron, transferrin, ferritin and haptoglobin were measured by immunoturbidimetric methods (Roche Cobas c702). Transferrin saturation was calculated by the formula serum iron/(25.2 × transferrin). Hepcidin (R&D), soluble transferrin receptor (sTfR) (Biovendor), erythroferrone (MyBioSource) and IL-6 levels (R&D) were measured by enzyme-linked immunosorbent assay kits.

### Statistical analysis

One-way ANOVA was used, or in case of non-normally distributed data, the Kruskal–Wallis. Categorical variables were compared with the Chi-square test or Fisher's exact tests.

First, it was investigated whether there were differences in iron metabolism between groups. Therefore, the predictive value of the explanatory groups for the iron metabolism variables was assessed. Since the observations over time are nested within patients, analysis was done by a linear mixed model, using the three different groups of ICU patients (AI, septic controls, non-septic controls) as a fixed effect. Patients, which include the repeated measures, were used as random effect. APACHE IV score and proton pump inhibitor (PPI) use were included in the model as potential confounders. The dependent variables in the model showed skewed distributions. The best data transformation from the Box–Cox family of power transformations [27] resulted in log transformations for all iron metabolism variables. The best model fit was investigated with the Linear and Nonlinear Mixed Effects Models package [28]. The modeling process is described in the supplement. Estimates from the log-transformed response scale predictions (levels of iron metabolism variables) were back-transformed and reported. Contrasts among predicted values for groups were tested by the Least-Square Means package [29]. Second, it was investigated whether there were significant

differences in levels of iron parameters between sample days using the Friedman test. Mean imputation was used to replace missing data (6 out of 270 data points were missing). Statistical significance was considered to be at $p = 0.05$. All tests were corrected by the Bonferroni method [29, 30]. When appropriate, statistical uncertainty is expressed by the 95% confidence levels. All analyses were performed in R statistics [31].

### Results

Patient selection algorithm is shown in Additional file 3: Fig. S1. Patients in the AI group did not differ from those in the control groups in age and sex, due to matching on these factors (Table 1). Patients with AI, however, tended to be sicker compared to septic and non-septic control groups, exemplified by higher Acute Physiology and Chronic Health Evaluation (APACHE) IV score ($p = 0.08$) and Sequential Organ Failure Assessment (SOFA) scores at admission ($p = 0.05$). However, SOFA scores did not differ between groups in follow-up sampling.

### Hemoglobin level

The course of Hb levels in the different groups is shown in Fig. 1. As per inclusion criteria, the patients in the AI group became anemic over time during the ICU course, but were not anemic when admitted to the ICU. The median time to become anemic in this group was 8 (4–11 interquartile range (IQR)) days. Also per inclusion criterion, the comparative groups (septic controls and non-septic controls) kept a high Hb level during the course of the study. The median sample days for these control groups were similar; admission day 3 (3–3 IQR) and day 5 (5–5 IQR). At admission, the mean Hb levels of the septic and the non-septic control groups were higher than the Hb level of AI patients ($p < 0.001$).

### Iron metabolism in patients with AI

In patients in the AI group, the levels of different regulators of iron metabolism were already largely deviating from reference values at ICU admission, even when anemia had not yet developed, and did not change further over time. Iron, transferrin and transferrin saturation were low in AI and did not decrease further over time (Fig. 2). Ferritin levels were increased in AI compared to the reference value and also hepcidin, and IL-6 levels were high, but did not increase further over time (Fig. 2). ERFE levels decreased over time in AI (Fig. 2). Haptoglobin levels were increased at admission compared to reference values and further increased over time (Fig. 2). Taken together, these parameters comply with the diagnosis of AI, characterized by high levels of hepcidin and ferritin and decreased levels of iron and transferrin. Of interest, in AI, iron metabolism was

**Table 1 Patient characteristics**

| Characteristics | AI (n = 30) | Septic controls, high Hb (n = 30) | Non-septic controls, high Hb (n = 30) | p value |
|---|---|---|---|---|
| Male, n (%) | 19 (63) | 19 (63) | 19 (63) | 1.00 |
| Age, years median (range) | 64.5 (20–85) | 65.5 (22–81) | 64 (21–79) | 0.99 |
| APACHE IV score median (range) | 82.5 (45–155) | 72 (45–128) | 71 (17–104) | 0.08 |
| Admission type, n (%) | | | | |
| Surgical ward | 7 (23) | 4 (13) | 7 (23) | 0.66 |
| Medical ward | 17 (57) | 16 (53) | 13 (43) | 0.75 |
| Neurological ward | 6 (20) | 10 (33) | 10 (33) | 0.72 |
| SOFA score median (range) | | | | |
| Sampling moment 1 | 7 (3–16) | 7 (3–10) | 5 (0–15) | 0.05 |
| Sampling moment 2 | 6 (3–17) | 6 (1–15) | 5 (2–12) | 0.09 |
| Sampling moment 3 | 5 (2–14) | 5 (1–15) | 4 (1–12) | 0.21 |
| Hemoglobin in mmol/L, mean SD | | | | |
| ICU admission | 7.2 (±0.7) | 8.6 (±0.8) | 8.4 (±0.7) | < 0.01 |
| Second sample | 5.6 (±0.3) | 8.1 (±0.8) | 8.1 (±0.6) | < 0.01 |
| Third sample | 5.3 (±0.3) | 8.1 (±0.7) | 8.0 (±0.6) | < 0.01 |
| ICU mortality, n (%) | 4 (13) | 2 (7) | 3 (10) | 0.69 |
| Hospital mortality, n (%) | 10 (33) | 6 (20) | 9 (30) | 0.49 |

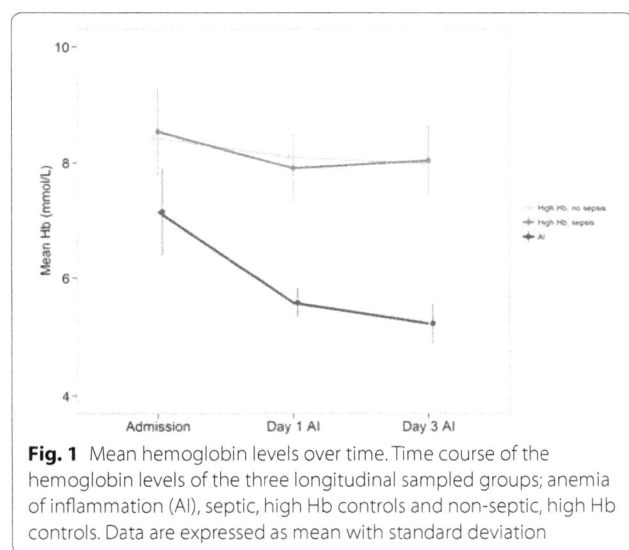

**Fig. 1** Mean hemoglobin levels over time. Time course of the hemoglobin levels of the three longitudinal sampled groups; anemia of inflammation (AI), septic, high Hb controls and non-septic, high Hb controls. Data are expressed as mean with standard deviation

already altered at ICU admission, when Hb levels were still normal.

## Iron metabolism in patients with AI compared to septic and non-septic controls with high Hb level

Table 2 shows the mean estimates derived from the linear mixed model of different parameters of iron metabolism for all patients per group at all time points. Patients in the AI group had a significantly lower iron level compared to septic controls with a high Hb level, as well as a lower transferrin level and a lower transferrin saturation

(Table 2). The haptoglobin concentration was significantly higher in AI patients compared to septic controls with a high Hb level. Hepcidin, ferritin, sTfR and ERFE levels were similar. The time course of iron parameters in AI shows a similar pattern as in septic patients with a high Hb level. The haptoglobin level increased over time in both groups and ERFE levels decreased over time, with an earlier decrease in AI compared to septic controls (Fig. 2). This comparison between AI patients and non-septic controls with a high Hb level is similar to the comparison of AI to septic controls with a high Hb level. However, the differences between AI and non-septic controls were more pronounced than the differences between AI and septic controls, suggesting that sepsis influences iron metabolism in AI. However, in the multivariate model, APACHE IV score as a measure of disease severity was not a confounder of results, except for the IL-6 model. Of note, proton pump inhibitors affect intestinal iron intake and are frequently administered to ICU patients [32]. However, the use of proton pump inhibitors was not a confounder of results either (see Additional file 4: Supplement).

## Contribution of iron deficiency to the development of anemia in patients on the ICU

To determine whether iron deficiency may have contributed to the development of anemia, the algorithm of Weiss [3] was applied to all anemic patients. According to this algorithm, none of the patients with AI were iron deficient.

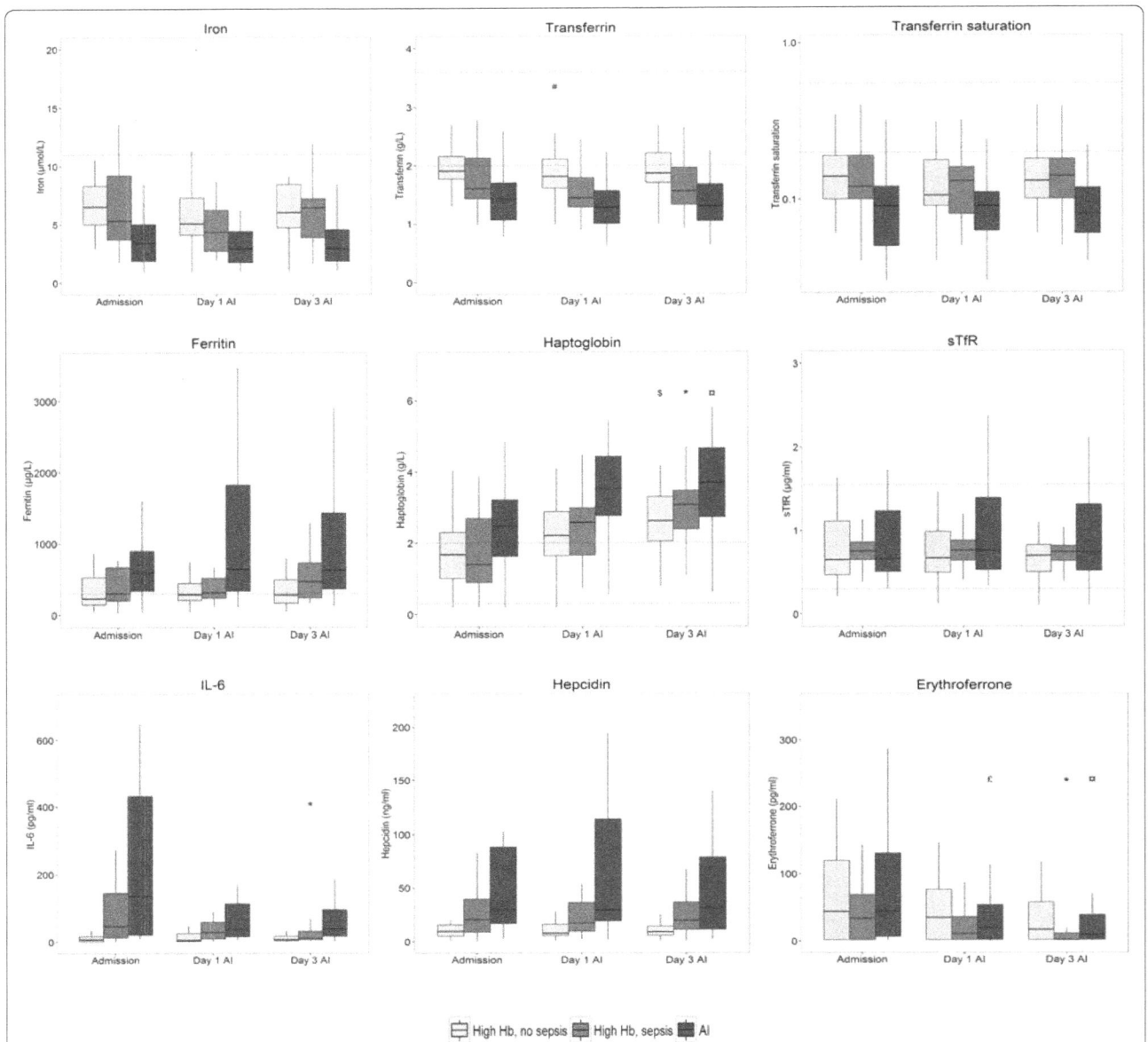

**Fig. 2** Iron parameters and IL-6 levels per group over time. Time course of observed plasma iron parameters of the three groups; anemia of inflammation (AI), Septic, high Hb controls, non-septic, high Hb controls. Dotted line represents reference values. Statistically significant differences within the groups over time are indicated with: £ $p < 0.05$ AI group 'Day 1 AI' compared to 'Admission', # $p < 0.05$ non-septic, high Hb group 'Day 1 AI' compared to 'Admission', $ $p < 0.05$ non-septic, high Hb group 'Day 3 AI' compared to 'Admission', * $p < 0.05$ Septic, high Hb group 'Day 3 AI' compared to 'Admission', ¤ $p < 0.05$ AI group 'Day 3 AI' compared to 'Admission'. Data are expressed as median with 25–75 interquartile ranges

## Discussion

The current study measured key players of iron metabolism over time in several critically ill patient populations. We show that iron metabolism is altered in ICU patients [20], regardless of the presence of anemia. However, alterations in iron metabolism are more pronounced in AI patients than in non-anemic controls. As patients with AI tended to be more severely ill, we investigated whether these changes could be related to disease severity. The

APACHE IV score did not influence outcome of the models, suggesting that not only disease severity drives the development of AI. Hepcidin, which is thought to be the main regulator of AI, was not different between AI and septic controls. ERFE, which regulates hepcidin, showed a rapid decrease in AI patients when compared to septic controls. Therefore, a decrease in ERFE levels may contribute to the development of AI. Haptoglobin levels increased over time in AI, suggesting that intravascular

**Table 2 Mean estimates of iron parameters derived from the linear mixed model**

| Iron parameter | AI | Septic controls, high Hb | Non-septic controls, high Hb |
|---|---|---|---|
| Iron (µmol/L) | 3.8 (3.2–4.5)*† | 5.6 (4.8–6.6) | 6.3 (5.4–7.3) |
| Transferrin (g/L) | 1.3 (1.2–1.5)*† | 1.6 (1.5–1.8) | 1.9 (1.7–2) |
| Transferrin saturation (%) | 10 (8–12)* | 14 (11–16) | 13 (11–15) |
| Ferritin (µg/L) | 1134 (548–2346)† | 473 (229–976) | 314 (152–648) |
| Haptoglobin (g/L) | 3.5 (3.2–3.9)*† | 2.7 (2.4–3) | 2.5 (2.2–2.8) |
| Hepcidin (pg/ml) | 20.7 (15.1–28.5)† | 12.9 (9.4–17.9) | 7.3 (5.4–9.8) |
| Erythroferrone (pg/ml) | 15.5 (9.3–26) | 9.6 (5.8–16) | 18.7 (11.2–31) |
| sTfR (µg/ml) | 0.83 (0.68–1.01) | 0.7 (0.55–0.87) | 0.70 (0.57–0.86) |
| IL-6 (pg/ml) | 14.4 (5.1–40.9)† | 8.0 (1.5–43.0) | 2.0 (0.4–10.9) |

Data are expressed as (back-transformed) mean estimates of iron parameters for all patients per group at all time points, with 95% confidence interval

Differences between mean estimates are tested by contrasts. * $p < 0.05$ AI compared to septic controls, † $p < 0.05$ AI compared to non-septic controls

hemolysis does not contribute to the development of anemia during sepsis. However, hemolysis could not be excluded, since increased haptoglobin levels can reflect inflammation, although IL-6 did not increase during AI development. Taken together, iron parameters are altered already at ICU admission. In those patients going on to develop AI, these disturbances are more pronounced compared to septic and non-septic controls, which is not solely due to disease severity.

Our finding that iron metabolism is already altered in AI prior to the development of anemia suggests a window of opportunity to prevent AI. Iron supplementation is an appealing approach. However, in our study, iron deficiency could not be detected in patients with AI. Although the algorithm used to detect iron deficiency has not been validated for ICU patients, AI may account for a large proportion of anemia in ICU patients. Therefore, it may not be surprising that studies on efficacy of iron therapy in critically ill patients showed conflicting results [13–15, 33–35]. Heterogeneity of causes of anemia in patients included in these studies could have contributed to conflicting outcomes. A possible exception is the recent IRONMAN study, which showed that iron supplementation resulted in an increased Hb level at hospital discharge compared to placebo [15]. In this study, patients with a low likelihood of iron deficiency (high ferritin, high transferrin saturation) were excluded, which may have yielded a more homogenous patient population. Given that our study indicates that absolute iron deficiency may not be present in a large proportion of the ICU patients that suffer from anemia, other treatment options may be to increase the amount of iron available for erythropoiesis, e.g. by inhibiting hepcidin activity. An anti-hepcidin antibody reduced the development of AI

in monkeys [18] and prevented a fall in iron levels in human endotoxemia [19]. However, the advantages of potential therapies to increase iron availability must be weighed against the risk of adverse events. Iron may promote bacterial growth [36] and increase the risk of infections in several patient populations [37–39]. In ICU patients, high levels of transferrin saturation, which reflects iron availability, has even shown to be a predictor of mortality in septic patients [40]. It is not known whether this association is due to a real pathogenic effect of abundant iron or only reflects a higher katabolic state. Notably, studies on iron therapy in ICU patients did not show an increased rate of in-hospital infections or mortality [13–15, 33, 34].

This study has limitations, the first of which is the small number of patients included. The finding that hepcidin levels were consistently higher in AI compared to septic controls without reaching statistical significance may reflect limited power. Secondly, to define AI patients, sepsis was used as inclusion criterion instead of inflammation, which hampers extrapolation of results to patients with inflammation due to other causes. Thirdly, as a result of the inclusion criteria, iron parameters were not measured at similar timepoints between groups. Finally, patients with liver cirrhosis and occult blood loss were not excluded. Strengths of our study are the case control design and the longitudinal sampling of ICU patients, using control groups which allow to determine the influence of the presence of sepsis on iron metabolism as well as the "background" influence of being critically ill. Also, strict exclusion criteria to limit external factors that influence iron metabolism were applied and strict definitions were used. Further, data and sample collection were performed by dedicated researchers leading to a complete follow-up.

## Conclusions

In conclusion, we have shown that iron metabolism is already changed in AI before anemia occurs, suggesting a window of opportunity for therapy to modulate iron metabolism. Levels of iron, transferrin and transferrin saturation are low in AI patients compared to septic controls, irrespective of disease severity, suggesting that AI is not solely determined by severity of inflammation. ERFE may play a role in the development of AI.

### Abbreviations
AI: Anemia of inflammation; APACHE IV score: Acute Physiology and Chronic Health Evaluation IV score; ERFE: Erythroferrone; Hb: Hemoglobin; ICU: Intensive care unit; IL-6: Interleukin 6; IQR: Interquartile range; MARS: Molecular Diagnosis and Risk Stratification of Sepsis; SOFA: Sequential Organ Failure Assessment; sTfR: Soluble transferrin receptor.

### Authors' contributions
MB, BN, RB, NJ were involved in the study design. MB, BN, JH, MS, KG, OC were contributed to the data. MB, JB, RB, NJ analyzed and interpreted the data. MB, RB, NJ wrote the manuscript. MB, BN, JB, JH, MS, KG, OC, PT, RB, NJ reviewed the manuscript and approved the final submitted version. All authors read and approved the final manuscript.

### Author details
[1] Department of Intensive Care Medicine, Academic Medical Center, University of Amsterdam, Meibergdreef 9, 1105 AZ Amsterdam, The Netherlands.
[2] Department of Blood Cell Research, Sanquin Research and Landsteiner Laboratory, Academic Medical Center, University of Amsterdam, Amsterdam, The Netherlands. [3] Department of Research Facilities, Sanquin Research and Landsteiner Laboratory, Academic Medical Center, University of Amsterdam, Amsterdam, The Netherlands. [4] Department of Intensive Care Medicine, University Medical Center Utrecht, Utrecht, The Netherlands. [5] Julius Center for Health Sciences and Primary Care, University Medical Center Utrecht, Utrecht, The Netherlands. [6] Department of Intensive Care Medicine, VU University Medical Center Amsterdam, University of Amsterdam, Amsterdam, The Netherlands.

### Acknowledgements
The authors thank all members of the MARS consortium for the participation in data collection and especially acknowledge: Friso M. de Beer, MD, Lieuwe D. J. Bos, MD, PhD Gerie J. Glas, MD, Roosmarijn T. M. van Hooijdonk, MD, PhD, Laura R. A. Schouten, MD, Marleen Straat, MD, Esther Witteveen, MD, and Luuk Wieske, MD, PhD (Department of Intensive Care Medicine, Academic Medical Center, University of Amsterdam), Arie J. Hoogendijk, PhD, Mischa A. Huson, MD, Brendon P. Scicluna, Tom van der Pol, MD, PhD, Lonneke A. van Vught, MD, PhD, Maryse A. Wiewel, MD, PhD, (Center for Experimental and Molecular Medicine, Academic Medical Center, University of Amsterdam), Marc J. M. Bonten, MD, PhD, Jos F. Frencken, MD, Peter M. C. Klein Klouwenberg, MD, PharmD, PhD, Maria E. Koster-Brouwer, MSc, David S. Y. Ong, MD, PharmD, Diana M. Verboom, MD (Department of Intensive Care Medicine, Julius Center for Health Sciences and Primary Care and Department of Medical Microbiology, University Medical Center Utrecht, Utrecht, The Netherlands).

### Competing interests
The authors declare that they have no competing interests.

### Funding
This study is financially supported by Sanquin (Grant No. PPOP-14-31).

### References
1. Corwin HL, Gettinger A, Pearl RG, Fink MP, Levy MM, Abraham E, et al. The CRIT Study: anemia and blood transfusion in the critically ill—current clinical practice in the United States. Crit Care Med. 2004;32:39–52.
2. Napolitano LM, Kurek S, Luchette FA, Anderson GL, Bard MR, Bromberg W, et al. Clinical practice guideline: red blood cell transfusion in adult trauma and critical care. J Trauma. 2009;67:1439–42.
3. Weiss G, Goodnough LT. Anemia of chronic disease. N Engl J Med. 2005;352:1011–23.
4. Prakash D. Anemia in the ICU: anemia of chronic disease versus anemia of acute illness. Crit Care Clin. 2012;28:333–43.
5. Pieracci FM, Barie PS. Diagnosis and management of iron-related anemias in critical illness. Crit Care Med. 2006;34:1898–905.
6. Sihler KC, Napolitano LM. Anemia of inflammation in critically ill patients. J Intensive Care Med. 2008;23:295–302.
7. Ganz T, Nemeth E. Iron sequestration and anemia of inflammation. Semin Hematol. 2009;46:387–93.
8. Krause A, Neitz S, Mägert HJ, Schulz A, Forssmann WG, Schulz-Knappe P, et al. LEAP-1, a novel highly disulfide-bonded human peptide, exhibits antimicrobial activity. FEBS Lett. 2000;480:147–50.
9. Park CH, Valore EV, Waring AJ, Ganz T. Hepcidin, a urinary antimicrobial peptide synthesized in the liver. J Biol Chem. 2001;276:7806–10.
10. Kautz L, Jung G, Valore EV, Rivella S, Nemeth E, Ganz T. Identification of erythroferrone as an erythroid regulator of iron metabolism. Nat Genet. 2014;46:678–84.
11. Chen H, Choesang T, Li H, Sun S, Pham P, Bao W, et al. Increased hepcidin in transferrin-treated thalassemic mice correlates with increased liver BMP2 expression and decreased hepatocyte ERK activation. Haematologica. 2015;101:297–308.
12. Libregts SF, Gutiérrez L, De Bruin AM, Wensveen FM, Papadopoulos P, Van Ijcken W, et al. Chronic IFN-γ production in mice induces anemia by reducing erythrocyte life span and inhibiting erythropoiesis through an IRF-1/PU. 1 axis. Blood. 2011;118:2578–88.
13. Pieracci FM, Stovall RT, Jaouen B, Rodil M, Cappa A, Burlew CC, et al. A multicenter, randomized clinical trial of IV iron supplementation for anemia of traumatic critical illness. Crit Care Med. 2014;42:2048–57.
14. Shah A, Roy NB, McKechnie S, Doree C, Fisher SA, Stanworth SJ. Iron supplementation to treat anaemia in adult critical care patients: a systematic review and meta-analysis. Crit Care. 2016;20:306.
15. Litton E, Baker S, Erber WN, Farmer S, Ferrier J, French C, et al. Intravenous iron or placebo for anaemia in intensive care: the IRONMAN multicentre randomized blinded trial. Intensive Care Med. 2016;42:1715–22.
16. Corwin HL, Gettinger A, Pearl RG, Fink MP, Levy MM, Shapiro MJ, Corwin MJ, Colton T. Efficacy of recombinant human erythropoietin in critically ill patients a randomized controlled trial. JAMA. 2002;288:2827–35.
17. Drueke TB, Locatelli F, Clyne N, Eckardt K, Macdougall IC, Tsakiris D, Burger HU, Scherhag A. Normalization of hemoglobin level in patients with chronic kidney disease and anemia. N Engl J Med. 2006;355:333–40.
18. Schwoebel F, van Eijk LT, Zboralski D, Sell S, Buchner K, Maasch C, et al. The effects of the anti-hepcidin Spiegelmer NOX-H94 on inflammation-induced anemia in cynomolgus monkeys. Blood. 2013;121:2311–5.
19. Van Eijk LT, John ASE, Schwoebel F, Summo L, Vauléon S, Zöllner S, et al. Effect of the antihepcidin Spiegelmer lexaptepid on inflammation-induced decrease in serum iron in humans. Blood. 2014;124:2643–6.
20. Piagnerelli M, Cotton F, Herpain A, Rapotec A, Chatti R, Gulbis B, et al. Time course of iron metabolism in critically ill patients. Acta Clin Belg. 2012;67:1–6.
21. Ho DE, Imai K, King G, Stuart EA. MatchIt: nonparametric preprocessing for parametric causal inference. J Stat Softw. 2011;42:1–28.
22. Garner JS, Jarvis WR, Emori TG, Horan TC, Hughes JM. CDC definitions for nosocomial infections, 1988. AJIC Am J Infect Control. 1988;16:128–40.
23. Calandra T, Cohen J. The international sepsis forum consensus conference on definitions of infection in the intensive care unit. Crit Care Med. 2005;33:1538–48.
24. Klein Klouwenberg PMC, Ong DSY, Bos LDJ, de Beer FM, van Hooijdonk RTM, Huson MA, et al. Interobserver agreement of centers for disease control and prevention criteria for classifying infections in critically ill patients. Crit Care Med. 2013;41:2373–8.

25. Levy MM, Fink MP, Marshall JC, Abraham E, Angus D, Cook D, et al. 2001 SCCM/ESICM/ACCP/ATS/SIS international sepsis definitions conference. Crit Care Med. 2003;31:1250–6.
26. Singer M, et al. The third international consensus definitions for sepsis and septic shock (sepsis-3). JAMA. 2016;315:801–10.
27. Box GEP, Cox DR. An analysis of transformations. J R Stat Soc Ser B. 1964;26:211–52.
28. Pinheiro J, Bates D, DebRoy S, Sarkar D, R Core Team. nlme: linear and nonlinear mixed effects models. R package version 3.1-128. 2016.
29. Lenth RV. Least-squares means: the R package lsmeans. J Stat Softw. 2016;69:1–33.
30. Searle SR, Speed FM, Milliken GA. Population marginal means in the linear model: an alternative to least squares means. Am Stat. 1980;34:216–21.
31. RC Team. R: A language and environment for statistical computing. Vienna, Austria: R Foundation for Statistical Computing; 2016.
32. Vanclooster A, van Deursen C, Jaspers R, Cassiman D, Koek G. Proton pump inhibitors decrease phlebotomy need in HFE hemochromatosis: double-blind randomized placebo-controlled trial. Gastroenterology. 2017;153:678e2–680e2.
33. Garrido-Martín P, Nassar-Mansur MI, de la Llana-Ducrós R, Virgos-Aller TM, Rodríguez Fortunez PM, Ávalos-Pinto R, et al. The effect of intravenous and oral iron administration on perioperative anaemia and transfusion requirements in patients undergoing elective cardiac surgery: a randomized clinical trial. Interact CardioVasc Thorac Surg. 2012;15:1013–8.
34. Pieracci FM, Henderson P, Rodney JRM, Holena DN, Genisca A, Ip I, et al. Randomized, double-blind, placebo-controlled trial of effects of enteral iron supplementation on anemia and risk of infection during surgical critical illness. Surg Infect (Larchmt). 2009;10:9–19.
35. Madi-Jebara SN, Sleilaty GS, Achouh PE, Yazigi AG, Haddad FA, Hayek GM, et al. Postoperative intravenous iron used alone or in combination with low-dose erythropoietin is not effective for correction of anemia after cardiac surgery. J Cardiothorac Vasc Anesth. 2004;18:59–63.
36. Patruta S, Walter HH. Iron and infection. Kidney Int. 1999;55:S125–30.
37. Hoen B. Iron and infection: clinical experience. Am J Kidney Dis. 1999;34:S30–4.
38. Sazawal S, Black R, Ramsan M, Chwaya H, Stoltzfus R, Dutta A, et al. Effect of routine prophylactic supplementation with iron and folic acid on admission to hospital and mortality in preschool children in a high malaria transmission setting: community based, randomised, placebo-controlled trial. Lancet. 2006;367:133–43.
39. Brookhart MA, Freburger JK, Ellis AR, Wang L, Winkelmayer WC, Kshirsagar AV. Infection risk with bolus versus maintenance iron supplementation in hemodialysis patients. J Am Soc Nephrol. 2013;24:1151–8.
40. Tacke F, Nuraldeen R, Koch A, Strathmann K, Hutschenreuter G, Trautwein C, et al. Iron parameters determine the prognosis of critically ill patients. Crit Care Med. 2016;44:1049–58.

# 20

# Vascular complications in adult postcardiotomy cardiogenic shock patients receiving venoarterial extracorporeal membrane oxygenation

Feng Yang, Dengbang Hou, Jinhong Wang, Yongchao Cui, Xiaomeng Wang, Zhichen Xing, Chunjing Jiang, Xing Hao, Zhongtao Du, Xiaofang Yang, Yu Jiang and Xiaotong Hou[*]

## Abstract

**Background:** The rate, prognostic impacts, and predisposing factors of major vascular complications (MVCs) in patients underwent venoarterial extracorporeal membrane oxygenation (VA-ECMO) by surgical cut-down are poorly understood. The purpose of this study was to identify these parameters in adult VA-ECMO patients.

**Methods:** Adult postcardiotomy cardiogenic shock (PCS) patients receiving VA-ECMO by femoral surgical cut-down cannulation from January 2004 to December 2015 were enrolled in this study. Patients were separated into two groups depending on the presence of MVCs. Multivariate logistic regression was performed to identify factors independently associated with MVCs.

**Results:** Of 432 patients with PCS treated with VA-ECMO, 252 patients (58.3%) were weaned off VA-ECMO and 153 patients (35.4%) survived to discharge. MVCs were seen in 72 patients (16.7%), including bleeding or hematoma in the cannulation site (8.6%), limb ischemia requiring fasciotomy (8.6%), femoral artery embolism (0.7%), and retroperitoneal bleeding (0.7%). The rate of survival to discharge was 16.7 and 39.2% in patients with or without MVCs, respectively ($p < 0.001$). Obesity, concomitant with intra-aortic balloon pump (IABP), Sequential Organ Failure Assessment (SOFA) score at 24 h post-ECMO, and hemostasis disorder were shown to be associated with MVCs. MVCs were an independent risk factor for in-hospital mortality by multivariate analysis (odds ratio 3.91; 95% confidence interval, 1.67–9.14; $p = 0.013$).

**Conclusions:** MVCs are common and associated with higher in-hospital mortality among adult PCS patients receiving peripheral VA-ECMO support. The obesity, concomitant with IABP, SOFA score at 24 h post-ECMO, and hemostasis disorder were independent risk factor of MVCs.

**Keywords:** Postcardiotomy cardiogenic shock, Venoarterial extracorporeal membrane oxygenation, Complications, Cannulation, Survival

## Background

Postcardiotomy cardiogenic shock (PCS) remains a clinical challenge, with high mortality rate [1]. Venoarterial extracorporeal membrane oxygenation (VA-ECMO) may provide a survival benefit for patients with PCS. Femoral VA-ECMO is less invasive and rapidly instituted at the bedside, especially in patients who have had a cardiac arrest [2]. The use of VA-ECMO for adult PCS has increased, with a survival rate of 16–42% [3–7].

Successful cannulation is the prerequisite and basis for VA-ECMO support for achieving good clinical results. Percutaneous and surgical cut-down vascular cannulations are commonly performed for VA-ECMO

*Correspondence: xt.hou@ccmu.edu.cn
Center for Cardiac Intensive Care, Beijing Institute of Heart, Lung, and Blood Vessels Diseases, Beijing Anzhen Hospital, Capital Medical University, No. 2 Anzhen Rd, Chaoyang District, Beijing 100029, China

implantation [8, 9]. Major vascular complications (MVCs) can occur from cannulation of the femoral vessels. However, the actual prevalence of MVCs and outcomes of PCS patients underwent VA-ECMO by surgical cut-down is still unclear. To date, only a few studies have reported on MVCs in PCS patients from single-center experience [10–12]. Therefore, we elucidated the prevalence of MVCs and their impact on in-hospital mortality in adult PCS patients receiving peripheral VA-ECMO by surgical cut-down. Furthermore, we also assessed the possible risk factors associated with the occurrence of MVCs.

## Methods

### Study population

Between January 2004 and December 2015, 43,192 adult patients underwent cardiac surgery. Of these patients, 451 patients (1.0%) required VA-ECMO support due to failure to wean from cardiopulmonary bypass (CPB) ($n = 231$) or a refractory PCS in the intensive care unit (ICU) ($n = 220$). For all patients receiving VA-ECMO, preoperative, perioperative, and postoperative clinical variables were prospectively recorded in the institutional database.

Patients who received VA-ECMO by femoral surgical cut-down cannulation for cardiac support ($n = 432$) were enrolled in this study. The patients implanted with VA-ECMO by either central ($n = 9$) or subclavian ($n = 10$) artery cannulation approach were excluded (Fig. 1). Patients were divided into two groups (MVCs group [$n = 72$] and no-MVCs group [$n = 360$]). The study was approved by the institutional ethics committee/review board of the Beijing Anzhen Hospital, and the requirement for informed patient consent was waived in view of the retrospective nature of the study.

### ECMO implantation techniques

VA-ECMO cannulas were surgically inserted by trained ECMO team members with femoral–femoral approach. The groin was incised, and the common femoral artery and vein were identified. A needle was inserted into the femoral vein using a subcutaneous tunnel. Following the Seldinger technique, a guidewire was advanced from the femoral vein toward the right atrium. The femoral vein was progressively dilated. A Bio-Medicus 19Fr-21Fr cannula was introduced over the guidewire, with placement of the tip just proximal to the right atrium. The common femoral artery was then similarly cannulated with Bio-Medicus 15Fr or 17Fr cannula. An additional 6F catheter was also performed at the time of ECMO initiation to preserve limb perfusion in most of patients (96.3%). All patients were cannulated and implanted the distal perfusion catheter under echocardiography guidance. In 246 patients (56.9%), a 7.5F IABP catheter (Datascope Corp., Fairfield, NJ, USA) was placed percutaneously through the contralateral femoral artery.

### Patient management

Detailed management strategies for patients were previously described [13]. ECMO blood flow was adjusted to maintain mixed venous oxygen saturation ($SvO_2$) level of 75%. The bleeding at the femoral cannulation site and the blood circulation of the lower limbs were observed continuously with trained ICU staff (bedside nurse) during ECMO support.

Heparin is the most commonly used anticoagulant. Previously given heparin was reversed with protamine prior to initiating VA-ECMO when patients had failed to wean from CPB. A heparin bolus (5000 IU) was injected before cannulation for PCS patients in the ICU. After VA-ECMO support, if surgical bleeding could be controlled, the patients were given continuous intravenous infusion of unfractionated heparin as early as possible to maintain an activated clotting time (ACT) of 160–180 s. Packed red blood cells were administered if the hemoglobin levels were less than 8 g/dL. Platelets were administered to maintain the platelet count at more than $50,000 \times 10^9$/L. When the patient had clinically improved, a weaning trial was performed using the protocol previously described [13]. All cannula removals were performed after exposing the femoral vessels. The femoral artery and vein were primarily repaired.

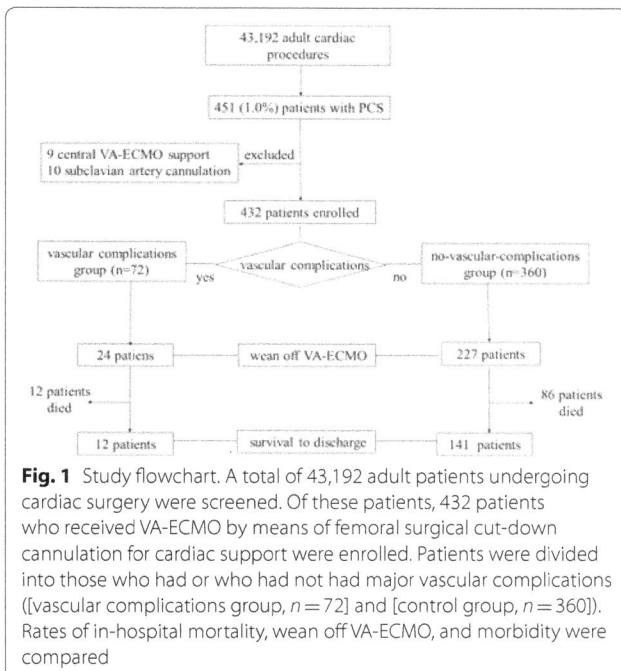

**Fig. 1** Study flowchart. A total of 43,192 adult patients undergoing cardiac surgery were screened. Of these patients, 432 patients who received VA-ECMO by means of femoral surgical cut-down cannulation for cardiac support were enrolled. Patients were divided into those who had or who had not had major vascular complications ([vascular complications group, $n = 72$] and [control group, $n = 360$]). Rates of in-hospital mortality, wean off VA-ECMO, and morbidity were compared

## Main aims and definitions

The primary endpoint was in-hospital mortality. The secondary endpoints were the proportion of patients weaned from VA-ECMO and major postoperative complications. In-hospital mortality was defined as death from any cause occurring in the hospital after surgery. Weaning off ECMO was considered successful when a patient survived VA-ECMO explantation for longer than 48 h [14].

MVCs related to cannulation were defined as those required surgical intervention by previous studies [7, 10, 11, 15]. Surgical indications included bleeding or hematoma at the VA-ECMO cannulation site, severe limb ischemia, femoral artery embolism, and retroperitoneal bleeding. Severe limb ischemia complications were defined as the deterioration of lower limb circulation ipsilateral to the cannulation site requiring surgical intervention (thrombectomy, fasciotomy, or amputation).

Postoperative renal failure was diagnosed in the presence of oliguria (< 30 mL/h) and a doubling of postoperative creatinine values requiring continuous renal replacement treatment (CRRT). Hemostasis disorders during ECMO included platelets < $20 \times 10^9$/L, fibrinogen < 1.5 g/L, and prothrombin time < 30% of the standard value [16]. Neurologic complications were recorded in the presence of clinical or radiologic evidence for a new neurologic deficit that was not present preoperatively. Diagnosis of acute extremity compartment syndrome is based on clinical symptoms and/or intra-compartmental pressure [17].

## Statistical analysis

Categorical variables and frequencies were presented as percentages and continuous variables as mean (range) or median (interquartile range) according to their distribution. Normality of distribution was tested with Kolmogorov–Smirnov test. The variables for patients with and without MVCs were compared using Student's $t$ test or the Mann–Whitney $U$ test for continuous variables, and Chi-square or Fisher's exact tests for categorical variables. The logistic regression analysis identified predictors of MVCs through the enter method. Survival rates were calculated using the Kaplan–Meier method. Analyses were performed using SPSS 20.0 (SPSS, Inc., Chicago, IL, USA) software and a two-sided $p < 0.05$ defined significance.

## Results

### Patient demographics, pre-ECMO characteristics, and ECMO variables

Demographics and pre-ECMO risk profiles of the 432 VA-ECMO patients are illustrated in Table 1. ECMO patients with MVCs had bigger body surface area (BSA),

higher body mass index (BMI), and higher inotrope scores at the beginning of VA-ECMO ($p < 0.05$). It is worth noting that the incidence of MVCs in patients with congenital heart disease was lower, but the difference was not statistically significant ($p = 0.068$).

Compared with the control group, blood lactate, and sequential organ failure assessment (SOFA) score at ECMO initiation, the ratio of severe bleeding (22.2 vs. 13.1%, $p = 0.044$) and repeat thoracotomy (51.4 vs. 36.7%, $p = 0.019$) in patients with MVCs were statistically higher. Therefore, patients with MVCs required a significantly higher number of red blood cell transfusion ($p = 0.002$). The duration of mechanical-assisted ventilation, ICU stay, and the length of stay in-hospital for MVCs patients were significantly shorter (Table 2).

### Occurrence rate of MVCs

A total of 72 patients (16.7%) had at least one episode of MVCs, including 37 patients (8.6%) with severe limb ischemia who progressed to compartment syndrome requiring prophylactic fasciotomy, 12 patients (2.8%) required limb amputation, 37 patients (8.6%) with significant bleeding or hematoma at the cannulation site that required surgical exploration, 3 patients (0.7%) with femoral artery embolism requirement surgical intervention, and 3 patients (0.7%) with retroperitoneal bleeding. Ten patients (2.3%) had both severe limb ischemia and bleeding in the cannulation site.

### Predisposing factors for MVCs

Table 3 reports the factors associated with the MVCs. The obesity, coronary artery disease, lactate and SOFA score at ECMO initiation, peak lactate during ECMO, SOFA score at 24 h post-ECMO, and concomitant with IABP were the risk factors significantly associated with the severe limb ischemia in the univariable analysis, whereas the multivariable logistic regression analysis retained obesity, SOFA score at 24 h post-ECMO, and VA-ECMO combined with IABP as the risk factors independently associated with the severe limb ischemia. In addition, the hemostasis disorders were significantly associated with cannulation site bleeding/hematoma during VA-ECMO support.

### Impact of MVCs on survival

The MVCs had a significant impact on in-hospital mortality (Fig. 2). Survival was 16.7% for patients with MVCs, compared with 39.2% for patients without MVCs ($p < 0.001$). The rates of weaning off VA-ECMO for the patients with MVCs were also lower than for those patients without MVCs (33.3 vs. 63.3%, $p < 0.001$).

**Table 1  Patient demographics, comorbidities, and surgical procedures**

| Variable | With vascular complications ($n = 72$) $n$ (%) | Without vascular complications ($n = 360$) $n$ (%) | P value |
|---|---|---|---|
| *Baseline characteristics* | | | |
| Male | 52 (72.2%) | 233 (64.7%) | 0.220 |
| Age (years) | 57(48.3, 65.0) | 57(47.3, 65.0) | 0.905 |
| Older age ($\geq$ 65 years) | 19 (26.4%) | 101 (28.1%) | 0.773 |
| BSA (m$^2$) | 1.9 (1.8, 2.0) | 1.8 (1.7, 2.0) | 0.009 |
| BMI (kg/m$^2$) | 25.0 $\pm$ 3.7 | 23.6 $\pm$ 3.4 | 0.002 |
| Smoking | 34 (47.2%) | 145 (40.3%) | 0.275 |
| *Comorbidities* | | | |
| Coronary artery disease | 42 (58.3%) | 176 (48.9%) | 0.143 |
| Peripheral vascular disease | 12 (16.7%) | 46 (12.8%) | 0.377 |
| Hypertension | 32 (44.4%) | 140 (38.9%) | 0.356 |
| Diabetes | 15 (20.8%) | 75 (20.8%) | 1.000 |
| Hypercholesterolemia | 61 (8.5%) | 260 (7.2%) | 0.718 |
| Chronic obstructive lung disease | 10 (1.4%) | 50 (1.4%) | 0.998 |
| Liver dysfunction | 10 (1.4%) | 2 (0.6%) | 0.437 |
| APACHE II score | 32.8 $\pm$ 5.2 | 30.8 $\pm$ 7.1 | 0.448 |
| *Type of surgery* | | | |
| CABG | 35 (48.6%) | 142 (39.4%) | 0.149 |
| Valve procedure | 17 (23.6%) | 105 (29.2%) | 0.339 |
| CABG + valve procedure | 8 (11.1%) | 37 (10.3%) | 0.833 |
| Congenital heart disease | 0 | 16 (4.4%) | 0.068 |
| Repair of acute aortic dissection | 4 (5.6%) | 18 (5.0%) | 0.845 |
| Repair of acute aortic dissection + CABG | 4 (5.6%) | 8 (2.2%) | 0.116 |
| Heart transplantation | 3 (4.2%) | 18 (5.0%) | 0.761 |
| Pulmonary embolectomy | 1 (1.4%) | 9 (2.5%) | 0.567 |
| Others | 0 | 6 (1.7%) | 0.270 |
| Reoperation | 20 (2.8%) | 12 (3.3%) | 0.808 |

*APACHE* acute physiologic and chronic health evaluation, *BSA* body surface area, *BMI* body mass index, *CABG* coronary artery bypass grafting, *CHD* congenital heart disease, *CPB* cardiopulmonary bypass, *CPR* cardiopulmonary resuscitation

Table 4 shows predisposing factors that influenced in-hospital mortality significantly by multivariate analysis. Presence of MVCs, renal dysfunction requiring CRRT, severe bleeding, and neurologic complications were independent risk factors associated with in-hospital mortality.

## Discussion

### Prevalence of MVCs in adult PCS patients

To our knowledge, this is the largest study on the MVCs in adult PCS patients receiving femoral–femoral VA-ECMO support by surgical cut-down. We observed that MVCs occurred in 16.7% of cases, including severe limb ischemia (8.6%) and bleeding in cannulation site (8.6%), which are in accordance with the literature on MVCs occurring in VA-ECMO patients (4.7–20.0%), largely due to lack of a clear definition [10, 11, 18–21].

Severe limb ischemia complications occurred in 8.6% of all our patients. In previous studies, others reported limb ischemia events among 2.3–52.0% of adult patients undergoing VA-ECMO [10–12, 21]. In a series of 84 adult patients, Tanaka and colleagues found that MVCs requiring surgical intervention were seen in 17 patients (20%), including 10 patients (12%) who had distal limb ischemia requiring prophylactic fasciotomy [11]. Similarly, another study in 93 adult PCS patients receiving peripheral VA-ECMO found that 15.1% of patients had severe limb ischemia [20]. In a meta-analysis of 1866 adult patients with CS, Cheng and colleagues [7] found that severe limb ischemia occurred in 10.3% of patients. Compared with these results, our observed limb ischemia rate of 8.6% is low, which may in part be explained by the potential advantages of surgically inserted with a distal perfusion catheter.

The mechanism of severe limb ischemia in PCS patients undergoing VA-ECMO is still unclear. A cannula in the common femoral artery has the potential of obstructing flow to the lower limb, and therefore reducing blood perfusion distal to the puncture site. VA-ECMO requires a

**Table 2 ECMO details and outcomes**

| Variable | With vascular complications (n = 72) n (%) | Without vascular complications (n = 360) n (%) | P value |
|---|---|---|---|
| *ECMO implantation* | | | |
| Failure to wean off CPB | 40 (55.6%) | 198 (55.0%) | 0.932 |
| LCOS in ICU | 32 (44.4%) | 162 (45.0%) | 0.932 |
| Inotrope scores | 52.5 ± 11.2 | 38.3 ± 12.9 | 0.008 |
| Lactate at ECMO initiation (mmol/L) | 11.0 (7.8, 14.3) | 9.5 (6.9, 12.8) | 0.035 |
| Peak lactate during ECMO (mmol/L) | 16.2 (13.6, 20.8) | 15.2 (11.5, 18.5) | 0.004 |
| SOFA score at ECMO initiation | 13.0 (12.0, 13.0) | 12.0 (11.0, 13.0) | <0.001 |
| SOFA score at 24 h post-ECMO | 11.0 (10.0, 11.0) | 9.0 (7.0, 11.0) | <0.001 |
| Arterial cannula size, Fr | 16.5 ± 0.6 | 16.1 ± 0.7 | 0.467 |
| Ongoing CPR | 13 (18.1%) | 56 (15.6%) | 0.597 |
| IABP support | 45 (62.5%) | 200 (55.6%) | 0.280 |
| *ECMO outcomes* | | | |
| Weaning from ECMO | 24 (33.3%) | 228 (63.3%) | <0.001 |
| Survival to discharge | 12 (16.7%) | 141 (39.2%) | <0.001 |
| Duration of ECMO (days) | 2.9 (1.6, 5.4) | 3.8 (2.2, 5.5) | 0.204 |
| *Complications* | | | |
| Renal failure required CRRT | 38 (52.1%) | 171 (47.6%) | 0.490 |
| Neurologic complications | 11 (15.3%) | 56 (15.6%) | 0.953 |
| DIC | 3 (4.2%) | 6 (1.7%) | 0.177 |
| Severe bleeding | 16 (22.2%) | 47 (13.1%) | 0.044 |
| Tracheostomy | 27 (37.5%) | 140 (39.0%) | 0.812 |
| Repeat thoracotomy | 37 (51.4%) | 132 (36.7%) | 0.019 |
| Femoral site infection | 6 (8.3%) | 25 (7.0%) | 0.681 |
| Sepsis | 13 (18.1%) | 84 (23.3%) | 0.335 |
| *Medical resources* | | | |
| PRBC transfusion (units) | 28.0 (19.3, 35.8) | 22.0 (14.0, 32.0) | 0.002 |
| FFP | 2400 (1600, 3600) | 2000 (1400, 3000) | 0.076 |
| Platelets | 3.0 (1.0, 5.0) | 3.0 (1.0, 5.0) | 0.578 |
| Duration of MV | 94.5 (38.8, 191.3) | 120.0 (51.0, 210.0) | 0.018 |
| ICU stay (days) | 107.0 (44.8, 237.4) | 168.0 (95.0, 255.8) | 0.007 |
| Post-ECMO hospital stay (days) | 0 (0, 7.8) | 7 (0, 15.8) | <0.001 |
| Hospital stay (days) | 17.0 (11.0, 25.8) | 23.0 (16.0, 34.8) | 0.001 |

Data presented as *n* (%) categorical variables and median (interquartile range) for non-parametric variable. Inotrope scores = dosage of dopamine (in μg/kg/min) + dosages of dobutamine (in μg/kg/min) + [dosages of epinephrine (in μg/kg/min + norepinephrine (in μg/kg/min)] × 100 + dosages of pituitrin (in u/min) × 100 + dosages of milrinone (in μg/kg/min) × 15

*CPR* cardiopulmonary resuscitation, *CRRT* continuous renal replacement therapy, *DIC* disseminated intravascular coagulation, *ECMO* extracorporeal membrane oxygenation, *FFP* fresh frozen plasma, *ICU* intensive care unit, *LCOS* low cardiac output syndrome, *MV* mechanical ventilation, *PRBC* packed red blood cells, *SOFA* sequential organ failure assessment

larger arterial cannula in the femoral artery for delivering oxygenated blood to the patient. There are several reports on prophylactic insertion of a small anterograde perfusion cannula into the superficial femoral artery, which can reduce the incidence of severe limb ischemia [13, 21, 22]. Although the incidence of severe limb ischemia was low, 8.6% of patients still needed decompression drainage, and 2.6% of patients required amputation in this study. There may be other reasons for the occurrence of limb ischemia complication, and further research is needed.

Another one of the most common MVCs is bleeding in the cannulation site, with a rate of 18.5% in peripheral VA-ECMO according to the extracorporeal life support registry [23]. A reduction in platelet count, hemolysis, and a consumptive coagulopathy along with systemic heparinization can further increase the hemorrhagic risk during VA-ECMO support. These patients required more blood transfusion; therefore, the effects of VA-ECMO support were severely affected.

**Table 3** Univariable and multivariable analyses of factors associated with major vascular complications (severe limb ischemia and cannulation site bleeding)

| Factor | Univariable analysis OR [95% CI], p value | Multivariable analysis OR [95% CI], p value |
|---|---|---|
| *Severe limb ischemia* | | |
| Peripheral artery disease | 0.73 [0.37–1.46] 0.378 | |
| Hypertension | 0.79 [0.47–1.31] 0.356 | |
| Hypercholesterolemia | 0.84 [0.33–2.13] 0.718 | |
| Smoking | 0.75 [0.45–1.25] 0.276 | |
| Obesity | 3.47 [1.20–10.03] 0.005 | 2.65 [1.26–5.56] 0.010 |
| Coronary artery disease | 2.47 [1.19–5.14] 0.022 | |
| Diabetes | 0.86 [0.68–3.14] 0.326 | |
| Combined with IABP | 2.97 [1.33–6.67] 0.018 | 2.49 [1.19–2.65] 0.025 |
| ECPR | 0.83 [0.43–1.63] 0.597 | |
| Lactate at ECMO initiation | 1.07 [0.98–1.14] 0.052 | |
| Peak lactate during ECMO | 1.10 [1.03–1.16] 0.002 | |
| SOFA score at ECMO initiation | 2.09 [1.60–2.23] < 0.001 | |
| SOFA score at 24 h post-ECMO | 1.67 [1.41–1.98] < 0.001 | 1.43 [1.08–1.86] 0.010 |
| *Cannulation site bleeding* | | |
| Hemostasis disorders during ECMO | 7.21 [2.28–22.77] < 0.001 | 6.11 [1.88–19.87] < 0.001 |

*CNS* central nervous system complications, *CRRT* continuous renal replacement treatment, *DIC* disseminated intravascular coagulation, *ECMO* extracorporeal membrane oxygenation, *ECPR* extracorporeal cardiopulmonary resuscitation, *IABP* intra-aortic balloon pump, *SOFA* sequential organ failure assessment

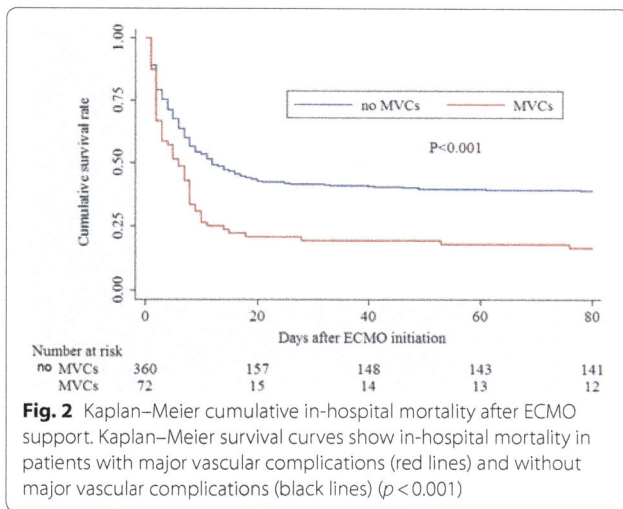

**Fig. 2** Kaplan–Meier cumulative in-hospital mortality after ECMO support. Kaplan–Meier survival curves show in-hospital mortality in patients with major vascular complications (red lines) and without major vascular complications (black lines) (p < 0.001)

**Table 4** Predisposing factors for in-hospital mortality (multivariate logistic regression)

| Variable | Odds ratio | 95% confidence interval | p value |
|---|---|---|---|
| Major vascular complications | 3.91 | 1.67–9.14 | 0.013 |
| Renal failure required CRRT | 10.98 | 6.21–19.41 | < 0.001 |
| Severe bleeding | 15.86 | 3.61–69.63 | < 0.001 |
| Neurologic complications | 13.68 | 5.38–34.80 | < 0.001 |

*CRRT* continuous renal replacement treatment

## Hospital outcome in adult VA-ECMO patients experiencing MVCs

There is still some controversy about the effect of MVCs on hospital outcomes. In this study, MVCs were an independent risk factor for in-hospital mortality in patients undergoing VA-ECMO support. This is in accordance with Tanaka [10] and colleagues, who demonstrated a strong relationship between vascular complications and in-hospital mortality. In contrast, in 143 patients receiving VA-ECMO support by femoral cannulation, of those 17 (11.9%) observed vascular complications. Two patients (1.4%) who had extremity ischemia required limb amputation. However, the MVCs were not associated with early mortality (65 vs. 61%, $p = 0.95$) [11]. The MVCs patients had increased transfusion requirements in this study as they are not only bleeding at the cannulation site, but they are also bleeding at the compartment syndrome decompression site. In previous studies, others found a strong relationship between red blood cell transfusion during VA-ECMO and in-hospital mortality [24, 25]. In agreement with other previous reports, we also found that neurologic complications, severe bleeding, ECPR, and renal failure requiring renal replacement therapy were associated with dismal prognoses [3, 4].

## Predictors of MVCs in adult VA-ECMO patients

Given the poor outcomes associated with MVCs, identifying the risk factors and actively preventing MVCs are very important for these patients. It is worth noting that obesity, concomitant IABP, and SOFA score at 24 h post-ECMO appeared to be significant risk factors for severe limb ischemia. Intriguingly, peripheral arterial disease was not associated with limb ischemia ($p = 0.38$) in this study. The peripheral arterial disease and absence of a distal perfusion catheter has been found to be predictors of severe limb ischemia in previous studies [10, 11]. All PCS patients receiving VA-ECMO support were implanted by surgical cut-down and conventional placement of a distal perfusion catheter in this study. Therefore, for the patients with femoral artery stenosis (moderate to severe), surgical cut-down combined with a distal perfusion tube for implantation of VA-ECMO is recommended. Although the incidence of limb ischemia was generally low, IABP has the risk of increasing the risk of limb ischemia [26]. A total of 246 patients (56.9%) received VA-ECMO combined with IABP support. A total of 235 of these patients (95.5%) received IABP first but were still unable to maintain hemodynamic stability, and were then given VA-ECMO. The other 11 patients (4.5%) underwent VA-ECMO first, and received IABP for that opening of the aortic valve were restricted. Therefore, it is necessary to pay attention to the occurrence of limb ischemia when the combined with IABP support is needed. It is worth noting that obesity was a significant risk factor for severe limb ischemia. Although the severe limb ischemia affects the clinical prognosis of those patients, there is still no suitable time for surgical decompression and drainage. In the present study, we found that higher SOFA score at 24 h post-ECMO was associated with increased incidence of MVCs. The clinical conditions of patients with higher SOFA score were more severe, and distal tissue hypoperfusion and thrombocytopenia seemed to be more common in those patients, which might account for our findings. In addition, we also demonstrated that the hemostasis disorders were independently associated with bleeding/hematoma in cannulation site during VA-ECMO support. Further research should focus on prevention and early management of MVCs to avoid devastating consequences.

Our study also has limitations. First, it is a retrospective, single-center study. Second, although the number of patients included in this study is small, our data report the largest series of adult PCS patients receiving VA-ECMO by surgical cut-down for evaluating the impact of MVCs on outcome and analysis of associated factors. The conclusions of this study can provide reference for peers. Third, we did not perform follow-up. Further studies focusing on this point are needed to support long-term safety of surgically inserted.

## Conclusions

The MVCs in adult PCS patients undergoing VA-ECMO support by surgical cut-down are common. Furthermore, the MVCs were associated with higher in-hospital mortality rates. The obesity, SOFA score at 24Â h post-ECMO, and the concomitant with IABP were independent risk factors for the occurrence of limb ischemia in VA-ECMO support. Surgical cut-down implantation of the VA-ECMO technique might be considered a valuable option for adult PCS patients, although more data and larger patient cohorts are needed to confirm the findings presented herein.

### Abbreviations
AMI: acute myocardial infarction; CABG: coronary artery bypass grafting; CAD: coronary artery disease; CI: confidence interval; CPB: cardiopulmonary bypass; CPR: cardiopulmonary resuscitation; ECMO: extracorporeal membrane oxygenation; ECPR: extracorporeal cardiopulmonary resuscitation; FFP: fresh frozen plasma; HR: hazard ratio; Htx: heart transplantation; IABP: intra-aortic balloon pump; LCOS: low cardiac output syndrome; LOS: length of stay; LV: left ventricular; LVEF: left ventricular ejection fraction; MVCs: major vascular complications; PLT: platelet; PRBC: packed red blood cells; VAD: ventricular assist device; SvO$_2$: mixed venous oxygen saturation; SOFA: sequential organ failure assessment; VA-ECMO: venoarterial extracorporeal membrane oxygenation.

### Authors' contributions
FY and DH designed the study, analyzed the data, and drafted the manuscript. JW, YC, and XW interpreted the data and revised the manuscript. ZX and CJ participated in the design of the study and performed the statistical analysis. X Hao, ZD, XY, and YJ participated in the data collection. X Hou conceived the study, participated in its design and coordination, and revised the manuscript. All authors read and approved the final manuscript.

### Acknowledgements
We acknowledge all participants for the effort they devoted to this study.

### Competing interests
The authors declare that they have no competing interests.

### Funding
This project has been funded by the Research Foundation of Beijing Lab for Cardiovascular Precision Medicine, Beijing, China (No. PXM2016_014226_000023) and with grants from Beijing Municipal Commission (No. Z161100000516017 to X Hou).

### References
1.  Reyentovich A, Barghash MH, Hochman JS. Management of refractory cardiogenic shock. Nat Rev Cardiol. 2016;13:481–92.
2.  Ouweneel DM, Schotborgh JV, Limpens J, Sjauw KD, Engström AE, Lagrand WK, et al. Extracorporeal life support during cardiac arrest and cardiogenic shock: a systematic review and meta-analysis. Intensive Care Med. 2016;42:1922–34.
3.  Rastan AJ, Dege A, Mohr M, Doll N, Falk V, Walther T, et al. Early and late outcomes of 517 consecutive adult patients treated with extracorporeal membrane oxygenation for refractory postcardiotomy cardiogenic shock. J Thorac Cardiovasc Surg. 2010;139:302–11.
4.  Khorsandi M, Dougherty S, Bouamra O, Pai V, Curry P, Tsui S, et al. Extracorporeal membrane oxygenation for refractory cardiogenic shock after

adult cardiac surgery: a systematic review and meta-analysis. J Cariot-horac Surg. 2017;12:55.

5.  Schmidt M, Burrell A, Roberts L, Bailey M, Sheldrake J, Rycus PT, et al. Predicting survival after ECMO for refractory cardiogenic shock: the survival after veno-arterial-ECMO (SAVE)-score. Eur Heart J. 2015;36:2246–56.

6.  Chang C, Chen H, Caffrey JL, Hsu J, Lin JW, Lai MS, et al. Survival analysis after extracorporeal membrane oxygenation in critically ill adults a nationwide cohort study. Circulation. 2016;133:2423–33.

7.  Cheng R, Hachamovitch R, Kittleson M, Patel J, Arabia F, Moriguchi J, et al. Complications of extracorporeal membrane oxygenation for treatment of cardiogenic shock and cardiac arrest: a meta-analysis of 1866 adult patients. Ann Thorac Surg. 2014;97:610–6.

8.  Roussel A, Al-Attar N, Alkhoder S, Radu C, Raffoul R, Alshammari M, et al. Outcomes of percutaneous femoral cannulation for venoarterial extracorporeal membrane oxygenation support. Eur Heart J Acute Cardiovasc Care. 2012;1:111–4.

9.  Conrad SA, Grier LR, Scott K, Green R, Jordan M. Percutaneous cannulation for extracorporeal membrane oxygenation by intensivists: a retrospective single-institution case series. Crit Care Med. 2015;43:1010–5.

10.  Tanaka D, Hirose H, Cavarocchi N, Entwistle JW. The impact of vascular complications on survival of patients on venoarterial extracorporeal membrane oxygenation. Ann Thorac Surg. 2016;101:1729–34.

11.  Bisdas T, Beutel G, Warnecke G, Hoeper MM, Kuehn C, Haverich A, et al. Vascular complications in patients undergoing femoral cannulation for extracorporeal membrane oxygenation support. Ann Thorac Surg. 2011;92:626–31.

12.  Lamb KM, DiMuzio PJ, Johnson A, Batista P, Moudgill N, McCullough M, et al. Arterial protocol including prophylactic distal perfusion catheter decreases limb ischemia complications in patients undergoing extracorporeal membrane oxygenation. J Vasc Surg. 2017;65:1074–9.

13.  Li CL, Wang H, Jia M, Ma N, Meng X, Hou XT. The early dynamic behavior of lactate is linked to mortality in postcardiotomy patients with extracorporeal membrane oxygenation support: a retrospective observational study. J Thorac Cardiovasc Surg. 2015;149:1445–50.

14.  Chang WW, Tsai FC, Tsai TY, Chang CH, Jeng CC, Chang MY, et al. Predictors of mortality in patients successfully weaned from extracorporeal membrane oxygenation. PLoS ONE. 2012;7:e42687.

15.  von Segesser L, Marinakis S, Berdajs D, Ferrari E, Wilhelm M, Maisano F. Prevention and therapy of limb ischemia in extracorporeal life support and extracorporeal membrane oxygenation with peripheral cannulation. Swiss Med Wkly. 2016;146:w14304.

16.  Luyt C, Bréchot N, Demondion P, Jovanovic T, Hékimian G, Lebreton G, et al. Brain injury during venovenous extracorporeal membrane oxygenation. Intensive Care Med. 2016;42:897–907.

17.  von Keudell AG, Weaver MJ, Appleton PT, Bae DS, Dyer GSM, Heng M, et al. Diagnosis and treatment of acute extremity compartment syndrome. Lancet. 2015;386:1299–310.

18.  Bakhtiary F, Keller H, Dogan S, Dzemali O, Oezaslan F, Meininger D, et al. Venoarterial extracorporeal membrane oxygenation for treatment of cardiogenic shock: clinical experiences in 45 adult patients. J Thorac Cardiovasc Surg. 2008;135:382–8.

19.  Park SJ, Kim JB, Jung SH, Choo SJ, Chung CH, Lee JW. Outcomes of extracorporeal life support for low cardiac output syndrome after major cardiac surgery. J Thorac Cardiovasc Surg. 2014;147:283–9.

20.  Gander JW, Fisher JC, Reichstein AR, Gross ER, Aspelund G, Middlesworth W, et al. Limb ischemia after common femoral artery cannulation for venoarterial extracorporeal membrane oxygenation: an unresolved problem. J Pediatr Surg. 2010;45:2136–40.

21.  Russo CF, Cannata A, Vitali E, Lanfranconi M. Prevention of limb ischemia and edema during peripheral venoarterial extracorporeal membrane oxygenation in adults. J Card Surg. 2009;24:185–7.

22.  Makdisi G, Makdisi T, Wang IW. Use of distal perfusion in peripheral extracorporeal membrane oxygenation. Ann Transl Med. 2017;5:103.

23.  Thiagarajan RR, Barbaro RP, Rycus PT, Mcmullan DM, Conrad SA, Fortemberry JD, et al. Extracorporeal life support organization registry international report 2016. ASAIO J. 2017;63:60–7.

24.  Aubron C, Cheng A, Pilcher D, Leong T, Magrin G, Cooper DJ, et al. Factors associated with outcomes of patients on extracorporeal membrane oxygenation support: a 5-year cohort study. Crit Care. 2013;17:R73.

25.  Mazzeffi M, Greenwood J, Tanaka K, Menaker J, Rector R, Herr D, et al. Bleeding, transfusion, and mortality on extracorporeal life support: eCLS working group on thrombosis and hemostasis. Ann Thorac Surg. 2016;101:682–9.

26.  de Jong MM, Lorusso R, Awami Al, Matteuci F, Parise O, Lozekoot P, et al. Vascular complications following intra-aortic balloon pump implantation: an updated review. Perfusion. 2018;33:96–104.

# 21

# Large-volume paracentesis effects plasma disappearance rate of indo-cyanine green in critically ill patients with decompensated liver cirrhosis and intraabdominal hypertension

Ulrich Mayr[*], Leonie Fahrenkrog-Petersen, Gonzalo Batres-Baires, Alexander Herner, Sebastian Rasch, Roland M. Schmid, Wolfgang Huber and Tobias Lahmer

**Abstract**

**Background:** Ascites is a major complication of decompensated liver cirrhosis. Intraabdominal hypertension and structural alterations of parenchyma involve decisive changes in hepatosplanchnic blood flow. Clearance of indo-cyanine green (ICG) is mainly dependent on hepatic perfusion and hepatocellular function. As a consequence, plasma disappearance rate of ICG (ICG-PDR) is rated as a useful dynamic parameter of liver function. This study primarily evaluates the impact of large-volume paracentesis (LVP) on ICG-PDR in critically ill patients with decompensated cirrhosis. Additionally, it describes influences on intraabdominal pressure (IAP), abdominal perfusion pressure (APP), hepatic blood flow, hemodynamic and respiratory function.

**Methods:** We analyzed LVP in 22 patients with decompensated liver cirrhosis. ICG-PDR was assessed by using noninvasive LiMON technology (Pulsion® Medical Systems; Maquet Getinge Group), and hepatic blood flow was analyzed by color-coded duplex sonography.

**Results:** Paracentesis of a median volume of 3450 mL ascites evoked significant increases of ICG-PDR from 3.6 (2.8–4.6) to 5.1 (3.9–6.2)%/min ($p < 0.001$). Concomitantly, we observed a raise in "ICG-Clearance" from 99 (73.5–124.5) to 104 (91–143.5) mL/min/m² ($p = 0.005$), while circulating blood volume index was unchanged [2412 (1983–3025) before paracentesis vs. 2409 (1997–2805) mL/m², $p = 0.734$]. Sonography revealed a significant impact of paracentesis on hepatic blood flow: Hepatic artery resistance index dropped from 0.74 (0.68–0.75) to 0.68 (0.65–0.71) ($p < 0.001$) and maximum flow velocity in hepatic vein increased from 24 (17–30) to 30 (22–36) cm/s ($p < 0.001$). Consistent with previous studies, paracentesis caused significant decreases in IAP from 19.0 (15.0–20.3) to 11.0 (8.8–12.3) mmHg ($p < 0.001$) and central venous pressure from 22.5 (17.8–29.0) to 17.5 (12.8–24.0) mmHg ($p < 0.001$) with inverse increases in APP from 63.0 (56.8–69.5) to 71.0 (65.5–78.5) mmHg ($p < 0.001$). Changes in ICG-PDR were concomitant with changes in IAP ($r = -0.602$) and APP ($r = 0.576$). Moreover, we found a substantial improvement in respiratory function. By contrast, hemodynamic parameters assessed by transpulmonary thermodilution, serum bilirubin and international normalized ratio did not change after paracentesis.

**Conclusion:** Critically ill patients with decompensated cirrhosis and elevated IAP showed dramatically impaired ICG-PDR. Paracentesis evoked an improvement in ICG-PDR in parallel with a decreased IAP and an increased APP, while conventional parameters of liver function did not change. This effect on ICG-PDR is mainly referable to a relief of intraabdominal hypertension and changes in hepatosplanchnic blood flow.

*Correspondence: mayr.ulrich@gmx.net
Klinik und Poliklinik für Innere Medizin II, Klinikum rechts der Isar,
Technische Universität München, Ismaninger Strasse 22, 81675 Munich,
Germany

**Keywords:** Indo-cyanine green (ICG), Plasma disappearance rate (PDR), Large-volume paracentesis (LVP), Intraabdominal hypertension (IAH), Intraabdominal pressure (IAP), Decompensated liver cirrhosis, Hepatosplanchnic blood flow, Transpulmonary thermodilution, Color-coded duplex sonography, Hepatic artery resistance index

## Background

Decompensated liver cirrhosis implies serious consequences for affected patients. Ascites is one major and highly frequently emerging complication [1, 2]. Intraabdominal hypertension (IAH) is associated with poor prognosis and high mortality [3, 4]. Increased intraabdominal pressure (IAP) involves multiple organ dysfunction regarding cardiovascular, respiratory, renal and abdominal impairment [5–8]. In particular, IAH interferes with proper abdominal perfusion, including hepatosplanchnic blood flow [9, 10].

Furthermore, advanced cirrhosis is accompanied by structural alterations leading to increased intrahepatic vascular resistance [11, 12]. Restrictions of intrahepatic blood flow cause portal hypertension, further aggravated by compensatory splanchnic arterial vasodilation [13]. Moreover, cirrhosis provokes impairment of blood flow in hepatic veins as well as increases in hepatic artery resistance index [14, 15]. Color-coded duplex sonography provides a subjective, but noninvasive diagnostic approach regarding vascular disorders in advanced liver disease [16].

Finally, end-stage liver disease is associated with progressive loss of functional liver capacity. Conventional laboratory assessment of liver function is mainly based on liver enzymes, bilirubin and the coagulation parameter international normalized ratio (INR) [17]. Dynamic tests of liver function at bedside might be more precise and objective relating to actual, short-term functional status [18]. Promising experiences were achieved with noninvasive measurement of plasma disappearance rate of indo-cyanine green (ICG-PDR). ICG is injected intravenously, distributed via blood circulation and excreted hepatobiliary [19]. ICG-PDR reflects both hepatosplanchnic blood flow and hepatocellular and excretory function [20, 21]. Some previous data described an interaction of ICG-PDR with intraabdominal pressure level [22–24]. Recently, one of these studies affirmed that ICG-PDR correlates inversely with IAP, suggesting that IAH restrains hepatosplanchnic and sinusoidal perfusion [25]. The abdominal perfusion pressure (APP), defined as difference between mean arterial pressure (MAP) and IAP, was positively correlated with ICG-PDR.

The accumulation of ascites is a typical complication of decompensated cirrhosis with elevated IAP and restricted organ perfusion [2, 10]. The evacuation of ascites by large-volume paracentesis (LVP) is one of the few nonsurgical treatment options [26]. ICG-PDR was already labeled as an accurate test for prediction of survival in advanced cirrhosis [27]. So far, none of the previous studies focused on the impact of LVP on dynamic liver assessment by ICG-PDR in this patient population. Consequently, the aim of our study was to investigate the effect of LVP on ICG-PDR in critically ill patients with decompensated liver cirrhosis (primary endpoint). This evaluation was supplemented by analyses of IAP, APP, hepatic blood flow by sonography, respiratory function as well as hemodynamic monitoring by using transpulmonary thermodilution.

## Methods

### Study design

This observational study was approved by the institutional review board (Ethikkommission Technische Universität München; Fakultät für Medizin; Project Number 5384/12), and informed consent was obtained by all patients.

Between April 2016 and July 2017, a total of 29 critically ill patients with decompensated liver cirrhosis on our university hospital general ICU were screened for the feasibility of LVP, analyses of ICG-PDR, IAP and hemodynamic monitoring via transpulmonary thermodilution. LVP was performed irrespective of the study based on the indication made by the treating ICU physician. We released a maximum of mobilizable ascites in each individual case of LVP; laboratory analyses of ascites revealed a cell count $< 500/\mu L$ and polymorphonuclear neutrophils $< 250/\mu L$ in every single patient. Due to potential influences on hepatosplanchnic blood flow, analysis was considered feasible only in patients without terlipressin treatment, portal vein thrombosis or transjugular intrahepatic portosystemic stent shunt. Therefore, 6 patients with terlipressin-treatment, 1 patient with portal vein thrombosis and 2 patients with portosystemic stent were restrained from the study. Finally, we analyzed a total of 22 critically ill patients with decompensated liver cirrhosis and tense ascites.

### Techniques

#### Assessment of ICG-PDR, BVI, CBI and laboratory tests

ICG-PDR, circulating blood volume index (BVI) and "ICG-Clearance" (CBI) were analyzed immediately before and after paracentesis by using noninvasive LiMON technology (Pulsion® Medical Systems; Maquet

Getinge Group) via a disposable finger color sensor as previously described [28]. We used ICG solubilized in distilled water and injected via a central venous catheter at a dose of 0.5 mg/kg of ICG-solution for measurement of ICG-PDR and additional assessment of BVI and CBI. Normally, ICG-PDR amounts to 18–25%/min [20]. Measurements of BVI and CBI were performed in parallel with ICG-PDR after manual input of current cardiac output and automatically indexed according to manufacturer's recommendations.

Main laboratory tests of excretory liver function and synthesis (Bilirubin, INR) were analyzed once a day—corresponding to current standard in our intensive care unit. Overall time interval between blood sampling was 24 h.

### LVP, IAP, abdominal compliance, APP and CVP

LVP was performed ultrasound guided after bringing the patient in supine position [29]. IAP was determined by intravesical measurement using a home-made technique according to The Abdominal Compartment Society (WSACS), and IAH was defined as IAP $\geq$ 12 mmHg [30, 31]. Abdominal compliance was expressed as the change of ascites volume per change in IAP (delta IAP) before and after paracentesis [32]. APP was calculated as MAP minus IAP by using concomitantly obtained values as explained previously [25, 31]. Substitution of albumin followed current guidelines and was performed after the final analyses [33]. Central venous pressure (CVP) was measured via jugular central venous catheters at end-expiration.

### Ventilator setting and respiratory function

Patients with spontaneous breathing received a demand-based application of oxygen. Mechanical ventilation was performed using the routine ventilator device EVITA XL of our ICU (Dräger, Lübeck, Germany). Parameters were set according to current ARDSNet recommendations, especially regarding positive end-expiratory pressure (PEEP) [34]. Ventilator setting was based on medical assessment by the treating ICU physician irrespective of the study. The EVITA XL ventilator continuously monitored levels of airway pressures and corresponding volumes. Routine ventilatory parameters such as PEEP, tidal volume (TV), mean airway pressure, dynamic respiratory system compliance ($C_{dyn}$) and fraction of inspired oxygen ($F_iO_2$) were recorded at baseline and at the end of LVP. $P_aO_2$ and $P_aCO_2$ were derived from a fully automatic blood gas analysis device (Rapid Point 400, Siemens Healthcare Diagnostic GmbH, Eschborn, Germany). Blood gas analysis and ventilatory parameters were used for calculation of Horowitz-index ($P_aO_2/F_iO_2$) and oxygenation index ($OI = F_iO_2$ * mean airway pressure * 100/$P_aO_2$) [35].

### Hemodynamic monitoring

With the exception of only a single subject, all patients were under hemodynamic monitoring irrespective of the study, by using transpulmonary thermodilution with the PiCCO-2-device (Pulsion Medical Systems SE, Maquet Getinge Group) as described previously [36]: A 5 Fr thermistor-tipped arterial line (Pulsiocath, Pulsion® Medical Systems; Maquet Getinge Group) inserted through a femoral artery and a hemodynamic monitor (PiCCO-2, Pulsion® Medical Systems, Maquet Getinge Group) served to derive and analyze the thermodilution curve after injection of a cold indicator bolus (15 ml of saline cooled down to 4 °C) through a jugular central venous catheter. Measurements were done in triplicate, averaged and automatically indexed according to manufacturer's recommendations.

### Color-coded duplex sonography

Transabdominal ultrasound examination was accomplished noninvasively at the bedside in a supine position of the patients. All analyses were performed by a single physician with 6 years of institutional experience in the field of abdominal ultrasound. We used the mobile ultrasound scanner ACUSON X300 (Siemens Healthcare GmbH, Erlangen, Germany) and a convex 3.5 MHz transducer with color Doppler capacity. The transducer was placed in the right intercostal space due to the intraabdominal fluid accumulation. Doppler-analyses of blood flow were performed of the portal vein, hepatic artery and right hepatic vein; middle hepatic vein was chosen only when analysis of right hepatic vein was insufficient [14].

### Data collection

Clinical and laboratory parameters for the calculation of APACHE II-, SOFA-, MELD- and Child–Pugh scores were recorded on the day of paracentesis. Measurements of ICG-PDR, BVI and CBI were done immediately before and after LVP, with a median time interval of 210 (180–255) min. Ventilatory parameters, hemodynamic profiles as well as IAP-assessment and ultrasound examinations were performed immediately before as well as after the maximal mobilizable release of ascites.

### Statistical analysis and primary endpoint

For primary outcome analysis, we investigated ICG-PDR at the end of LVP compared to baseline. All analyses and graphs were generated using GraphPad Prism 7.0 (GraphPad Software, La Jolla, CA, USA). Correlations were calculated using Pearson's correlation coefficient $r$ and linear regressions using the coefficient $R^2$. Continuous variables are expressed as median and interquartile range (IQR). Categorical variables are expressed as percentages. To compare continuous variables, we used nonparametric Wilcoxon test for paired samples. Significance was assumed at a $p$ value < 0.05.

## Results

### Patients' baseline characteristics

Patients' baseline characteristics and clinical scores are presented in Table 1.

We performed LVP procedures in a total of 22 patients (7 female, 15 male) with decompensated liver cirrhosis and tense ascites. APACHE-, SOFA-, MELD- and Child–Pugh scores are explainable by advanced hepatic impairment and critical illness. The etiology of cirrhosis was predominantly alcoholic-toxic. About 75% of patients were mechanically ventilated and about 25% were spontaneously breathing. Regarding mechanically ventilated patients, PEEP-setting was unchanged during LVP and study measurements.

### LVP, ICG-PDR, BVI, CBI and laboratory tests

Twenty-two LVP procedures with a median volume of 3450 (3075–4700) mL removed ascites ($\geq$ 3000 mL for every paracentesis) were analyzed. We noticed a median ascitic cell count of 180 (100–310)/μL ($\leq$ 500/μL in all patients), with polymorphonuclear neutrophils < 250/μL in each patient to exclude spontaneous bacterial peritonitis and to justify a release of a maximum of mobilizable ascites volume.

ICG-PDR at baseline was decreased substantially to 3.6 (2.8–4.6)%/min compatible with dramatic hepatic impairment of advanced liver cirrhosis. LVP provoked a significant increase of ICG-PDR to 5.1 (3.9–6.2)%/min ($p$ < 0.001) (Fig. 1). Median change of ICG-PDR (delta ICG-PDR) induced by LVP was 1.2 (1.0–2.1)%/min.

Circulating blood volume index (BVI) was unchanged after LVP [2412 (1983–3025) before paracentesis vs. 2409 (1997–2805) mL/m$^2$, $p$ = 0.734], while "ICG-Clearance" (CBI) increased from 99 (73.5–124.5) to 104 (91–143.5) mL/min/m$^2$ ($p$ = 0.005) (Fig. 2).

In comparison, main laboratory tests of liver function showed no significant changes after an overall time interval of 24 h: Parameter of liver excretion function bilirubin as well as plasmatic coagulation parameter INR remained stable (Table 2).

### IAP, abdominal compliance, APP and CVP

Paracentesis caused a distinct relief of IAH: At the end of LVP, pressure levels of IAP had lowered from 19.0 (15.0–20.3) to 11.0 (8.8–12.3) mmHg ($p$ < 0.001). Grading of IAH before and after LVP is listed in Table 3, according to the definition established by the WSACS [31]. Median abdominal compliance based on paracentesis of 3450 (3075–4700) mL was 461 (383–659) mL/mmHg.

Consecutively, we noticed a marked improvement of APP from 63.0 (56.8–69.5) to 71.0 (65.5–78.5)

**Table 1 Patients baseline characteristics and clinical scores**

| Patients characteristics | |
|---|---|
| Male sex [n/total (%)] | 15/22 (68%) |
| Age (years) | 55 (52–69.3) |
| Body weight (kg) | 82.5 (70–100) |
| Body height (cm) | 180 (170–183) |
| APACHE II | 24 (19–29.3) |
| SOFA | 12 (9.8–16) |
| MELD | 27.5 (23.8–36.3) |
| Child–Pugh | 12 (10–13) |
| Child C [n/total (%)] | 19/22 (86%) |
| Etiology of cirrhosis [n/total (%)] | Alcoholic 16/22 (72%) |
| | Viral 3/22 (14%) |
| | Cryptogenic 3/22 (14%) |
| Admission diagnoses [n/total (%)] | Sepsis/Pneumonia 10/22 (45%) |
| | Acute kidney failure 7/22 (32%) |
| | Hepatic encephalopathy 5/22 (23%) |
| Mode of ventilation [n/total (%)] | Spontaneous breathing 6/22 (27%) |
| | Pressure-supported 6/22 (27%) |
| | Pressure-controlled 10/22 (46%) |
| Ascites volume (mL) | 3450 (3075–4700) |
| Total cell count (n/μL) | 180 (100–310) |
| PEEP-level (cmH$_2$O) | 8 (8–10) |
| Baseline F$_i$O$_2$ (%) | 45 (35–60) |

*APACHE* acute physiology and chronic health evaluation, *SOFA* sequential organ failure assessment, *MELD* model of end-stage liver disease, *PEEP* positive end-expiratory pressure, *F$_i$O$_2$* fraction of inspired oxygen

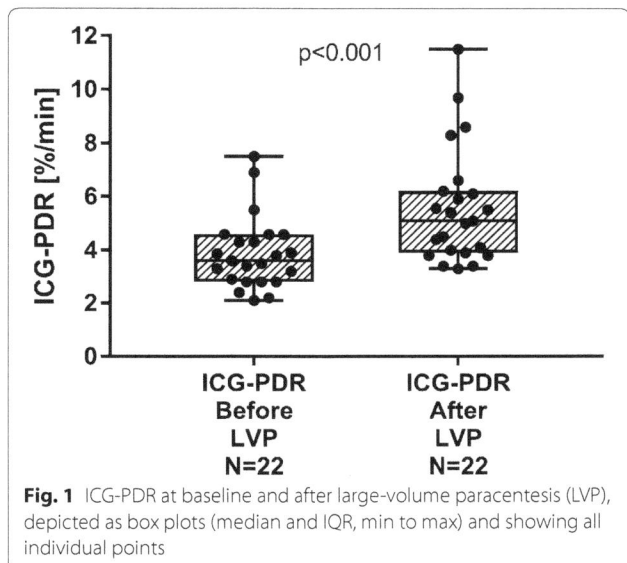

**Fig. 1** ICG-PDR at baseline and after large-volume paracentesis (LVP), depicted as box plots (median and IQR, min to max) and showing all individual points

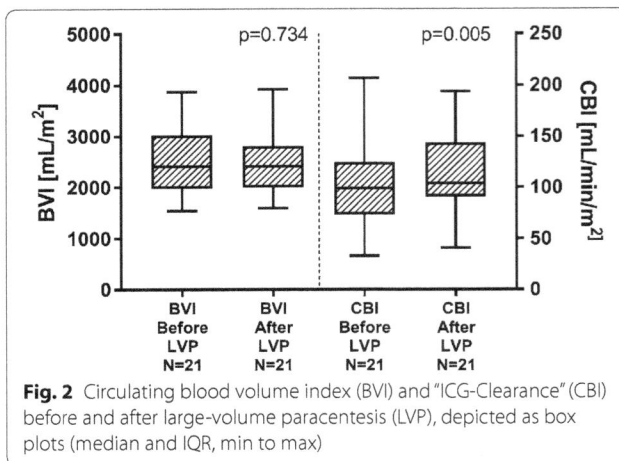

**Fig. 2** Circulating blood volume index (BVI) and "ICG-Clearance" (CBI) before and after large-volume paracentesis (LVP), depicted as box plots (median and IQR, min to max)

**Table 2 Main conventional laboratory parameters of liver function before and after paracentesis (overall time interval of 24 h)**

Conventional laboratory tests of hepatic function

| | Before paracentesis | After paracentesis | p value |
|---|---|---|---|
| | Median (IQR) | Median (IQR) | |
| Bilirubin (mg/dL) | 7.8 (3.3–19.0) | 7.6 (2.5–21.4) | 0.868 |
| INR | 1.8 (1.4–2.2) | 1.8 (1.4–2.5) | 0.094 |

*INR* international normalized ratio

**Table 3 Grading of intraabdominal hypertension before and after paracentesis**

Grading of IAH according to WSACS definition

| | Before LVP | After LVP |
|---|---|---|
| | n/total (%) | n/total (%) |
| No IAH, IAP ≤ 11 mmHg | 1/22 (5%) | 13/22 (59%) |
| IAH Grade I, IAP 12–15 mmHg | 5/22 (23%) | 6/22 (27%) |
| IAH Grade II, IAP 16–20 mmHg | 11/22 (50%) | 2/22 (9%) |
| IAH Grade III, IAP 21–25 mmHg | 3/22 (13%) | 1/22 (5%) |
| IAH Grade IV, IAP > 25 mmHg | 2/22 (9%) | 0/22 (0%) |

*IAH* intraabdominal hypertension, *WSACS* The Abdominal Compartment Society, *LVP* large-volume paracentesis, *IAP* Intraabdominal pressure

mmHg ($p < 0.001$). Pressure levels of IAP and APP are depicted in Fig. 3. In parallel with the decline of IAP, LVP induced a significant decrease of CVP from 22.5 (17.8–29.0) to 17.5 (12.8–24.0) mmHg ($p = 0.001$).

Median changes in IAP (delta IAP) and APP (delta APP) caused by paracentesis were -8.0 (−5.0 to −10.0) mmHg and 8.5 (5.8–10.3) mmHg, respectively.

Furthermore, LVP provoked a median change in CVP (delta CVP) of −5.0 (−3.0 to −7.0) mmHg.

**Correlations and regression plots**

Analyses according to Pearson as well as linear regressions are illustrated in Fig. 4. Paracentesis of a median volume of 3450 (3075–4700) mL in a total of 22 patients provoked concomitant changes of ICG-PDR (delta ICG-PDR) with changes in IAP (panel A, $r = -0.602$, $p = 0.003$). In parallel, delta ICG-PDR correlated significantly with delta APP (panel B, $r = 0.576$, $p = 0.005$). In contrast, delta ICG-PDR was not significantly associated with evacuated ascites volume (panel C, $r = 0.281$, $p = 0.205$). Concerning concomitant changes of IAP and CVP after LVP, correlation analyses outlined an association of delta IAP and delta CVP (panel D, $r = 0.637$, $p = 0.001$).

**Color-coded duplex sonography**

By sonographic examination, we registered a significant impact of LVP on hepatic blood flow: Hepatic artery resistance index dropped from 0.74 (0.68–0.75) to 0.68 (0.65–0.71) ($p < 0.001$). This reduction was mainly reflected in an increase of diastolic hepatic arterial flow velocity, while systolic arterial flow velocity was steady. Furthermore, LVP provoked an increase of maximum hepatic vein flow velocity. In contrast, maximum flow velocity in portal vein was mainly unaffected by paracentesis (Table 4).

**Respiratory and ventilatory parameters**

Respiratory function improved by paracentesis without changes of PEEP-level, outlined in Table 5. Horowitz-index ($P_aO_2/F_iO_2$) increased and oxygenation index (OI) improved. Furthermore, we registered a significant raise in TV and $C_{dyn}$. We also recorded a decrease in respiratory rate and $P_aCO_2$, but results were not statistically significant.

**Hemodynamic parameters**

Hemodynamic assessment by transpulmonary thermodilution and pulse contour analysis revealed overall unchanged parameters of hemodynamic function after LVP: Mean arterial pressure MAP, cardiac Index CI, cardiac output CO, global end-diastolic volume index GEDVI, extravascular lung water index EVLWI and systemic vascular resistance index SVRI did not change significantly (Table 6).

**Discussion**

The present study shows that large-volume paracentesis (LVP) induced an improvement in ICG-PDR in critically ill patients with decompensated liver cirrhosis. This effect comes along with a relief of intraabdominal hypertension

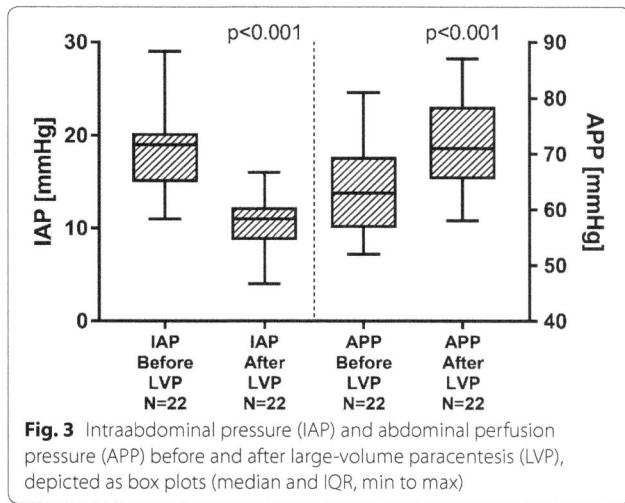

**Fig. 3** Intraabdominal pressure (IAP) and abdominal perfusion pressure (APP) before and after large-volume paracentesis (LVP), depicted as box plots (median and IQR, min to max)

(IAH) reflected in a decrease in intraabdominal pressure (IAP) and an inverse raise of abdominal perfusion pressure (APP).

ICG-PDR represents a useful dynamic liver test in addition to conventional laboratory parameters [17]. On the one hand, ICG-PDR is dependent on hepatocellular function [18–20, 37, 38]. On the other hand, it is highly influenced by sufficient hepatosplanchnic blood flow and sinusoidal perfusion [18, 21, 39]. Normal range of ICG-PDR is between 18 and 25%/min. Advanced liver cirrhosis involves severe decreases of ICG-PDR with consecutively grave consequences on patients outcome [20].

This dramatic impairment of ICG-PDR in case of end-stage liver disease is confirmed in our study. Median baseline ICG-PDR was reduced markedly to 3.6%/min. Large-volume paracentesis (LVP) provoked a significant increase in ICG-PDR. Additionally, we noticed an increase in "ICG-Clearance" in contrast to unchanged circulating blood volume index, but data on the relevance of these parameters are rare so far. As opposed to this, paracentesis had no influence on main laboratory parameters of hepatic function. In this context, it should be pointed out that an earlier study found no correlation

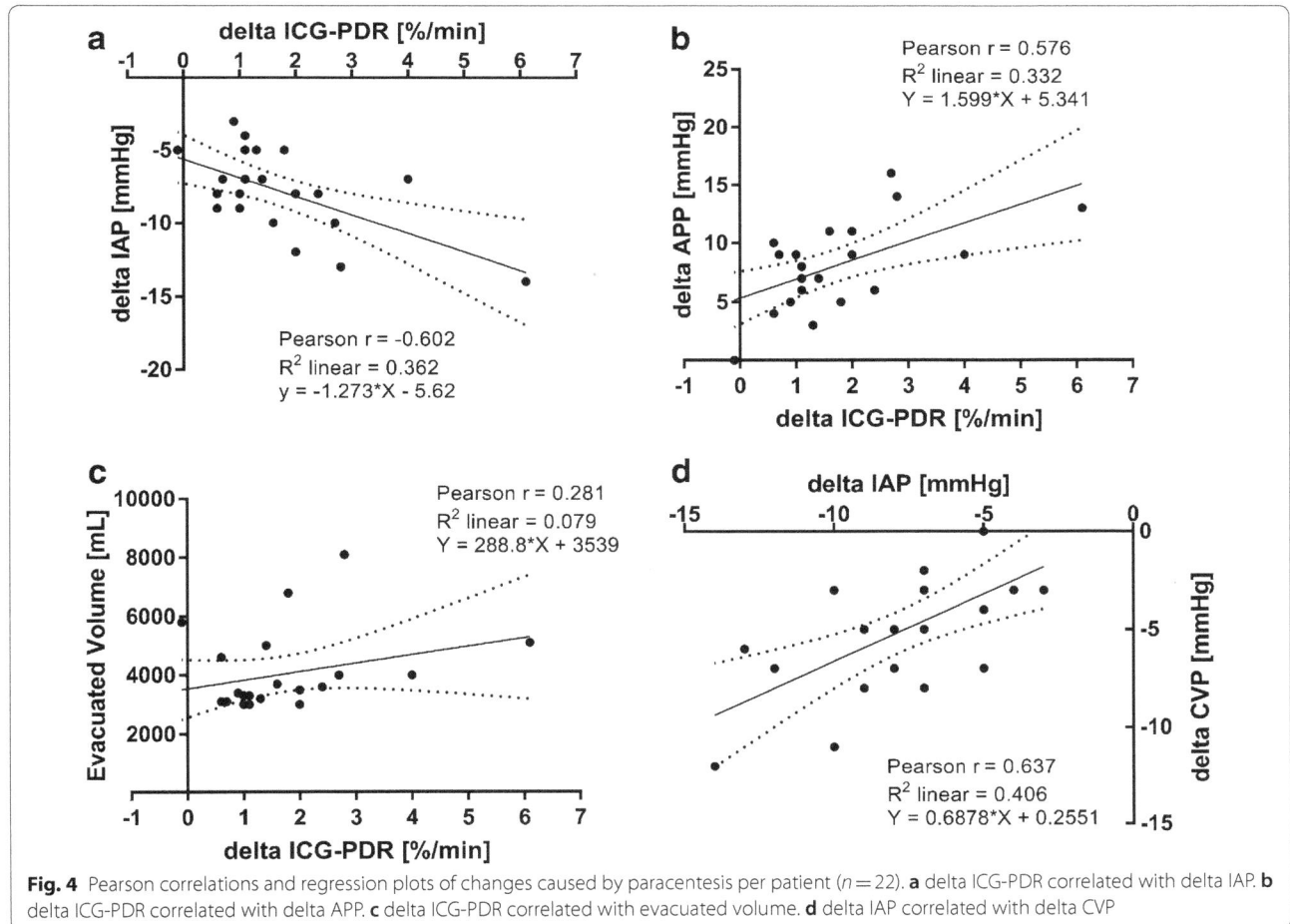

**Fig. 4** Pearson correlations and regression plots of changes caused by paracentesis per patient (n = 22). **a** delta ICG-PDR correlated with delta IAP. **b** delta ICG-PDR correlated with delta APP. **c** delta ICG-PDR correlated with evacuated volume. **d** delta IAP correlated with delta CVP

**Table 4** Ultrasound examination of hepatic blood flow by color-coded duplex sonography of hepatic artery, portal vein and hepatic vein before and after paracentesis

Color-coded duplex sonography of hepatic blood flow

| | Before paracentesis | After paracentesis | p value |
|---|---|---|---|
| | Median (IQR) | Median (IQR) | |
| HARI | 0.74 (0.68–0.75) | 0.68 (0.65–0.71) | < 0.001 |
| Systolic HAF (cm/s) | 129 (115–145) | 123 (114–140) | 0.100 |
| Diastolic HAF (cm/s) | 35 (24–48) | 40 (31–50) | 0.009 |
| PVF (cm/s) | 20 (16–28) | 21 (15–32) | 0.753 |
| HVF (cm/s) | 24 (17–30) | 30 (22–36) | < 0.001 |

*HARI* hepatic artery resistance index, *HAF* maximum hepatic arterial flow velocity, *PVF* maximum portal vein flow velocity, HVF: Maximum hepatic vein flow velocity

**Table 5** Respiratory and ventilatory parameters before and after paracentesis

Respiratory and ventilatory parameters

| | Before paracentesis | After paracentesis | p value |
|---|---|---|---|
| | Median (IQR) | Median (IQR) | |
| $P_aO_2/F_iO_2$ | 220 (126–271) | 247 (138–321) | < 0.001 |
| OI (cmH$_2$O/mmHg) | 8.0 (4.8–12.3) | 5.8 (3.8–11.1) | < 0.001 |
| TV (mL) | 491 (337–542) | 530 (414–590) | 0.001 |
| $C_{dyn}$ (mL/cmH$_2$O) | 41 (21–46) | 49 (24–65) | < 0.001 |
| Respiratory rate (min$^{-1}$) | 24 (18–26) | 22 (16–26) | 0.062 |
| $P_aCO_2$ | 36.7 (32.6–46.4) | 37.0 (32.7–41.2) | 0.115 |

*OI* oxygenation index, *TV* tidal volume, $C_{dyn}$ dynamic respiratory system compliance, $P_aCO_2$ arterial partial pressure of carbon dioxide

**Table 6** Parameters of hemodynamic monitoring before and after paracentesis

Hemodynamic parameters assessed by transpulmonary thermodilution

| | Before paracentesis | After paracentesis | p value |
|---|---|---|---|
| | Median (IQR) | Median (IQR) | |
| MAP (mmHg) | 82 (76–91) | 79 (74–91) | 0.134 |
| CI (L/min/m$^2$) | 4.5 (3.8–6.5) | 5.0 (3.8–6.6) | 0.522 |
| CO (L/min) | 8.9 (7.5–13.1) | 10.3 (7.3–13.4) | 0.579 |
| GEDVI (mL/m$^2$) | 880 (788–1021) | 902 (758–1021) | 0.437 |
| EVLWI (mL/kg) | 12 (9.5–15) | 12 (9.5–14.5) | 0.918 |
| SVRI (dyn * s * cm$^{-5}$ * m$^{-2}$) | 978 (725–1254) | 1064 (713–1236) | 0.772 |
| CVP (mmHg) | 22.5 (17.8–29.0) | 17.5 (12.8–24) | 0.001 |

*CI* cardiac index, *CO* cardiac output, *GEDVI* global end-diastolic volume index, *EVLWI* extravascular lung water index, *SVRI* systemic vascular resistance index, *CVP* central venous pressure

between ICG-PDR and standard laboratory liver tests [25].

The improvement in ICG-PDR is in parallel with a decline of IAP after evacuation of ascites. Correlation analyses revealed a statistically significant association of changes in ICG-PDR with changes in IAP. Previously, a few studies described a relationship between ICG-PDR and IAP. Some of them focused on the effect of prone positioning on IAP and ICG-PDR in patients with respiratory failure [22, 40, 41]. Two studies characterized the inverse correlation of ICG-PDR with the dimension of IAP in critically ill patients [24, 25]. Sakka presented a case of abdominal compartment syndrome with impaired ICG-PDR and a significant increase after surgical relief [42]. Not less interesting is another report from the same author describing the beneficial effect of paracentesis on ICG-PDR in a woman with ascites due to chronic heart failure; while IAP dropped from 18 to 12 mmHg, ICG-PDR rose from 11.6 to 15.6%/min [23]. The basic rationale behind all these findings seems to be that IAH compromises APP and consecutively restrains hepatosplanchnic blood flow and sinusoidal perfusion [25]. According to this, decompression of abdomen with a decrease in IAP improves hepatic blood flow and increases ICG-PDR [23].

The results of our study reaffirmed previous trials concerning a significant and immediate drop of IAP after LVP in patients with decompensated cirrhosis and tense ascites [27, 30, 43]. The relief of IAH is paralleled by a significant raise of APP, suggesting a substantial effect on hepatic perfusion. In the present study, we used color-coded duplex sonography for analyses of liver blood flow. At baseline, we found an elevated hepatic artery resistance index. This observation is in line with former ultrasound examinations showing increased resistance index in case of advanced liver fibrosis and cirrhosis [15, 44–46]. The alterations of intrahepatic circulation in cirrhosis with endothelial dysfunction and increased vasoconstrictor activity are well established [13, 47]. We recognized a significant decrease in hepatic artery resistance index after LVP, mainly referable to a change in diastolic blood flow. The hypothesis behind this finding is that LVP reduces hepatic vascular resistance and enhances sinusoidal perfusion. Moreover, sonography revealed a raise in maximum blood flow velocity in hepatic vein after LVP. Damping of hepatic venous waveform is a frequent observation in advanced cirrhosis, but the significance of blood flow velocity in hepatic vein alone is not investigated so far [14, 48]. In contrast, there was no relevant change of portal vein flow after paracentesis, indicating an obvious portal hypertension in the studied population with advanced liver cirrhosis.

Considered as secondary endpoints of this study, we analyzed the impact of LVP on respiratory and circulatory function in case of decompensated cirrhosis. We registered an overall beneficial effect on parameters of oxygenation and ventilation. Several studies underlined that respiratory improvement was particularly attributable to decreases in IAP, enhanced ventilatory mechanics with increased compliance as well as alveolar recruitment with increased end-expiratory lung volume [43, 49–51]. Concerning hemodynamic function, previous studies yielded diverging results about the existing threat of paracentesis-induced cardiocirculatory dysfunction [52–54]. Nevertheless, a recent study demonstrated that LVP did not impair hemodynamic parameters assessed by transpulmonary thermodilution [43]. Our analyses via transpulmonary thermodilution reconfirmed this favorable situation with steady parameters of hemodynamic function after LVP. However, we noticed a significant decrease in central venous pressure after LVP, most probably due to the decrease in IAP and therefore extra-thoracic pressure level. In line with this, we found a significant association of changes in IAP with changes in central venous pressure.

Altogether, the present study emphasizes the inverse correlation of ICG-PDR with IAP and the far-reaching effects of IAH in critically ill patients with decompensated cirrhosis. Hydropic decompensation evokes harmful increases of IAP with negative effects on abdominal perfusion and liver blood flow. LVP immediately lowers IAP in combination with an increase in ICG-PDR. According to ultrasound examination, this beneficial effect on ICG-PDR is mainly referable to improved arterial liver perfusion and decreased hepatic vascular resistance. By implication, our study to some extent questions the significance of ICG-PDR for an exclusive evaluation of hepatocellular function in case of IAH.

## Strengths and limitations

To our knowledge, this is the first study evaluating the effects of LVP on ICG-PDR in a characterized population of critically ill patients with decompensated cirrhosis and tense ascites. The study combines ICG-PDR with assessments of IAP and APP, ultrasound examinations as well as respiratory and advanced hemodynamic monitoring. Despite the overall modest beneficial effect of paracentesis on ICG-PDR, the results are conclusive with high levels of statistical significance.

However, this is a single-center study with consecutively a very limited number of patients. Paracentesis was performed with a maximum release of mobilizable ascites instead of a stepwise release of predefined fluid amounts. Therefore, our data allowed only the calculation of an "overall" abdominal compliance with limited validity considering its evolution during progressive, stepwise evacuation of ascites [32]. Moreover, this study provides no further information about a possible influence of LVP on kidney function. In light of highly frequently occurring hepatorenal syndrome in case of decompensated liver cirrhosis, further studies would be interesting to investigate the impact of paracentesis on renal perfusion. In consideration of a relatively high baseline EVLWI in our patients, hemodynamic monitoring via transpulmonary thermodilution would have been even more accurate when performed with a higher saline bolus [55]. Ultrasound examinations via color-coded duplex sonography are operator-dependent and were performed only by one physician. Beside ICG-PDR, reliable data on additional parameters CBI and BVI provided by LiMON technology are rare.

## Conclusion

Decompensated cirrhosis is associated with a marked decrease of dynamic liver test ICG-PDR, reflecting reduced hepatocellular capacity as well as impaired hepatosplanchnic blood flow. LVP evokes a modest but significant improvement in ICG-PDR, primarily referable to a decline in IAP and an inverse increase in APP. While conventional laboratory parameters of liver function did not change, the increase in ICG-PDR is mainly attributable to changes in hepatic perfusion.

Moreover, LVP induced substantial improvement in respiratory parameters, while hemodynamic profiles remained stable.

## Abbreviations

IAH: intraabdominal hypertension; IAP: intraabdominal pressure; INR: international normalized ratio; ICG: indo-cyanine green; PDR: plasma disappearance rate; APP: abdominal perfusion pressure; MAP: mean arterial pressure; LVP: large-volume paracentesis; ICU: intensive care unit; BVI: circulating blood volume index; CBI: "ICG-Clearance"; WSACS: The Abdominal Compartment Society; CVP: central venous pressure; ARDS: acute respiratory distress syndrome; PEEP: positive end-expiratory pressure; TV: tidal volume; $C_{dyn}$: dynamic respiratory system compliance; $F_iO_2$: fraction of inspired oxygen; $P_aO_2$: arterial partial pressure of oxygen; $P_aCO_2$: arterial partial pressure of carbon dioxide; OI: oxygenation Index; APACHE: acute and physiology chronic health evaluation; SOFA: sequential organ failure assessment; MELD: model of end-stage liver disease; IQR: interquartile range; HARI: hepatic artery resistance index; HAF: maximum hepatic arterial flow; PVF: maximum portal vein flow; HVF: maximum hepatic vein flow; CI: cardiac index; CO: cardiac output; GEDVI: global end-diastolic volume index; EVLWI: extravascular lung water index; SVRI: systemic vascular resistance index.

## Authors' contributions

UM, WH and TL designed the study. UM, LF and TL collected data, performed statistical analysis and drafted the manuscript. GB, AH, SR and RS also collected data, participated in the analysis of the data and helped to draft the manuscript. All authors read and approved the final manuscript.

**Acknowledgements**
None.


**Competing interests**
Wolfgang Huber collaborates with Pulsion Medical Systems SE, Feldkirchen, Germany, as member of the Medical Advisory Board. All other authors have no competing interests to disclose.


**Funding**
Funding was provided by Pulsion Medical Systems SE, Feldkirchen, Germany.


**References**

1. Gines P, Quintero E, Arroyo V, Teres J, Bruguera M, Rimola A, et al. Compensated cirrhosis: natural history and prognostic factors. Hepatology. 1987;7(1):122–8.
2. Bernardi M, Moreau R, Angeli P, Schnabl B, Arroyo V. Mechanisms of decompensation and organ failure in cirrhosis: from peripheral arterial vasodilation to systemic inflammation hypothesis. J Hepatol. 2015;63(5):1272–84. https://doi.org/10.1016/j.jhep.2015.07.004.
3. Malbrain ML, Chiumello D, Pelosi P, Bihari D, Innes R, Ranieri VM, et al. Incidence and prognosis of intraabdominal hypertension in a mixed population of critically ill patients: a multiple-center epidemiological study. Crit Care Med. 2005;33(2):315–22.
4. Malbrain ML, Chiumello D, Pelosi P, Wilmer A, Brienza N, Malcangi V, et al. Prevalence of intra-abdominal hypertension in critically ill patients: a multicentre epidemiological study. Intensive Care Med. 2004;30(5):822–9. https://doi.org/10.1007/s00134-004-2169-9.
5. Rouby JJ, Constantin JM, De Roberto AGC, Zhang M, Lu Q. Mechanical ventilation in patients with acute respiratory distress syndrome. Anesthesiology. 2004;101(1):228–34.
6. Barnes GE, Laine GA, Giam PY, Smith EE, Granger HJ. Cardiovascular responses to elevation of intra-abdominal hydrostatic pressure. Am J Physiol. 1985;248(2 Pt 2):R208–13.
7. Malbrain ML, Cheatham ML, Kirkpatrick A, Sugrue M, Parr M, De Waele J, et al. Results from the international conference of experts on intra-abdominal hypertension and abdominal compartment syndrome. I. Definitions. Intensive Care Med. 2006;32(11):1722–32. https://doi.org/10.1007/s00134-006-0349-5.
8. von Delius S, Karagianni A, Henke J, Preissel A, Meining A, Frimberger E, et al. Changes in intra-abdominal pressure, hemodynamics, and peak inspiratory pressure during gastroscopy in a porcine model. Endoscopy. 2007;39(11):962–8. https://doi.org/10.1055/s-2007-966973.
9. Malbrain ML, Deeren D, De Potter TJ. Intra-abdominal hypertension in the critically ill: it is time to pay attention. Curr Opin Crit Care. 2005;11(2):156–71.
10. Cresswell AB, Wendon JA. Hepatic function and non-invasive hepatosplanchnic monitoring in patients with abdominal hypertension. Acta Clin Belg. 2007;62(Suppl 1):113–8.
11. Bosch J. Vascular deterioration in cirrhosis: the big picture. J Clin Gastroenterol. 2007;41(Suppl 3):S247–53. https://doi.org/10.1097/MCG.0b013e3181572357.
12. Iwakiri Y, Groszmann RJ. The hyperdynamic circulation of chronic liver diseases: from the patient to the molecule. Hepatology. 2006;43(2 Suppl 1):S121–31. https://doi.org/10.1002/hep.20993.
13. Iwakiri Y. Pathophysiology of portal hypertension. Clin Liver Dis. 2014;18(2):281–91. https://doi.org/10.1016/j.cld.2013.12.001.
14. Scheinfeld MH, Bilali A, Koenigsberg M. Understanding the spectral Doppler waveform of the hepatic veins in health and disease. Radiographics. 2009;29(7):2081–98. https://doi.org/10.1148/rg.297095715.
15. Zekanovic D, Ljubicic N, Boban M, Nikolic M, Delic-Brkljacic D, Gacina P, et al. Doppler ultrasound of hepatic and system hemodynamics in patients with alcoholic liver cirrhosis. Dig Dis Sci. 2010;55(2):458–66. https://doi.org/10.1007/s10620-009-0760-1.
16. Zwiebel WJ. Sonographic diagnosis of hepatic vascular disorders. Semin Ultrasound CT MRI. 1995;16(1):34–48.
17. Sakka SG. Assessing liver function. Curr Opin Crit Care. 2007;13(2):207–14. https://doi.org/10.1097/MCC.0b013e328012b268.
18. Sakka SG, Klein M, Reinhart K, Meier-Hellmann A. Prognostic value of extravascular lung water in critically ill patients. Chest. 2002;122(6):2080–6.
19. Stehr A, Ploner F, Traeger K, Theisen M, Zuelke C, Radermacher P, et al. Plasma disappearance of indocyanine green: a marker for excretory liver function? Intensive Care Med. 2005;31(12):1719–22. https://doi.org/10.1007/s00134-005-2826-7.
20. Faybik P, Hetz H. Plasma disappearance rate of indocyanine green in liver dysfunction. Transplant Proc. 2006;38(3):801–2. https://doi.org/10.1016/j.transproceed.2006.01.049.
21. Seibel A, Muller A, Sakka SG. Indocyanine green plasma disappearance rate for monitoring hepatosplanchnic blood flow. Intensive Care Med. 2011;37(2):357–9. https://doi.org/10.1007/s00134-010-2063-6.
22. Michelet P, Roch A, Gainnier M, Sainty JM, Auffray JP, Papazian L. Influence of support on intra-abdominal pressure, hepatic kinetics of indocyanine green and extravascular lung water during prone positioning in patients with ARDS: a randomized crossover study. Crit Care. 2005;9(3):R251–7. https://doi.org/10.1186/cc3513.
23. Sakka SG. Indocyanine green plasma disappearance rate during relief of increased abdominal pressure. Intensive Care Med. 2006;32(12):2090–1. https://doi.org/10.1007/s00134-006-0411-3.
24. Inal MT, Memis D, Sezer YA, Atalay M, Karakoc A, Sut N. Effects of intra-abdominal pressure on liver function assessed with the LiMON in critically ill patients. Can J Surg. 2011;54(3):161–6. https://doi.org/10.1503/cjs.042709.
25. Malbrain ML, Viaene D, Kortgen A, De Laet I, Dits H, Van Regenmortel N, et al. Relationship between intra-abdominal pressure and indocyanine green plasma disappearance rate: hepatic perfusion may be impaired in critically ill patients with intra-abdominal hypertension. Ann Intensive Care. 2012;2(Suppl 1):S19. https://doi.org/10.1186/2110-5820-2-S1-S19.
26. Zipprich A, Kuss O, Rogowski S, Kleber G, Lotterer E, Seufferlein T, et al. Incorporating indocyanin green clearance into the Model for End Stage Liver Disease (MELD-ICG) improves prognostic accuracy in intermediate to advanced cirrhosis. Gut. 2010;59(7):963–8. https://doi.org/10.1136/gut.2010.208595.
27. Cheatham ML. Nonoperative management of intraabdominal hypertension and abdominal compartment syndrome. World J Surg. 2009;33(6):1116–22. https://doi.org/10.1007/s00268-009-0003-9.
28. Sakka SG, Reinhart K, Meier-Hellmann A. Comparison of invasive and noninvasive measurements of indocyanine green plasma disappearance rate in critically ill patients with mechanical ventilation and stable hemodynamics. Intensive Care Med. 2000;26(10):1553–6.
29. Umgelter A, Reindl W, Wagner KS, Franzen M, Stock K, Schmid RM, et al. Effects of plasma expansion with albumin and paracentesis on haemodynamics and kidney function in critically ill cirrhotic patients with tense ascites and hepatorenal syndrome: a prospective uncontrolled trial. Crit Care. 2008;12(1):R4. https://doi.org/10.1186/cc6765.
30. Malbrain ML. Different techniques to measure intra-abdominal pressure (IAP): time for a critical re-appraisal. Intensive Care Med. 2004;30(3):357–71. https://doi.org/10.1007/s00134-003-2107-2.
31. Kirkpatrick AW, Roberts DJ, De Waele J, Jaeschke R, Malbrain ML, De Keulenaer B, et al. Intra-abdominal hypertension and the abdominal compartment syndrome: updated consensus definitions and clinical practice guidelines from the World Society of the Abdominal Compartment Syndrome. Intensive Care Med. 2013;39(7):1190–206. https://doi.org/10.1007/s00134-013-2906-z.
32. Malbrain ML, Peeters Y, Wise R. The neglected role of abdominal compliance in organ–organ interactions. Crit Care. 2016;20:67. https://doi.org/10.1186/s13054-016-1220-x.
33. Gines A, Fernandez-Esparrach G, Monescillo A, Vila C, Domenech E, Abecasis R, et al. Randomized trial comparing albumin, dextran 70, and polygeline in cirrhotic patients with ascites treated by paracentesis. Gastroenterology. 1996;111(4):1002–10.
34. Bein T, Grasso S, Moerer O, Quintel M, Guerin C, Deja M, et al. The standard of care of patients with ARDS: ventilatory settings and rescue therapies for refractory hypoxemia. Intensive Care Med. 2016;42(5):699–711. https://doi.org/10.1007/s00134-016-4325-4.
35. Bone RC, Maunder R, Slotman G, Silverman H, Hyers TM, Kerstein MD, et al. An early test of survival in patients with the adult respiratory distress syndrome. The $P_aO_2/F_iO_2$ ratio and its differential response to conventional therapy. Prostaglandin E1 Study Group. Chest. 1989;96(4):849–51.

36. Huber W, Umgelter A, Reindl W, Franzen M, Schmidt C, von Delius S, et al. Volume assessment in patients with necrotizing pancreatitis: a comparison of intrathoracic blood volume index, central venous pressure, and hematocrit, and their correlation to cardiac index and extravascular lung water index. Crit Care Med. 2008;36(8):2348–54. https://doi.org/10.1097/CCM.0b013e3181809928.

37. Hemming AW, Scudamore CH, Shackleton CR, Pudek M, Erb SR. Indocyanine green clearance as a predictor of successful hepatic resection in cirrhotic patients. Am J Surg. 1992;163(5):515–8.

38. Scheingraber S, Richter S, Igna D, Flesch S, Kopp B, Schilling MK. Indocyanine green disappearance rate is the most useful marker for liver resection. Hepatogastroenterology. 2008;55(85):1394–9.

39. Inal MT, Memis D, Kargi M, Sut N. Prognostic value of indocyanine green elimination assessed with LiMON in septic patients. J Crit Care. 2009;24(3):329–34. https://doi.org/10.1016/j.jcrc.2008.11.012.

40. Hering R, Vorwerk R, Wrigge H, Zinserling J, Schroder S, von Spiegel T, et al. Prone positioning, systemic hemodynamics, hepatic indocyanine green kinetics, and gastric intramucosal energy balance in patients with acute lung injury. Intensive Care Med. 2002;28(1):53–8. https://doi.org/10.1007/s00134-001-1166-5.

41. Kirkpatrick AW, Pelosi P, De Waele JJ, Malbrain ML, Ball CG, Meade MO, et al. Clinical review: intra-abdominal hypertension: does it influence the physiology of prone ventilation? Crit Care. 2010;14(4):232. https://doi.org/10.1186/cc9099.

42. Sakka SG. Indocyanine green plasma disappearance rate as an indicator of hepato-splanchnic ischemia during abdominal compartment syndrome. Anesth Analg. 2007;104(4):1003–4. https://doi.org/10.1213/01.ane.0000256097.61730.cc.

43. Phillip V, Saugel B, Ernesti C, Hapfelmeier A, Schultheiss C, Thies P, et al. Effects of paracentesis on hemodynamic parameters and respiratory function in critically ill patients. BMC Gastroenterol. 2014;14:18. https://doi.org/10.1186/1471-230X-14-18.

44. Sacerdoti D, Merkel C, Bolognesi M, Amodio P, Angeli P, Gatta A. Hepatic arterial resistance in cirrhosis with and without portal vein thrombosis: relationships with portal hemodynamics. Gastroenterology. 1995;108(4):1152–8.

45. Lutz HH, Gassler N, Tischendorf FW, Trautwein C, Tischendorf JJ. Doppler ultrasound of hepatic blood flow for noninvasive evaluation of liver fibrosis compared with liver biopsy and transient elastography. Dig Dis Sci. 2012;57(8):2222–30. https://doi.org/10.1007/s10620-012-2153-0.

46. Glisic TM, Perisic MD, Dimitrijevic S, Jurisic V. Doppler assessment of splanchnic arterial flow in patients with liver cirrhosis: correlation with ammonia plasma levels and MELD score. J Clin Ultrasound. 2014;42(5):264–9. https://doi.org/10.1002/jcu.22135.

47. Gracia-Sancho J, Lavina B, Rodriguez-Vilarrupla A, Garcia-Caldero H, Bosch J, Garcia-Pagan JC. Enhanced vasoconstrictor prostanoid production by sinusoidal endothelial cells increases portal perfusion pressure in cirrhotic rat livers. J Hepatol. 2007;47(2):220–7. https://doi.org/10.1016/j.jhep.2007.03.014.

48. Kim MY, Baik SK, Park DH, Lim DW, Kim JW, Kim HS, et al. Damping index of Doppler hepatic vein waveform to assess the severity of portal hypertension and response to propranolol in liver cirrhosis: a prospective nonrandomized study. Liver Int. 2007;27(8):1103–10. https://doi.org/10.1111/j.1478-3231.2007.01526.x.

49. Levesque E, Hoti E, Jiabin J, Dellamonica J, Ichai P, Saliba F, et al. Respiratory impact of paracentesis in cirrhotic patients with acute lung injury. J Crit Care. 2011;26(3):257–61. https://doi.org/10.1016/j.jcrc.2010.08.020.

50. Byrd RP Jr, Roy TM, Simons M. Improvement in oxygenation after large volume paracentesis. South Med J. 1996;89(7):689–92.

51. Wauters J, Claus P, Brosens N, McLaughlin M, Hermans G, Malbrain M, et al. Relationship between abdominal pressure, pulmonary compliance, and cardiac preload in a porcine model. Crit Care Res Pract. 2012;2012:763181. https://doi.org/10.1155/2012/763181.

52. Cabrera J, Falcon L, Gorriz E, Pardo MD, Granados R, Quinones A, et al. Abdominal decompression plays a major role in early postparacentesis haemodynamic changes in cirrhotic patients with tense ascites. Gut. 2001;48(3):384–9.

53. Nasr G, Hassan A, Ahmed S, Serwah A. Predictors of large volume paracantesis induced circulatory dysfunction in patients with massive hepatic ascites. J Cardiovasc Dis Res. 2010;1(3):136–44. https://doi.org/10.4103/0975-3583.70914.

54. Peltekian KM, Wong F, Liu PP, Logan AG, Sherman M, Blendis LM. Cardiovascular, renal, and neurohumoral responses to single large-volume paracentesis in patients with cirrhosis and diuretic-resistant ascites. Am J Gastroenterol. 1997;92(3):394–9.

55. Hofkens PJ, Verrijcken A, Merveille K, Neirynck S, Van Regenmortel N, De Laet I, et al. Common pitfalls and tips and tricks to get the most out of your transpulmonary thermodilution device: results of a survey and state-of-the-art review. Anaesthesiol Intensive Ther. 2015;47(2):89–116. https://doi.org/10.5603/AIT.a2014.0068.

# 22

# Principles of fluid management and stewardship in septic shock: it is time to consider the four D's and the four phases of fluid therapy

Manu L. N. G. Malbrain[1,2*], Niels Van Regenmortel[3], Bernd Saugel[4], Brecht De Tavernier[3], Pieter-Jan Van Gaal[3], Olivier Joannes-Boyau[5], Jean-Louis Teboul[6], Todd W. Rice[7], Monty Mythen[8] and Xavier Monnet[6]

## Abstract

In patients with septic shock, the administration of fluids during initial hemodynamic resuscitation remains a major therapeutic challenge. We are faced with many open questions regarding the type, dose and timing of intravenous fluid administration. There are only four major indications for intravenous fluid administration: aside from resuscitation, intravenous fluids have many other uses including maintenance and replacement of total body water and electrolytes, as carriers for medications and for parenteral nutrition. In this paradigm-shifting review, we discuss different fluid management strategies including early adequate goal-directed fluid management, late conservative fluid management and late goal-directed fluid removal. In addition, we expand on the concept of the "four D's" of fluid therapy, namely drug, dosing, duration and de-escalation. During the treatment of patients with septic shock, four phases of fluid therapy should be considered in order to provide answers to four basic questions. These four phases are the resuscitation phase, the optimization phase, the stabilization phase and the evacuation phase. The four questions are "When to start intravenous fluids?", "When to stop intravenous fluids?", "When to start de-resuscitation or active fluid removal?" and finally "When to stop de-resuscitation?" In analogy to the way we handle antibiotics in critically ill patients, it is time for fluid stewardship.

**Keywords:** Fluids, Fluid therapy, Fluid management, Fluid stewardship, Four D's, Four indications, Four hits, Four phases, Four questions, Resuscitation, Antibiotics, Drug, Dose, Duration, De-escalation, De-resuscitation, Maintenance, Replacement, Goal-directed therapy, Monitoring, Fluid responsiveness, Passive leg raising

## Background

In patients with septic shock, hemodynamic stabilization using intravenous fluids remains a major therapeutic challenge as numerous questions remain regarding the type, dose and timing of fluid administration. In these patients, fluids play an important role beyond hemodynamic stabilization and resuscitation. Intravenous fluids should be prescribed as any other drug we give to our patients: we should take into account the indications and contraindications for different types of fluids [2–8]. We should only prescribe fluids when they are clearly indicated and should balance the risk of not administering enough with the increasingly apparent risks of too much fluid.

In this review, we will expand on the concept of the "four D's" of fluid therapy (drug, duration, dosing and de-escalation). We will also focus on the recent concept defining four different phases in the time course of septic shock (resuscitation, optimization, stabilization and evacuation). Each phase requires a different therapeutic attitude regarding fluid administration. Taking into account both of these concepts in combination with other suggested ideas may promote more rational fluid

*Correspondence: manu.malbrain@uzbrussel.be
[1] Intensive Care Unit, University Hospital Brussels (UZB), Laarbeeklaan 101, 1090 Jette, Belgium
Full list of author information is available at the end of the article

administration aimed at avoiding both too little and too much. In analogy to the way we handle antibiotic usage in the critically ill, it is now time for fluid stewardship.

## The risk of fluid overload

Treating a patient with septic shock inevitably results in some degree of salt and water overload. First and foremost, this is the result of the initial fluid resuscitation with the aim of restoring intravascular volume, increasing cardiac output, augmenting oxygen delivery and improving tissue oxygenation. Salt and water overload can also result from the administration of large volumes of fluid as drug diluents, artificial nutrition and maintenance fluids. The capillary leak that is inherent to sepsis promotes the extravasation of large amounts of fluid, inducing relative central hypovolemia that often requires further fluid administration, despite interstitial oedema. Capillary leak represents the maladaptive, often excessive, and undesirable loss of fluid and electrolytes with or without protein into the interstitium that generates anasarca and end-organ oedema causing organ dysfunction and eventually failure [9]. Fluid overload should be avoided in this setting.

> ### Fluid overload
> As often described in paediatric populations, the percentage of fluid accumulation is calculated by dividing the cumulative fluid balance in litres by the patient's baseline body weight and multiplying by 100%. Fluid overload at any stage is defined by a cut-off value of 10% of fluid accumulation, as this is associated with worse outcomes [14, 76, 88].

Studies demonstrate an association between fluid overload, illustrated by the increase in the cumulative fluid balance, with worse patient centred outcomes [1] in critically ill patients with septic shock [10, 11] and/or acute respiratory distress syndrome [12]. Fluid administration potentially induces a vicious cycle, where interstitial oedema induces organ dysfunction that contributes to fluid accumulation (Fig. 1). Peripheral and generalized oedema is not only of cosmetic concern, as believed by some [13], but harmful to the patient as a whole as it can cause organ oedema and dysfunction [1, 14]. Figure 2 details all the potential harmful consequences of fluid overload on different end-organ systems, with consequential effects on patient morbidity and mortality. As such, fluid therapy can be considered a double-edged sword [1, 15].

Therefore, current treatment of septic shock should include every effort to reduce the cumulative fluid balance. We must always bear in mind that fluids are drugs and oedema is akin to a drug overdose. Their characteristics,

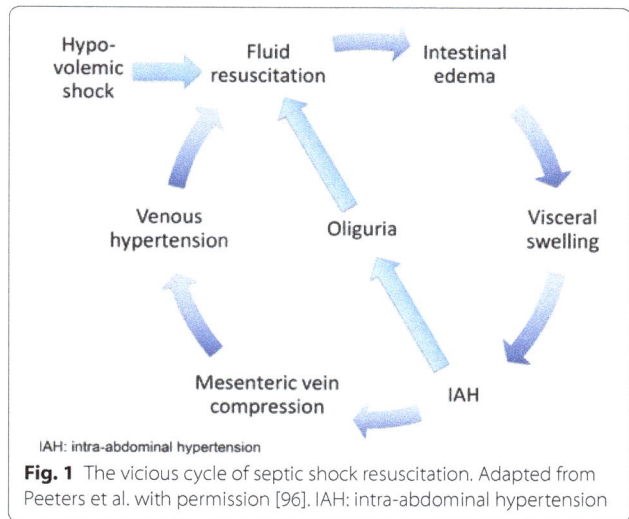

**Fig. 1** The vicious cycle of septic shock resuscitation. Adapted from Peeters et al. with permission [96]. IAH: intra-abdominal hypertension

indications and contraindications should be carefully considered when choosing their type, their dose, the timing of their administration and the timing for their removal. In parallel, a reasoned fluid strategy requires that we do not consider septic shock as a single "one size fits all" disease, but rather that it is made of different phases, each implying a different therapeutic attitude [16].

## The four D's of fluid therapy

When prescribing fluids in patients with septic shock, we must take into account their composition and their pharmocodynamic and pharmacokinetic properties. In practice, we should consider the "four D's" of fluid therapy: drug, dosing, duration and de-escalation (Table 1) [5]. Many clinicians already use these four D's for the prescription of antibiotics (Table 1).

### Drug

We should consider the different compounds: crystalloids versus colloids, synthetic versus blood derived, balanced versus unbalanced, intravenous versus oral. The osmolality, tonicity, pH, electrolyte composition (chloride, sodium, potassium, etc.) and levels of other metabolically active compounds (lactate, acetate, malate, etc.) are all equally important. Clinical factors (underlying conditions, kidney or liver failure, presence of capillary leak, acid–base equilibrium, albumin levels, fluid balance, etc.) must all be taken into account when choosing the type and amount of fluid for a given patient at a given time. Moreover, the type of fluid is different depending on the reason why they are administered. There are only four indications for fluid administration, namely resuscitation, maintenance, replacement and nutrition, or a combination.

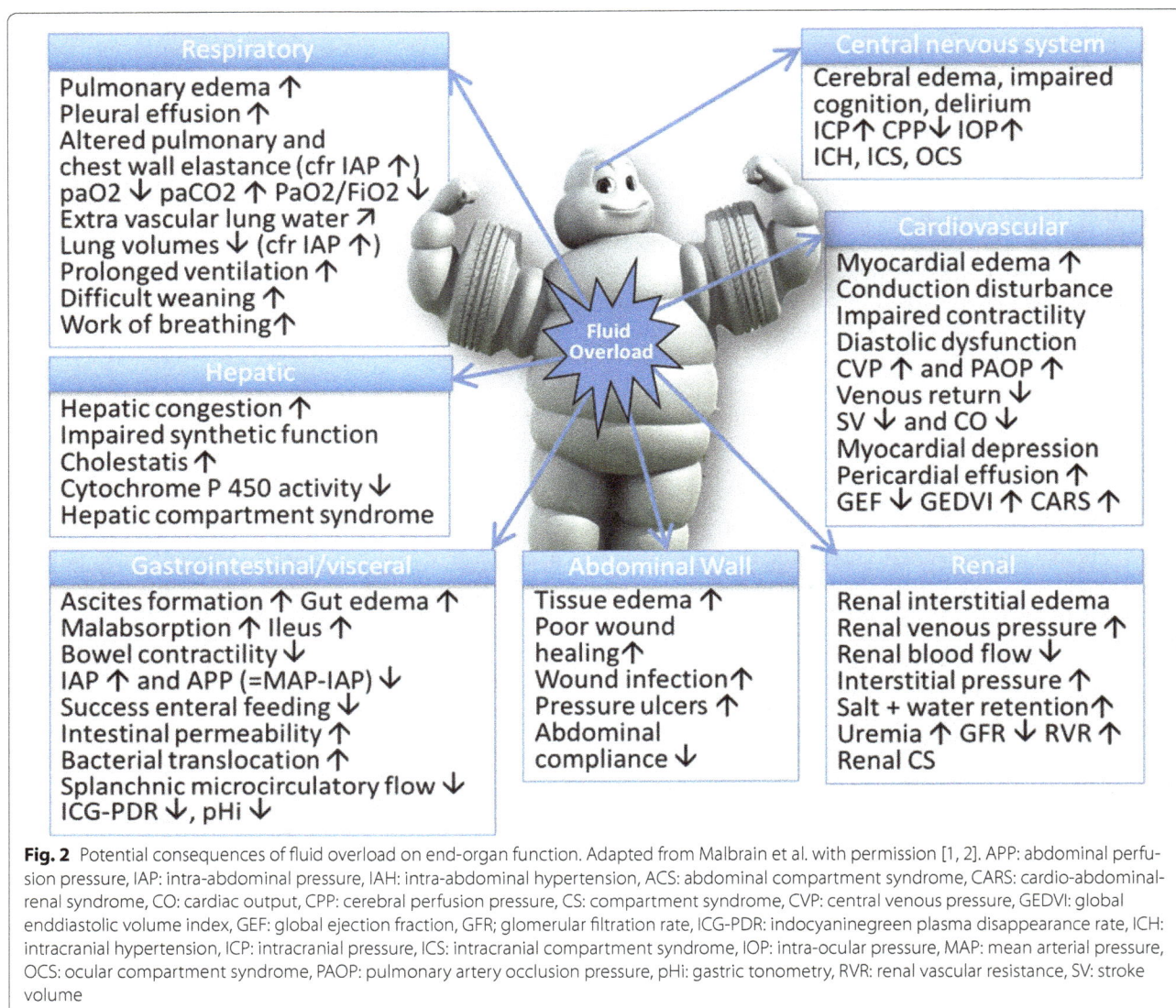

**Respiratory**
Pulmonary edema ↑
Pleural effusion ↑
Altered pulmonary and
chest wall elastance (cfr IAP ↑)
paO2 ↓ paCO2 ↑ PaO2/FiO2 ↓
Extra vascular lung water ↗
Lung volumes ↓ (cfr IAP ↑)
Prolonged ventilation ↑
Difficult weaning ↑
Work of breathing↑

**Hepatic**
Hepatic congestion ↑
Impaired synthetic function
Cholestatis ↑
Cytochrome P 450 activity ↓
Hepatic compartment syndrome

**Gastrointestinal/visceral**
Ascites formation ↑ Gut edema ↑
Malabsorption ↑ Ileus ↑
Bowel contractility ↓
IAP ↑ and APP (=MAP-IAP) ↓
Success enteral feeding ↓
Intestinal permeability ↑
Bacterial translocation ↑
Splanchnic microcirculatory flow ↓
ICG-PDR ↓, pHi ↓

**Fluid Overload**

**Central nervous system**
Cerebral edema, impaired
cognition, delirium
ICP↑ CPP↓ IOP↑
ICH, ICS, OCS

**Cardiovascular**
Myocardial edema ↑
Conduction disturbance
Impaired contractility
Diastolic dysfunction
CVP ↑ and PAOP ↑
Venous return ↓
SV ↓ and CO ↓
Myocardial depression
Pericardial effusion ↑
GEF ↓ GEDVI ↑ CARS ↑

**Abdominal Wall**
Tissue edema ↑
Poor wound
healing↑
Wound infection↑
Pressure ulcers ↑
Abdominal
compliance ↓

**Renal**
Renal interstitial edema
Renal venous pressure ↑
Renal blood flow ↓
Interstitial pressure ↑
Salt + water retention↑
Uremia ↑ GFR ↓ RVR ↑
Renal CS

Fig. 2 Potential consequences of fluid overload on end-organ function. Adapted from Malbrain et al. with permission [1, 2]. APP: abdominal perfusion pressure, IAP: intra-abdominal pressure, IAH: intra-abdominal hypertension, ACS: abdominal compartment syndrome, CARS: cardio-abdominal-renal syndrome, CO: cardiac output, CPP: cerebral perfusion pressure, CS: compartment syndrome, CVP: central venous pressure, GEDVI: global enddiastolic volume index, GEF: global ejection fraction, GFR; glomerular filtration rate, ICG-PDR: indocyaninegreen plasma disappearance rate, ICH: intracranial hypertension, ICP: intracranial pressure, ICS: intracranial compartment syndrome, IOP: intra-ocular pressure, MAP: mean arterial pressure, OCS: ocular compartment syndrome, PAOP: pulmonary artery occlusion pressure, pHi: gastric tonometry, RVR: renal vascular resistance, SV: stroke volume

*Resuscitation fluids*
Resuscitation fluids are given to correct an intravascular volume deficit in the case of absolute or relative hypovolemia. In theory, the choice between colloids and crystalloids should take into account the revised Starling equation and the glycocalyx model of transvascular fluid exchange [17]. When capillary pressure (or transendothelial pressure difference) is low, as in hypovolemia or sepsis and especially septic shock, or during hypotension (after induction and anaesthesia), albumin or plasma substitutes have no advantage over crystalloid infusions, since they all remain intravascular. However, the glycocalyx layer is a fragile structure and is disrupted by surgical trauma-induced systemic inflammation or sepsis, but also by rapid infusion of fluids (especially saline). Under these circumstances, transcapillary flow (albumin leakage

and risk of tissue oedema) is increased, as is the risk to evolve to a state of global increased permeability syndrome (GIPS) [17].

*Global increased permeability syndrome*
Some patients will not transgress to the "flow" phase spontaneously and will remain in a persistent state of *global increased permeability syndrome* and ongoing fluid accumulation [9]. The global increased permeability syndrome can hence be defined as fluid overload in combination with new onset organ failure. This is referred to as "the third hit of shock" [41].

Because of their potential risk, *hydroxyethyl starches* are contraindicated in case of septic shock, burns,

**Table 1** Analogy between the four D's of antibiotic and fluid therapy. Adapted from Malbrain et al. with permission [5]

| Description | Terminology | Antibiotics | Fluids |
|---|---|---|---|
| Drug | Inappropriate therapy | More organ failure, longer ICU LOS, longer hospital LOS, longer MV | Hyperchloremic metabolic acidosis, more AKI, more RRT, increased mortality |
| | Appropriate therapy | Key factor in empiric AB selection is consideration of patient risk factors (e.g. prior AB, duration MV, corticosteroids, recent hospitalization, residence in nursing home) | Key factor in empiric fluid therapy is consideration of patient risk factors (e.g. fluid balance, fluid overload, capillary leak, kidney and other organ function). Do not use glucose as resuscitation fluid |
| | Combination therapy | Possible benefits: e.g. broader spectrum, synergy, avoidance of emergency of resistance, less toxicity | Possible benefits: e.g. specific fluids for different indications (replacement vs. maintenance vs. resuscitation), less toxicity |
| | Class | Broad-spectrum or specific, beta-lactam or glycopeptide, additional compounds as tazobactam. The choice has a real impact on efficacy and toxicity | Hypo- or hypertonic, high or low chloride and sodium level, lactate or bicarbonate buffer, glucose containing or not. This will impact directly acid–base equilibrium, cellular hydration and electrolyte regulation |
| | Appropriate timing | Survival decreases with 7% per hour delay. Needs discipline and practical organization | In refractory shock, the longer the delay, the more microcirculatory hypoperfusion |
| Dosing | Pharmacokinetics | Depends on distribution volume, clearance (kidney and liver function), albumin level, tissue penetration | Depends on type of fluid: glucose 10%, crystalloids 25%, versus colloids 100% IV after 1 h, distribution volume, osmolality, oncoticity, kidney function |
| | Pharmacodynamics | Reflected by the minimal inhibitory concentration. Reflected by "kill" characteristics, time ($T$ > MIC) versus concentration (Cmax/MIC) dependent | Depends on type of fluid and desired location: IV (resuscitation), IS versus IC (cellular dehydration) |
| | Toxicity | Some ABs are toxic to kidneys, advice on dose adjustment needed. However, not getting infection under control is not helping the kidney either | Some fluids (HES) are toxic for the kidneys. However, not getting shock under control is not helping the kidney either |
| Duration | Appropriate duration | No strong evidence but trend towards shorter duration. Do not use AB to treat fever, CRP or chest X-ray infiltrates but use AB to treat infections | No strong evidence but trend towards shorter duration. Do not use fluids to treat low CVP, MAP or UO, but use fluids to treat shock |
| | Treat to response | Stop AB when signs and symptoms of active infection resolves. Future role for biomarkers (PCT) | Fluids can be stopped when shock is resolved (normal lactate). Future role for biomarkers (NGAL, cystatin C, citrullin, L-FABP) |
| De-escalation | Monitoring | Take cultures first and have the guts to change a winning team | After stabilization with EAFM (normal PPV, normal CO, normal lactate) stop ongoing resuscitation and move to LCFM and LGFR (=de-resuscitation) |

*AB* antibiotic, *AKI* acute kidney injury, *Cmax* maximal peak concentration, *CO* cardiac output, *CRP* C reactive protein, *CVP* central venous pressure, *EAFM* early adequate fluid management, *EGDT* early goal-directed therapy, *IC* intracellular, *ICU* intensive care unit, *IS* interstitial, *IV* intravascular, *LCFM* late conservative fluid management, *L-FABP* L-type fatty acid binding protein, *LGFR* late goal-directed fluid removal, *LOS* length of stay, *MAP* mean arterial pressure, *MIC* mean inhibitory concentration, *MV* mechanical ventilation, *NGAL* neutrophil gelatinase-associated lipocalin, *PCT* procalcitonin, *PPV* pulse pressure variation, *RRT* renal replacement therapy, *UO* urine output

patients with acute or chronic kidney injury or in case of oliguria not responsive to fluids (within 6 h) [18]. In other circumstances (post-operative phase, trauma and haemorrhagic shock), starches may still be able to be used as resuscitation fluids, although this remains controversial. Recently, the Coordination Group for Mutual Recognition and Decentralised Procedures-Human (CMDh) has endorsed the European Medicine's Agency PRAC (Pharmacovigilance Risk Assessment Committee) recommendation to suspend the marketing authorisations of hydroxyethyl starch solutions for infusion across the European Union. This suspension is due to the fact that hydroxyethyl starch solutions have continued to be used in critically ill patients and patients with sepsis, despite the introduction in 2013 of restrictions on use in these patient populations in order to reduce the risk of kidney injury and death (http://www.ema.europa.eu).

---

**Septic shock phases**

Septic shock starts with an *ebb phase*, which refers to the phase when the patient shows hyperdynamic shock with decreased systemic vascular resistance due to vasodilation, increased capillary permeability, and severe absolute or relative intravascular hypovolemia. The Surviving Sepsis Campaign guidelines mandate the administration of IV fluids at a dose of 30 mL/kg given within the first 3 h, as a possible life-saving procedure in this phase, although there is no randomized controlled trial to support this statement [18]. The *flow phase* refers to the phase after initial stabilization where the patient will mobilize the excess fluid spontaneously. A classic example is when a patient enters a polyuric phase recovering from acute kidney injury. In this post-shock phase, the metabolic turnover is increased, the innate immune system is activated, and a hepatic acute-phase response is induced. This hypercatabolic metabolic state is characterized by an increase in oxygen consumption and energy expenditure [95].

---

It is justified to use *albumin* as a resuscitation fluid in patients with hypoalbuminemia [18, 19]. *Glucose* should never be used in resuscitation fluid. Surprisingly, *normal saline,* which does not contain potassium, will result in a higher increase in potassium levels in patients with renal impairment compared to a balanced solution (lactated Ringer's) containing 5 mmol/L of potassium, owing to concomitant metabolic acidosis due to a decreased strong ion difference (SID) [20, 21].

(Ab)normal saline as resuscitation fluid should not be administered in large amounts as it carries the risk of hypernatremic hyperchloremic metabolic acidosis, acute kidney injury and death. The use of *balanced solutions* may avoid these complications. Recent evidence shows

the association between fluid-induced chloride loading/hyperchloremia and worse outcomes, probably due to an impact on renal function [22, 23]. In a recent clinical study in human volunteers, a reduction in iatrogenic chloride loading was associated with a decreased incidence of acute kidney injury [24]. Nevertheless, the SALT trial found no significant difference between both types of fluid [25]. Similarly, the recent SPLIT trial also failed to demonstrate a significant difference between saline and a balanced solution (Plasma-Lyte) in critically ill patients [26], although this study has been subject to a lot of criticisms [21]. Recently, as follow-up on the SALT trial, the same authors published the SMART study results [25, 27]. In this pragmatic, cluster-randomized, multiple-crossover trial, the authors assigned 15,802 adults to receive saline (0.9% sodium chloride) or balanced crystalloids (lactated Ringer's solution or Plasma-Lyte A) and they demonstrated that the use of balanced crystalloids resulted in a lower rate of the composite outcome of death from any cause, new renal replacement therapy, or persistent renal dysfunction than the use of saline [27]. In a companion study at the same institution, noncritically ill adults treated with intravenous fluids in the emergency department had similar numbers of hospital-free days between treatment with balanced crystalloids and treatment with saline [28]. However, similar to the SMART trial, administration of balanced crystalloids resulted in less composite death, new renal replacement therapy or persistent renal dysfunction.

The context-sensitive half-time of crystalloids and colloids may change and vary over time depending on the patient's condition (Fig. 3). In fact, as long as crystalloids or colloids are infused, they will exert a similar volume expansion effect and their *distribution* and/or *elimination* and excretion will be slowed in case of shock, hypotension, sedation or general anaesthesia [29, 30]. This may explain why crystalloids have a much better short-term effect on the plasma volume than previously believed. Their efficiency (i.e. the plasma volume expansion divided by the infused volume) is 50–80% as long as *infusion* continues and even increases to 100% when the arterial pressure has dropped. Elimination is very slow during surgery and amounts to only 10% of that recorded in conscious volunteers. *Capillary refill* further reduces the need for crystalloid fluid when bleeding occurs. These four factors (distribution–elimination–infusion–capillary refill) limit the need for large volumes of crystalloid fluid during surgery [30].

### Maintenance fluids

Maintenance fluids are given, specifically, to cover the patient's daily basal requirements of water, glucose and electrolytes. As such, they are intended to cover daily needs. The basic daily needs are water, in an amount of

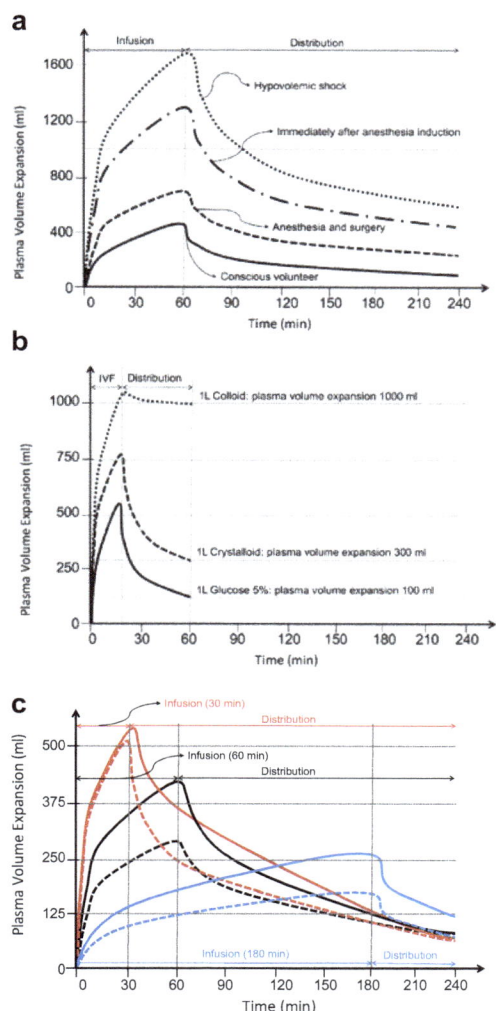

**Fig. 3** Pharmacokinetics and pharmacodynamics fluids. Original artwork based on the work of Hahn R [29, 43]. **a** Volume kinetic simulation. Expansion of plasma volume (in mL) after intravenous infusion of 2 L of Ringer's acetate over 60 min in an adult patient (average weight 80 kg), depending on normal condition as conscious volunteer (solid line), during anaesthesia and surgery (dashed line), immediately after induction of anaesthesia due to vasoplegia and hypotension with decrease in arterial pressure to 85% of baseline, (mixed line) and after bleeding during haemorrhagic shock with mean arterial pressure below 50 mmHg (dotted line) (see text for explanation). **b** Volume kinetic simulation. Expansion of plasma volume (in mL) is 100, 300 and 1000 mL, respectively, after 60 min following intravenous infusion of 1 L of glucose 5% over 20 min in an adult patient (solid line), versus 1 L of crystalloid (dashed line), versus 1 L of colloid (dotted line) (see text for explanation). **c** Volume kinetic simulation. Expansion of plasma volume (in mL) after intravenous infusion of 500 mL of hydroxyethyl starch 130/0.4 (Volulyte, solid line) versus 1 L of Ringer's acetate (dashed line) when administered in an adult patient (average weight 80 kg), over 30 min (red) versus 60 min (black), versus 180 min (blue). When administered rapidly and as long as infusion is ongoing, the volume expansion kinetics are similar between crystalloids and colloids, especially in case of shock, after induction and anaesthesia and during surgery (see text for explanation)

25–30 mL/kg of body weight, 1 mmol/kg potassium, 1–1.5 mmol/kg sodium per day and glucose or dextrose 5 or 10% 1.4–1.6 g/kg (to avoid starvation ketosis) [31].

Some specific maintenance solutions are commercially available, but they are far from ideal. There is a lot of debate whether isotonic or hypotonic maintenance solutions should be used. Data in children showed that hypotonic solutions carry the risk of hyponatremia and neurologic complications [32, 33]. However, studies in adults are scarce and indicate that administration of isotonic solutions will result in a more positive fluid balance as compared to hypotonic solutions [34]. This was confirmed in a recent pilot study in healthy volunteers showing that isotonic solutions caused lower urine output, characterized by decreased aldosterone concentrations indicating (unintentional) volume expansion, than hypotonic solutions. Despite their lower sodium and potassium content, hypotonic fluids were not associated with hyponatremia or hypokalemia [24].

### Replacement fluids
Replacement fluids are administered to correct fluid deficits that cannot be compensated by oral intake. Such fluid deficits have a number of potential origins, like drains or stomata, fistulas, hyperthermia, open wounds, polyuria (salt-wasting nephropathy, cerebral salt wasting, osmotic diuresis or diabetes insipidus) [4].

Data on replacement fluids are also scarce. Several recent guidelines advise matching the amount and composition of fluid and electrolytes as closely as possible to the fluid that is being or has been lost [35, 36]. An overview of the composition of the different body fluids can be found in the NICE guidelines [35]. Replacement fluids are usually isotonic balanced solutions. In patients with fluid deficit due to a loss of chloride-rich gastric fluid, high-chloride solutions, like saline (0.9% NaCl), might be used as replacement fluid.

### Nutrition fluids
Often overlooked, it is about time to consider parenteral nutrition as another source of intravenous fluids that may contribute to fluid overload. Likewise, nutritional therapy in the critically ill should be seen as "medication" helping the healing process. As such, we might consider also the four D's of nutritional therapy in analogy to how we deal with antibiotics and fluids [5]: drug (type of feeding), dose (caloric and protein load), duration (when and how long) and de-escalation (stop enteral nutrition and/or parenteral nutrition when oral intake improves) [37].

### Combination of fluids
A combination of different types of fluids is often justified. For example, numerous combinations may be used

in daily practice with regard to resuscitation fluids: blood and crystalloids (trauma), crystalloids early (post-operative hypovolemia), albumin late (sepsis). Similarly, maintenance fluids are often a combination of enteral and parenteral nutrition, other glucose-containing solutions, saline and/or balanced crystalloids to dissolve medications.

## Duration

The longer the delay in fluid administration, the more microcirculatory hypoperfusion and subsequent organ damage related to ischaemia–reperfusion injury. In patients with sepsis [38], Murphy and colleagues compared outcomes related to early adequate versus early conservative and late conservative versus late liberal fluid administration and found that the combination of early adequate and late conservative fluid management carried the best prognosis [38] (Fig. 4). Combined data from other studies confirm that late conservative is maybe more important than early adequate fluid therapy [39–41].

## Dosing

As Paracelsus nicely stated: "All things are poison, and nothing is without poison; only the dose permits something not to be poisonous" Like other drugs, it is the dose of fluids that make them poisonous. As stated before, the risk of excessive fluid overload is well established.

Similar to other drugs, choosing the right dose implies that we take into account the pharmacokinetics and pharmacodynamics of intravenous fluids (Table 1). *Pharmacokinetics* describes how the body affects a drug resulting in a particular plasma and effect site concentration [42]. Pharmacokinetics of intravenous fluids depends on distribution volume, osmolality, tonicity, oncoticity and kidney function. Eventually, the half-time depends on the type of fluid, but also on the patient's condition and the clinical context (Table 2). When administering 1 L of fluid only, 10% of glucose solution, versus 25–30% of an isotonic crystalloid solution, versus 100% of a colloid solution will remain intravascularly after 1 h, but as stated above the half-life is dependent on other conditions (like infection, inflammation, sedation, surgery, anaesthesia, blood pressure) (Fig. 3) [29, 43].

Volume kinetics is an adaptation of pharmacokinetic theory that makes it possible to analyse and simulate the distribution and elimination of infusion fluids [29]. Applying this concept, it is possible, by simulation, to determine the infusion rate that is required to reach a predetermined plasma volume expansion. Volume kinetics may also allow the quantification of changes in the distribution and elimination of fluids (and calculation of

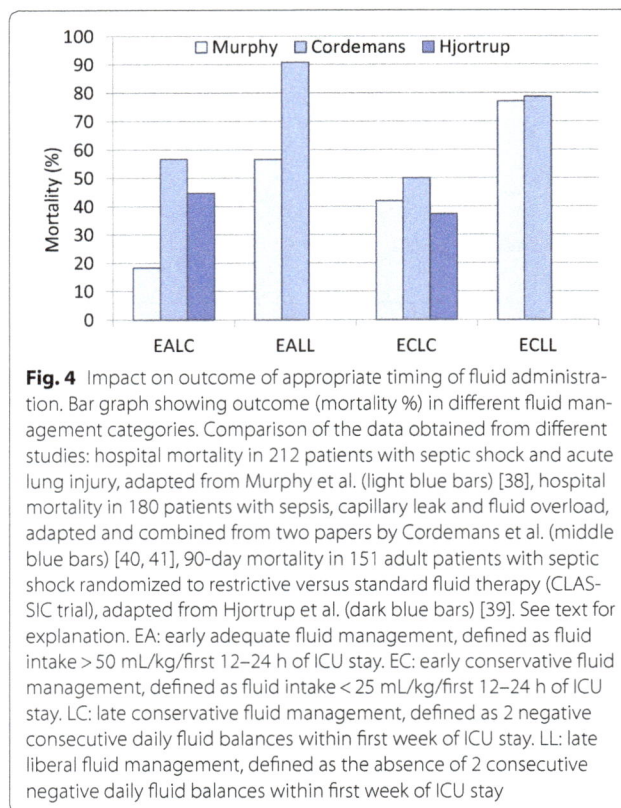

**Fig. 4** Impact on outcome of appropriate timing of fluid administration. Bar graph showing outcome (mortality %) in different fluid management categories. Comparison of the data obtained from different studies: hospital mortality in 212 patients with septic shock and acute lung injury, adapted from Murphy et al. (light blue bars) [38], hospital mortality in 180 patients with sepsis, capillary leak and fluid overload, adapted and combined from two papers by Cordemans et al. (middle blue bars) [40, 41], 90-day mortality in 151 adult patients with septic shock randomized to restrictive versus standard fluid therapy (CLAS-SIC trial), adapted from Hjortrup et al. (dark blue bars) [39]. See text for explanation. EA: early adequate fluid management, defined as fluid intake > 50 mL/kg/first 12–24 h of ICU stay. EC: early conservative fluid management, defined as fluid intake < 25 mL/kg/first 12–24 h of ICU stay. LC: late conservative fluid management, defined as 2 negative consecutive daily fluid balances within first week of ICU stay. LL: late liberal fluid management, defined as the absence of 2 consecutive negative daily fluid balances within first week of ICU stay

the half-life) that result from stress, hypovolemia, anaesthesia and surgery [43].

*Pharmacodynamics* relates the drug concentrations to its specific effect. For fluids, the Frank–Starling relationship between cardiac output and cardiac preload is the equivalent of the dose effect curve for standard medications. Because of the shape of the Frank–Starling relationship, the response of cardiac output to the fluid-induced increase in cardiac preload is not constant [44]. The effective dose 50 (ED50), in pharmacology, is the dose or amount of drug that produces a therapeutic response or desired effect in 50% of the subjects receiving it, whereas lethal dose 50 (LD50) will result in death of 50% of recipients. Translated to IV fluids, this would be the dose of fluid that induces, respectively, a therapeutic response or death in 50% of the patients. The problem is that the therapeutic response varies from one patient to another. Fluid administration can be toxic (or even lethal) at a high enough dose, as demonstrated in 2007 when a California woman died of water intoxication (and hyponatremia) in a contest organized by a radio station (http://articles.latimes.com/2007/jan/14/local/me-water14). The difference between toxicity and efficacy is dependent upon the particular patient

**Table 2 Overview of half-life (T1/2) of Ringer's, glucose and colloid solutions as reported in different studies. Adapted from Hahn R [43]**

| Category | Study population | n | Fluid studied | T1/2 (min) |
|---|---|---|---|---|
| Volunteers | Healthy adults | 24 | Glucose 2.5% | 19 |
| | Healthy adults | 9 | Glucose 5% | 13 |
| | Healthy adults | 6 | Ringer's acetate | 22–46 |
| | Healthy adults | 8 | dextran 70 | 175 |
| | Healthy adults | 15 | Plasma | 197 |
| | Healthy adults | 15 | Albumin 5% | 110 |
| | Healthy adults | 20 | HES 130/0.4 | 110 |
| | Dehydrated adults | 20 | Ringer's acetate | 76 |
| | Healthy children | 14 | Ringer's lactate | 30 |
| Pregnancy | Normal | 8 | Ringer's acetate | 71 |
| | Pre-eclampsia | 8 | Ringer's acetate | 12 |
| | Before caesarean section | 10 | Ringer's acetate | 175 |
| Surgery | Before surgery | 29 | Ringer's acetate | 23 |
| | Before surgery | 15 | Ringer's lactate | 169 |
| | Thyroid | 29 | Ringer's acetate | 327–345 |
| | Laparoscopic cholecystectomy | 12 | Glucose 2.5% | 492 |
| | Laparoscopic cholecystectomy | 12 | Ringer's acetate | 268 |
| | Gynaecological laparoscopy | 20 | Ringer's lactate | 346 |
| | Open abdominal | 10 | Ringer's lactate | 172 |
| | After hysterectomy | 15 | Glucose 2.5% | 14 |
| | After laparoscopy | 20 | Ringer's lactate | 17 |

*HES* hydroxyethyl starch

and the specific condition of that patient, although the amount of fluids administered by a physician should fall into the predetermined therapeutic window. Unanswered questions remain: what is an effective dose of IV fluids? What is the exact desired therapeutic effect? What is the therapeutic window? In some patients, volume expansion increases the mean systemic filling pressure (the backward pressure of venous return), but it increases the right atrial pressure (the forward pressure of venous return) to the same extent, such that venous return and, hence, cardiac output do not increase [45]. Hence, venous congestion and backward failure may even play a more important and currently underestimated role [46]. The probability of the heart to "respond" to fluid by a significant increase in cardiac preload varies along the shock time course, and thus, pharmacodynamics of fluids must be regularly evaluated. At the very early phase, fluid responsiveness is constant. After the very initial fluid administration, only one half of patients with circulatory failure respond to an increase in cardiac output [47].

### Fluid responsiveness

Fluid responsiveness indicates a condition in which a patient will respond to fluid administration by a significant increase in stroke volume and/or cardiac output or their surrogates. A *threshold of 15%* is most often used for this definition, as it is the least significant change of measurements of the techniques that are often used to estimate cardiac output [80, 91]. Physiologically, fluid responsiveness means that cardiac output depends on cardiac preload, i.e. the slope of the Frank–Starling relationship is steep. Many studies have shown that fluid responsiveness, which is a normal physiologic condition, exists in only half of the patients receiving a fluid challenge in intensive care units [47].

The adverse effects of fluids must also be considered in their pharmacodynamics. Depending on the degree of vascular permeability, the oedema resulting from fluid administration is highly variable. At the maximum, disruption of the capillary barrier leads to global increased permeability syndrome (GIPS). This pharmacodynamic aspect is also very important in patients with acute respiratory distress syndrome (ARDS), as the effect of a given amount of fluid on the lung function basically depends on the pulmonary vascular permeability [48]. Therefore, even two litres of saline may induce severe respiratory deterioration in a patient with severe ARDS.

### De-escalation

As we will discuss below, the final step in fluid therapy is to consider withholding or withdrawing resuscitation fluids when they are no longer required [1, 14, 15].

Like for antibiotics (Table 1), the duration of fluid therapy must be as short as possible, and the volume must be tapered when shock is resolved. However, many clinicians use certain triggers to start, but are unaware of triggers to stop fluid resuscitation, increasing the potential for fluid overload. As with duration of antibiotics, although there is no strong evidence, there is a trend towards shorter duration of intravenous fluids [39].

### The four phases of fluid therapy

Not only are the characteristics of fluids important, but also the strategy for their administration. This strategy fundamentally changes along with the time course of septic shock. Recently a three-hit, or even four-hit model of septic shock was suggested trying to answer four basic questions, in which we can recognize four distinct dynamic phases of fluid therapy [40]: resuscitation, optimization, stabilization and evacuation (de-resuscitation) (the acronym ROSE) (Table 3, Fig. 5). The four questions that will be discussed in the next section are "When to start intravenous fluids?", "When to stop intravenous fluids?", "When to start de-resuscitation or active fluid removal?" and finally "When to stop de-resuscitation?"

### First phase: Resuscitation

After the *first hit* which can be sepsis, but also burns, pancreatitis or trauma, the patient will enter the "ebb" phase of shock. This life-threatening phase of severe circulatory shock can occur within minutes and is characterized by a strong vasodilation leading to a low mean arterial pressure and microcirculatory impairment (Table 3). It may be accompanied by high (hyperdynamic circulatory shock as seen in sepsis, burns, severe acute pancreatitis, liver cirrhosis, thiamine deficiency, etc.) or low cardiac output (e.g. septic shock with severe hypovolemia or septic shock with sepsis-induced cardiomyopathy).

At this initial phase, usually during the first 3–6 h after the initiation of therapy, fluid resuscitation is commonly administered according to an *early, adequate, goal-directed, fluid management* strategy. The modalities of fluid administration at this early phase have been a matter of great debate. In the study by Rivers et al. [49], a protocol-based fluid management called early goal-directed therapy (EGDT) was associated with a significant reduction in mortality compared to standard care. Since this publication, similar outcome benefits have been reported in over 70 observational and randomized controlled studies comprising over 70,000 patients [50]. As a result, EGDT was incorporated as a "resuscitation bundle" into the first 6 h of sepsis management adopted by the Surviving Sepsis Campaign. As such, it has been disseminated internationally as the standard of care for early sepsis management. Recently, a trio of trials (ProCESS [51], ARISE [52] and ProMISe [53]), while reporting an all-time low sepsis mortality, showed no improvement in outcomes with EGDT, questioning the need and pointing towards the potential dangers of protocolized care for patients with severe and septic shock [54, 55]. A recent study employing a combined Bayesian and frequentist methodological approach to evaluate 12 randomized trials and 31 observational studies found that EGDT was potentially harmful in the patients with the highest disease severity [56]. In addition, although conducted in sub-Saharan Africa, three recent trials have demonstrated worse outcomes when administering fluid boluses for resuscitation in patients with septic shock [57–59]. What remains from the EGDT debate is that the rapidity of fluid administration and of the achievement of hemodynamic goals for initial resuscitation is important, even though this aspect has also recently been called into question [60].

In fact, rather than infusing a predefined given amount of fluid, the goal should be individualized for every patient, based on the evaluation of the need for fluids and on the patient's premorbid conditions [16, 55, 61–64]. In this phase, on an individual basis for each patient, we try to find an answer to the first question: "When to start fluid therapy?"

At the very initial phase of septic shock, answering the question is easy: fluid administration will significantly increase cardiac output in almost all cases. Nevertheless, after the first boluses of fluid, the likelihood of preload unresponsiveness is high. Therefore, at this stage, fluid administration should be conditioned to the positivity of indices and tests predicting fluid responsiveness. However, it must be noted that the state of responsiveness can only be determined a posteriori (after the intervention with administration of fluid bolus) and when a hemodynamic monitoring device is in place to estimate or calculate cardiac output. Therefore, we advocate the use of specific tests to increase the a priori probability and likelihood for a favourable event/outcome, as fluid administration should be limited to responders.

---

**Fluid bolus**

A fluid bolus is the rapid infusion of fluids over a short period of time. In clinical practice, a fluid bolus is usually given to correct hypovolemia, hypotension, inadequate blood flow or impaired microcirculatory perfusion. The volume of fluid bolus is heterogeneous among clinicians [68, 89], typically 500–1000 mL [68]. The minimal fluid volume that is able to increase the backward pressure of venous return is 4 mL/kg [90].

---

Several of these tests are available today [44]. Instead of using static markers of cardiac preload, which do not reliably predict fluid responsiveness, one should use dynamic indices to predict fluid responsiveness. The principle of these indices is to observe the effect on cardiac output of changes in cardiac preload, either spontaneously induced during mechanical ventilation or provoked by some manoeuvres. If changes are larger than a given threshold, preload responsiveness is present, and the positive response to fluid is likely. Fluid challenge, which has been described years ago [65], is a reliable test for fluid responsiveness, but, since it requires the irreversible administration of fluid, it contributes to excessive fluid administration. The passive leg raise test, which mimics fluid administration [66], has been extensively studied and is now recommended by the Surviving Sepsis Campaign [18]. Other tests utilize the changes in cardiac preload induced by mechanical ventilation. The respiratory changes of pulse pressure and stroke volume, or of the diameter of the venae cava are limited because they cannot be used in many circumstances in critically ill patients [44]. The end-expiratory occlusion test is easy

**Table 3 The ROSE concept avoiding fluid overload. Adapted from Malbrain et al. with permission [1]**

| | Resuscitation | Optimization | Stabilization | Evacuation |
|---|---|---|---|---|
| Hit sequence | First hit | Second hit | Second hit | Third hit |
| Time frame | Minutes | Hours | Days | Days to weeks |
| Underlying mechanism | Inflammatory insult | Ischaemia and reperfusion | Ischaemia and reperfusion | Global increased permeability syndrome |
| Clinical presentation | Severe shock | Unstable shock | Absence of shock or threat of shock | Recovery from shock, possible global increased permeability syndrome |
| Goal | Early adequate goal-directed fluid management | Focus on organ support and maintaining tissue perfusion | Late conservative fluid management | Late goal-directed fluid removal (de-resuscitation) |
| Fluid therapy | Early administration with fluid boluses, guided by indices of fluid responsiveness | Fluid boluses guided by fluid responsiveness indices and indices of the risk of fluid administration | Only for normal maintenance and replacement | Reversal of the positive fluid balance, either spontaneous or active |
| Fluid balance | Positive | Neutral | Neutral to negative | Negative |
| Primary result of treatment | Salvage or patient rescue | Organ rescue | Organ support (homeostasis) | Organ recovery |
| Main risk | Insufficient resuscitation | Insufficient resuscitation and fluid overload (e.g. pulmonary oedema, intra-abdominal hypertension) | Fluid overload (e.g. pulmonary oedema, intra-abdominal hypertension) | Excessive fluid removal, possibly inducing hypotension, hypoperfusion, and a "fourth hit" |

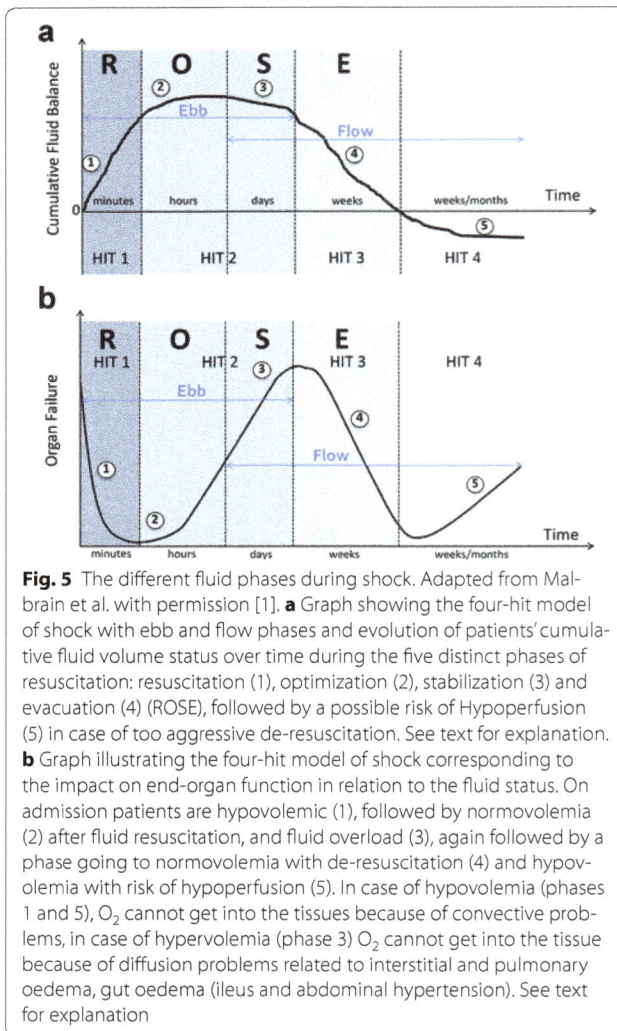

**Fig. 5** The different fluid phases during shock. Adapted from Malbrain et al. with permission [1]. **a** Graph showing the four-hit model of shock with ebb and flow phases and evolution of patients' cumulative fluid volume status over time during the five distinct phases of resuscitation: resuscitation (1), optimization (2), stabilization (3) and evacuation (4) (ROSE), followed by a possible risk of Hypoperfusion (5) in case of too aggressive de-resuscitation. See text for explanation. **b** Graph illustrating the four-hit model of shock corresponding to the impact on end-organ function in relation to the fluid status. On admission patients are hypovolemic (1), followed by normovolemia (2) after fluid resuscitation, and fluid overload (3), again followed by a phase going to normovolemia with de-resuscitation (4) and hypovolemia with risk of hypoperfusion (5). In case of hypovolemia (phases 1 and 5), $O_2$ cannot get into the tissues because of convective problems, in case of hypervolemia (phase 3) $O_2$ cannot get into the tissue because of diffusion problems related to interstitial and pulmonary oedema, gut oedema (ileus and abdominal hypertension). See text for explanation

to perform in patients under mechanical ventilation who can tolerate 15-s respiratory holds [67]. However, a cognitive dissonance exists between the fact that most fluid boluses are given to treat hypotension (in 59% of cases in the FENICE trial), while fluid responsiveness can only be defined post-factum by a change in cardiac output [68]. Furthermore, not all that glitters is gold when it comes to predicting fluid responsiveness and some patients may even exhibit an increase in blood pressure with a concomitant decrease in cardiac output after passive leg raising, while others may show the opposite. This relates to the baseline and changing compliance of the aorta over time [69].

---

**Prediction of fluid responsiveness**

This is a process that consists of predicting before fluid administration whether or not subsequent fluid

---

administration will increase cardiac output. It avoids unnecessary fluid administration and contributes to reducing the cumulative fluid balance. It also allows one to undertake fluid removal as it informs that such removal will not result in a hemodynamic impairment [44]. Prediction of fluid responsiveness is based on dynamic tests and indices, which observe the effect on cardiac output of changes in cardiac preload, either spontaneously induced during mechanical ventilation or provoked by some manoeuvres [44]. The threshold to define fluid responsiveness depends on the change in cardiac preload induced by the test (e.g. 15% for fluid challenge, 10% for the PLR test, 5% for the end-expiratory occlusion test).

**Fluid challenge**

A fluid challenge is a dynamic test to assess fluid responsiveness by giving a fluid bolus and simultaneously monitoring the hemodynamic effect (e.g. the evolution of barometric or volumetric preload indices). A fluid challenge is therefore also a fluid bolus, which means that it tests the response to treatment by administering the treatment itself up to the level where the treatment has no longer a response. This is why repeated fluid challenges may potentially lead to fluid overload. Recently, it has been shown that in clinical practice there is a marked variability in how fluid challenge tests are performed [68].

---

## Second phase: Optimization

The *second hit* occurs within hours and refers to ischaemia and reperfusion (Table 3). At this phase, fluid accumulation reflects the severity of illness and might be considered a "biomarker" for it [70]. The greater the fluid requirement, the sicker the patient and the more likely organ failure (e.g. acute kidney injury) may occur [71, 72].

In this phase, we must try to find an answer to the second question: "When to stop fluid therapy?" avoiding fluid overload. Indices of fluid responsiveness are again of utmost importance, since fluid administration should be stopped when these indices become negative [73]. Second, the clinical context must be taken into account. Obviously, more fluid is needed in septic shock from peritonitis than from pneumonia. Third, the decision to refrain from fluid administration should be based on indices that indicate the risk of excessive fluid administration. The presence of lung impairment is the condition that is most likely to be associated with the worst consequences of fluid overload. To estimate the pulmonary risk of further fluid infusion, one may consider the pulmonary artery occlusion pressure measured with the Swan–Ganz catheter. Nonetheless, this does not take into account the degree of lung permeability, which is a key factor in the mechanisms of pulmonary oedema formation [48]. Extravascular lung water measured by transpulmonary thermodilution, as well as the pulmonary vascular permeability index which is inferred from it, might reflect the pulmonary risk of fluid infusion more directly [40, 48, 74]. Intra-abdominal hypertension is also a potential consequence of too much fluid administration [40]. The intra-abdominal pressure should be cautiously monitored in patients at risk [75].

---

### Passive leg raising test

This test predicting fluid responsiveness consists of moving a patient from the semi-recumbent position to a position where the legs are lifted at 45° and the trunk is horizontal. The transfer of venous blood from the inferior limbs and the splanchnic compartment towards the cardiac cavities mimics the increase in cardiac preload induced by fluid infusion [66]. In general, the threshold to define fluid responsiveness with the passive leg raising test is a 10% increase in stroke volume and/or cardiac output.

### End-expiratory occlusion test

This is a test of fluid responsiveness that consists of stopping mechanical ventilation at end expiration for 15 s and measuring the resultant changes in cardiac output [92–94]. The test increases cardiac preload by stopping the cyclic impediment of venous return that occurs at each insufflation of the ventilator. An increase in cardiac output above the *threshold of 5%* indicates preload/fluid responsiveness [92–94]. When the test is performed with echocardiography, it is better to add the effects of an end-inspiratory occlusion, because the diagnostic threshold of changes in stroke volume is more compatible with precision of echocardiography [67].

---

### Third phase: Stabilization

With successful treatment, stabilization should follow the optimization phase (homoeostasis), evolving over the next few days (Table 3). It is distinguished from the prior two by the absence of shock or the imminent threat of shock. As previously described, the focus is now on organ support and this phase reflects the point at which a patient is in a stable steady state [1, 76] (Table 3).

Fluid therapy is now only needed for ongoing maintenance in the setting of normal fluid losses (i.e. renal, gastrointestinal, insensible) and replacement fluids if the patient is experiencing ongoing losses because of unresolved pathologic conditions [1, 76]. Since persistence of a positive daily fluid balance over time is strongly

associated with a higher mortality rate in septic patients [11, 77], clinicians should also be aware of the hidden obligatory fluid intake, as it may contribute more than a litre daily [78].

---

### Fluid balance

Daily fluid balance is the sum of all fluid intakes and outputs over 24 h, and the cumulative fluid balance is the sum of daily fluid balances over a set period of time [76, 87]. Intakes include resuscitation, but also maintenance fluids. Outputs include urine, ultrafiltration fluids, third space or gastrointestinal losses and should ideally also include insensible losses, even though they are difficult to quantify.

---

Maintenance fluids should be used only to cover daily needs, and their prescription should take these other sources of fluids and electrolytes into account. Therefore, when a patient already receives daily needs of water, glucose and electrolytes via other means (enteral or parenteral nutrition, medication solutions, etc.), specific intravenous maintenance fluids should be stopped.

### Fourth phase: Evacuation

After the second hit, the patient may either further recover, entering the "flow" phase with spontaneous evacuation of the excess fluids that have been administrated previously, or, as is the case in many critically ill patients, the patient remains in a "no-flow" state followed by a *third hit*, usually resulting from global increased permeability syndrome with ongoing fluid accumulation due to capillary leak [17, 79]. In any case, the patient enters a phase of "de-resuscitation" (Table 3). This term was first suggested in 2012 [41] and finally coined in 2014 [1]. It specifically refers to *late goal-directed fluid removal* and *late conservative fluid management.*

*Late goal-directed fluid removal* involves aggressive and active fluid removal using diuretics and renal replacement therapy with net ultrafiltration. It is characterized by the discontinuation of invasive therapies and a transition to a negative fluid balance [40]. *Late conservative fluid management* describes a moderate fluid management strategy following the initial treatment in order to avoid (or reverse) fluid overload. Recent studies showed that two consecutive days of negative fluid balance within the first week of the intensive care unit stay is a strong and independent predictor of survival [1].

In this de-resuscitation phase, we try to find an answer to the third and fourth question: "When to start fluid removal?" and "When to stop fluid removal?" in order to find the balance between the benefits (reduction in second and third space fluid accumulation and tissue oedema) and risk (hypoperfusion) of fluid removal. To answer these questions, testing preload responsiveness may still be useful. Indeed, if no preload responsiveness is detected, it is reasonable to assume that fluid removal will not induce a reduction in cardiac output [80]. On the opposite, positive indices of preload responsiveness might indicate the limit of fluid removal and could even be a target to reach when removing fluids.

Obviously, the risk at this phase is to be too aggressive with fluid removal and to induce hypovolemia, which may trigger a "fourth hit" for hemodynamic deterioration and hypoperfusion (Fig. 5). If fluid is needed at this phase, the use of albumin seems to have positive effects on vessel wall integrity facilitates achieving a negative fluid balance in hypoalbuminemia and may be less likely to cause nephrotoxicity [81].

This four-phase approach should be better characterized by some epidemiological studies. Its prognostic impact might be significant, because it may lead to a reduction in the cumulative fluid balance, which by itself is clearly associated with poor prognosis (Fig. 4). Similar principles have also been suggested by others, confirming the need for a multicenter prospective clinical trial with a biphasic fluid therapy approach, starting with initial early adequate goal-directed treatment followed by late conservative fluid management in those patients not transgressing spontaneously from the ebb to the flow phase [14, 15, 70, 76, 82–86]. The RADAR (Role of Active De-resuscitation After Resuscitation) trial may help to find such answers (http://www.hra.nhs.uk/news/research-summaries/radar-icu/).

## Conclusions

There are only four major *indications* for fluid administration in the critically ill: resuscitation, maintenance, replacement and nutrition (enteral or parenteral). In this review, a conceptual framework is presented looking at fluids as drugs by taking into account the four *D's* (drug selection, dose, duration and de-escalation) and the four *phases* of fluid therapy within the ROSE concept (resuscitation, optimization, stabilization and evacuation). The four *hits* model is presented herein. This will provide answers to the four basic *questions* surrounding fluid therapy: (1) When to start IV fluids? (2) When to stop fluid administration? (3) When to start fluid removal and finally (4) When to stop fluid removal? In analogy to the way we deal with antibiotics in critically ill patients, it is time for fluid stewardship.

## Abbreviations
EGDT: early goal-directed therapy; GIPS: global increased permeability syndrome; ROSE: acronym for resuscitation–optimization–stabilization–evacuation.

## Authors' contributions
MLNGM designed the initial version of the paper, BDT, PJVG, BS, XM, OJB participated in drafting the second version of the paper, MLNGM, BS, BDT, PJVG, OJB, JLT, XM, TWR and MM participated in drafting the final manuscript, and all authors read and approved the final manuscript.

## Author details
[1] Intensive Care Unit, University Hospital Brussels (UZB), Laarbeeklaan 101, 1090 Jette, Belgium. [2] Faculteit Geneeskunde en Farmacie, Vrije Universiteit Brussel (VUB), Brussels, Belgium. [3] Intensive Care Unit, ZiekenhuisNetwerk Antwerpen, ZNA Stuivenberg, Lange Beeldekensstraat 267, 2060 Antwerpen 6, Belgium. [4] Department of Anesthesiology, Centre of Anesthesiology and Intensive Care Medicine, University Medical Centre Hamburg-Eppendorf, Hamburg, Germany. [5] Service d'Anesthésie-Réanimation 2, CHU Bordeaux, 33000 Bordeaux, France. [6] Medical Intensive Care Unit, Hopitaux universitaires Paris-Sud, AP-HP, Université Paris-Sud, Le Kremlin-Bicetre, France. [7] University College London Hospitals, National Institute of Health Research Biomedical Research Centre, London, UK. [8] Division of Allergy, Pulmonary and Critical Care Medicine, Vanderbilt University School of Medicine, Nashville, TN, USA.

## Acknowledgements
This article is endorsed by the International Fluid Academy (IFA). The mission statement of the IFA is to foster education, promote research on fluid management and hemodynamic monitoring, and thereby improve survival of critically ill by bringing together physicians, nurses and others from throughout the world and from a variety of clinical disciplines. The IFA is integrated within the not-for-profit charitable organization iMERiT, International Medical Education and Research Initiative, under Belgian law. The IFA website (http://www.fluidacademy.org) is now an official SMACC-affiliated site (Social Media and Critical Care), and its content is based on the philosophy of FOAM (Free Open Access Medical education—#FOAMed). The site recently received the HONcode quality label for medical education (https://www.healthonnet.org/HONcode/Conduct.html?HONConduct519739).

## Competing interests
Manu Malbrain is founding President of WSACS (the Abdominal Compartment Society, www.wsacs.org) and current Treasurer. He is also member of the medical advisory Board of Getinge (Pulsion Medical Systems) and consults for Baxter, Maltron, ConvaTec, Acelity, Spiegelberg and Holtech Medical. Niels Van Regenmortel has received honoraria for giving lectures from Baxter Belgium and resided in a medical advisory board organized by Baxter Healthcare, USA. Manu Malbrain and Niels Van Regenmortel are co-founders of the International Fluid Academy (IFA, www.fluidacademy.org). Bernd Saugel is a member of the medical advisory board of Getinge (Pulsion Medical Systems). He received honoraria for giving lectures from Pulsion Medical Systems and CNSystems Medizintechnik AG. He received refund of travel expenses from Pulsion Medical Systems, Tensys Medical Inc and CNSystems Medizintechnik AG. He received research grants and unrestricted research grants from Tensys Medical Inc and received research support from Edwards Lifesciences. Olivier Joannes-Boyau is consultant for Baxter and BBraun. Jean-Louis Teboul and Xavier Monnet are members of the medical advisory board of Pulsion Medical Systems (part of Maquet Getinge group). They received honoraria for giving lectures from Pulsion Medical Systems, Edwards Lifesciences, Cheetah Medical and Masimo. Monty Mythen is Director of the UCL Discovery Lab. His University Chair is sponsored by Smiths Medical. He is Co-Director Duke-UCL Consortium (The Morpheus Project); a paid Consultant for Deltex Medical and Edwards Lifesciences; a Director of the Bloomsbury Innovation Group (BiG); a Director and Chair of Evidence Based Perioperative Medicine (EBPOM) Community Interest Company; Share holder and Scientific Advisor Medical Defense Technologies LLC (Gastrostim and Entarik); Share holder and Director Clinical Hydration Solutions ltd (Patent holder "QUENCH"); GIFTASUP guidelines—Senior Author; NICE—Expert Advsior IV Fluids—Guideline 174. The other authors have no potential conflict of interest with regard to the content of this review paper.

**Funding**
Not applicable.

**References**

1. Malbrain ML, Marik PE, Witters I, Cordemans C, Kirkpatrick AW, Roberts DJ, Van Regenmortel N. Fluid overload, de-resuscitation, and outcomes in critically ill or injured patients: a systematic review with suggestions for clinical practice. Anaesthesiol Intensive Ther. 2014;46(5):361–80.

2. Guidet B, Martinet O, Boulain T, Philippart F, Poussel JF, Maizel J, Forceville X, Feissel M, Hasselmann M, Heininger A, et al. Assessment of hemodynamic efficacy and safety of 6% hydroxyethylstarch 130/0.4 vs. 0.9% NaCl fluid replacement in patients with severe sepsis: the CRYSTMAS study. Crit Care. 2012;16(3):R94.

3. Perner A, Haase N, Guttormsen AB, Tenhunen J, Klemenzson G, Aneman A, Madsen KR, Moller MH, Elkjaer JM, Poulsen LM, et al. Hydroxyethyl starch 130/0.42 versus Ringer's acetate in severe sepsis. N Engl J Med. 2012;367(2):124–34.

4. Van Regenmortel N, Jorens PG, Malbrain ML. Fluid management before, during and after elective surgery. Curr Opin Crit Care. 2014;20(4):390–5.

5. Malbrain ML, Van Regenmortel N, Owczuk R. It is time to consider the four D's of fluid management. Anaesthesiol Intensive Ther. 2015;47:1–5.

6. Myburgh JA, Finfer S, Bellomo R, Billot L, Cass A, Gattas D, Glass P, Lipman J, Liu B, McArthur C, et al. Hydroxyethyl starch or saline for fluid resuscitation in intensive care. N Engl J Med. 2012;367(20):1901–11.

7. Annane D, Siami S, Jaber S, Martin C, Elatrous S, Declere AD, Preiser JC, Outin H, Troche G, Charpentier C, et al. Effects of fluid resuscitation with colloids vs crystalloids on mortality in critically ill patients presenting with hypovolemic shock: the CRISTAL randomized trial. JAMA. 2013;310(17):1809–17.

8. Myburgh JA, Mythen MG. Resuscitation fluids. N Engl J Med. 2013;369(25):2462–3.

9. Duchesne JC, Kaplan LJ, Balogh ZJ, Malbrain ML. Role of permissive hypotension, hypertonic resuscitation and the global increased permeability syndrome in patients with severe hemorrhage: adjuncts to damage control resuscitation to prevent intra-abdominal hypertension. Anaesthesiol Intensive Ther. 2015;47(2):143–55.

10. Vincent JL, Sakr Y, Sprung CL, Ranieri VM, Reinhart K, Gerlach H, Moreno R, Carlet J, Le Gall JR, Payen D. Sepsis in European intensive care units: results of the SOAP study. Crit Care Med. 2006;34(2):344–53.

11. Sakr Y, Rubatto Birri PN, Kotfis K, Nanchal R, Shah B, Kluge S, Schroeder ME, Marshall JC, Vincent JL, Intensive Care Over Nations I. Higher fluid balance increases the risk of death from sepsis: results from a large international audit. Crit Care Med. 2017;45(3):386–94.

12. Jozwiak M, Silva S, Persichini R, Anguel N, Osman D, Richard C, Teboul JL, Monnet X. Extravascular lung water is an independent prognostic factor in patients with acute respiratory distress syndrome. Crit Care Med. 2013;41(2):472–80.

13. Pinsky MR. Hemodynamic evaluation and monitoring in the ICU. Chest. 2007;132(6):2020–9.

14. O'Connor ME, Prowle JR. Fluid overload. Crit Care Clin. 2015;31(4):803–21.

15. Benes J, Kirov M, Kuzkov V, Lainscak M, Molnar Z, Voga G, Monnet X. Fluid therapy: double-edged sword during critical care? Biomed Res Int. 2015;2015:729075.

16. Vandervelden S, Malbrain ML. Initial resuscitation from severe sepsis: one size does not fit all. Anaesthesiol Intensive Ther. 2015;47:44–55.

17. Woodcock TE, Woodcock TM. Revised Starling equation and the glycocalyx model of transvascular fluid exchange: an improved paradigm for prescribing intravenous fluid therapy. Br J Anaesth. 2012;108(3):384–94.

18. Rhodes A, Evans LE, Alhazzani W, Levy MM, Antonelli M, Ferrer R, Kumar A, Sevransky JE, Sprung CL, Nunnally ME, et al. Surviving sepsis campaign: international guidelines for management of sepsis and septic shock: 2016. Intensive Care Med. 2017;43(3):304–77.

19. Caironi P, Tognoni G, Masson S, Fumagalli R, Pesenti A, Romero M, Fanizza C, Caspani L, Faenza S, Grasselli G, et al. Albumin replacement in patients with severe sepsis or septic shock. N Engl J Med. 2014;370(15):1412–21.

20. Khajavi MR, Etezadi F, Moharari RS, Imani F, Meysamie AP, Khashayar P, Najafi A. Effects of normal saline vs. lactated ringer's during renal transplantation. Ren Fail. 2008;30(5):535–9.

21. Langer T, Santini A, Scotti E, Van Regenmortel N, Malbrain ML, Caironi P. Intravenous balanced solutions: from physiology to clinical evidence. Anaesthesiol Intensive Ther. 2015;47:78–88.

22. Yunos NM, Bellomo R, Hegarty C, Story D, Ho L, Bailey M. Association between a chloride-liberal vs chloride-restrictive intravenous fluid administration strategy and kidney injury in critically ill adults. JAMA. 2012;308(15):1566–72.

23. Chowdhury AH, Cox EF, Francis ST, Lobo DN. A randomized, controlled, double-blind crossover study on the effects of 2-L infusions of 0.9% saline and plasma-lyte(R) 148 on renal blood flow velocity and renal cortical tissue perfusion in healthy volunteers. Ann Surg. 2012;256(1):18–24.

24. Van Regenmortel N, De Weerdt T, Van Craenenbroeck AH, Roelant E, Verbrugghe W, Dams K, Malbrain M, Van den Wyngaert T, Jorens PG. Effect of isotonic versus hypotonic maintenance fluid therapy on urine output, fluid balance, and electrolyte homeostasis: a crossover study in fasting adult volunteers. Br J Anaesth. 2017;118:892–900.

25. Semler MW, Wanderer JP, Ehrenfeld JM, Stollings JL, Self WH, Siew ED, Wang L, Byrne DW, Shaw AD, Bernard GR, et al. Balanced crystalloids versus saline in the intensive care unit. The SALT randomized trial. Am J Respir Crit Care Med. 2017;195(10):1362–72.

26. Young JB, Utter GH, Schermer CR, Galante JM, Phan HH, Yang Y, Anderson BA, Scherer LA. Saline versus Plasma-Lyte A in initial resuscitation of trauma patients: a randomized trial. Ann Surg. 2014;259(2):255–62.

27. Semler MW, Self WH, Wanderer JP, Ehrenfeld JM, Wang L, Byrne DW, Stollings JL, Kumar AB, Hughes CG, Hernandez A, et al. Balanced crystalloids versus saline in critically ill adults. N Engl J Med. 2018;378(9):829–39.

28. Self WH, Semler MW, Wanderer JP, Wang L, Byrne DW, Collins SP, Slovis CM, Lindsell CJ, Ehrenfeld JM, Siew ED, et al. Balanced crystalloids versus saline in noncritically ill adults. N Engl J Med. 2018;378(9):819–28.

29. Hahn RG. Volume kinetics for infusion fluids. Anesthesiology. 2010;113(2):470–81.

30. Hahn RG. Why crystalloids will do the job in the operating room. Anaesthesiol Intensive Ther. 2014;46(5):342–9.

31. Herrod PJ, Awad S, Redfern A, Morgan L, Lobo DN. Hypo- and hypernatraemia in surgical patients: is there room for improvement? World J Surg. 2010;34(3):495–9.

32. McNab S, Duke T, South M, Babl FE, Lee KJ, Arnup SJ, Young S, Turner H, Davidson A. 140 mmol/L of sodium versus 77 mmol/L of sodium in maintenance intravenous fluid therapy for children in hospital (PIMS): a randomised controlled double-blind trial. Lancet. 2015;385(9974):1190–7.

33. Moritz ML, Ayus JC. Maintenance intravenous fluids in acutely ill patients. N Engl J Med. 2015;373(14):1350–60.

34. Lobo DN, Stanga Z, Simpson JA, Anderson JA, Rowlands BJ, Allison SP. Dilution and redistribution effects of rapid 2-litre infusions of 0.9% (w/v) saline and 5% (w/v) dextrose on haematological parameters and serum biochemistry in normal subjects: a double-blind crossover study. Clin Sci (Lond). 2001;101(2):173–9.

35. Padhi S, Bullock I, Li L, Stroud M, National Institute for H, Care Excellence Guideline Development G. Intravenous fluid therapy for adults in hospital: summary of NICE guidance. BMJ. 2013;347:f7073.

36. Soni N. British consensus guidelines on intravenous fluid therapy for adult surgical patients (GIFTASUP): Cassandra's view. Anaesthesia. 2009;64(3):235–8.

37. De Waele E, Honore PM, Malbrain M. Does the use of indirect calorimetry change outcome in the ICU? Yes it does. Curr Opin Clin Nutr Metab Care. 2018;21(2):126–9.

38. Murphy CV, Schramm GE, Doherty JA, Reichley RM, Gajic O, Afessa B, Micek ST, Kollef MH. The importance of fluid management in acute lung injury secondary to septic shock. Chest. 2009;136(1):102–9.

39. Hjortrup PB, Haase N, Bundgaard H, Thomsen SL, Winding R, Pettila V, Aaen A, Lodahl D, Berthelsen RE, Christensen H, et al. Restricting volumes of resuscitation fluid in adults with septic shock after initial management: the CLASSIC randomised, parallel-group, multicentre feasibility trial. Intensive Care Med. 2016;42(11):1695–705.

40. Cordemans C, De Laet I, Van Regenmortel N, Schoonheydt K, Dits H, Huber W, Malbrain MLNG. Fluid management in critically ill patients: the role of extravascular lung water, abdominal hypertension, capillary leak and fluid balance. Annals Intensive Care. 2012;2(Supplem 1):S1.

41. Cordemans C, De Laet I, Van Regenmortel N, Schoonheydt K, Dits H, Martin G, Huber W, Malbrain ML. Aiming for a negative fluid balance in patients with acute lung injury and increased intra-abdominal pressure: a pilot study looking at the effects of PAL-treatment. Ann Intensive Care. 2012;2(Suppl 1):S15.

42.  Elbers PW, Girbes A, Malbrain ML, Bosman R. Right dose, right now: using big data to optimize antibiotic dosing in the critically ill. Anaesthesiol Intensive Ther. 2015;47(5):457–63.

43.  Hahn RG, Lyons G. The half-life of infusion fluids: an educational review. Eur J Anaesthesiol. 2016;33(7):475–82.

44.  Monnet X, Marik P, Teboul JL. Prediction of fluid responsiveness: an update. Ann Intensive Care. 2017;6(1):111.

45.  Guerin L, Teboul JL, Persichini R, Dres M, Richard C, Monnet X. Effects of passive leg raising and volume expansion on mean systemic pressure and venous return in shock in humans. Crit Care. 2015;19:411.

46.  Verbrugge FH, Dupont M, Steels P, Grieten L, Malbrain M, Tang WH, Mullens W. Abdominal contributions to cardiorenal dysfunction in congestive heart failure. J Am Coll Cardiol. 2013;62(6):485–95.

47.  Bentzer P, Griesdale DE, Boyd J, MacLean K, Sirounis D, Ayas NT. Will this hemodynamically unstable patient respond to a bolus of intravenous fluids? JAMA. 2016;316(12):1298–309.

48.  Jozwiak M, Teboul JL, Monnet X. Extravascular lung water in critical care: recent advances and clinical applications. Ann Intensive Care. 2015;5(1):38.

49.  Rivers E, Nguyen B, Havstad S, Ressler J, Muzzin A, Knoblich B, Peterson E, Tomlanovich M. Early goal-directed therapy in the treatment of severe sepsis and septic shock. N Engl J Med. 2001;345(19):1368–77.

50.  Osborn TM. Severe sepsis and septic shock trials (ProCESS, ARISE, ProM-ISe): what is optimal resuscitation? Crit Care Clin. 2017;33(2):323–44.

51.  Pro CI, Yealy DM, Kellum JA, Huang DT, Barnato AE, Weissfeld LA, Pike F, Terndrup T, Wang HE, Hou PC, et al. A randomized trial of protocol-based care for early septic shock. N Engl J Med. 2014;370(18):1683–93.

52.  Investigators A, Group ACT, Peake SL, Delaney A, Bailey M, Bellomo R, Cameron PA, Cooper DJ, Higgins AM, Holdgate A, et al. Goal-directed resuscitation for patients with early septic shock. N Engl J Med. 2014;371(16):1496–506.

53.  Mouncey PR, Osborn TM, Power GS, Harrison DA, Sadique MZ, Grieve RD, Jahan R, Tan JC, Harvey SE, Bell D et al. Protocolised Management In Sepsis (ProMISe): a multicentre randomised controlled trial of the clinical effectiveness and cost-effectiveness of early, goal-directed, protocolised resuscitation for emerging septic shock. Health Technol Assess. 2015;19(97):i–xxv, 1–150.

54.  Marik PE. Iatrogenic salt water drowning and the hazards of a high central venous pressure. Ann Intensive Care. 2014;4:21.

55.  Marik PE, Malbrain M. The SEP-1 quality mandate may be harmful: how to drown a patient with 30 mL per kg fluid! Anaesthesiol Intensive Ther. 2017;49(5):323–8.

56.  Kalil AC, Johnson DW, Lisco SJ, Sun J. Early goal-directed therapy for sepsis: a novel solution for discordant survival outcomes in clinical trials. Crit Care Med. 2017;45(4):607–14.

57.  Maitland K, Kiguli S, Opoka RO, Engoru C, Olupot-Olupot P, Akech SO, Nyeko R, Mtove G, Reyburn H, Lang T, et al. Mortality after fluid bolus in African children with severe infection. N Engl J Med. 2011;364(26):2483–95.

58.  Andrews B, Semler MW, Muchemwa L, Kelly P, Lakhi S, Heimburger DC, Mabula C, Bwalya M, Bernard GR. Effect of an early resuscitation protocol on in-hospital mortality among adults with sepsis and hypotension: a randomized clinical trial. JAMA. 2017;318(13):1233–40.

59.  Andrews B, Muchemwa L, Kelly P, Lakhi S, Heimburger DC, Bernard GR. Simplified severe sepsis protocol: a randomized controlled trial of modified early goal-directed therapy in Zambia. Crit Care Med. 2014;42(11):2315–24.

60.  Seymour CW, Gesten F, Prescott HC, Friedrich ME, Iwashyna TJ, Phillips GS, Lemeshow S, Osborn T, Terry KM, Levy MM. Time to treatment and mortality during mandated emergency care for sepsis. N Engl J Med. 2017;376(23):2235–44.

61.  Perel A, Saugel B, Teboul JL, Malbrain ML, Belda FJ, Fernandez-Mondejar E, Kirov M, Wendon J, Lussmann R, Maggiorini M: The effects of advanced monitoring on hemodynamic management in critically ill patients: a pre and post questionnaire study. J Clin Monit Comput. 2016;30(5):511–8.

62.  Saugel B, Trepte CJ, Heckel K, Wagner JY, Reuter DA. Hemodynamic management of septic shock: is it time for "individualized goal-directed hemodynamic therapy" and for specifically targeting the microcirculation? Shock. 2015;43(6):522–9.

63.  Saugel B, Malbrain ML, Perel A. Hemodynamic monitoring in the era of evidence-based medicine. Crit Care. 2016;20(1):401.

64.  Muckart DJJ, Malbrain M. The future of evidence-based medicine: is the frog still boiling? Anaesthesiol Intensive Ther. 2017;49(5):329–35.

65.  Weil MH, Henning RJ. New concepts in the diagnosis and fluid treatment of circulatory shock. Thirteenth annual Becton, Dickinson and Company Oscar Schwidetsky Memorial Lecture. Anesth Analg. 1979;58(2):124–32.

66.  Monnet X, Teboul JL. Passive leg raising: five rules, not a drop of fluid! Crit Care. 2015;19:18.

67.  Jozwiak M, Depret F, Teboul JL, Alphonsine JE, Lai C, Richard C, Monnet X. Predicting fluid responsiveness in critically ill patients by using combined end-expiratory and end-inspiratory occlusions with echocardiography. Crit Care Med. 2017;45(11):e1131–8.

68.  Cecconi M, Hofer C, Teboul JL, Pettila V, Wilkman E, Molnar Z, Della Rocca G, Aldecoa C, Artigas A, Jog S, et al. Fluid challenges in intensive care: the FENICE study: a global inception cohort study. Intensive Care Med. 2015;41(9):1529–37.

69.  Hofkens PJ, Verrijcken A, Merveille K, Neirynck S, Van Regenmortel N, De Laet I, Schoonheydt K, Dits H, Bein B, Huber W, et al. Common pitfalls and tips and tricks to get the most out of your transpulmonary thermodilution device: results of a survey and state-of-the-art review. Anaesthesiol Intensive Ther. 2015;47(2):89–116.

70.  Bagshaw SM, Brophy PD, Cruz D, Ronco C. Fluid balance as a biomarker: impact of fluid overload on outcome in critically ill patients with acute kidney injury. Crit Care. 2008;12(4):169.

71.  Wang N, Jiang L, Zhu B, Wen Y, Xi XM, Beijing Acute Kidney Injury Trial W. Fluid balance and mortality in critically ill patients with acute kidney injury: a multicenter prospective epidemiological study. Crit Care. 2015;19:371.

72.  Bellomo R, Cass A, Cole L, Finfer S, Gallagher M, Lee J, Lo S, McArthur C, McGuiness S, Norton R, et al. An observational study fluid balance and patient outcomes in the randomized evaluation of normal vs. augmented level of replacement therapy trial. Crit Care Med. 2012;40(6):1753–60.

73.  Teboul JL, Monnet X. Detecting volume responsiveness and unresponsiveness in intensive care unit patients: two different problems, only one solution. Crit Care. 2009;13(4):175.

74.  Monnet X, Teboul JL. Transpulmonary thermodilution: advantages and limits. Crit Care. 2017;21(1):147.

75.  Malbrain ML, Peeters Y, Wise R. The neglected role of abdominal compliance in organ-organ interactions. Crit Care. 2016;20(1):67.

76.  Hoste EA, Maitland K, Brudney CS, Mehta R, Vincent JL, Yates D, Kellum JA, Mythen MG, Shaw AD, Group AXI. Four phases of intravenous fluid therapy: a conceptual model. Br J Anaesth. 2014;113(5):740–7.

77.  Acheampong A, Vincent JL. A positive fluid balance is an independent prognostic factor in patients with sepsis. Crit Care. 2015;19:251.

78.  Bashir MU, Tawil A, Mani VR, Farooq U, DeVita A. Hidden obligatory fluid intake in critical care patients. J Intensive Care Med. 2017;32(3):223–7.

79.  Malbrain ML, De Laet I. AIDS is coming to your ICU: be prepared for acute bowel injury and acute intestinal distress syndrome. Intensive Care Med. 2008;34(9):1565–9.

80.  Monnet X, Marik PE, Teboul JL. Prediction of fluid responsiveness: an update. Ann Intensive Care. 2016;6(1):111.

81.  Vincent JL, De Backer D, Wiedermann CJ. Fluid management in sepsis: the potential beneficial effects of albumin. J Crit Care. 2016;35:161–7.

82.  McDermid RC, Raghunathan K, Romanovsky A, Shaw AD, Bagshaw SM. Controversies in fluid therapy: type, dose and toxicity. World J Crit Care Med. 2014;3(1):24–33.

83.  Rivers EP. Fluid-management strategies in acute lung injury—liberal, conservative, or both? N Engl J Med. 2006;354:2598–600.

84.  Bellamy MC. Wet, dry or something else? Br J Anaesth. 2006;97(6):755–7.

85.  Bagshaw SM, Bellomo R. The influence of volume management on outcome. Curr Opin Crit Care. 2007;13(5):541–8.

86.  Vincent JL, De Backer D. Circulatory shock. N Engl J Med. 2013;369(18):1726–34.

87.  Macedo E, Bouchard J, Soroko SH, Chertow GM, Himmelfarb J, Ikizler TA, Paganini EP, Mehta RL, Program to Improve Care in Acute Renal Disease S. Fluid accumulation, recognition and staging of acute kidney injury in critically-ill patients. Crit Care. 2010;14(3):R82.

88.  Vaara ST, Korhonen AM, Kaukonen KM, Nisula S, Inkinen O, Hoppu S, Laurila JJ, Mildh L, Reinikainen M, Lund V, et al. Fluid overload is associated with an increased risk for 90-day mortality in critically ill patients with renal replacement therapy: data from the prospective FINNAKI study. Crit Care. 2012;16(5):R197.

89. Taylor CB, Hammond NE, Laba TL, Watts N, Thompson K, Saxena M, Micallef S, Finfer S, Myburgh J, Fluid Trips DCE. Drivers of choice of resuscitation fluid in the intensive care unit: a discrete choice experiment. Crit Care Resusc. 2017;19(2):134–41.

90. Aya HD, Rhodes A, Chis Ster I, Fletcher N, Grounds RM, Cecconi M. Hemodynamic effect of different doses of fluids for a fluid challenge: a quasi-randomized controlled study. Crit Care Med. 2017;45(2):e161–8.

91. Monnet X, Persichini R, Ktari M, Jozwiak M, Richard C, Teboul JL. Precision of the transpulmonary thermodilution measurements. Crit Care. 2011;15(4):R204.

92. Monnet X, Osman D, Ridel C, Lamia B, Richard C, Teboul JL. Predicting volume responsiveness by using the end-expiratory occlusion in mechanically ventilated intensive care unit patients. Crit Care Med. 2009;37(3):951–6.

93. Monnet X, Dres M, Ferre A, Le Teuff G, Jozwiak M, Bleibtreu A, Le Deley MC, Chemla D, Richard C, Teboul JL. Prediction of fluid responsiveness by a continuous non-invasive assessment of arterial pressure in critically ill patients: comparison with four other dynamic indices. Br J Anaesth. 2012;109(3):330–8.

94. Biais M, Larghi M, Henriot J, de Courson H, Sesay M, Nouette-Gaulain K. End-expiratory occlusion test predicts fluid responsiveness in patients with protective ventilation in the operating room. Anesth Analg. 2017;125(6):1889–95.

95. Cuthbertson DP. Post-shock metabolic response. Lancet. 1942;1:433–7.

96. Peeters Y, Lebeer M, Wise R, Malbrain ML. An overview on fluid resuscitation and resuscitation endpoints in burns: past, present and future. Part 2—avoiding complications by using the right endpoints with a new personalized protocolized approach. Anaesthesiol Intensive Ther. 2015;47:15–26.

# 23

# ICU physicians' and internists' survival predictions for patients evaluated for admission to the intensive care unit

Monica Escher[1,2]* iD, Bara Ricou[3], Mathieu Nendaz[2,4], Fabienne Scherer[1], Stéphane Cullati[1], Patricia Hudelson[5] and Thomas Perneger[6]

## Abstract

**Background:** A higher chance of survival is a key justification for admission to the intensive care unit (ICU). This implies that physicians should be able to accurately estimate a patient's prognosis, whether cared for on the ward or in the ICU. We aimed to determine whether physicians' survival predictions correlate with the admission decisions and with patients' observed survival. Consecutive ICU consultations for internal medicine patients were included. The ICU physician and the internist were asked to predict patient survival with intensive care and with care on the ward using 5 categories of probabilities (< 10%, 10–40%, 41–60%, 61–90%, > 90%). Patient mortality at 28 days was recorded.

**Results:** Thirty ICU physicians and 97 internists assessed 201 patients for intensive care. Among the patients, 140 (69.7%) were admitted to the ICU. Fifty-eight (28.9%) died within 28 days. Admission to intensive care was associated with predicted survival gain in the ICU, particularly for survival estimates made by ICU physicians. Observed survival was associated with predicted survival, for both groups of physicians. The discrimination of the predictions for survival with intensive care, measured by the area under the ROC curve, was 0.63 for ICU physicians and 0.76 for internists; for survival on the ward the areas under the ROC curves were 0.69 and 0.74, respectively.

**Conclusions:** Physicians are able to predict survival probabilities when they assess patients for intensive care, albeit imperfectly. Internists are more accurate than ICU physicians. However, ICU physicians' estimates more strongly influence the admission decision. Closer collaboration between ICU physicians and internists is needed.

**Keywords:** Intensive care, Survival, Prediction, Patient admission, Triage

## Background

The decision to admit or not a patient to the intensive care unit (ICU) is often complex and is based on a combination of criteria [1]. They include a patient's need for life-sustaining therapies, but also patient prognosis, pre-hospital functional status, patient preferences, and available clinical expertise and resources. Since expected survival benefit is one of the main justifications for ICU admission, physicians must estimate and compare the patient's prognosis according to two scenarios: continued care on the ward, and care in the ICU. Most scoring systems apply to patients once admitted to the ICU and the low performance of the few existing triage scores limits their use [2]. Moreover, even validated scoring systems are not accurate enough in predicting an individual's mortality and they should not be used alone to determine level of care [1, 3, 4].

Previous research has shown that physicians predict patient survival more accurately than scoring systems [5]. However, their accuracy in prediction was generally assessed for patients already admitted to the ICU. In one French study, ICU physicians estimated patient mortality at the time of the admission decision [6]. Their predictions were higher than the observed mortality rates both for non-admitted and for admitted patients.

*Correspondence: monica.escher@hcuge.ch
[1] Pain and Palliative Care Consultation, Division of Clinical Pharmacology and Toxicology, Geneva University Hospitals, Rue Gabrielle-Perret-Gentil 4, 1211 Geneva, Switzerland
Full list of author information is available at the end of the article

Furthermore, the requesting physicians and the ICU physicians sometimes disagree about the appropriateness of an ICU admission [7, 8]. Whether this is due to differences in survival estimates or to other reasons is currently unknown.

When medical in-patients become critically ill, the need for intensive care is first assessed by the internists. They will then request an ICU consultation. The final decision about the patient's admission to the ICU belongs to the ICU physician. The ICU physician is not involved in the patient's care if he is not admitted to the ICU. The objective of this study was to compare internists' and ICU physicians' predictions of patient survival if cared on the ward or in the ICU, i.e., expected survival benefit from intensive care, and to determine whether the survival estimates correlated with the admission decisions and with observed survival. We hypothesized that agreement between the physicians would be weak to moderate, that expected survival would be greater in admitted than in non-admitted patients, and that observed survival would be associated with predicted survival. We also hypothesized that ICU physicians, who are used to care for acutely ill patients, would be more accurate in their predictions than internists.

## Methods
### Setting
The study took place at the Geneva University Hospitals, a tertiary care hospital of 1741 beds, including 156 internal medicine beds and 34 adult ICU beds, between August 2014 and August 2015. It was approved by the Geneva Research Ethics Committee.

### Participants
All consecutive ICU consultations for patients hospitalized in the Division of General Internal Medicine were identified. The internist and the ICU physician directly involved were eligible. Upon first contact, all physicians provided written consent to participate and socio-demographic data.

### Data collection
Internists and ICU physicians were contacted by phone within 12 h of the request for ICU consultation and were asked to complete a questionnaire. Questionnaires were administered orally, by phone, or by email, according to physicians' preferences. Reminders were sent 3 days later when necessary. Physicians were asked to predict patient survival (i.e., "probability that the patient survives the acute health problem") if admitted in the ICU and if staying on the ward using 5 predetermined categories of probabilities (< 10%, 10–40%, 41–60%, 61–90%, > 90%). They also rated how confident they were

in their estimates on a Likert scale ranging from 1 (not at all confident) to 5 (fully confident). Internists were asked about the reason for requesting the ICU consultation and whether the patient was admitted or not. The ICU consultation was included and patient data were recorded only if both physicians completed the questionnaire. Patient data (gender, age, comorbidities) and mortality at 28 days were collected from the electronic patient file.

### Sample size and statistical analysis
Sample size was driven by the main objective of the study, i.e., modeling of the decision to admit a patient to intensive care. Assuming 8 potential predictors of the decision to admit the patient, we intended to enroll 80 patients in the smaller of the 2 groups (admitted or not), and aimed for 160 patients if the admission rate was 50%. As the observed admission rate was 70%, the sample size was increased to 200.

Each patient was assigned 4 survival estimates (2 by each of the physicians: survival on the ward and in the ICU) on a 5-point ordinal scale. We compared survival predictions on the ward versus in the ICU for each physician, and survival predictions by the internist versus the intensivist for each location, using paired Wilcoxon tests. We also obtained Spearman correlation coefficients between survival predictions.

To capture the expected survival benefit of an ICU admission, we computed the difference, in survival categories, between predicted survival in the ICU and on the ward, for each physician (thus 0 indicated the same survival category in both locations, and 4 a survival > 90% in the ICU and < 10% on the ward). We cross-tabulated this expected survival benefit with the admission to the ICU, expecting that patients with the highest expected benefit would be the most likely to be admitted (Table 3).

To clarify which physician's opinion weighed more in the decision to admit the patient, we used a logistic regression model, with admission as the dependent variable, and expected survival benefit estimated by each physician as covariates (because of sparse data, expected survival benefit was grouped as − 1 or 0, 1 or 2, and 3 or 4).

To assess the accuracy of physicians' predictions, we cross-tabulated predicted survival with observed survival at 28 days, stratifying on the admission decision, separately for the 2 categories of physicians. Because expected survival was on an ordinal scale, we obtained $P$ values for linear trend (Table 4). We also obtained areas under the receiver operating characteristic (ROC) curves. The area represents the probability that predicted survival would be lower for a randomly selected patient who died than for a randomly selected patient who survived; 0.5 corresponds to a coin toss, and 1.0 to perfect discrimination. To clarify which physician's survival prediction was more accurate, we used a logistic regression model with actual survival as the dependent variable, and the 2 physicians' predictions as independent variables.

Finally, we computed mean ratings of confidence (on a 1–5 scale) in the four survival estimates and compared them across levels of survival using Kruskal–Wallis tests.

## Results

During the study period, 219 patients were assessed for intensive care admission and 201 situations were included. They involved 128 men and 73 women (Table 1). Mean age was 64.9 years (SD 14.3). Among the patients, 140 (69.7%) were admitted to the ICU and 58 (28.9%) died within 28 days.

In total, 30 ICU physicians (1–14 assessments per physician) and 97 internists (1–11 assessments per physician) participated in the study (Additional file 1: Table S1). ICU physicians were mostly men (66%) and internists mostly women (61%). ICU physicians were older than internists (mean age 38 vs. 30 years, respectively). They were more experienced: mean years from graduation were 12 and 7, respectively, and mean years of experience in medical specialty were 7 and 3.5, respectively. The delay between the admission decision and physicians' prediction of survival was one day or less for 143 (71.1%) of the internists and 127 (63.2%) of the ICU physicians (McNemar test, $P = 0.11$).

### Predicting survival

The physicians used all five categories of survival probabilities (Table 2). Both physician groups rated expected patient survival significantly higher with care in the ICU rather than on the ward, e.g., the ICU physicians assigned 59.2% of patients to the 2 highest categories of survival (> 60%) if in the ICU, but only 24.8% to the same categories of survival on the ward. For the internists, the corresponding proportions were 67.9% and 13.9%. The internists were more optimistic about the patients'

chances of survival with intensive care than the ICU physicians ($P = 0.006$) and somewhat more pessimistic about survival on the ward, but the latter difference

### Table 1 Patient characteristics

| Characteristics | Patients, N (%)[a] (n = 201) |
|---|---|
| Men | 128 (63.7) |
| Age, median (IQR) (year) | 67 (56–77) |
| Living place | |
|   Home | 191 (95) |
|   Nursing home | 10 (5) |
| Advanced disease | 105 (52.2) |
| Type of disease in patients with advanced disease[b] | (n = 105) |
|   Metastatic cancer or active hematologic malignancy | 37 (35.2) |
|   Chronic obstructive pulmonary disease (FEV ≤ 50% or non-invasive ventilation or oxygenotherapy) | 38 (36.2) |
|   Chronic heart failure (NYHA III and IV and/or LVEF ≤ 20%) | 7 (6.6) |
|   Chronic renal failure (GFR ≤ 30 ml/min) | 20 (19.0) |
|   Cirrhosis Child B or C | 18 (17.1) |
| Number of hospitalizations in previous 12 months | |
|   0 | 107 (53.2) |
|   1 | 39 (19.4) |
|   > 1 | 55 (27.4) |
| Number of days between admission to general internal medicine wards and ICU consultation, median (IQR) | 3 (1–8) |
| Code status (2 missing): full code | 104 (51.7) |
| Reason for calling ICU[c] | |
|   Respiratory failure | 111 (55.2) |
|   Cardiac failure or shock (including sepsis) | 55 (27.4) |
|   Neurological symptoms | 32 (15.9) |
|   Cardiac arrest or arrhythmia | 16 (8) |
|   ICU physician's advice | 48 (23.9) |
|   Other | 18 (8.9) |

[a] Data are N (%) of patients unless otherwise indicated

[b] Total > 100% because more than one advanced disease per patient

[c] Total > 100% because more than one reason possible

### Table 2 Physicians' estimated probabilities of survival for 201 patients evaluated for intensive care

| Estimate | Prediction by intensive care physician | | Prediction by internist | |
|---|---|---|---|---|
| | Survival if care in the ICU N (%) | Survival if care on the ward N (%) | Survival if care in the ICU (2 missing) N (%) | Survival if care on the ward N (%) |
| < 10% | 15 (7.5) | 72 (35.8) | 8 (4.0) | 62 (30.8) |
| 10–40% | 34 (16.9) | 47 (23.4) | 19 (9.5) | 62 (30.8) |
| 41–60% | 33 (16.4) | 32 (15.9) | 37 (18.6) | 49 (24.4) |
| 61–90% | 54 (26.9) | 28 (13.9) | 72 (36.2) | 24 (11.9) |
| > 90% | 65 (32.3) | 22 (10.9) | 63 (31.7) | 4 (2.0) |
| Within physician* | P < 0.001 | | P < 0.001 | |

* Wilcoxon paired test

was not statistically significant ($P = 0.079$). As expected, the survival estimates were correlated with each other, both within physician (Spearman r correlation coefficient 0.69 for the ICU physician and 0.61 for the internist) and between physicians (0.48 for survival if in the ICU, 0.44 for survival on the ward).

### Estimated survival benefit

We examined the difference in expected survival categories between care in the ICU and on the ward (Table 3). For the ICU physicians, 31.4% of the patients would not increase their chances of survival if admitted to the ICU. The other patients would gain between 1 and 4 categories on the 5-level survival scale. Internists were globally more optimistic than intensive care physicians ($P < 0.001$) and classified only 11.9% of the patients as not increasing their chances of survival if admitted to the ICU.

### Survival benefit and admission to the ICU

Ratings by both physicians were associated with observed proportions of admitted patients (Table 3). The probability of admission was below 40% for patients who were not expected to improve their survival if admitted, but exceeded 80% if the patient was predicted to gain 2 categories of survival or more. The linear association between survival gain and admission was highly significant for both physicians. However, ICU physicians' estimates had a greater influence on the admission decision: the adjusted odds ratios of admission were 7.6 (95% confidence interval 3.6–15.8) for a gain of 1–2 categories, and 30.8 (95% CI 3.8–247) for a gain of 3–4 categories, compared to no gain. The corresponding adjusted odds ratios for estimates made by the internist were 2.3 (95% CI 0.8–6.5) and 4.2 (95% CI 1.1–16.4).

### Patient survival

Of the 140 patients admitted to the ICU, 40 (28.6%) had died at 28 days of follow-up, and of the 61 patients who were not admitted to the ICU, 18 (29.5%) had died. Observed survival was associated with predicted survival, for both groups of physicians (Table 4). Patient survival in the ICU ranged from 33.3 to 91.4% across categories of survival predicted by ICU physicians, and from 0 to 95.1% across predictions made by internists. The discrimination of the predictions, measured by the area under the ROC curve, was 0.63 and 0.76, respectively. The predictions for the patients who stayed on the ward were of similar accuracy. The gradients of observed proportions of survivors ran from 40.0 to 85.0% across estimates made by ICU physicians, and from 25.0 to 100% across estimates made by internists. The areas under the ROC curves were 0.69 and 0.74, respectively.

We compared the predictions made by the two groups of physicians in mutually adjusted logistic regression models (Table 5). For both groups of patients—those admitted to the ICU and those who stayed on the ward—the prediction of the internists was more accurate. In fact, once the opinion of the internists was taken into account, the ICU physicians' estimates did not increase the accuracy in predicting survival.

On the whole, physicians felt rather confident about their survival estimates, ICU physicians more so than internists (in the ICU: mean 4.2 vs. 3.9, on the ward 4.2 vs. 3.8, both $P < 0.001$). Physicians' confidence differed according to the survival probabilities (Additional file 2: Table S2). It was higher for extreme probabilities (i.e., < 10% or > 90%) than for mid-range probabilities.

### Discussion

In this study we found that physicians involved in decisions to admit patients to the ICU were able to predict short term survival for admitted and non-admitted patients. The physicians perceived a survival benefit from

**Table 3** Estimated gain in survival attributable to intensive care, and observed proportion of patients admitted

| Difference in survival categories* between ICU and ward | Intensive care physician | | Internist | |
|---|---|---|---|---|
| | N (%) | Proportion admitted (%) | N (%) | Proportion admitted (%) |
| Loss of 1 | 5 (2.5) | 80.0 | – | |
| Even | 58 (28.9) | 32.8 | 24 (11.9) | 37.5 |
| Gain of 1 | 62 (30.8) | 79.0 | 75 (37.3) | 61.3 |
| Gain of 2 | 50 (24.9) | 88.0 | 65 (32.3) | 86.2 |
| Gain of 3 | 22 (10.9) | 90.9 | 29 (14.4) | 82.8 |
| Gain of 4 | 4 (2.0) | 100 | 6 (3.0) | 83.3 |
| Test for linear trend | | <0.001 | | <0.001 |

*Survival was categorized as < 10%, 10–40%, 41–60%, 61–90%, > 90%

**Table 4 Patients' observed 28 day survival according to physicians' survival predictions**

| Predicted survival if care in the ICU | Patients admitted to intensive care ($N = 140$) | | | | |
|---|---|---|---|---|---|
| | Intensive care physicians | | Internists | | |
| | N (column %) | Survived (row %) | N (column %) | Survived (row %) | |
| <10% | 6 (4.3) | 2 (33.3) | 2 (1.4) | 0 (0) | |
| 10–40% | 30 (21.4) | 18 (60.0) | 16 (11.4) | 4 (25.0) | |
| 41–60% | 27 (19.3) | 18 (66.7) | 28 (20.0) | 17 (60.7) | |
| 61–90% | 42 (30.0) | 30 (71.4) | 53 (37.9) | 40 (75.5) | |
| >90% | 35 (25.0) | 32 (91.4) | 41 (29.3) | 39 (95.1) | |
| P for linear trend | $P = 0.001$ | | $P < 0.001$ | | |
| Area under ROC curve | 0.63 (0.53–0.73) | | 0.76 (0.67–0.84) | | |
| **Predicted survival if care on the ward** | **Patients NOT admitted to intensive care ($N = 61$)** | | | | |
| | Intensive care physicians | | Internists | | |
| | N (column %) | Survived (row %) | N (column %) | Survived (row %) | |
| <10% | 10 (16.4) | 4 (40.0) | 12 (19.7) | 3 (25.0) | |
| 10–40% | 11 (18.0) | 7 (63.6) | 14 (23.0) | 11 (78.6) | |
| 41–60% | 9 (14.8) | 7 (77.8) | 19 (31.1) | 15 (78.9) | |
| 61–90% | 11 (18.0) | 8 (72.7) | 13 (21.3) | 11 (84.4) | |
| >90% | 20 (32.8) | 17 (85.0) | 3 (4.9) | 3 (100) | |
| P for linear trend | $P = 0.016$ | | $P = 0.001$ | | |
| Area under ROC curve | 0.69 (0.54–0.84) | | 0.74 (0.61–0.89) | | |

**Table 5 Multivariate regression model of survival at 28 days, according to physicians' baseline predictions**

| Physicians' predictions | Odds ratio[*] | 95% CI | P value |
|---|---|---|---|
| | *Patients admitted to ICU* | | |
| Intensive care physicians | 1.32 | 0.90–1.93 | 0.15 |
| Internists | 3.05 | 1.87–4.95 | <0.001 |
| | *Patients on ward* | | |
| Intensive care physicians | 1.23 | 0.78–1.96 | 0.37 |
| Internists | 2.23 | 1.14–4.34 | 0.019 |

*The odds ratios are for a 1 category increase on the 5-point survival prediction scale. Predictions made by internists and by ICU physicians are adjusted for each other

an admission to intensive care for a majority of patients. Internists' estimates of survival were higher than ICU physicians', but globally there was a substantial agreement between the 2 groups of physicians. Physicians showed high levels of confidence in their estimates.

The estimated survival benefit was associated with the decision to admit a patient to the ICU: most patients with a high expected benefit were admitted compared to a minority of patients with a low expected benefit. The ICU admission decision was more strongly

influenced by the ICU physician's survival prediction than by the internist's. However internists predicted patient survival more accurately than ICU physicians, both for patients admitted to the ICU and for those who remained on the ward.

Our results expand on available data. In a small study based on scenarios, good agreement about ICU survival prediction was also found between internists and ICU physicians, but their prediction accuracy varied [9]. In our study higher accuracy in prediction is likely explained by the fact that physicians estimated survival for patients they had actually assessed. We could not compare physicians' performance with a scoring system as no validated score exists for estimating patient prognosis at the time of triage [10, 11]. However, physicians' clinical judgment has been shown to be at least as accurate as objective risk scores for predicting mortality in patients admitted to the ICU [5] and for predicting medical in-patients' deterioration [12]. Values of the ROC curves in our study were similar to those published for ICU physicians' survival estimates for patients admitted to intensive care. Our findings also show that both internists and ICU physicians are accurate about patient prognosis under different circumstances, i.e., at the time of triage and for continued care on the ward or for care in the ICU.

In keeping with recommendations about ICU admission [1], physicians' predicted gain in survival was associated with admission decisions. Interestingly, some patients with no expected survival benefit were admitted. It suggests that physicians are aware of their limited ability in predicting survival for individuals and prefer to err toward overtriage, an attitude supported by current guidelines [1]. Considerations other than survival may also be deemed important enough for physicians to propose intensive care. Notably, during the updating process of a consensus statement about triage principles, ICU experts could not agree about a survival cutoff precluding ICU admission, not even for a chance of survival of 0.1% or less [13]. Furthermore, ICU physicians seem to use less stringent admission criteria when more ICU beds are available [14–16].

Not surprisingly the ICU physicians' opinions weighed more than the internists' in the decision to admit a patient to the ICU. ICU physicians are considered experts and most capable in estimating the benefit of intensive care for patients. Our findings however challenge this assumption, as internists were more accurate in predicting patient survival for both care on the ward and in the ICU. In this respect, the influence of ICU physicians on the admission decision may not be entirely justified, all the more so that they sometimes assume a dismissive behavior toward requesting physicians and potentially disregard their assessment [8, 17, 18]. Because considerations other than survival benefit influence ICU admission decisions, increased collaborative decision making between ICU physicians and internists seems advisable.

Our study has several limitations. The involved physicians were contacted after they had discussed intensive care for a patient. So their opinions were not independent as they had had the opportunity to come to a shared assessment of the situation. It may partially explain the high level of agreement between the physicians. In some cases, the patient may have died by the time the physicians completed the questionnaire, in which case survival predictions would have been meaningless. However, it would not change the main findings of this study, as it would concern a minority of patients. Moreover, only the physician caring for the patient would know about his death, and for patients assessed during night shifts and week-ends he would not necessarily be the physician in charge at the time of death. Delay between admission decision and completion of the questionnaire may cause an overestimation of physicians' accuracy in prediction, as the physician in charge had the opportunity to observe how the patient's condition evolved. We minimized this risk by contacting physicians twice a day, and by offering them to complete the questionnaire on the phone, thus keeping delays as short as possible.

Moreover, on average, the delays were longer for ICU physicians, whose predictions were less accurate than those of the internists. Hence, if delays caused a bias, it should be conservative.

## Conclusions

Physicians are able to predict survival probabilities for patients assessed for admission to intensive care, albeit imperfectly. Internists are more accurate than ICU physicians. However, ICU physicians' estimates more strongly influence the admission decision. These results highlight the need for objective risk scores in support to physicians' judgment and for closer collaboration between internists and ICU physicians. Strategies to improve the decision making process should focus on the development of valid triage scoring systems and address potential communication gaps between physicians.

**Authors' contributions**
Conceived and designed the study: ME, BR, MN, SC, PH, TP. Collected the data: FS. Analyzed the data: ME, BR, MN, TP. Drafted the manuscript: ME. Read and commented the paper: ME, BR, MN, FS, SC, PH, TP. All authors read and approved the final manuscript.

**Author details**
[1] Pain and Palliative Care Consultation, Division of Clinical Pharmacology and Toxicology, Geneva University Hospitals, Rue Gabrielle-Perret-Gentil 4, 1211 Geneva, Switzerland. [2] Unit of Development and Research in Medical Education, Faculty of Medicine, University of Geneva, Geneva, Switzerland. [3] Division of Intensive Care, Geneva University Hospitals, Geneva, Switzerland. [4] Division of General Internal Medicine, Geneva University Hospitals, Geneva, Switzerland. [5] Division of Primary Care Medicine, Geneva University Hospitals, Geneva, Switzerland. [6] Division of Clinical Epidemiology, Geneva University Hospitals, Geneva, Switzerland.

**Competing interests**
All the authors declare that they have no conflict of interest.

**Funding**
This study was funded by the Swiss National Science Foundation, National Research Program "End of Life" (NRP 67), Grant No. 139304. The Swiss National Science Foundation did not contribute to the design of the study, to the collection, analysis, and interpretation of data and to the writing of the manuscript.

## References

1. Nates JL, Nunnally M, Kleinpell R, Blosser S, Goldner J, Birriel B, et al. ICU admission, discharge, and triage guidelines: a framework to enhance clinical operations, development of institutional policies, and further research. Crit Care Med. 2016;44:1553–602.
2. Jansen JO, Cuthbertson BH. Detecting critical illness outside the ICU: the role of track and trigger systems. Curr Opin Crit Care. 2010;16:184–90.
3. Vincent J, Moreno R. Scoring systems in the critically ill. Crit Care. 2010;14:207.
4. Christian MD, Fowler R, Muller MP, Gomersall C, Sprung CL, Hupert N, et al. Critical care resource allocation: trying to PREEDICCT outcomes without a crystal ball. Crit Care. 2013;17:107.
5. Sinuff T, Adhikari NK, Cook DJ, Schunemann HJ, Griffith LE, Rocker G, et al. Mortality predictions in the intensive care unit: comparing physicians with scoring systems. Crit Care Med. 2006;34:878–85.
6. Garrouste-Orgeas M, Montuclard L, Timsit JF, Misset B, Christias M, Carlet J. Triaging patients to the ICU: a pilot study of factors influencing admission decisions and patient outcomes. Intensive Care Med. 2003;29:774–81.
7. Boumendil A, Angus DC, Guitonneau AL, Menn AM, Ginsburg C, Takun K, et al. Variability of intensive care admission decisions for the very elderly. PLoS ONE. 2012;7:e34387.
8. Fassier T, Valour E, Colin C, Danet F. Who am I to decide whether this person is to die today? Physicians' life-or-death decisions for elderly critically ill patients at the emergency department-ICU interface: a qualitative study. Ann Emerg Med. 2016;68(28–39):e3.
9. Dahine J, Mardini L, Jayaraman D. The perceived likelihood of outcome of critical care patients and its impact on triage decisions: a case-based survey of intensivists and internists in a Canadian, Quaternary Care Hospital Network. PLoS ONE. 2016;11:e0149196.
10. Sprung CL, Baras M, Iapichino G, Kesecioglu J, Lippert A, Hargreaves C, et al. The Eldicus prospective, observational study of triage decision making in European intensive care units: part I-European Intensive Care Admission Triage Scores. Crit Care Med. 2012;40:125–31.
11. Ramos JG, Perondi B, Dias RD, Miranda LC, Cohen C, Carvalho CR, et al. Development of an algorithm to aid triage decisions for intensive care unit admission: a clinical vignette and retrospective cohort study. Crit Care. 2016;20:81.
12. Patel AR, Zadravecz FJ, Young RS, Williams MV, Churpek MM, Edelson DP. The value of clinical judgment in the detection of clinical deterioration. JAMA Intern Med. 2015;175:456–8.
13. Sprung CL, Danis M, Iapichino G, Artigas A, Kesecioglu J, Moreno R, et al. Triage of intensive care patients: identifying agreement and controversy. Intensive Care Med. 2013;39:1916–24.
14. Sinuff T, Kahnamoui K, Cook DJ, Luce JM, Levy MM, Values E, et al. Rationing critical care beds: a systematic review. Crit Care Med. 2004;32:1588–97.
15. Stelfox HT, Hemmelgarn BR, Bagshaw SM, Gao S, Doig CJ, Nijssen-Jordan C, et al. Intensive care unit bed availability and outcomes for hospitalized patients with sudden clinical deterioration. Arch Intern Med. 2012;172:467–74.
16. Gooch RA, Kahn JM. ICU bed supply, utilization, and health care spending: an example of demand elasticity. JAMA. 2014;311:567–8.
17. Oerlemans AJ, van Sluisveld N, van Leeuwen ES, Wollersheim H, Dekkers WJ, Zegers M. Ethical problems in intensive care unit admission and discharge decisions: a qualitative study among physicians and nurses in the Netherlands. BMC Med Ethics. 2015;16:9.
18. Escher M, Cullati S, Hudelson P, Nendaz M, Ricou B, Perneger T, et al. Admission to intensive care: a qualitative study of triage and its determinants. Health Serv Res. 2018. https://doi.org/10.1111/1475-6773.13076.

# Prediction of chronic kidney disease after acute kidney injury in ICU patients: study protocol for the PREDICT multicenter prospective observational study

Guillaume Geri[1,2,3]* , Bénédicte Stengel[2,3], Christian Jacquelinet[2,4], Philippe Aegerter[5,6], Ziad A. Massy[2,3,7] and Antoine Vieillard-Baron[1,2,3] on behalf of the PREDICT investigators

## Abstract

**Background:** Acute kidney injury (AKI) is frequent and associated with poor outcome in intensive care unit (ICU) patients. Besides the association with short- and long-term mortality, the increased risk of chronic kidney disease (CKD) has been recently highlighted in non-ICU patients. This study aims to describe the incidence and determinants of CKD after AKI and to develop a prediction score for CKD in ICU patients.

**Methods:** Prospective multicenter ($n = 17$) observational study included 1200 ICU patients who suffered from AKI (defined by an AKIN stage $\geq 1$) during their ICU stay and were discharged alive from ICU. Preexisting end-stage renal disease (ESRD) and immunosuppressant treatments are the main exclusion criteria. Patients will be monitored by a nephrologist at day 90 and every year for 3 years. The main outcome is the occurrence of CKD defined by a creatinine-based estimated glomerular filtration rate (eGFR) lower than 60 mL/min/1.73 m$^2$ or renal replacement therapy for ESRD in patients whose eGFR will be normalized ($\geq 60$ mL/min/1.73 m$^2$) at day 90. Secondary outcomes include albuminuria changes, eGFR decline slope and ESRD risk in patients with preexisting CKD, cardiovascular and thrombo-embolic events and health-related quality of life.

**Discussion:** This is the first study prospectively investigating kidney function evolution in ICU patients who suffered from AKI. Albuminuria and eGFR monitoring will allow to identify ICU patients at risk of CKD who may benefit from close surveillance after recovering from AKI. Major patient and AKI-related determinants will be tested to develop a prediction score for CKD in this population.

*Trial registration* ClinicalTrials.gov, NCT03282409. Registered on September 14, 2017

**Keywords:** Chronic kidney disease, Acute kidney injury, Intensive care unit, End-stage renal disease

## Background

Acute kidney injury (AKI) occurs very frequently in patients admitted to an intensive care unit (ICU). The prevalence of AKI in ICU patients has been estimated between 5 and 15% [1–3]. It is strongly and independently associated with short- and long-term mortality

*Correspondence: guillaume.geri@aphp.fr
[1] Medico-Surgical ICU, Service de Réanimation médico-chirurgicale, Ambroise Paré Hospital, APHP, 92100 Boulogne Billancourt, France
Full list of author information is available at the end of the article

[4]. While acute tubular necrosis is the most frequently reported cause of AKI in ICU patients, numerous patho-logical patterns have been observed in autopsy of kidneys in patients who died in the ICU following a septic shock [5]. This highlights the complexity of AKI in ICU, related to many harmful factors from ischemia–reperfusion lesions to sepsis-specific injuries. This may explain the association with AKI occurrence in the ICU and long-term mortality as some of these injuries are not as able to regenerate as tubular cells [3]. Moreover, endothelial dys-function may be a worsening factor impacting long-term

renal recovery and so the occurrence of chronic kidney disease.

Besides an association between AKI occurrence and long-term arterial hypertension, AKI has also been associated with chronic kidney disease (CKD), even if glomerular filtration rate (GFR) rose back to normal range [6, 7]. However, most of these data come from administrative registries and mostly include non-ICU patients. In the ICU setting, Wald et al. [8] reported an incidence of end-stage renal disease (ESRD) of 2.63 and 0.91 cases per 100 ICU person-year in patients with AKI requiring dialysis during the ICU stay, and in matched controls without AKI, respectively. While it is well recognized that an early management of CKD patients may slow GFR decline, the identification of AKI patients at risk to develop CKD is uneasy.

Thus, we aim to develop a prediction score for CKD in patients who suffered from AKI during their ICU stay and were discharged alive using a prospective multicenter observational study.

## Methods/design

### Design and setting

The prediction of chronic kidney disease after acute kidney injury in the intensive care unit (PREDICT) study is a multicenter observational prospective study promoted by the Assistance Publique—Hôpitaux de Paris. The study aims to evaluate factors associated with CKD risk in patients discharged alive from ICU and who suffered from AKI during ICU stay. The study was designed by both the medico-surgical intensive care unit and the department of clinical research and public health of Ambroise Paré Hospital (Boulogne-Billancourt, France) and the INSERM (French National Institute of Medical Research) Unit 1018 (Villejuif, France).

Patients who comply with the inclusion criteria will be monitored by a nephrologist at day 90 after ICU discharge and annually thereafter during 3 years: creatinine-based GFR estimation (eGFR), albuminuria measurement, cardiovascular events as well as health-related quality of life will be collected at each time point as shown in the Standard Protocol Items: Recommendations for Interventional Trials (SPIRIT) 2013 diagram (Fig. 1).

### Ethical considerations

This study follows the principles of the Helsinki Declaration 2008. The whole protocol has been reviewed and approved by the *Comité de Protection des Personnes—Sud-Est III* (no. 2017-053B).

### Registration

The study is registered on Clinical Trials (NCT03282409) and on the European Clinical Trials Database (*EudraCT 2017-A02649-44*).

### Participants

The study will enroll adults (18 years or older) discharged alive from ICU and who suffered from AKI during ICU stay. Participants will be eligible if they meet the acute kidney injury network (AKIN) classification stage 1 or higher [9]. All patients will have to be able to read and understand the patient information form and provide written informed consent. Patients will not be eligible for enrollment if (1) they suffer ESRD (defined by an eGFR below 15 mL/min/1.73 $m^2$ or renal replacement therapy, i.e., dialysis or renal transplantation) before the index hospitalization, (2) they require renal replacement therapy at ICU discharge, (3) if they were prescribed immunosuppressive agents before index hospitalization or (4) there was no extra-renal failure at the time of acute kidney injury (defined by a SOFA score without the renal component equal to 0). Other exclusion criteria are expected life expectancy less than 90 days, inability to perform follow-up (homeless patients, main address far away from the nephrology center, etc.), pregnancy, privation of liberty by administrative or judicial decision, no affiliation to the national social security scheme and refusal to participate in the study.

### Recruitment, inclusion and consent

Patients will be recruited at ICU discharge. After a first screening with regard to the inclusion and exclusion criteria, patients who fulfill the inclusion criteria and are willing to participate will be included in the study after providing written informed consent. Patients will be recruited from 17 ICU (15 in the Greater Paris area, 1 in

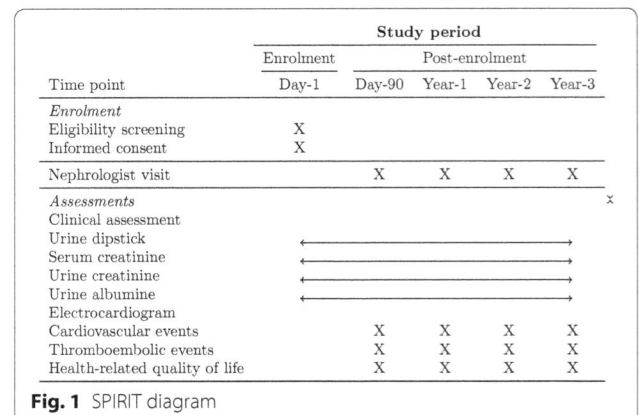

| | | Study period | | | |
|---|---|---|---|---|---|
| | Enrolment | Post-enrolment | | | |
| Time point | Day-1 | Day-90 | Year-1 | Year-2 | Year-3 |
| *Enrolment* | | | | | |
| Eligibility screening | X | | | | |
| Informed consent | X | | | | |
| Nephrologist visit | | X | X | X | X |
| *Assessments* | | | | | x |
| Clinical assessment | | | | | |
| Urine dipstick | | ←——————————————→ | | | |
| Serum creatinine | | ←——————————————→ | | | |
| Urine creatinine | | ←——————————————→ | | | |
| Urine albumine | | ←——————————————→ | | | |
| Electrocardiogram | | | | | |
| Cardiovascular events | | X | X | X | X |
| Thromboembolic events | | X | X | X | X |
| Health-related quality of life | | X | X | X | X |

**Fig. 1** SPIRIT diagram

Clermont-Ferrand and 1 in Amiens) and monitored in 10 nephrology centers.

### Confidentiality

All original records will be kept on file at the trial sites or the coordinating data center for 15 years. The frozen trial database file will be kept on file for 15 years.

### Sample size

The sample size was calculated based on the primary outcome, namely the occurrence of de novo CKD at 3 years. Assuming an attrition bias of 10% and a competing risk of death of 20%, we calculated that 1200 patients fulfilling the inclusion criteria should be included according to the following distribution: 700 AKI patients who would fully recover kidney function at ICU discharge, 150 with impaired kidney function at ICU discharge and 350 with preexisting CKD. According to epidemiological data provided by the multicenter prospective observational study CUB-REA [10] and assuming an inclusion rate of 50% of the patients fulfilling the inclusion criteria, we estimated that the inclusion pace could be 5 patients/center/month leading to study completion within 24 months.

### Nephrologist active follow-up

Every patient will be monitored by a nephrologist at day 90 after ICU discharge and then every year for 3 years. As shown in the SPIRIT diagram, CKD will be evaluated by creatinine-based eGFR and urinary albumin (protein)-to-creatinine ratio. Cardiovascular and thromboembolic events will be collected as well as health-related quality of life.

### Primary and secondary outcomes

The main outcome of the study will be the incidence of CKD defined by an eGFR lower than 60 mL/min/1.73 m$^2$ for at least 3 months or chronic dialysis initiation or renal transplantation, as previously published (KDIGO) in patients who recovered kidney function at day 90, defined by an eGFR $\geq$ 60 mL/min/1.73 m$^2$.

The secondary outcomes will include:

- CKD progression defined by an eGFR decline greater than 30% at 3 years or the occurrence of ESRD (defined by an eGFR lower than 15 mL/min/1.73 m$^2$ or chronic dialysis initiation or renal transplantation) in patients with preexisting CKD
- Evolution of urinary protein-to-creatinine ratio (mg/mmol)
- Prevalence of patients discharged from ICU with end-stage renal disease

- Occurrence of cardiovascular (acute coronary syndrome, ischemic stroke, peripheral artery disease, ventricular rhythm disorders, sudden death) and/or thromboembolic (deep-vein thrombosis or pulmonary embolism) events
- All-cause and cardiovascular long-term mortality
- Health-related quality of life using the KDQOL-SF-12 [11] and the EQ-5D-5L [12] questionnaires.

### Biological sampling

We plan to sample 10 mL of plasma at inclusion. This biobank will be stored at *the Centre de Ressources Biologiques* (Hôpital Ambroise Paré, APHP) and will be used to assess the association between biomarkers of kidney injury and long-term outcomes.

### Pre-planned ancillary analysis: 10-year follow-up

We plan to extend patient follow-up up to 10 years through record linkage between the PREDICT database and the following datasets:

- The national Renal Epidemiology and Information Network (REIN) registry to identify ESRD events (dialysis and kidney transplantation) [13]
- The national death registry (RNIPP, Registre national d'identité des personnes physiques) to assess vital status and identify cause(s) of death.
- The national health insurance information system (SNIIR-AM) to collect data about patient use of health resources.

Patient consent for this ancillary study will be requested at inclusion in the main study.

### Data collection, monitoring and data analysis

During the visits, data will be collected in an electronic case report form (eCRF) using CleanWEB software (TéléMédecine®, Boulogne, France). This data management system allows direct data entry. Data entry will be monitored by an independent researcher according to a predefined monitoring plan. Patient confidentiality will be ensured by using identification numbers.

Patient baseline characteristics will be compared between AKIN categories at inclusion using analysis of variance or Mann–Whitney test and Pearson's Chi-square test for continuous and categorical data, respectively. Factors associated with main outcome will be evaluated using a competing risk survival analysis. Factors associated with the main outcome in univariate analysis with a $p$ value lower than 0.10 will be included in the multivariate model. Clinically relevant interactions will be studied (especially with age, gender and preexisting diabetes). Factors associated with long-term mortality will be evaluated using the same methodology.

Yearly eGFR assessment will allow to describe the evolution of GFR over time and the evaluation of factors associated with eGFR decline. This analysis will be performed using mixed models with random intercepts and slopes.

The score aiming at predicting the occurrence of CKD at 3 years will be built as follows: (1) evaluation of factors associated with the main outcome using competing risk analysis, (2) assessment of the selection of the variables using the least absolute shrinkage and selection operator (LASSO) method, (3) evaluation of score performance, (4) assessment of the internal validity using bootstrapping. Such a score will be developed using two-thirds of the entire cohort and validated (external validation) using the remaining one-third.

The findings of this study will be published in national and international journals.

## Discussion

The PREDICT study is a multicenter observational prospective study aiming at describing the occurrence of CKD at 3 years in patients who suffered AKI during their ICU stay. It will be the first prospective study including a large sample of patients discharged alive from ICU able to provide CKD incidence after AKI in ICU and to highlight factors associated with CKD occurrence in this specific setting.

Several observational studies performed in medicine wards using administrative billing codes have reported an increased risk of CKD occurrence after AKI. While pathogenesis of such a mid- and long-term complication remains unclear, several hypotheses have been raised to explain such an outcome. Ischemia–reperfusion phenomena as well as tubular injuries, renal arteriolar injuries and endothelial dysfunction might explain the occurrence of long term of CKD after AKI [5]. All these phenomena widely occur in ICU patients, much more often than in non-ICU patients, and this could lead to a higher risk of CKD in this very specific subgroup of patients. Although clinically relevant, data about CKD after AKI in ICU patients remain scarce and specifically focused on ESRD occurrence and renal replacement therapy [14–16]. The present study may provide interesting insights in the early identification of these patients who could benefit from long-term prophylactic measures.

We will specifically focus on patients who recovered a normal eGFR. Kidney function recovery is difficult to define as eGFR may only be a part of such an evaluation. "De novo" CKD after AKI highlights the lack of discrimination of eGFR in CKD prediction in these patients and

the need for new tools to identify patients who could benefit from prophylactic treatments [17]. Accordingly, the present study will provide two major information: (1) the proportion of patients who recover a normal eGFR and who will suffer CKD after ICU discharge and the factors (during and after the ICU stay) associated with this complication and (2) the kinetics of eGFR decline and more importantly of albuminuria, which may be an earlier biomarker of kidney injury. Thus, we aim to provide tools to help physicians to identify patients who will suffer CKD and who could be difficult to early target with the blood creatinine assessment. Furthermore, we could get some interesting results in the clinical, biological and pathological description of AKI injuries in ICU patients. Besides tubular injuries, numerous other lesions could be observed and could help to better understand chronic kidney injury pathogenesis.

Finally, we will also include patients with previously known CKD and will be able to describe eGFR decline slope after AKI in ICU. This could help nephrologists and transplantation specialists to model the kidney function worsening and prepare patients to dialysis or renal transplantation.

In conclusion, the PREDICT study will evaluate CKD incidence and its determinants in ICU patients who suffered AKI during their ICU stay. It will provide a score able to predict CKD and help to identify patients who could benefit from early management and potential prophylactic treatments.

## Trial status

Patient recruitment has started on April 26, 2018.

### Abbreviations

AKI: acute kidney injury; ICU: intensive care unit; CKD: chronic kidney disease; ESRD: end-stage renal disease; GFR: glomerular filtration rate.

### Author details

[1] Medico-Surgical ICU, Service de Réanimation médico-chirurgicale, Ambroise Paré Hospital, APHP, 92100 Boulogne Billancourt, France. [2] Inserm U1018, Center for Research in Epidemiology and Population Health (CESP), Univ Paris Sud, Univ Paris Saclay, Villejuif, France. [3] Versailles Saint Quentin University, Montigny le Bretonneux, France. [4] Biomedicine Agency, Saint Denis, France. [5] Department of Clinical Research and Public Health, Ambroise Paré Hospital, APHP, Boulogne Billancourt, France. [6] UVSQ-INSERM U1168, University Paris Saclay, Villejuif, France. [7] Department of Nephrology, Ambroise Paré Hospital, APHP, Boulogne Billancourt, France.

### Acknowledgements

*List of coinvestigators* Stéphane Legriel (service de réanimation, Versailles), Virginie Laurent (service de réanimation, Versailles), Jean-Louis Teboul (service de réanimation médicale, Bicêtre), Virginie Tarazona (service de réanimation chirurgicale, Bicêtre), Armand Mekontso-Dessap (service de réanimation médicale, Henri Mondor), Jean-Paul Mira (service de réanimation médicale, Cochin), Jean-Luc Diehl (service de réanimation médicale, HEGP), Romain Pirracchio (service de réanimation chirurgicale, HEGP), Naike Bigé (service de réanimation médicale, Saint Antoine), Claire Dupuis (service de réanimation médicale, Bichat), Stéphane Gaudry (service de réanimation, Louis Mourier),

Julien Maizel (service de réanimation, Amiens), Bertrand Souweine (service de réanimation, Clermont-Ferrand), Lara Zafrani (service de réanimation médicale, Saint Louis), Bruno Mégarbane (service de réanimation médicale, Lariboisière), Alexandre Mebazaa (service de réanimation chirurgicale, Lariboisière), Antoine Durbach (service de néphrologie, Bicêtre), Vincent Audard (service de néphrologie, Henri Mondor), Eric Thervet (service de néphrologie, HEGP), Jean-Jacques Boffa (service de néphrologie, Tenon), Guillaume Hanouna (service de néphrologie, Bichat), Dimitri Titeca (service de néphrologie, Amiens), Carole Philiponnet (service de néphrologie, Clermont-Ferrand), Denis Glotz (service de néphrologie, Saint Louis).

## Authors' contributions

GG, BS, CJ, ZM, PA and AVB designed the study. GG, PA and BS designed the statistical analysis plan. GG and AVB drafted the manuscript. BS, CJ and ZM carefully reviewed the manuscript. All authors read and approved the final manuscript.

## Competing interests

The authors declare that they have no competing interests.

## Funding

The study was funded by a grant from Programme Hospitalier de Recherche Clinique—PHRC 2016 (contract AOR16089—French Ministry of Health). The study is promoted by the Greater Paris Hospitals (Assistance Publique—Hôpitaux de Paris). The research unit Paris Ile de France Ouest (URC Paris Ile de France Ouest) organizes the study.

## References

1. Uchino S, Kellum JA, Bellomo R, Doig GS, Morimatsu H, Morgera S, et al. Acute renal failure in critically ill patients: a multinational, multicenter study. JAMA. 2005;294:813–8.

2. Bagshaw SM, Uchino S, Cruz D, Bellomo R, Morimatsu H, Morgera S, et al. A comparison of observed versus estimated baseline creatinine for determination of RIFLE class in patients with acute kidney injury. Nephrol Dial Transplant. 2009;24:2739–44.

3. Horkan CM, Purtle SW, Mendu ML, Moromizato T, Gibbons FK, Christopher KB. The association of acute kidney injury in the critically ill and postdischarge outcomes: a cohort study*. Crit Care Med. 2015;43:354–64.

4. Vaara ST, Pettilä V, Kaukonen K-M, Bendel S, Korhonen A-M, Bellomo R, et al. The attributable mortality of acute kidney injury. Crit Care Med. 2014;42:878–85.

5. Lerolle N, Nochy D, Guerot E, Bruneval P, Fagon J-Y, Diehl J-L, et al. Histopathology of septic shock induced acute kidney injury: apoptosis and leukocytic infiltration. Intensive Care Med. 2010;36:471–8.

6. Spurgeon-Pechman KR, Donohoe DL, Mattson DL, Lund H, James L, Basile DP. Recovery from acute renal failure predisposes hypertension and secondary renal disease in response to elevated sodium. Am J Physiol Renal Physiol. 2007;293:F269–78.

7. Ishani A, Xue JL, Himmelfarb J, Eggers PW, Kimmel PL, Molitoris BA, et al. Acute kidney injury increases risk of ESRD among elderly. J Am Soc Nephrol. 2009;20:223–8.

8. Wald R, Quinn RR, Luo J, Li P, Scales DC, Mamdani MM, et al. Chronic dialysis and death among survivors of acute kidney injury requiring dialysis. JAMA. 2009;302:1179–85.

9. Mehta RL, Kellum JA, Shah SV, Molitoris BA, Ronco C, Warnock DG, et al. Acute kidney injury network: report of an initiative to improve outcomes in acute kidney injury. Crit Care. 2007;11:R31.

10. Nguyen Y-L, Milbrandt EB, Weissfeld LA, Kahn JM, Chiche J-D, Aegerter P, et al. Intensive care unit renal support therapy volume is not associated with patient outcome. Crit Care Med. 2011;39:2470–7.

11. Hays RD, Kallich JD, Mapes DL, Coons SJ, Amin N, Carter WB, et al. Kidney disease quality of life short form, version 1.3: a manual for use and scoring. Santa Monica: RAND; 1997. p. 1–41.

12. Herdman M, Gudex C, Lloyd A, Janssen M, Kind P, Parkin D, et al. Development and preliminary testing of the new five-level version of EQ-5D (EQ-5D-5L). Qual Life Res. 2011;20:1727–36.

13. Couchoud C, Stengel B, Landais P, Aldigier J-C, de Cornelissen F, Dabot C, et al. The renal epidemiology and information network (REIN): a new registry for end-stage renal disease in France. Nephrol Dial Transplant. 2005;21:411–8.

14. An JN, Hwang JH, Kim DK, Lee H, Ahn SY, Kim S, et al. Chronic kidney disease after acute kidney injury requiring continuous renal replacement therapy and its impact on long-term outcomes: a multicenter retrospective Cohort Study in Korea. Crit Care Med. 2017;45:47–57.

15. Rimes-Stigare C, Frumento P, Bottai M, Mårtensson J, Martling C-R, Walther SM, et al. Evolution of chronic renal impairment and long-term mortality after de novo acute kidney injury in the critically ill; a Swedish Multi-centre Cohort Study. Crit Care. 2015;19:221.

16. Rimes-Stigare C, Frumento P, Bottai M, Mårtensson J, Martling C-R, Bell M. Long-term mortality and risk factors for development of end-stage renal disease in critically ill patients with and without chronic kidney disease. Crit Care. 2015;19:383.

17. Bucaloiu ID, Kirchner HL, Norfolk ER, Hartle JE, Perkins RM. Increased risk of death and de novo chronic kidney disease following reversible acute kidney injury. Kidney Int. 2012;81:477–85.

# Inflammatory and coagulatory parameters linked to survival in critically ill children with sepsis

Christian Niederwanger[1], Mirjam Bachler[2]*, Tobias Hell[3], Caroline Linhart[4], Andreas Entenmann[1], Agnes Balog[1], Katharina Auer[5] and Petra Innerhofer[6]

## Abstract

**Background:** Sepsis is associated with a deflection of inflammatory and coagulative parameters, since some clotting factors are known to be involved in the host's defense against infection and inflammation. These parameters could play a crucial role in the course of sepsis and be used as prognostic markers in critically ill children.

**Methods:** A total of 250 critically ill pediatric patients diagnosed with sepsis were retrospectively analyzed to identify routinely measured predictors for in-hospital mortality at the peak level of C-reactive protein. Those parameters entered multivariate logistic regression analysis as well as a decision tree for survival.

**Results:** Multivariate logistic regression analysis revealed fibrinogen, platelets and activated partial thromboplastin time (aPTT) at the peak level of C-reactive protein to be predictors for survival ($p = 0.03$, $p = 0.01$ and $p = 0.02$, respectively). An increase in fibrinogen and platelets is linked to survival, whereas an aPTT prolongation is associated with higher mortality; adjusted odds ratios (95% CI) for an increase of 100 mg/dl in fibrinogen are 1.35 (1.04–1.82) per 50 G/l platelets 1.94 (1.3–3.29) and 0.83 (0.69–0.96) for an aPTT prolongation of 10 s. Decision tree analysis shows that a fibrinogen level below 192 mg/dl (90.9% vs. 13% mortality) is most distinctive in non-survivors.

**Conclusions:** High levels of fibrinogen and platelets as well as a non-overshooting aPTT are associated with a higher survival rate in pediatric patients with diagnosed sepsis. In particular, hypofibrinogenemia is distinctive for a high mortality rate in septic critically ill children.

**Keywords:** Fibrinogen, Sepsis, Children, Survival, Inflammation, Coagulation, Platelets

## Introduction

Although the number of deaths caused by sepsis has drastically decreased in the last couple of decades [1], sepsis remains one of the main causes of mortality in infants and toddlers worldwide [1–3]. Sepsis in children peaks in the neonatal period and symptoms may be non-specific in those patients [4], while older children may show hyperthermia, tachycardia, tachypnea, hypotension

and disorders in hemostasis up to the clinical picture of disseminated intravascular coagulation (DIC).

Sepsis is initially characterized by excessive production of pro-inflammatory cytokines, leukocyte activation and tissue damage, followed by release of anti-inflammatory cytokines, leukocyte deactivation and immunosuppression [5]. In the later phase of sepsis, compensatory release of anti-inflammatory molecules is thought to mediate a state of immunosuppression associated with significant impairment of immune cell function (immunoparalysis) [6].

The systemic inflammation during sepsis is observed by measuring leukocytes, procalcitonin, C-reactive protein and others. Leukocyte count is part of the definition of sepsis, but only at extreme levels are leukocytes

*Correspondence: mirjam.bachler@tirol-kliniken.at
[2] Institute for Sports Medicine, Alpine Medicine and Health Tourism, UMIT - University for Health Sciences, Medical Informatics and Technology, Eduard Wallnöfer Zentrum 1, 6060 Hall in Tirol, Austria
Full list of author information is available at the end of the article

associated with the progression of sepsis [7]. Data confirm that procalcitonin, which specifically increases in bacterial processes [8], is suitable as a diagnostic parameter in many cases in adults due to its high specificity [9, 10]. However, limited data are available for use in pediatric patients [11]. C-reactive protein reflects the inflammatory process and is widely used in clinical routine. Many studies have described an interrelation between an elevated C-reactive protein level and sepsis [12–15]. Thus, in clinical routine, daily C-reactive protein measurements might be used to assess the efficacy of treatment [16]. C-reactive protein can also be an indicator of organ failure [17–21] and therefore has potential for the surveillance of sepsis severity.

Systemic inflammation is followed by activation of the coagulation system, and conversely, components of the coagulation system significantly affect the inflammatory response [22]. This cross-link occurs on several levels: Pro-inflammatory cytokines stimulate the production of coagulation factors and coagulation factors mediate inflammation via binding to receptors of endothelium and immune cells [23]. The coagulation factors also play a direct role in host defense. For example, fibrinogen modulates the immune system [24, 25] and acts as a chemotactical factor for monocytes and neutrophils [26]. Furthermore, as part of the innate immune system, it limits bacterial spreading by forming fiber nets in which the pathogens become immobilized [24].

With few exceptions, such as antithrombin or platelets, the role of coagulation parameters in sepsis is largely ignored. New diagnostic, prognostic and therapeutic strategies can be deduced by observing coagulating laboratory data and, where appropriate, modifying them in the event of excessive activation or dysregulation of the system [27, 28]. An increase in the pro-coagulatory parameters to high level is seen rather negatively in the inflammatory process because of their pro-thrombotic potential [29], although elevation of the pro-coagulatory parameters might be beneficial during sepsis due to their role in host defense.

Therefore, it is worthwhile to examine the behavior and influence of coagulation parameters in combination with the typical inflammatory parameters during sepsis. Correct interpretation of these could facilitate assessment of the course of sepsis in critically ill children.

## Methods

This retrospective analysis comprises clinical data and routine laboratory parameters from 250 pediatric patients at the Pediatric Intensive Care Unit of Innsbruck Medical University Hospital.

### Inclusion of patients

All medical files of patients younger than 18 years of age who were treated at the pediatric intensive care unit (PICU) between January 1, 2000, and December 31, 2014, with the diagnosis of sepsis or systemic infection were reviewed. A total of 250 patients met the sepsis criteria of Goldstein [1]. There was no need to obtain oral and written informed consent from the study participants since the data were processed anonymously. The study protocol was approved by the institutional review board of the Medical University of Innsbruck (AN2013-0044).

### Data collection

We collected the demographic variables age, sex and the diagnosed underlying disease that triggered hospitalization. Septic shock was defined as the need for a vasoactive drug to maintain blood pressure in the normal range during the septic episode [1]. The C-reactive protein level was used to objectify the progression of sepsis, because it is an established parameter of sepsis [12–16] and is used in our clinic in children of all ages as opposed to IL-6 and procalcitonin.

The day on which C-reactive protein peaked was defined as day 0 in the report. The available routine parameters (fibrinogen, platelets, antithrombin, PT, aPTT, leukocytes) were observed from 3 days before until 3 days after day 0. In-hospital mortality was chosen as the outcome parameter.

To evaluate changes in therapy and outcome due to the protracted study period, we grouped patients into four time cohorts (2000–2004, 2005–2007, 2008–2010 and 2011–2014).

### Statistical analysis

A mathematician not involved in the study procedures or patient assessment (TH) was responsible for the statistical analyses using R, version 3.4.1. All statistical assessments were two sided, and a significance level of 5% was used. The hypothesis of a normal distribution was not reasonable for most of the continuous variables (Shapiro–Wilk normality test). The Wilcoxon rank sum test and Fisher's exact test were applied to assess differences between survivors and non-survivors. We present continuous data as medians (25th–75th percentile) and binary variables as no./total no. (%). We show effect size and precision with estimated median differences between survivors and non-survivors for continuous data and odds ratios (OR) for binary variables, with 95% CIs.

Stratified by survival, the progression of inflammation- and coagulation-related parameters from 3 days prior to 3 days after the peak of C-reactive protein is illustrated by the sequence of the median with corresponding 95% CIs in a purely descriptive manner.

In the univariate analysis, significant predictors at the peak of C-reactive protein as well as the respective patient's characteristics for survival were identified. Those variables entered a forward–backward stepwise selection by Akaike information criterion (AIC) to fit a logistic regression model for survival [30]. We provide adjusted odds ratios for the remaining predictors with 95% CIs. Receiver operating characteristic (ROC curves) analysis was performed, and ROC AUC is provided with 95% CIs. In addition, with the variables that entered the stepwise model selection, a recursive partitioning tree for survival was fitted using the R package rpart (version 4.1-11). All analyses were performed in a purely exploratory fashion.

## Results
### Patient characteristics
In total, 250 patients met the eligibility criteria for study inclusion and final analysis. Of those septic children, 41 (16.4%) did not survive while in hospital. Of the critically ill children, 53.2% suffered from sepsis and 26.4% from severe sepsis. Septic shock was reported in 51/250 (20.4%) children, of whom 21/51 (41.2%) died. Patients' baseline characteristics stratified for survival and non-survival are presented in Table 1.

The population consisted of 134/250 (53.6%) male patients, and median (25th–75th percentile) age was 35

(6–109) months. The 22/249 (8.8%) neonates showed a significantly higher ($p = 0.02$) mortality rate, because 8/22 (36.4%) neonates as compared to 33/227 (14.5%) children older than 1 month did not survive the septic episode. The most commonly affected organ systems resulting in ICU admission were the respiratory system in 51/250 (20.4%) and the central nervous system in 46/250 (18.4%) children.

To rule out possible confounding due to the protracted study period (2000–2014), we grouped patients into four time cohorts: 80 patients were included in 2000–2004, 56 in 2005–2007, 68 in 2008–2010 and 46 in 2011–2014. Mortality was 12.5%, 28.6%, 13.2% and 13%, respectively, and was not significantly associated with the time periods (Fisher's exact test: $p = 0.07$).

### Univariate analysis of parameters at the peak level of C-reactive protein
As presented in Table 2, no significant difference was observed in C-reactive protein or leukocyte levels between survivors and non-survivors at the peak level of C-reactive protein. There was a difference in the timing between hospital admission and C-reactive protein peak between survivors and non-survivors ($p < 0.0001$) with non-survivors having a longer time period to reach the C-reactive protein peak. In contrast, fibrinogen, platelets and antithrombin significantly differ. This is also the case for aPTT and PT.

**Table 1 Characteristics of patients stratified for survival and non-survival**

| Characteristics[a] | Total (n = 250) | Survivors (n = 209) | Non-survivors (n = 41) | Estimate with 95% CI[b] | p value[c] |
|---|---|---|---|---|---|
| Female gender | 116/250 (46.4%) | 97/209 (46.4%) | 19/41 (46.3%) | 1 (0.48 to 2.06) | 1 |
| Age[d] (months) | 34.83 (6.47–108.63) | 35.5 (7.16–111.45) | 23.8 (1.43–81.97) | 3.33 (−6.55 to 18.07) | 0.2725 |
| Neonates < 1 month | 22/249 (8.8%) | 14/208 (6.7%) | 8/41 (19.5%) | 3.34 (1.12 to 9.34) | 0.0149 |
| Infants 1–3 months | 24/249 (9.6%) | 20/208 (9.6%) | 4/41 (9.8%) | 1.02 (0.24 to 3.28) | 1 |
| *Diagnosed underlying disease* | | | | | |
| Central nervous system· | 46/250 (18.4%) | 34/209 (16.3%) | 12/41 (29.3%) | 2.12 (0.89 to 4.82) | 0.075 |
| Cardiovascular | 39/250 (15.6%) | 31/209 (14.8%) | 8/41 (19.5%) | 1.39 (0.51 to 3.45) | 0.4808 |
| Digestive tract | 41/250 (16.4%) | 32/209 (15.3%) | 9/41 (22%) | 1.55 (0.59 to 3.74) | 0.3546 |
| Respiratory system | 51/250 (20.4%) | 41/209 (19.6%) | 10/41 (24.4%) | 1.32 (0.53 to 3.05) | 0.5258 |
| Oncologic | 37/250 (14.8%) | 31/209 (14.8%) | 6/41 (14.6%) | 0.98 (0.31 to 2.64) | 1 |
| Kidney | 30/250 (12%) | 22/209 (10.5%) | 8/41 (19.5%) | 2.05 (0.73 to 5.31) | 0.1169 |
| Liver | 18/250 (7.2%) | 15/209 (7.2%) | 3/41 (7.3%) | 1.02 (0.18 to 3.87) | 1 |
| Skin | 11/250 (4.4%) | 10/209 (4.8%) | 1/41 (2.4%) | 0.5 (0.01 to 3.68) | 1 |
| Other diagnosis | 30/250 (12%) | 25/209 (12%) | 5/41 (12.2%) | 1.02 (0.29 to 2.97) | 1 |

[a] Binary data are presented as no./total no. (%) and continuous data as medians (25th–75th percentile)

[b] Odds ratio for binary variables and estimated median difference for continuous variables

[c] Differences between survivors and non-survivors assessed with Fisher's exact test for binary variables and Wilcoxon rank sum test for continuous variables

[d] For one survivor, the exact age in months is not known

**Table 2 Parameters at the peak level of C-reactive protein stratified for survival and non-survival**

| Parameters[a] | Total (n = 250) | Survivors (n = 209) | Non-survivors (n = 41) | Estimate with 95% CI[b] | p value[c] | Not known[d] |
|---|---|---|---|---|---|---|
| C-reactive protein (mg/dl) | 18.5 (9.8–28.4) | 18.6 (10–28) | 17.6 (7.9–31.9) | −0.13 (−5.3 to 4.55) | 0.9491 | 0/0 |
| Fibrinogen (mg/dl) | 506 (329–675) | 518 (383–685) | 279 (173–514) | 206 (118 to 289) | <0.0001 | 56/9 |
| Platelets (G/l) | 124 (50–232) | 147 (62.5–247) | 63 (29–98) | 74 (37 to 111) | <0.0001 | 5/0 |
| aPTT (s) | 47 (38–56) | 46 (36–53) | 64 (53.5–83) | −20 (−28 to −13) | <0.0001 | 59/15 |
| PT (%) | 71 (51–84) | 74 (55–85) | 49 (36–71.5) | 20 (10 to 30) | 0.0001 | 59/14 |
| Antithrombin (%) | 63 (47–81) | 65.5 (50–82) | 51 (40–66) | 14 (5 to 23) | 0.0045 | 75/10 |
| Leukocytes (G/l) | 10.4 (4.6–17.8) | 11.1 (5.3–17.5) | 8.2 (3–20) | 1.4 (−1.6 to 5.1) | 0.3342 | 4/5 |

[a] Data are presented as medians (25th–75th percentile)

[b] Estimated median difference

[c] Differences between survivors and non-survivors assessed with Wilcoxon rank sum test for continuous variables

[d] Number of missing measurements in survivors/non-survivors

## Progression of parameters around the peak level of C-reactive protein

The course of fibrinogen and antithrombin seems to be associated with the progression of C-reactive protein (Figs. 1, 2). Fibrinogen concentration followed the progression of C-reactive protein in survivors, but not in non-survivors. Note that for the main portion of the survivors, fibrinogen levels increased distinctly above the norm values around day 0.

Antithrombin levels were constantly higher in survivors than in non-survivors, but, in contrast to fibrinogen, irrespective of the progression of C-reactive protein. In survivors, platelets decreased slightly over time, while patients who did not survive showed a sharp decline in platelets already 2 days before the peak level of C-reactive protein was reached. Survivors showed significantly higher PT levels and shorter aPTT around the peak of C-reactive protein. Progression of leukocytes between survivors and non-survivors is comparable up to day 2.

CRP, fibrinogen, platelets, aPTT, PT and antithrombin levels were comparable between time cohorts (Kruskal–Wallis test: $p = 0.40$, $p = 0.32$, $p = 0.58$, $p = 0.90$, $p = 0.17$ and $p = 0.22$, respectively). Leukocyte count significantly differed between time cohorts (Kruskal–Wallis test: $p = 0.04$). Median leukocyte counts in G/l were 12.3 (6.13–20) in 2000–2004, 12.1 (6.8–17.1) in 2005–2007, 10.3 (3.1–16.4) in 2008–2010 and 7.7 (2.8–12) in 2011–2014.

## Multivariate logistic regression analysis for survival

The following significant univariate predictors for survival entered a stepwise model selection: fibrinogen, platelets, antithrombin, aPTT, PT and age. The resulting logistic regression model for survival includes fibrinogen, platelets and aPTT as variables, all of them being significant predictors for survival ($p = 0.03$, $p = 0.01$ and $p = 0.02$, respectively).

Figure 3 shows the adjusted odds ratios (95% CI) retrieved from logistic regression. An increase in fibrinogen and platelets is linked to survival, whereas aPTT prolongation is associated with higher mortality. An increase of 100 mg/dl in fibrinogen increases the survival chance by 26%, per 50 G/l platelets by 48.4%, and aPTT prolongation of 10 s increases the mortality risk by 20.8%.

Adding the time cohort or the year of CRP peak as input variables resulted in the identical logistic regression model after stepwise model selection.

The ROC analysis (Additional file 1) for survival predicted by fibrinogen, platelets and aPTT resulted in an AUC of 0.74 (0.63–0.85), 0.71 (0.63–0.79) and 0.81 (0.73–0.90), respectively.

## Decision tree for survival

To gain a deeper insight into the interplay of coagulation parameters leading to death in septic children, a decision tree was fitted using the univariate predictors at the peak level of C-reactive protein and age to explore these interrelations.

The obtained classification tree (see Fig. 4) shows that most distinctive in non-survivors is a fibrinogen level below 192 mg/dl [90.9% (58.7–99.8%) vs. 13% (8.1–18.5%) mortality]. For patients presenting with a fibrinogen level of at least 192 mg/dl, an aPTT of less than 58 s is associated with better outcome [8.4% (5.0–13.1%) vs. 37.8% (22.5–55.2%) mortality]. If, in addition, patients show a platelet count of at least 80 G/l, a low mortality rate is observed [4.1% (1.5–8.7%) vs. 20% (10.4–33.0%) mortality]. Patients with a platelet count below 80 G/l and younger than 1.2 months show high mortality as compared to older [57.1% (18.4–90.1%) vs. 14.6% (6.1–27.8%)].

In the case of a fibrinogen level of at least 192 mg/dl and an aPTT prolongation of 58 s or more, antithrombin levels below 58% led to lower mortality [25% (9.8–46.7%)

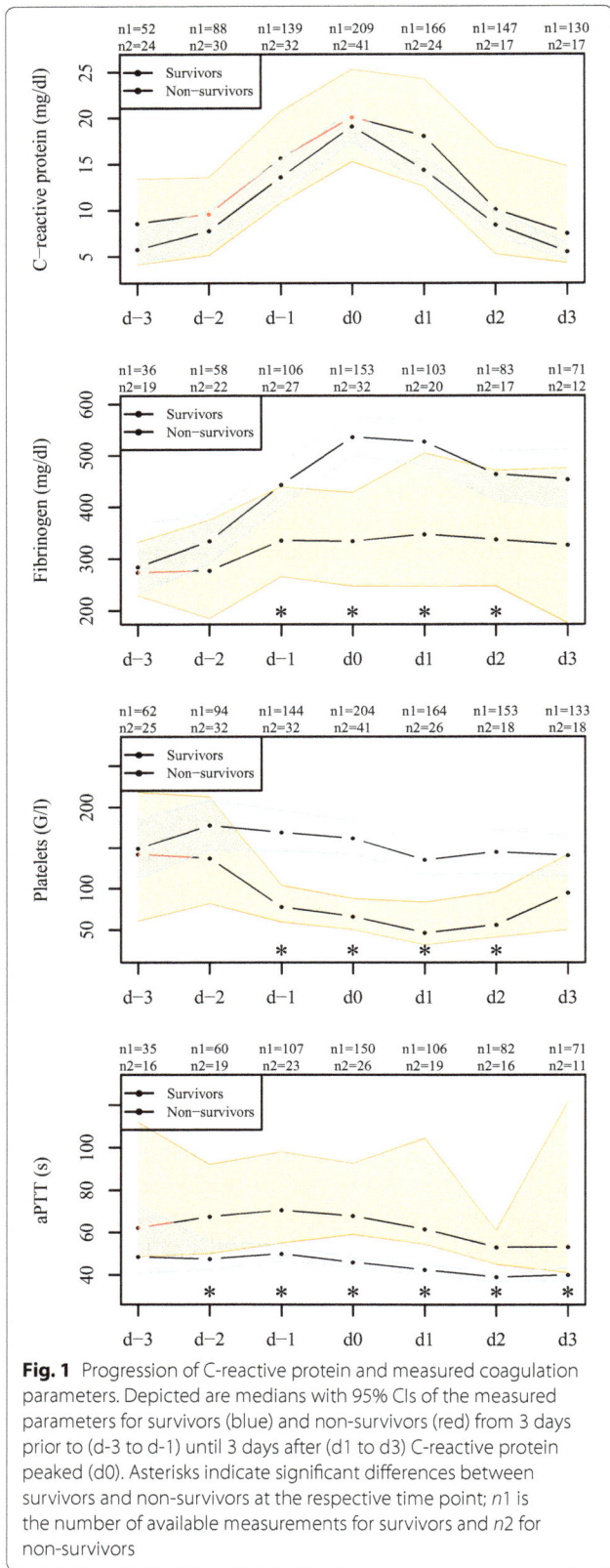

**Fig. 1** Progression of C-reactive protein and measured coagulation parameters. Depicted are medians with 95% CIs of the measured parameters for survivors (blue) and non-survivors (red) from 3 days prior to (d-3 to d-1) until 3 days after (d1 to d3) C-reactive protein peaked (d0). Asterisks indicate significant differences between survivors and non-survivors at the respective time point; n1 is the number of available measurements for survivors and n2 for non-survivors

vs. 61.5% (31.6–86.1%)], especially in patients exceeding an aPTT of 66 s [0% (0.0–24.7%) vs. 54.5% (23.4–83.3%) mortality].

The identical decision tree was obtained when the time cohort or the year of C-reactive protein peak was added as predictors for survival, indicating that there was no confounding due to the protracted study period (2000–2014).

In order to predict mortality with fibrinogen < 192 mg/ dl, platelets < 80 G/l and aPTT > 58 s, sensitivity and specificity were calculated (Additional file 2).

**Age-adjusted hypofibrinogenemia**
The fibrinogen level of each child was classified as hypo-, normo- or hyperfibrinogenemia according to the age-dependent norm value ranges. For normal fibrinogen values, please see the table in Additional file 3.

Patients presenting with hypofibrinogenemia have a significantly higher mortality rate than do patients with normo- or hyperfibrinogenemia: OR 28.42 (5.42–284.81), $p < 0.0001$. As depicted in Fig. 5, 82% of the patients with low fibrinogen levels died, whereas the mortality rate in patients with fibrinogen levels within the normal range was 22% and 10% in children with an elevated fibrinogen level.

No significant difference in the occurrence of a diagnosed thromboembolic event was observed for the 5/128 (3.9%) children with hyperfibrinogenemia as compared to the 4/56 (7.1%) patients with fibrinogen within the normal values or below: OR 0.53 (0.11–2.78), $p = 0.46$.

**Discussion**
In this study, we investigated the impact of routinely measured coagulation and inflammation parameters on in-hospital survival in pediatric patients diagnosed with sepsis. The main result is that C-reactive protein at its peak level does not significantly differ between survivors and non-survivors, whereas fibrinogen, platelets and aPTT are predictors of survival. An increase in fibrinogen and platelets is linked to survival, whereas aPTT prolongation is associated with higher mortality. Most distinctive for mortality are fibrinogen levels below 192 mg/dl. Especially in children younger than 1.2 months, isolated thrombocytopenia is associated with poor outcome. In general, age-adjusted hypofibrinogenemia is significantly associated with a poor chance of survival.

In some points, these results stand in contrast to findings reported in the literature. Several studies claim that C-reactive protein is of prognostic value in sepsis [12–15]. However, in our study focusing on mortality, C-reactive protein levels did not allow any differentiation between survivors and non-survivors during the observation period of 7 days. Most likely, in children as

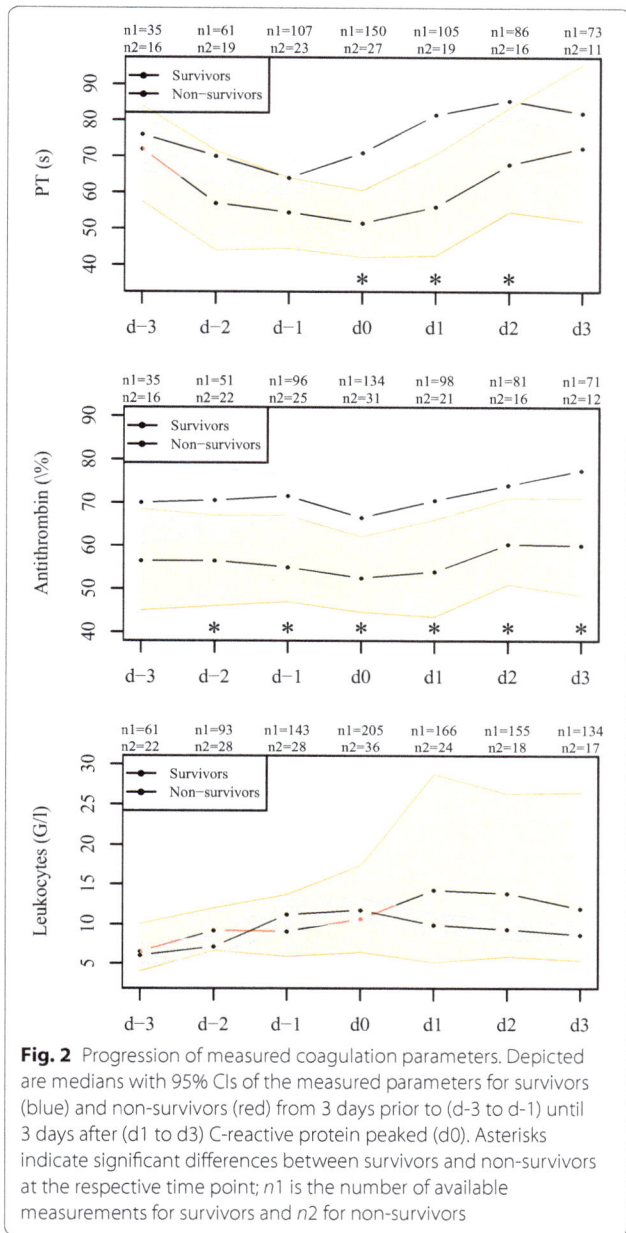

**Fig. 2** Progression of measured coagulation parameters. Depicted are medians with 95% CIs of the measured parameters for survivors (blue) and non-survivors (red) from 3 days prior to (d-3 to d-1) until 3 days after (d1 to d3) C-reactive protein peaked (d0). Asterisks indicate significant differences between survivors and non-survivors at the respective time point; n1 is the number of available measurements for survivors and n2 for non-survivors

well as in adults with diagnosed sepsis C-reactive protein levels are highly elevated without predicting final outcome.

Among the variables routinely measured in our study at the peak level of C-reactive protein, multivariate analysis revealed that only three of these coagulation parameters are essential for the prediction of survival in septic children: An increase in fibrinogen and platelets lowers the mortality risk, while a prolongation of aPTT increases the risk.

We found that hypofibrinogenemia is associated with very high mortality. This is in accordance with Esroy et al., who also confirm in their study that deceased patients exhibited significantly lower fibrinogen levels than did survivors [31]. Moreover, in baboons, survivors had higher fibrinogen levels than did non-survivors after induced sepsis [32]. This was also found in several earlier studies with fibrinogen-deficient mice following induced sepsis [33, 34].

The reason why fibrinogen is associated with survival in sepsis could be that it helps the immune system limit bacterial growth and enhance bacterial clearance [35]. The fibrin net captures and immobilizes invasive bacteria [24], thus restricting local spreading [24, 36]. Once the fibrinolysis sets in, plasminogen releases fibrinogen-derived so-called antimicrobial peptides (AMPs), thus causing an antimicrobial environment to arise within the clot. Such a peptide is the Bß15–42 fragment, and an unambiguous antimicrobial effect of this protein was already proven by S. aureus, group A Streptococcus (GAS) and group B Streptococcus (GBS) [25]. Besides that, this peptide binds to the VE cadherin of the endothelial cells and thus reinforces the tight junctions, which has a positive effect on organ failure and survival during sepsis [37, 38]. The importance of fibrinogen, fibrinolysis and the consequently released peptides during sepsis and their beneficial impact on infection, multiple-organ dysfunction and reduced mortality have already been proven in several studies [39–41].

In our study, age-adjusted hyperfibrinogenemia is associated with increased survival in sepsis. In studies of adult patients, this connection between acute and transient fibrinogen levels in the context of sepsis and survival was also observed [42]. In this context of high levels of pro-thrombotic factors, the fear of a hypercoagulatory state during sepsis is present and justified, since this could contribute to the development of thrombosis. In our study, the incidence rate of thromboembolic events was not significantly increased in patients with hyperfibrinogenemia.

Low fibrinogen levels may reflect ongoing consumption and deposition, development of DIC and MODS [43, 44]. Sepsis itself also causes severe damage to the liver, via hemodynamic changes as well as the direct or indirect destruction of hepatocytes or both [45]. The destroyed hepatocytes are no longer able to synthesize a sufficient amount of fibrinogen, which might be another reason for the low fibrinogen levels in non-survivors.

High concentrations of fibrinogen before the C-reactive protein peak in our study rarely coincided with platelet concentrations below the critical limit of 100 G/l. Low platelets in addition to low fibrinogen levels result in weak clot firmness, which is known to lead

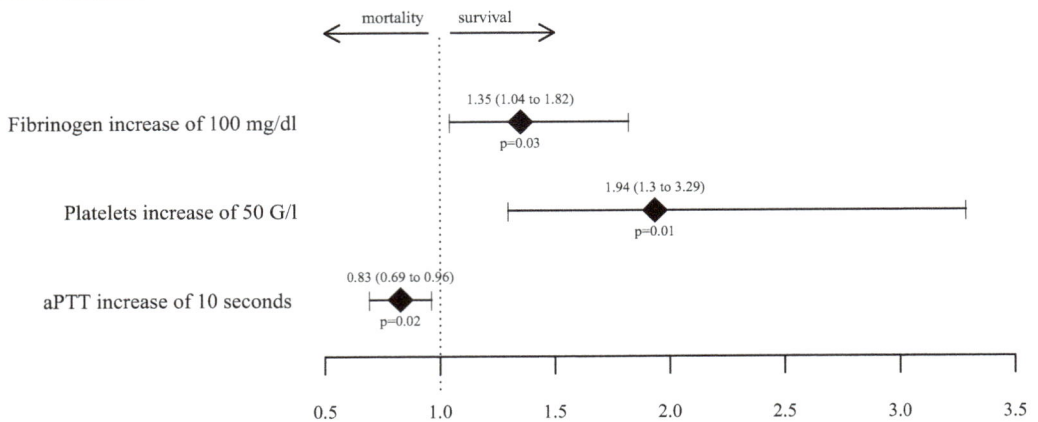

**Fig. 3** Adjusted odds ratios (95% CI) for survival retrieved from logistic regression. For an odds ratio greater than 1, an increase in the parameter decreases the mortality risk

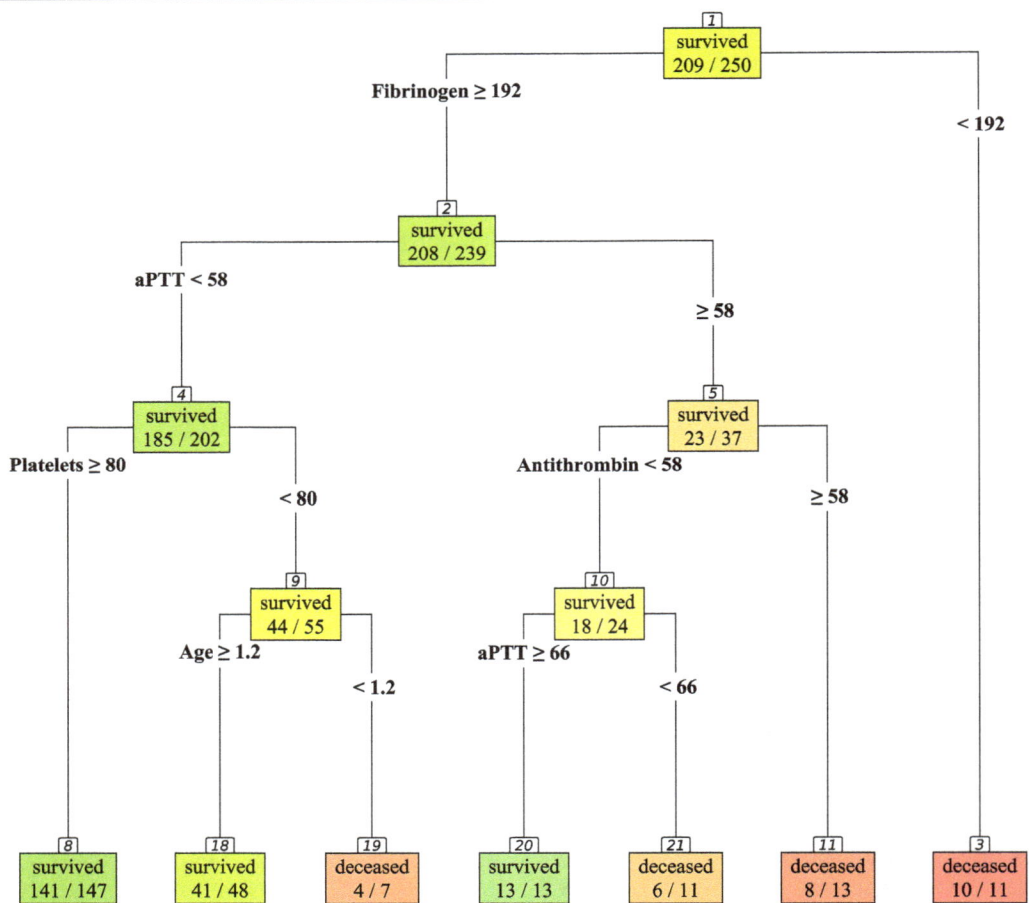

**Fig. 4** Decision tree for survival. The classification tree was fitted with univariate predictors at the peak of C-reactive protein and age

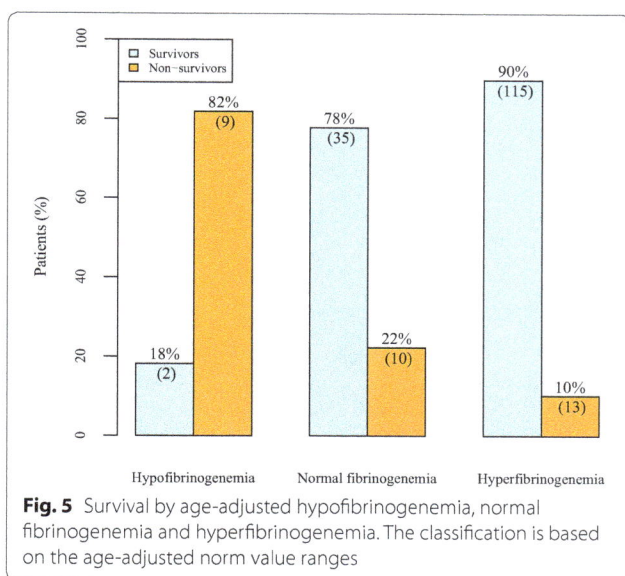

**Fig. 5** Survival by age-adjusted hypofibrinogenemia, normal fibrinogenemia and hyperfibrinogenemia. The classification is based on the age-adjusted norm value ranges

to poor outcome [4, 46]. Especially in neonates, isolated thrombocytopenia leads to increased mortality. This may be explained by the fact that during the first 6 weeks after birth, the plasmatic coagulation cascade is not fully developed and therefore hemostatic competence heavily relies on platelet function [47].

Overall, a decreased platelet count is associated with mortality. This might be due to the fact that thrombocytes are also an important part of the innate immune system. Whenever pathogens are present, platelets bind to them via the glycoprotein receptor IIb/IIIa and Toll-like receptors. That either happens directly, or it is mediated by plasma proteins like fibrinogen [48]. The activated platelets release antimicrobial peptides like defensins, kinocidins and thrombocidins to kill bacteria. In addition, they release members of the chemokine family like platelet factor 4 (PF4, CXCL-4) in order to attract other immune cells [49, 50].

The third coagulation parameter essential for the prediction of mortality in septic children in our study was aPTT. Prolongation leads to poorer outcome. A long aPTT might reflect the most severe cases of sepsis due to consumption of coagulation factors or high-dose heparin therapy, but may also be caused by a FXII deficiency. In septic patients, FXII deficiency can be protective via attenuation of the FXII-dependent bradykinin generation, complement activation and further contact pathway activation. This consequence of low FXII levels might explain why 13/13 children with fibrinogen levels above 192 mg/dl and an aPTT above 66 s survived, despite an antithrombin level below 58.

Compared with developed countries, at 16.4% the overall mortality of our children was in the upper frame [51, 52]. Due to the tertiary care status of our university hospital, the study included a large number of seriously ill children. Of them, 20.4% developed septic shock with a mortality rate of 41.2%. The literature reports a mortality rate of 20–30% in the presence of septic shock [53, 54], which increases to 52% in the case of additional MODS.

The limitations of our study have to be mentioned. The retrospective design of the study precludes assessment of causal relationships. Nevertheless, the main finding that high fibrinogen levels are beneficial in sepsis can be well explained by recently reported pathophysiological mechanisms. Further, not all the considered parameters were available throughout the observation period of 7 days. Especially for children who died rapidly or were transferred to another hospital soon after C-reactive protein peaked, data are lacking and a bias could be present in the consecutive days due to the smaller sample size. Therefore, the main analyses were performed solely on the day of C-reactive protein peak. The number of 250 sepsis cases diagnosed in children over a period of 14 years could be considered low. A deeper insight might be gained in a prospective setting.

Interpretation of the results of the multivariate logistic regression analysis for survival and decision tree analysis should be done carefully, since it cannot be concluded that these coagulation parameters are independently associated with survival because major well-known risk factors for death such as organ dysfunction or lactate were not taken into account. These analyses were used solely in an explorative fashion to describe the relation of the inflammatory and coagulatory parameters to survival. Therefore, this study is mainly descriptive and cannot determine the predictive value of coagulation parameters for outcome after sepsis. Another limitation is the fact that some values, such as low fibrinogen or low platelets, might have led to interventions that were not captured by this retrospective study. This could have influenced the magnitude of the associations. Despite all limitations, this study gives new insight into the course of sepsis and provides a good basis for a prospective study using these parameters as proxy for mortality, like organ dysfunction resolution or new and progressive MODS.

## Conclusion

The link between inflammation and coagulation plays a crucial role in children with sepsis. C-reactive protein does not allow discrimination between survivors and non-survivors. In contrast, increased levels of fibrinogen and platelets are linked to survival and distinctively reflect the inflammatory process. Prolonged aPTT is associated with lower survival, which might reflect therapy-related measures needed due to disease severity.

## Abbreviations

AIC: Akaike information criterion; AMP: antimicrobial peptides; aPTT: activated partial thromboplastin time; CRP: C-reactive protein; DIC: disseminated intravascular coagulopathy; FXII: coagulation factor XII; GAS: group A Streptococci; GBS: group B Streptococci; ICD: International Statistical Classification of Diseases and Related Health Problems; MODS: multiple organ dysfunction syndrome; OR: odds ratio; PF4: platelet factor 4; PICU: pediatric intensive care unit; PT: prothrombin time.

## Authors' contributions

CN conceived the study, developed the study design, contributed to the acquisition and interpretation of data and drafted and edited the manuscript. MB conceived the study, developed the study design and contributed to the acquisition and interpretation of data. She also drafted and edited the manuscript. She was responsible for ensuring that this study was reported honestly, accurately and transparently and also for the overall work by ensuring that questions pertaining to the accuracy or integrity of any portion of the work were appropriately investigated and resolved (corresponding author). TH performed the statistical analysis and gave support in interpretation of the data. He also contributed significantly to the drafting and editing the manuscript. CL gave support in development of the study design and contributed to the statistical analysis. She contributed to the drafting and editing the manuscript. AE contributed to the interpretation of data. He also gave support in drafting and editing the manuscript. AB helped with the English translation and assisted with drafting and editing the manuscript. KA contributed to the acquisition and interpretation of data. She also assisted with drafting and editing the manuscript. KA contributed to the acquisition and interpretation of data. She also assisted with drafting and editing the manuscript. PI contributed to the interpretation of data and gave major support in drafting and editing the manuscript. All authors read and approved the final manuscript.

## Author details

[1] Department of Pediatrics, Pediatrics I, Medical University of Innsbruck, Anichstrasse 35, 6020 Innsbruck, Austria. [2] Institute for Sports Medicine, Alpine Medicine and Health Tourism, UMIT - University for Health Sciences, Medical Informatics and Technology, Eduard Wallnöfer Zentrum 1, 6060 Hall in Tirol, Austria. [3] Department of Mathematics, Faculty of Mathematics, Computer Science and Physics, University of Innsbruck, Technikerstraße 13, 6020 Innsbruck, Austria. [4] Department of Medical Statistics, Informatics and Health Economics, Medical University of Innsbruck, Anichstrasse 35, 6020 Innsbruck, Austria. [5] Department of General and Surgical Critical Care Medicine, Medical University of Innsbruck, Anichstrasse 35, 6020 Innsbruck, Austria. [6] Department of Anaesthesiology and Critical Care Medicine, Medical University of Innsbruck, Anichstrasse 35, 6020 Innsbruck, Austria.

## Acknowledgements

We thank Dr. Sophie Hofer, Dr. Christina Schoner, Dr. Daniela Hainz, Dr. Ahmed Fideh, Martin Wagner, Dr. Thomas Varga and Dr. Dietmar Fries for their assistance in executing this project.

## Competing interests

The authors state that they have no competing interests in regard to this study. MB has received personal fees from LFB Biomedicaments, Baxter GmbH, CSL Behring GmbH and Mitsubishi Tanabe and non-financial support from TEM International outside the submitted work. PI has received personal fees from Baxter GmbH, personal fees from CSL Behring GmbH, personal fees from Fresenius Kabi GmbH Austria, personal fees from Bayer GmbH Austria and personal fees from LFB and non-financial support from TEM International outside the submitted work.

## Funding

There is no funding to declare.

## References

1. Goldstein B, Giroir B, Randolph A. International pediatric sepsis consensus conference: definitions for sepsis and organ dysfunction in pediatrics. Pediatr Crit Care Med. 2005;6(1):2–8.
2. Randolph AG, McCulloh RJ. Pediatric sepsis: important considerations for diagnosing and managing severe infections in infants, children, and adolescents. Virulence. 2014;5(1):179–89.
3. Hartman ME, Linde-Zwirble WT, Angus DC, Watson RS. Trends in the epidemiology of pediatric severe sepsis*. Pediatr Crit Care Med. 2013;14(7):686–93.
4. Sokou R, Giallouros G, Konstantinidi A, Pantavou K, Nikolopoulos G, Bonovas S, et al. Thromboelastometry for diagnosis of neonatal sepsis-associated coagulopathy: an observational study. Eur J Pediatr. 2018;177(3):355–62.
5. van der Poll T, van Deventer SJ. Cytokines and anticytokines in the pathogenesis of sepsis. Infect Dis Clin North Am. 1999;13(2):413–26.
6. Reddy RC, Chen GH, Tekchandani PK, Standiford TJ. Sepsis-induced immunosuppression. Immunol Res. 2001;24(3):273–87.
7. Levy MM, Fink MP, Marshall JC, Abraham E, Angus D, Cook D, et al. 2001 SCCM/ESICM/ACCP/ATS/SIS international sepsis definitions conference. Crit Care Med. 2003;31(4):1250–6.
8. Schneider HG, Lam QT. Procalcitonin for the clinical laboratory: a review. Pathology. 2007;39(4):383–90.
9. Castelli GP, Pognani C, Meisner M, Stuani A, Bellomi D, Sgarbi L. Procalcitonin and C-reactive protein during systemic inflammatory response syndrome, sepsis and organ dysfunction. Crit Care. 2004;8(4):R234–42.
10. Clec'h C, Ferriere F, Karoubi P, Fosse JP, Cupa M, Hoang P, et al. Diagnostic and prognostic value of procalcitonin in patients with septic shock. Crit Care Med. 2004;32(5):1166–9.
11. Chiesa C, Natale F, Pascone R, Osborn JF, Pacifico L, Bonci E, et al. C reactive protein and procalcitonin: reference intervals for preterm and term newborns during the early neonatal period. Clin Chim Acta. 2011;412(11):1053–9.
12. Schentag JJ, O'Keeffe D, Marmion M, Wels PB. C-reactive protein as an indicator of infection relapse in patients with abdominal sepsis. Arch Surg. 1984;119(3):300–4.
13. Maury CP. Monitoring the acute phase response: comparison of tumour necrosis factor (cachectin) and C-reactive protein responses in inflammatory and infectious diseases. J Clin Pathol. 1989;42(10):1078–82.
14. Povoa P, Almeida E, Moreira P, Fernandes A, Mealha R, Aragao A, et al. C-reactive protein as an indicator of sepsis. Intensive Care Med. 1998;24(10):1052–6.
15. Presterl E, Staudinger T, Pettermann M, Lassnigg A, Burgmann H, Winkler S, et al. Cytokine profile and correlation to the APACHE III and MPM II scores in patients with sepsis. Am J Respir Crit Care Med. 1997;156(3 Pt 1):825–32.
16. Yentis SM, Soni N, Sheldon J. C-reactive protein as an indicator of resolution of sepsis in the intensive care unit. Intensive Care Med. 1995;21(7):602–5.
17. Pinilla JC, Hayes P, Laverty W, Arnold C, Laxdal V. The C-reactive protein to prealbumin ratio correlates with the severity of multiple organ dysfunction. Surgery. 1998;124(4):799–805 (discussion-6).
18. Waydhas C, Nast-Kolb D, Trupka A, Zettl R, Kick M, Wiesholler J, et al. Posttraumatic inflammatory response, secondary operations, and late multiple organ failure. J Trauma. 1996;40(4):624–30 (discussion 630-1).
19. Ikei S, Ogawa M, Yamaguchi Y. Blood concentrations of polymorphonuclear leucocyte elastase and interleukin-6 are indicators for the occurrence of multiple organ failures at the early stage of acute pancreatitis. J Gastroenterol Hepatol. 1998;13(12):1274–83.
20. de Beaux AC, Goldie AS, Ross JA, Carter DC, Fearon KC. Serum concentrations of inflammatory mediators related to organ failure in patients with acute pancreatitis. Br J Surg. 1996;83(3):349–53.
21. Rau B, Steinbach G, Baumgart K, Gansauge F, Grunert A, Beger HG. Serum amyloid A versus C-reactive protein in acute pancreatitis: clinical value of an alternative acute-phase reactant. Crit Care Med. 2000;28(3):736–42.

22. Levi M, van der Poll T. Inflammation and coagulation. Crit Care Med. 2010;38(2 Suppl):S26–34.

23. van der Poll T, Levi M. Crosstalk between inflammation and coagulation: the lessons of sepsis. Curr Vasc Pharmacol. 2012;10(5):632–8.

24. Berends ET, Kuipers A, Ravesloot MM, Urbanus RT, Rooijakkers SH. Bacteria under stress by complement and coagulation. FEMS Microbiol Rev. 2014;38(6):1146–71.

25. Pahlman LI, Morgelin M, Kasetty G, Olin AI, Schmidtchen A, Herwald H. Antimicrobial activity of fibrinogen and fibrinogen-derived peptides—a novel link between coagulation and innate immunity. Thromb Haemost. 2013;109(5):930–9.

26. Senior RM, Skogen WF, Griffin GL, Wilner GD. Effects of fibrinogen derivatives upon the inflammatory response. Studies with human fibrinopeptide B. J Clin Invest. 1986;77(3):1014–9.

27. Lauterbach R, Pawlik D, Radziszewska R, Wozniak J, Rytlewski K. Plasma antithrombin III and protein C levels in early recognition of late-onset sepsis in newborns. Eur J Pediatr. 2006;165(9):585–9.

28. Semeraro F, Colucci M, Caironi P, Masson S, Ammollo CT, Teli R, et al. Platelet drop and fibrinolytic shutdown in patients with sepsis. Crit Care Med. 2018;46(3):e221–8.

29. Esmon CT. The interactions between inflammation and coagulation. Br J Haematol. 2005;131(4):417–30.

30. Akaike H. A new look at the statistical model identification. IEEE Trans Autom Control. 1974;19(6):716–23.

31. Ersoy B, Nehir H, Altinoz S, Yilmaz O, Dundar PE, Aydogan A. Prognostic value of initial antithrombin levels in neonatal sepsis. Indian Pediatr. 2007;44(8):581–4.

32. Taylor FB Jr, Kinasewitz GT, Lupu F. Pathophysiology, staging and therapy of severe sepsis in baboon models. J Cell Mol Med. 2012;16(4):672–82.

33. Luo D, Szaba FM, Kummer LW, Plow EF, Mackman N, Gailani D, et al. Protective roles for fibrin, tissue factor, plasminogen activator inhibitor-1, and thrombin activatable fibrinolysis inhibitor, but not factor XI, during defense against the gram-negative bacterium *Yersinia enterocolitica*. J Immunol. 2011;187(4):1866–76.

34. Mullarky IK, Szaba FM, Berggren KN, Parent MA, Kummer LW, Chen W, et al. Infection-stimulated fibrin deposition controls hemorrhage and limits hepatic bacterial growth during listeriosis. Infect Immun. 2005;73(7):3888–95.

35. Davalos D, Akassoglou K. Fibrinogen as a key regulator of inflammation in disease. Semin Immunopathol. 2012;34(1):43–62.

36. McAdow M, Missiakas DM, Schneewind O. *Staphylococcus aureus* secretes coagulase and von Willebrand factor binding protein to modify the coagulation cascade and establish host infections. J Innate Immun. 2012;4(2):141–8.

37. Jennewein C, Mehring M, Tran N, Paulus P, Ockelmann PA, Habeck K, et al. The fibrinopeptide bbeta15–42 reduces inflammation in mice subjected to polymicrobial sepsis. Shock. 2012;38(3):275–80.

38. Wolf T, Kann G, Becker S, Stephan C, Brodt HR, de Leuw P, et al. Severe Ebola virus disease with vascular leakage and multiorgan failure: treatment of a patient in intensive care. Lancet. 2015;385(9976):1428–35.

39. Wada H, Mori Y, Okabayashi K, Gabazza EC, Kushiya F, Watanabe M, et al. High plasma fibrinogen level is associated with poor clinical outcome in DIC patients. Am J Hematol. 2003;72(1):1–7.

40. Renckens R, Roelofs JJ, Stegenga ME, Florquin S, Levi M, Carmeliet P, et al. Transgenic tissue-type plasminogen activator expression improves host defense during Klebsiella pneumonia. J Thromb Haemost. 2008;6(4):660–8.

41. Asakura H, Ontachi Y, Mizutani T, Kato M, Saito M, Kumabashiri I, et al. An enhanced fibrinolysis prevents the development of multiple organ failure in disseminated intravascular coagulation in spite of much activation of blood coagulation. Crit Care Med. 2001;29(6):1164–8.

42. Mihajlovic D, Lendak D, Mitic G, Cebovic T, Draskovic B, Novakov A, et al. Prognostic value of hemostasis-related parameters for prediction of organ dysfunction and mortality in sepsis. Turk J Med Sci. 2015;45(1):93–8.

43. Semeraro N, Ammollo CT, Semeraro F, Colucci M. Coagulopathy of acute sepsis. Semin Thromb Hemost. 2015;41(6):650–8.

44. Parker RI. Coagulopathies in the PICU: DIC and liver disease. Crit Care Clin. 2013;29(2):319–33.

45. Nesseler N, Launey Y, Aninat C, Morel F, Malledant Y, Seguin P. Clinical review: the liver in sepsis. Crit Care. 2012;16(5):235.

46. Ostrowski SR, Haase N, Muller RB, Moller MH, Pott FC, Perner A, et al. Association between biomarkers of endothelial injury and hypocoagulability in patients with severe sepsis: a prospective study. Crit Care. 2015;19(191):015–0918.

47. Andrew M, Vegh P, Johnston M, Bowker J, Ofosu F, Mitchell L. Maturation of the hemostatic system during childhood. Blood. 1992;80(8):1998–2005.

48. Yeaman MR. Platelets in defense against bacterial pathogens. Cell Mol Life Sci. 2010;67(4):525–44.

49. Clemetson KJ. The role of platelets in defence against pathogens. Hamostaseologie. 2011;31(4):264–8.

50. Saloga J, Klimek L, Buhl R, Mann W, Knop J, Grabbe S. Allergologie-Handbuch: Grundlagen und klinische Praxis. Stuttgart: Schattauer Verlag; 2012.

51. Taori RN, Lahiri KR, Tullu MS. Performance of PRISM (pediatric risk of mortality) score and PIM (pediatric index of mortality) score in a tertiary care pediatric ICU. Indian J Pediatr. 2010;77(3):267–71.

52. Kutko MC, Calarco MP, Flaherty MB, Helmrich RF, Ushay HM, Pon S, et al. Mortality rates in pediatric septic shock with and without multiple organ system failure. Pediatr Crit Care Med. 2003;4(3):333–7.

53. Hatherill M, Tibby SM, Turner C, Ratnavel N, Murdoch IA. Procalcitonin and cytokine levels: relationship to organ failure and mortality in pediatric septic shock. Crit Care Med. 2000;28(7):2591–4.

54. Wilkinson JD, Pollack MM, Ruttimann UE, Glass NL, Yeh TS. Outcome of pediatric patients with multiple organ system failure. Crit Care Med. 1986;14(4):271–4.

# Permissions

# List of Contributors

**Irene Lamanna, Ilaria Belloni, Jacques Creteur, Jean-Louis Vincent and Fabio Silvio Taccone**
Department of Intensive Care, Erasme Hospital, Université Libre de Bruxelles, Route de Lennik 808, 1070 Brussels, Belgium

**Antonio Maria Dell'Anna**
Department of Intensive Care, Erasme Hospital, Université Libre de Bruxelles, Route de Lennik 808, 1070 Brussels, Belgium
Department of Anesthesiology and Intensive Care, Catholic University School of Medicine, Largo Agostino Gemelli 8, 00168 Rome, Italy

**Claudio Sandroni**
Department of Anesthesiology and Intensive Care, Catholic University School of Medicine, Largo Agostino Gemelli 8, 00168 Rome, Italy

**Katia Donadello**
Department of Intensive Care, Erasme Hospital, Université Libre de Bruxelles, Route de Lennik 808, 1070 Brussels, Belgium
Anaesthesia and Intensive Care B, Department of Surgery, Dentistry, Paediatrics and Gynaecology, University of Verona, AOUIUniversity Hospital Integrated Trust of Verona, P.le L.A. Scuro 10, 37134 Verona, Italy

**Song-qiao Liu, Qin Sun, Jian-feng Xie, Jing-yuan Xu, Qing Li, Chun Pan, Ling Liu and Ying-zi Huang**
Department of Critical Care Medicine, Zhongda Hospital, School of Medicine, Southeast University, No. 87, Dingjiaqiao Road, Gulou District, Nanjing 210009, China

**Yi Zheng**
Department of Critical Care Medicine, Zhongda Hospital, School of Medicine, Southeast University, No. 87, Dingjiaqiao Road, Gulou District, Nanjing 210009, China
Department of Critical Care Medicine, The First Affiliated Hospital of Medical School of Zhejiang University, 79 Qingchun Road, Shangcheng District, Hangzhou 310003, China

**Kay Choong See, Jeffrey Ng, Wen Ting Siow, Venetia Ong and Jason Phua**
Division of Respiratory and Critical Care Medicine, University Medicine Cluster, National University Health System, 1E Kent Ridge Road, NUHS TowerBlock Level 10, Singapore 119228, Singapore. Department of Medicine, Yong Loo Lin School of Medicine, National University of Singapore, Singapore

**Laura Van Coile**
Faculty of Medicine and Health Sciences, Ghent University, Ghent, Belgium

**Alexander Decruyenaere**
Faculty of Medicine and Health Sciences, Ghent University, Ghent, Belgium
Department of Internal Medicine, Ghent University Hospital, Ghent, Belgium

**Astrid Van den broecke, Kirsten Colpaert, Dominique Benoit and Johan Decruyenaere**
Faculty of Medicine and Health Sciences, Ghent University, Ghent, Belgium
Department of Intensive Care Medicine, Ghent University Hospital, De Pintelaan 185, 9000 Ghent, Belgium

**Hans Van Vlierberghe**
Faculty of Medicine and Health Sciences, Ghent University, Ghent, Belgium
Department of Hepatology and Gastro-Enterology, Ghent University Hospital, Ghent, Belgium

**Nicolas Terzi**
INSERM, Université Grenoble-Alpes, U1042, HP2, 38000 Grenoble, France
CHU Grenoble Alpes, Service de réanimation médicale, 38000 Grenoble, France
Service de réanimation médicale, Centre Hospitalier Universitaire Grenoble - Alpes, CS10217, Grenoble Cedex 09, France

**Romain Masson, Cédric Daubin and Jennifer Brunet**
Service de réanimation médicale, Centre Hospitalier Universitaire Grenoble - Alpes, CS10217, Grenoble Cedex 09, France

**Frédéric Lofaso**
Université de Versailles Saint Quentin en Yvelines, INSERM U1179, Garches, France
CIC 1429, INSERM, AP-HP, Hôpital Raymond Poincaré, 92380 Garches, France
Service d'Explorations Fonctionnelles Respiratoires, AP-HP, Hôpital Raymond Poincaré, 92380 Garches, France

**Pascal Beuret**
Service de Réanimation, Centre Hospitalier de Roanne, 42300 Roanne, France

**Hervé Normand**
INSERM, U1075, 14000 Caen, France
Université de Caen, 14000 Caen, France
CHRU Caen, Service d'Explorations Fonctionnelles Respiratoire, 14000 Caen, France

**Edith Dumanowski**
CHRU Caen, Service d'Explorations Fonctionnelles Respiratoire, 14000 Caen, France

**Line Falaize**
INSERM U 1179, Université de Versailles-Saint Quentin en Yvelines, 104 Bd Raymond Poincaré, 92380 Garches, France
CIC 1429, Inserm-APHP, Hôpital Raymond Poincaré, 104 Bd Raymond Poincaré, 92380 Garches, France

**Bertrand Sauneuf**
Service de réanimation médicale, Centre Hospitalier Universitaire Grenoble - Alpes, CS10217, Grenoble Cedex 09, France
Service de Réanimation Médicale Polyvalente, Centre Hospitalier Public du Cotentin, BP 208, 50102 Cherbourg-en-Cotentin, France

**Djillali Annane**
General Intensive Care Unit, Raymond Poincaré Hospital (AP-HP), Laboratory of Inflammation and Infection, U1173, INSERM and University of Versailles SQY, 92380 Garches, France

**Jacques Parienti**
Unité de Biostatistique et de Recherche Clinique, Centre Hospitalier Universitaire de Caen, Avenue de la Côte de Nacre, 14033 Caen, France

**Jean- and David Orlikowski**
Université de Versailles Saint Quentin en Yvelines, INSERM U1179, Garches, France

CIC 1429, INSERM, AP-HP, Hôpital Raymond Poincaré, 92380 Garches, France
Pôle de ventilation à domicile, AP-HP, Hôpital Raymond Poincaré, 92380 Garches, France
Service de Santé Publique, AP-HP, Hôpital Raymond Poincaré, 92380 Garches, France

**Lu Chen and Laurent Brochard**
Interdepartmental Division of Critical Care Medicine, University of Toronto, Toronto, ON, Canada
Keenan Research Centre and Li Ka Shing Knowledge Institute, St. Michael's Hospital, 30 Bond St, Toronto, ON M5B 1W8, Canada

**Nuttapol Rittayamai**
Interdepartmental Division of Critical Care Medicine, University of Toronto, Toronto, ON, Canada
Keenan Research Centre and Li Ka Shing Knowledge Institute, St. Michael's Hospital, 30 Bond St, Toronto, ON M5B 1W8, Canada
Division of Respiratory Diseases and Tuberculosis, Department of Medicine, Faculty of Medicine Siriraj Hospital, Bangkok, Thailand

**François Beloncle**
Interdepartmental Division of Critical Care Medicine, University of Toronto, Toronto, ON, Canada
Keenan Research Centre and Li Ka Shing Knowledge Institute, St. Michael's Hospital, 30 Bond St, Toronto, ON M5B 1W8, Canada
Medical Intensive Care Unit, Hospital of Angers, University of Angers, Angers, France

**Ewan C. Goligher**
Interdepartmental Division of Critical Care Medicine, University of Toronto, Toronto, ON, Canada
Department of Medicine, University of Toronto, Toronto, Canada
Department of Physiology, University of Toronto, Toronto, Canada
Division of Respirology, Department of Medicine, University Health Network and Mount Sinai Hospital, Toronto, Canada

**Jordi Mancebo**
Centre de recherche du Centre Hospitalier de l, Université de Montréal (CRCHUM), University of Montreal', Montreal, Canada

Servei de Medicina Intensiva, Hospital Sant Pau, Barcelona, Spain

**Jean-Christophe M. Richard**
Emergency Department, General Hospital of Annecy, Annecy, France
INSERM UMR 955 eq 13,Créteil, France

**Hernan Aguirre-Bermeo, Marta Turella, Maddalena Bitondo, Juan Grandjean, Stefano Italiano, Olimpia Festa, Indalecio Morán and Jordi Mancebo**
Servei de Medicina Intensiva, Hospital de la Santa Creu i Sant Pau, Universitat Autònoma de Barcelona (UAB), Sant Quintí, 89, 08041 Barcelona, Spain

**Carolin F. Manthey and Ansgar W. Lohse**
First Department of Internal Medicine and Gastroenterology, University Hospital Hamburg-Eppendorf, Martinistr. 52, 20246 Hamburg, Germany

**Darja Dranova, Stefan Kluge and Valentin Fuhrmann**
Department of Intensive Care Medicine, University Hospital Hamburg-Eppendorf, Hamburg, Germany

**Martin Christner and Laura Berneking**
Department of Microbiology, University Hospital Hamburg-Eppendorf, Hamburg, Germany

**M. Gardette, L. Reydellet, V. Blasco, A. Lannelongue, F. Sayagh, S. Wiramus and J. Albanèse**
Department of Anesthesia and Intensive Care Medicine, University Hospital of Marseille, la Timone Hospital, Marseille, France

**L. Zieleskiewicz and F. Antonini**
Department of Anaesthesia and Intensive Care Medicine, University Hospital of Marseille, North Hospital, Marseille, France

**M. Leone**
Department of Anaesthesia and Intensive Care Medicine, University Hospital of Marseille, North Hospital, Marseille, France
Centre d'Investigation Clinique, Aix-Marseille University, AP-HM, 14901 Marseille, France

**C. Nafati**
Department of Anesthesia and Intensive Care Medicine, University Hospital of Marseille, la Timone Hospital, Marseille, France

Service d'anesthésie et de réanimation, CHU de la Timone, 264 rue Saint Pierre, 13005 Marseille, France

**Kent W. Stewart, J. Geoffrey Chase and Christopher G. Pretty**
Department of Mechanical Engineering, Centre for Bio-Engineering, University of Canterbury, Private Bag 4800, Christchurch 8140, New Zealand.

**Geoffrey M. Shaw**
Department of Intensive Care, Christchurch Hospital, Christchurch, New Zealand

**Kevin Roedl, Andreas Drolz, Thomas Horvatits, Karoline Rutter and Valentin Fuhrmann**
Department of Intensive Care Medicine, University Medical Center Hamburg-Eppendorf, Martinistraße 52, 20246 Hamburg, Germany
Division of Gastroenterology and Hepatology, Department of Internal Medicine 3, Medical University of Vienna, Vienna, Austria

**Dominik Jarczak**
Department of Intensive Care Medicine, University Medical Center Hamburg-Eppendorf, Martinistraße 52, 20246 Hamburg, Germany

**Christian Wallmüller, Peter Stratil, Pia Hubner, Christoph Weiser, Harald Herkner and Fritz Sterz**
Department of Emergency Medicine, Medical University of Vienna, Vienna, Austria

**Julia Ortbauer and Jasmin Katrin Motaabbed**
Division of Gastroenterology and Hepatology, Department of Internal Medicine 3, Medical University of Vienna, Vienna, Austria

**Alexander Spiel**
Department of Intensive Care Medicine, University Medical Center Hamburg-Eppendorf, Martinistraße 52, 20246 Hamburg, Germany
Department of Emergency Medicine, Medical University of Vienna, Vienna, Austria

**Océane Garnier, Julie Carr and Albert Prades**
Department of Anaesthesia and Critical Care Medicine, University of Montpellier Saint Eloi Hospital, 80, avenue Augustin Fliche, 34295 Montpellier Cedex 5, France

**Samir Jaber, Gérald Chanques and Audrey de Jong**
Department of Anaesthesia and Critical Care Medicine, University of Montpellier Saint Eloi Hospital, 80, avenue Augustin Fliche, 34295 Montpellier Cedex 5, France
PhyMedExp, INSERM U1046, CNRS, UMR 9214, University of Montpellier, Montpellier, France

**Christine M. Rowan**
Department of Medicine, Division of Allergy, Pulmonary, and Critical Care Medicine and the Center for Health Services Research, Vanderbilt University School of Medicine, Nashville, TN, USA.

**E. Wesley Ely**
Department of Medicine, Division of Allergy, Pulmonary, and Critical Care Medicine and the Center for Health Services Research, Vanderbilt University School of Medicine, Nashville, TN, USA Geriatric Research Education Clinical Center (GRECC), Department of Veterans Affairs, Tennessee Valley Healthcare System, Nashville, TN, USA

**Fanny Perrigault and Anaïs Eloi**
Department of Speech and Language Therapy, School of Medicine, University of Montpellier, Montpellier, France

**Sylvie Moritz-Gasser**
Department of Speech and Language Therapy, School of Medicine, University of Montpellier, Montpellier, France
Institute of Neurosciences of Montpellier, INSERM U105, University of Montpellier, Montpellier, France

**Nicolas Molinari**
Department of Statistics, University of Montpellier Hospitals, Montpellier, France

**Ryo Matsuura, Yohei Komaru, Teruhiko Yoshida, Rei Isshiki, Kengo Mayumi, Tetsushi Yamashita and Eisei Noiri**
Department of Nephrology and Endocrinology, The University of Tokyo Hospital, 7-3-1 Hongo, Bunkyo-ku, Tokyo 113-8655, Japan

**Kohei Yoshimoto, Naoto Morimura and Kent Doi**
Department of Emergency and Critical Care Medicine, The University of Tokyo Hospital, 7-3-1 Hongo, Bunkyo-ku, Tokyo 113-8655, Japan

**Yoshihisa Miyamoto and Yoshifumi Hamasaki**
Department of Dialysis and Apheresis, The University of Tokyo Hospital, 7-3-1 Hongo, Bunkyo-ku, Tokyo 113-8655, Japan

**Masaomi Nangaku**
Department of Nephrology and Endocrinology, The University of Tokyo Hospital, 7-3-1 Hongo, Bunkyo-ku, Tokyo 113-8655, Japan
Department of Dialysis and Apheresis, The University of Tokyo Hospital, 7-3-1 Hongo, Bunkyo-ku, Tokyo 113-8655, Japan

**Achille Kouatchet, Nicolas Lerolle, Rafael Mahieu and Thomas Reydel**
Département de réanimation médicale et médecine hyperbare, CHU Angers et faculté de santé Angers, 49933 Angers, France
Adel Maamar and Jean-Marc Tadié
Service des Maladies Infectieuses et Réanimation Médicale, Maladies Infectieuses et Réanimation Médicale, CHU Rennes, 35033 Rennes, France

**Angeline Jamet and Arnaud W. Thille**
Service de Réanimation Médicale, CHU de Poitiers, 2, rue de la Milétrie, 86021 Poitiers, France

**Nicolas Chudeau**
Département d'anesthésie-réanimation, LUNAM université, université d'Angers, CHU d'Angers, 49933 Angers, France

**Julien Huntzinger**
Service de réanimation, Centre hospitalier Bretagne Atlantique, 56017 Vannes Cedex, France

**Steven Grangé and Gaetan Beduneau**
Medical Intensive Care Unit, Rouen University Hospital, Rouen, France

**Anne Courte**
Medical-surgical ICU, Hospital of Saint-Brieuc, 10 rue Marcel Proust, 22000 Saint-Brieuc, France

**Stephane Ehrmann**
Médecine Intensive Réanimation, Centre Hospitalier Régional et Universitaire de Tours, 37044 Tours, France

**Jérémie Lemarié and Sébastien Gibot**
9 Service de Réanimation Médicale, CHRU Nancy, Hôpital Central, Nancy, France

**Michael Darmon**
Medical-Surgical ICU, Saint-Etienne University Hospital, Saint-Priest-en-Jarez, France

**Christophe Guitton**
Medical intensive care unit, Nantes academic hospital, Nantes university, Nantes, France

**Julia Champey and Carole Schwebel**
Intensive Care Medicine, CHU de Grenoble, BP 218, 38043 Grenoble Cedex 9, France

**Jean Dellamonica**
Service de Réanimation, Centre Hospitalier-Universitaire, Nice, France

**Thibaut Wipf and Ferhat Meziani**
Service de Réanimation Médicale, Nouvel Hôpital Civil, Centre Hospitalo-Universitaire, Strasbourg, France

**Damien Du Cheyron**
Intensive Care Unit, University Hospital of Caen, Caen, France

**Christian Ertmer and Hugo Van Aken**
Department of Anaesthesiology, Intensive Care and Pain Medicine, University Hospital Münster, 48149 Münster, Germany

**Bernhard Zwißler**
Department of Anaesthesiology, University Hospital, LMU Munich, 80337 Munich, Germany.

**Michael Christ3**
3 Department of Emergency and Critical Care Medicine, Paracelsus Medical University, 90419 Nuremberg, Germany

**Fabian Spöhr**
Department of Anaesthesiology and Intensive Care Medicine, Sana Kliniken Stuttgart, 70174 Stuttgart, Germany
Department of Anaesthesiology and Intensive Care Medicine, University of Cologne, 50937 Cologne, Germany

**Axel Schneider**
Department of Anaesthesiology, Krankenhaus Barmherzige Brueder, 54292 Trier, Germany

**Robert Deisz**
Department of Intensive Care and Intermediate Care, RWTH University Hospital Aachen, 52074 Aachen, Germany

**Matthias Jacob**
Department of Anaesthesiology, University Hospital, LMU Munich, 80337 Munich, Germany
Department of Anaesthesiology, Surgical Intensive Care and Pain Medicine, St. Elisabeth Hospital, St.-Elisabeth-Str. 23, 94315 Straubing, Germany

**Jean Ripoche**
INSERM U1026, BioTis, Univ. Bordeaux, 33000 Bordeaux, France

**Antoine Dewitte**
INSERM U1026, BioTis, Univ. Bordeaux, 33000 Bordeaux, France
Department of Anaesthesia and Critical Care II, Magellan Medico-Surgical Center, CHU Bordeaux, 33000 Bordeaux, France

**Sébastien Lepreux**
INSERM U1026, BioTis, Univ. Bordeaux, 33000 Bordeaux, France
Department of Pathology, CHU Bordeaux, 33000 Bordeaux, France

**Julien Villeneuve**
Cell and Developmental Biology Department, Centre for Genomic Regulation, The Barcelona Institute for Science and Technology, 08003 Barcelona, Spain

**Claire Rigothier and Christian Combe**
INSERM U1026, BioTis, Univ. Bordeaux, 33000 Bordeaux, France
Department of Nephrology, Transplantation and Haemodialysis, CHU Bordeaux, 33000 Bordeaux, France

**Alexandre Ouattara**
Department of Anaesthesia and Critical Care II, Magellan Medico-Surgical Center, CHU Bordeaux, 33000 Bordeaux, France
INSERM U1034, Biology of Cardiovascular Diseases, Univ. Bordeaux, 33600 Pessac, France

**Ricardo Castro, Leyla Alegría and Glenn Hernández**
Departamento de Medicina Intensiva, Facultad de Medicina, Pontificia Universidad Católica de Chile, Diagonal Paraguay 362, Santiago, Chile

**Alexandre Biasi Cavalcanti and Fernando Godinho Zampieri**
Research Institute HCor, Hospital do Coração, R. Des. Eliseu Guilherme, 147 - Paraíso, São Paulo, Brazil

**Gustavo Ospina-Tascón**
Department of Intensive Care Medicine, Fundación Valle del Lili, Universidad ICESI, Carrera 98 # 18-49, Cali, Colombia

**Arnaldo Dubin**
Servicio de Terapia Intensiva, Sanatorio Otamendi y Miroli, Azcuénaga 894, Ciudad Autónoma deBuenos Aires, Argentina

**F. Javier Hurtado**
Centro de Tratamiento Intensivo, Hospital Español, Escuela de Medicina, Universidad de la República, Avda. Gral. Garibaldi, 1729 esq. Rocha, Montevideo, Uruguay

**Gilberto Friedman**
Departamento de Medicina Interna, Faculdade de Medicina, Universidade Federal do Rio Grande do Sul, R. Ramiro Barcelos 2350 – Santa Cecilia, Porto Alegre, Brazil

**Maurizio Cecconi**
St George's University Hospitals NHS Foundation Trust, Rd, London SW17 0QT, UK.

**Jean-Louis Teboul**
Service de Réanimation médicale, Hôpitaux universitaires Paris-Sud, Assistance Publique-Hôpitaux de Paris, Paris, France

**Jan Bakker**
Departamento de Medicina Intensiva, Facultad de Medicina, Pontificia Universidad Católica de Chile, Diagonal Paraguay 362, Santiago, Chile
Division of Pulmonary, Allergy and Critical Care Medicine, Columbia University Medical Center, 630 W 168th St, New York, USA
Department Intensive Care Adults, Erasmus MC University Medical Center, Rotterdam, CA, The Netherlands
Division of Pulmonary, and Critical Care Medicine, New York University-Langone, New York, USA

**Woo Jin Jang, Woo Jung Chun and Ju Hyeon Oh**
Division of Cardiology, Department of Internal Medicine, Samsung Changwon
Hospital, Sungkyunkwan University School of Medicine, Changwon, Republic of Korea

**Yang Hyun Cho**
Department of Thoracic and Cardiovascular Surgery, Samsung Medical Center, Sungkyunkwan University School of Medicine, Seoul, Republic of Korea

**Taek Kyu Park, Young Bin Song, Jin-Oh Choi, Joo-Yong Hahn, Seung-Hyuk Choi, Hyeon-Cheol Gwon, Eun-Seok Jeon and Jeong Hoon Yang**
Division of Cardiology, Department of Critical Care Medicine and Medicine, Heart Vascular Stroke Institute, Samsung Medical Center, Sungkyunkwan University School of Medicine, 81, Irwon-dong, Gangnam-gu, Seoul 135-710, Republic of Korea

**Margit Boshuizen**
Department of Intensive Care Medicine, Academic Medical Center, University of Amsterdam, Meibergdreef 9, 1105 AZ Amsterdam, The Netherlands
Department of Blood Cell Research, Sanquin Research and Landsteiner Laboratory, Academic Medical Center, University of Amsterdam, Amsterdam, The Netherlands

**Jan M. Binnekade, Janneke Horn, Marcus J. Schultz and Nicole P. Juffermans**
Department of Intensive Care Medicine, Academic Medical Center, University of Amsterdam, Meibergdreef 9, 1105 AZ Amsterdam, The Netherlands

**Robin van Bruggen**
Department of Blood Cell Research, Sanquin Research and Landsteiner Laboratory, Academic Medical Center, University of Amsterdam, Amsterdam, The Netherlands

**Benjamin Nota**
Department of Research Facilities, Sanquin Research and Landsteiner Laboratory, Academic Medical Center, University of Amsterdam, Amsterdam, The Netherlands

**Kirsten van de Groep**
Department of Intensive Care Medicine, University Medical Center Utrecht, Utrecht, The Netherlands
Julius Center for Health Sciences and Primary Care, University Medical Center Utrecht, Utrecht, The Netherlands

**Olaf L. Cremer**
Department of Intensive Care Medicine, University Medical Center Utrecht, Utrecht, The Netherlands

**Pieter R. Tuinman**
Department of Intensive Care Medicine, VU University Medical Center Amsterdam, University of Amsterdam, Amsterdam, The Netherlands

**Feng Yang, Dengbang Hou, Jinhong Wang, Yongchao Cui, Xiaomeng Wang, Zhichen Xing, Chunjing Jiang, Xing Hao, Zhongtao Du, Xiaofang Yang, Yu Jiang and Xiaotong Hou**
Center for Cardiac Intensive Care, Beijing Institute of Heart, Lung, and Blood Vessels Diseases, Beijing Anzhen Hospital, Capital Medical University, No. 2 Anzhen Rd, Chaoyang District, Beijing 100029, China

**Ulrich Mayr, Leonie Fahrenkrog-Petersen, Gonzalo Batres-Baires, Alexander Herner, Sebastian Rasch, Roland M. Schmid, Wolfgang Huber and Tobias Lahmer**
Klinik und Poliklinik für Innere Medizin II, Klinikum rechts der Isar, Technische Universität München, Ismaninger Strasse 22, 81675 Munich,Germany

**Manu L. N. G. Malbrain**
Intensive Care Unit, University Hospital Brussels (UZB), Laarbeeklaan 101, 1090 Jette, Belgium
Faculteit Geneeskunde en Farmacie, Vrije Universiteit Brussel (VUB), Brussels, Belgium

**Niels Van Regenmortel, Brecht De Tavernier and Pieter-Jan Van Gaal**
Intensive Care Unit, ZiekenhuisNetwerk Antwerpen, ZNA Stuivenberg, Lange Beeldekensstraat 267, 2060 Antwerpen 6, Belgium

**Bernd Saugel**
Department of Anesthesiology, Centre of Anesthesiology and Intensive Care Medicine, University Medical Centre Hamburg-Eppendorf, Hamburg, Germany

**Olivier Joannes-Boyau**
Service d'Anesthésie-Réanimation 2, CHU Bordeaux, 33000 Bordeaux, France

**Jean-Louis Teboul and Xavier Monnet**
Medical Intensive Care Unit, Hopitaux universitaires Paris-Sud, AP-HP, Université Paris-Sud, Le Kremlin-Bicetre, France

**Todd W. Rice**
University College London Hospitals, National Institute of Health Research Biomedical Research Centre, London, UK

**Monty Mythen**
Division of Allergy, Pulmonary and Critical Care Medicine, Vanderbilt University School of Medicine, Nashville, TN, USA

**Fabienne Scherer and Stéphane Cullati**
Pain and Palliative Care Consultation, Division of Clinical Pharmacology and Toxicology, Geneva University Hospitals, Rue Gabrielle-Perret-Gentil 4, 1211 Geneva, Switzerland

**Monica Escher**
Pain and Palliative Care Consultation, Division of Clinical Pharmacology and Toxicology, Geneva University Hospitals, Rue Gabrielle-Perret-Gentil 4, 1211 Geneva, Switzerland
Unit of Development and Research in Medical Education, Faculty of Medicine, University of Geneva, Geneva, Switzerland

**Bara Ricou**
Division of Intensive Care, Geneva University Hospitals, Geneva, Switzerland

**Mathieu Nendaz**
Unit of Development and Research in Medical Education, Faculty of Medicine, University of Geneva, Geneva, Switzerland
Division of General Internal Medicine, Geneva University Hospitals, Geneva, Switzerland

**Patricia Hudelson**
Division of Primary Care Medicine, Geneva University Hospitals, Geneva, Switzerland

**Thomas Perneger**
Division of Clinical Epidemiology, Geneva University Hospitals, Geneva, Switzerland

**Guillaume Geri and Antoine Vieillard-Baron**
Medico-Surgical ICU, Service de Réanimation médico-chirurgicale, Ambroise Paré Hospital, APHP, 92100 Boulogne Billancourt, France
Inserm U1018, Center for Research in Epidemiology and Population Health (CESP), Univ Paris Sud, Univ Paris Saclay, Villejuif, France
Versailles Saint Quentin University, Montigny le Bretonneux, France

**Bénédicte Stengel**
Inserm U1018, Center for Research in Epidemiology and Population Health (CESP), Univ Paris Sud, Univ Paris Saclay, Villejuif, France
Versailles Saint Quentin University, Montigny le Bretonneux, France

**Christian Jacquelinet**
Inserm U1018, Center for Research in Epidemiology and Population Health (CESP), Univ Paris

Sud, Univ Paris Saclay, Villejuif, France
Biomedicine Agency, Saint Denis, France

**Philippe Aegerter**
Department of Clinical Research and Public Health, Ambroise Paré Hospital, APHP, Boulogne Billancourt, France
UVSQ-INSERM U1168, University Paris Saclay, Villejuif, France

**Ziad A. Massy**
Inserm U1018, Center for Research in Epidemiology and Population Health (CESP), Univ Paris Sud, Univ Paris Saclay, Villejuif, France
Versailles Saint Quentin University, Montigny le Bretonneux, France
Department of Nephrology, Ambroise Paré Hospital, APHP, Boulogne Billancourt, France

**Christian Niederwanger, Andreas Entenmann and Agnes Balog**
Department of Pediatrics, Pediatrics I, Medical University of Innsbruck, Anichstrasse 35, 6020 Innsbruck, Austria

**Mirjam Bachler**
Institute for Sports Medicine, Alpine Medicine and Health Tourism, UMIT - University for Health Sciences, Medical Informatics and Technology, Eduard Wallnöfer Zentrum 1, 6060 Hall in Tirol, Austria

**Tobias Hell**
Department of Mathematics, Faculty of Mathematics, Computer Science and Physics, University of Innsbruck, Technikerstraße 13, 6020 Innsbruck, Austria

**Caroline Linhart**
Department of Medical Statistics, Informatics and Health Economics, Medical University of Innsbruck, Anichstrasse 35, 6020 Innsbruck, Austria

**Katharina Auer**
Department of General and Surgical Critical Care Medicine, Medical University of Innsbruck, Anichstrasse 35, 6020 Innsbruck, Austria

**Petra Innerhofer**
Department of Anaesthesiology and Critical Care Medicine, Medical University of Innsbruck, Anichstrasse 35, 6020 Innsbruck, Austria

# Index

www.ingramcontent.com/pod-product-compliance
Lightning Source LLC
Chambersburg PA
CBHW061304190326
41458CB00011B/3757